W9-CDS-318

ANGIOGRAPHY and PLAQUE IMAGING

Advanced Segmentation Techniques

Biomedical Engineering Series

Edited by Michael R. Neuman

Published Titles

Electromagnetic Analysis and Design in Magnetic Resonance Imaging, Jianming Jin

Endogenous and Exogenous Regulation and Control of Physiological Systems, Robert B. Northrop

Artificial Neural Networks in Cancer Diagnosis, Prognosis, and Treatment, Raouf N.G. Naguib and Gajanan V. Sherbet

Medical Image Registration, Joseph V. Hajnal, Derek Hill, and David J. Hawkes

Introduction to Dynamic Modeling of Neuro-Sensory Systems, Robert B. Northrop

Noninvasive Instrumentation and Measurement in Medical Diagnosis, Robert B. Northrop

Handbook of Neuroprosthetic Methods, Warren E. Finn and Peter G. LoPresti

Signals and Systems Analysis in Biomedical Engineering, Robert B. Northrop

Angiography and Plaque Imaging: Advanced Segmentation Techniques, Jasjit S. Suri and Swamy Laxminarayan

The **BIOMEDICAL ENGINEERING** Series

Series Editor Michael Neuman

ANGIOGRAPHY and PLAQUE IMAGING

Advanced Segmentation Techniques

EDITED BY

Jasjit S. Suri, Ph.D.
Swamy Laxminarayan, D.Sc.

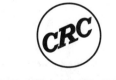

CRC PRESS

Boca Raton   London   New York   Washington, D.C.

Library of Congress Cataloging-in-Publication Data

Angiography and plaque imaging : a segmentation perspective / edited by
Jasjit S. Suri and Swamy Laxminarayan.
      p. ; cm.– (Biomedical engineering series)
  Includes bibliographical references and index.
  ISBN 0-8493-1740-1 (alk. paper)
  1. Angiography. 2. Atherosclerotic plaque. 3.
Blood-vessels–Diseases–Diagnosis. 4. Blood-vessels–Imaging.
  [DNLM: 1. Blood Vessels–pathology. 2. Imaging,
Three-Dimensional–methods. 3. Magnetic Resonance Angiography–methods.
4. Vascular Diseases–diagnosis. WG 500 A5862 2003] I. Suri, Jasjit
S. II. Laxminarayan, Swamy. III. Series: Biomedical engineering series (Boca Raton, Fla.).
RC691.6.A53A54 2003
616.1'30754—dc21
                                          2003046074

Visit the CRC Press Web site at www.crcpress.com

Dedication

Jasjit Suri would like to dedicate this book to his son, Harman, who led to a family bond; to his parents, especially his late mother for her immortal softness and encouragement; his sister Angela, his family, and his wife Malvika.

Swamy Laxminarayan would like to dedicate this book to the many distinguished peers with whom he had the privilege to interact and learn from and to all his students who gave him the opportunity to impart in some small measure the benefits of his research endeavors.

Preface

The art of imaging blood vessels in the human body is called angiography. Since its inception, physicians have benefited from the field of angiography imaging. This has helped them to diagnostically treat patients with various kinds of vascular diseases. Recently, because of the technology growth in fields of acquisition techniques, such as magnetic resonance, computer tomography, digital subtraction angiography, and ultrasound, the vascular imaging research community has become very interested. But acquisition is just one side of the coin. Given the high resolution acquired with angiographic volumetric data, the art of blood vessel extraction is another side of the coin. The recent growth in mathematical engineering and applied mathematics has opened the door to solve complex problems in angiographic imaging, such as detection, segmentation, tracking, display, and quantification of blood vessels. By fusing together different branches of engineering and medicine, such as physics, computer engineering, electrical engineering, biomedical engineering, and medicine, it has become possible to understand not only the needs of today's fast-growing technology, but also to solve difficult problems in angiographic imaging. This book is an attempt to present, for the first time, different medical imaging modalities such as MR, CT, x-ray, and ultrasound for performing angiography and its analysis.

The art of angiography imaging has penetrated several fields of medicine, such as ophthalmology, neurology, cardiology and pulmonology. Keeping this in mind, we address the state-of-the-art issues of angiography, pre- and post-angiographic imaging, and applications. This includes intravascular ultrasound (IVUS) and x-ray fusion, plaque imaging, and morphology analysis. The angiographic imaging covers different body parts such as retinal, neuro, renal, coronary, and run-off based on the above four medical imaging modalities.

Readers who will benefit from this book include researchers in the field of medicine, imaging sciences, biomedical engineering, physics, and applied mathematics, algorithmic developers, and researchers who are beginners in the field of image processing and graphics but are interested in shape analysis. This book is a collection of chapters in the area of angiography acquisition and postprocessing of angiography volumetric data sets and applications of vascular segmentation techniques.

The contributors to this book consist of pioneers in the field of engineering, imaging sciences, biomedical engineering, computer engineering, image processing, computer vision, deformable models, and partial differential equations. This book is also a classic example of a buffer between industry and academics, because the contributors are from both sides of engineering and mathematics.

Chapter 1 presents a long survey of vascular image processing techniques. It divides the techniques into two broad classes: skeleton vs. non-skeleton-based techniques. The major part of this chapter focuses on skeleton (indirect) and non-skeleton (direct) based techniques. We present more than five different skeleton or indirect techniques, along with their mathematical foundations, algorithms, and their pros and cons. Then, the chapter presents eight different techniques in the class of non-skeleton or direct methods. A full section is dedicated to a discussion of Fuzzy connectedness vs. geometric techniques, their pros and cons, skeleton versus non-skeleton approaches, and the major dominance of scale-spaces. This chapter concludes with a clinical discussion of automated vascular segmentation algorithms for MR data sets, possible extensions for improving the segmentation system, and the future of vascular segmentation techniques.

Chapter 2 focuses on scale-space filtering of the white- and black-blood angiography imaging. This chapter presents a system where the raw MR angiographic volume is first converted to isotropic volume, followed by three-dimensional, higher-order, separable Gaussian derivative convolution with known scales to generate edge volume. The edge volume is then run by the directional processor at each voxel where the eigenvalues of the three-dimensional ellipsoid are computed. The vessel score per voxel is then estimated based on these three eigenvalues, which suppress the nonvasculature and background structures yielding the filtered volume. The filtered volume is ray-cast to generate the maximum intensity projection images for display. This chapter then presents the performance evaluation system by computing the mean, variance, signal-to-noise ratio, and contrast-to-noise ratio images. The system shows the results of 20 patient studies from different areas of the body, including the brain, abdomen, kidney, knee, and ankle. This chapter also discusses the timing issues and compares its strategy with other MR filtering algorithms.

Chapter 3 focuses on segmentation tools from an industrial point of view. Vessel View is an interactive postprocessing application for three-dimensional magnetic resonance angiography (MRA) and computed tomography angiography (CTA) images. The application provides simple interactive point-and-click localization and quantification of vessels. Behind the scenes, there are several robust and efficient segmentation algorithms that operate at interactive speeds. For three-dimensional localization of vessels, a variant of Dijkstra's algorithm grows a segmenting surface from initial seeds and connects them with a minimal path computation. The technique is local and does not require any preprocessing of the volume. The propagation is controlled by iterative computation of border probabilities. As expanding regions meet, the statistics collected during propagation are passed to an active minimal-path generation module that links the associating points through the vessel tree. Once the vessel tree is obtained, local, high-precision segmentation techniques, employing mean-shift-modulated ray propagation, are used for quantifying selected pathologies, such as aneurysm and stenosis. This chapter describes in detail these algorithms and also explains why these particular techniques were chosen based on clinical workflow. The costliest element of the diagnosis is the time spent by doctors and technicians. Optimization of user time leads to a simple set of design criteria: algorithms must be fast, robust, give immediate visual feedback, and respond intuitively to user guidance. These demands require a system in which visualization and segmentation are tightly coupled. Integral visualization and navigation techniques are developed in conjunction with the content extraction methods.

Chapter 4 focuses on black-blood angiography. It introduces different kinds of masking strategies such as Bayesian, fuzzy, recursive mathematical morphology, and connected components analysis for mask generation for black-blood angiographic volumes. One section of the chapter presents the filtering/segmentation algorithms for black-blood angiography. Here is discussed the role of scale-spaces for vessel detection and display techniques for black-blood vessels. The last section of this chapter presents a clinical discussion on automated vascular segmentation algorithms for MR data sets, possible extensions for improving the black-blood segmentation system, and the future of black-blood vascular segmentation techniques.

Chapter 5 reports on techniques for automatic analysis of retinal angiographic images. In particular, we focus on the segmentation of the blood vessels in these images and subsequent shape analysis of the segmented branching structures. We describe a recently proposed approach based on the continuous wavelet transform using the Morlet wavelet. The main advantage of the latter, with respect to retinal images, relies on its capability of tuning to specific frequencies, thus allowing noise filtering and blood vessel enhancement in a single step. Furthermore, because of the importance of using shape analysis techniques for the detection and quantitative characterization of the blood vessel vascular branching pattern in the retina, the wavelets can also be explored to extract shape features for image analysis. The chapter concludes with an exploration of the fractal analysis of the segmented vessels for characterization of the branching pattern using the correlation dimension.

Chapter 6 focuses on retinal vascular image processing. This chapter provides a detailed review of algorithms for extracting the retinal vasculature from clinical instruments such as the fundus microscope. Also described are methods for extracting key points, such as bifurcations and crossovers, and methods for performing vessel morphometry. Tracing of retinal vessels has a number of applications, including support for clinical trials, real-time instrumentation for computer-assisted surgery, computer-assisted diagnosis, and fundamental science. Examples of applications are provided. Depending on the intended application, different algorithmic and implementation choices can be made. This chapter describes the rationale behind these choices, using several examples.

Chapters 7, 8, and 9 discuss the MRI of atherosclerosis. These three chapters describe the imaging techniques, morphologic index, and tissue characterization approaches for the visualization and characteristics of atherosclerosis. Noninvasive magnetic resonance imaging is ideally suited for such purposes. Plaque characteristics may be useful in determining high risk, or "vulnerable" plaques. Chapter 7 focuses on plaque imaging techniques useful in imaging basic plaque tissues and specific plaque features with magnetic resonance imaging.

Traditionally, the degree of lumen stenosis is used as a marker for high-risk (vulnerable) plaques. Clinically, x-ray, CT, ultrasound, and MR angiography are used to determine lumen stenosis. Stenosis, however, is just one simple feature in morphology analysis. We believe that complex morphology markers can provide more information for vulnerable plaques. A set of carotid shape descriptors developed to distinguish the different types of plaque morphology based on carotid wall thickness to assist in determining the vulnerable plaque is presented in Chapter 8.

Knowing the composition and distribution of atherosclerotic plaque components within the walls of arteries can be valuable for surgical planning, assessing disease severity, and monitoring response to treatment. Chapter 9 details techniques for the segmentation of artery walls into distinct tissue regions, measurement of compositional indexes, and three-dimensional display of plaque distribution. The methods focus on magnetic resonance images of the carotid arteries, but can be extended for use in other vessels and with other methods for vessel wall imaging.

Chapter 10 addresses the problem of constructing volumetric dynamic models of coronary vessels. The growing appreciation of the pathophysiological and prognostic importance of arterial morphology has led to the realization of the importance of volumetric analysis of coronary vessels for a reliable diagnosis and choice of therapeutic procedure. The problem of real three-dimensional reconstruction of dynamic vessels is a complex task that needs to incorporate data from different medical image modalities. Today, angiograms represent the most-used image modality for diagnosis during clinical practice. However, due to the projective nature of x-ray images, direct quantitative measurements are prone to errors. A three-dimensional reconstruction of the vessels could estimate vessel lesions and aid in the process of determining the reliable therapy more precisely (length of stent, etc.). In this chapter, different computer vision approaches for two-dimensional analysis and three-dimensional reconstruction of vessels on (biplane) angiogram systems is discussed, focusing on their performance and need for user interaction.

On the other hand, angiograms, visualizing just the vessel lumen, are inherently limited in defining the distribution and extension of coronary wall disease. As a perfect complement, intravascular ultrasound (IVUS) images represent a unique interoperative image modality that allows physicians to obtain a picture of the composition of the vessel in detail. IVUS images contain valuable geometric information (diameters, area, etc.) about plaque, vessel lumen, mutual position with stent, etc. Given the huge amount of IVUS data, the problem of (semi)-automatic segmentation and extraction of geometric measurements arouses increasing interest by cardiac caregivers in order to avoid the tedious and time-consuming process of manual segmentation. Moreover, image processing and computer vision techniques allow for an automatic texture characterization of vessel morphology (plaque, calcium deposits, etc.), which represents essential help to cardiologists during the process of diagnosis and therapy. Chapter 10 discusses the current state-of-the-art of automatic analysis (segmentation, statistical description of vessel composition, dynamics, etc.) of IVUS images. The chapter finishes with current work on fusing IVUS and angiogram data to obtain a real volumetric vessel model, thereby making easier the arduous task of mental conceptualization of vessel shape and analysis of real spatial extension, distribution, and treatment of the coronary diseases.

Chapter 11 presents the issues and problems that computer-assisted analysis of images of vasculature pose to medical image processing researchers. Methods that are appropriate for the analysis of images of tissues are not always appropriate for vascular images. For example, vessels generally form sparse networks in which each vessel's cross-section is nearly circular and varies smoothly along its tortuous path. If ignored, these geometric properties confound standard image segmentation and registration methods. However, if these geometric properties are specifically exploited, the resulting vascular image processing methods can gain accuracy, consistency, and ease-of-use. In this chapter we review several prominent methods for characterizing and viewing vascular images for surgical planning as well as methods for registering vascular images for surgical guidance and treatment monitoring. These reviews focus on the current and potential clinical use of the methods. Special attention is given to the role of vascular image processing methods for neurosurgical planning, liver transplant planning, liver shunt placement, and liver lesion ablation guidance. The utility of these and other clinical applications are shown to often be related to the degree to which the underlying image processing methods exploit the geometric properties of vessels.

Chapter 12 focuses on the future aspects of vasculature image processing. Here we summarize the acquisition of MR, CT, and ultrasound modalities. Postprocessing issues such as separation are also presented.

Acknowledgments

This book is the result of collective endeavours from several noted engineering and computer scientists, mathematicians, physicists, and radiologists. The authors are indebted to all of their efforts and outstanding scientific contributions. The editors are particularly grateful to Drs. Sameer Singh, Petia Reveda, James Williams, Roberto M. Cesar, Jr., Badrinath Roysam, Chun Yuan, Stephen Alyward, and all their team members for working with us so closely in meeting all of the deadlines of the book.

We would like to express our appreciation to CRC Press for helping create this book. We are particularly thankful to Susan Farmer, Helena Redshaw, and Susan Fox for their excellent coordination of the book at every stage.

Dr. Suri would like to thank Philips Medical Systems, Inc., for the MR data sets and encouragement during his experiments and research. Special thanks are due to Dr. Larry Kasuboski and Dr. Elaine Keeler from Philips Medical Systems, Inc., for their support and motivation. Thanks are also due to past Ph.D. committee research professors, particularly Professors Linda Shapiro, Robert M. Haralick, Dean Lytle, and Arun Somani, for their encouragement.

We extend our appreciation to Dr. George Thoma, Chief, Imaging Science Division from the National Institutes of Health; and Dr. Sameer Singh, University of Exeter, U.K. for their motivation. Special thanks go to Michael Neuman, Series Editor of the Biomedical Engineering Series, for advising us on all aspects of the book.

We thank IEEE Press, Academic Press, Springer-Verlag Publishers, and several medical and engineering journals for permitting us to use some of the images previously published in these journals.

Finally, Jasjit Suri would like to thank his wife Malvika Suri for all the love and support she has shown over the years and our baby Harman whose presence is always a constant source of pride and joy. Dr. Suri also expresses his gratitude to his father, a mathematician, who inspired him throughout his life and career, and to his late mother, who passed away a few days before his Ph.D. graduation. Special thanks to Pom Chadha, a true salesperson, who taught me that life is not just books. He is one of my best friends. I would like to also thank my in-laws who have a special place for me in their hearts and have shown lots of love and care for me.

Swamy Laxminarayan would like to express his profound appreciation to the senior author, Dr. Jasjit Suri, for his highest level of collaborative spirit and warm scientific interactions during the course of editing this book. A book of this complexity and content is a collective venture with excellent contributions by authors whose scholarly work will always be an intellectual reference resource to the biomedical community. We are most grateful to them. I have had the pleasure of numerous technical and scientific discussions with Dr. Beth Stamm and Dr. Neil Piland of the Institute of Rural Health at the Idaho State University. This has been especially important to the critical evaluation of the book, for which I owe them and my colleagues at the Institute of Rural Health a great debt of gratitude and thanks. Two mathematical scientists, Lakshminarayan Rajaram and Ramanath Laxminarayan, have served as "non-imaging" oriented gold standards by providing feedback about the worth and value of the book to the non-medical applied scientific community. These are important considerations and I thank them. My active participation over the years in the technical programs of the IEEE Engineering in Medicine and Biology Society and especially my tenure as the Founding Editor-in-Chief of the IEEE Transactions on Information Technology has had a significant influence on my in-depth appreciation of the practical applications of diagnostic imaging. I want to recognize the Society, some of the medical imaging gurus in the Society and other leaders such as Charles Robinson, Yongmin Kim, Michael Vannier, Willis Tompkins, Christian Roux, Joseph Bronzino, Jean Louis Coatrieux, Banu Onaral, Jerry Harris, and others. To Joe Bronzino, our special thanks for his ever encouraging words of wisdom. I also want to recognize the deep sense of sacrifice of our families, during all the long hours we spent on the book. My loving thanks to my wife, Marijke, and my children, Vinod and Malini, for sharing with me the frustrations of my long absences from the regular schedule of life. Projects like this always remind me of my sister Ramaa, a musical genius, whose death at the tender age of 16 from epileptic complications inspired my biomedical engineering career.

The Editors

Jasjit S. Suri, Ph.D., received a B.S. in computer engineering with distinction from Maulana Azad College of Technology, Bhopal, India, an M.S. in computer sciences from the University of Illinois, Chicago, and a Ph.D. in electrical engineering from the University of Washington, Seattle. He has been working in the field of computer engineering/imaging sciences for more than 19 years. He has published more than 100 papers in the area of image sciences and medical engineering and has filed several U.S. patents.

He is a lifetime member of various research engineering societies including Tau Beta Pi, and Eta Kappa Nu, Sigma Xi, New York Academy of Sciences, Engineering in Medicine and Biology Society (EMBS), SPIE, ACM, and also a Senior Member of IEEE. He is on the editorial board/reviewer of several international journals, including *Real Time Imaging, Pattern Analysis and Applications, Engineering in Medicine and Biology Society, Radiology, Journal of Computer Assisted Tomography, IEEE Transactions on Information Technology in Biomedicine,* and *IASTED*. He has chaired image processing sessions at several international conferences and has given more than 40 international presentations.

Dr. Suri has published two books; the first book is in the area of medical imaging covering cardiology, neurology, pathology, and mammography imaging, primarily in collaboration with University of Exeter, England. The second book is in the area of mathematical imaging techniques applied to static and motion imagery. Dr. Suri has been listed in Who's Who five times (World, Executive, and Mid-West), is a recipient of the President's Gold Medal in 1980, and has been awarded more than 50 scholarly and extra-curricular awards during his career.

Dr. Suri has worked with Siemens and Philips. Currently, Dr. Suri is also completing his EMBA from Weatherhead School of Management, Case Western Reserve University, Cleveland, Ohio. He is also working as a Senior Research Scientist/Associate at Case Western Reserve University, Professor of Computer Science at University of Exeter, Exter, UK, and a Director of Biomedical Engineering Division, Jebra Wells and Technology, Inc., Cleveland, Ohio. Dr. Suri's major interests are imaging sciences, various fields in biomedical engineering, engineering management, software engineering, and the role of engineering in medicine management.

Swamy Laxminarayan is currently on the faculty of the Idaho State University and serves as the Chief of Biomedical Information Engineering at the Institute of Rural Health. Prior to joining ISU, he held several senior positions in both industry and academia. These have included serving as the Chief Information Officer at the National Louis University in Chicago, Director of the Pharmaceutical and Health Care Information Services at NextGen Internet (the premier Internet organization that spun off from the NSF-sponsored John von Neuman National Supercomputer Center in Princeton, NJ), Program Director of Biomedical Engineering and Research Computing at the University of Medicine and Dentistry in New Jersey, Director of Computational Biology, Vice-Chair of Advanced Medical Imaging Center, and Director of Clinical Computing at the Montefiore Hospital and Medical Center and the Albert Einstein College of Medicine in New York, Director of the VocalTec High Tech Corporate University in New Jersey, and the Director of the Bay Networks Authorized Center in Princeton. Prior to his immigration to the U.S., he was a faculty member as a Senior Research Investigator at the Physiology Laboratory of the Free University in Amsterdam, and at the Thorax Center of the Erasmus University in Rotterdam, the Netherlands. He also served as a Research Physicist at the Christian Medical College in Vellore and later became an Aerodynamicist and a Flight Test Engineer in Germany before he switched careers to biomedical engineering. Dr. Laxminarayan has had a long tenure as an Adjunct Professor of Biomedical Engineering at the New Jersey Institute of Technology, a Clinical Associate Professor of Health Informatics, a Visiting Professor at the University of Brno in the Czech Republic and an Honorary Professor of Health Sciences at Tsinghua University in China.

As an educator, researcher, technologist, and executive, Dr. Laxminarayan has been involved in biomedical engineering and information technology applications in medicine and healthcare for over 25 years and has published over 250 articles in international journals, books, and conferences. He has had the privilege of giving invitational keynote addresses at a number of international conferences. His expertise is in the areas of biomedical information technology, high performance computing, digital signals and image processing, bioinformatics, and physiological systems analysis. He has been actively involved in the technical activities of the IEEE Engineering in Medicine and Biology Society for over 20 years. He is the Founding Editor-in-Chief and an Editor Emeritus of the *IEEE Transactions on Information Technology in Biomedicine*. He also currently serves as an elected member at large on the IEEE Publications and Products Board. His technical and scientific contributions to the field of biomedical engineering and information technology have earned him numerous national and international awards. He is a Fellow of the American Institute of Medical and Biological Engineering, a recipient of the IEEE 3rd Millennium Medal, and a recipient of the Purkynje Award, one of the highest awards in Europe given to an American scientist by the Czech Academy of Medical Societies. Dr. Laxminarayan can be reached at s.n.laxminarayan@ieee.org.

Contributors

Brian Avants University of Pennsylvania, Philadelphia, Pennsylvania

Stephen R. Aylward University of North Carolina, Chapel Hill, North Carolina

Elizabeth Bullitt University of North Carolina, Chapel Hill, North Carolina

Ali Can Woods Hole Oceanographic Institute, Woods Hole, Massachusetts

Roberto Marcond Cesar, Jr. University of Sao Paulo, Sao Paulo, Brazil

Dorin Comaniciu Siemens Corporate Research, Princeton, New Jersey

Kenneth H. Fritzsche Rensselaer Polytechnic Institute, Troy, New York

Chao Han University of Washington, Seattle, Washington

Herbert Jelinek Charles Sturt University, Albury, NSW, Australia

William S. Kerwin University of Washington, Seattle, Washington

Swamy Laxminarayan Idaho State University, Pocatello, Idaho

Kecheng Liu Zhejiang University, Shen Zhen, China

Zachary Miller University of Washington, Seattle, Washington

Petia Radeva Universitat Autonoma de Barcelona, Barcelona, Spain

Badrinath Roysam Rensselaer Polytechnic Institute, Troy, New York

Hong Shen Siemens Corporate Research, Princeton, New Jersey

Sameer Singh University of Exeter, Exeter, England

Charles V. Stewart Rensselaer Polytechnic Institute, Troy, New York

Jasjit S. Suri   Case Western Reserve University, Cleveland, Ohio

Howard Tanenbaum   The Center for Sight, Albany, New York

Hüseyin Tek   Siemens Corporate Research, Princeton, New Jersey

Chia-Ling Tsai   Rensselaer Polytechnic Institute, Troy, New York

James N. Turner   Wadsworth Center, Albany, New York

James P. Williams   Siemens Corporate Research, Princeton, New Jersey

Chun Yuan   University of Washington, Seattle, Washington

Contents

1

Non-Skeleton- and Skeleton-Based Segmentation Techniques from Angiography Data Sets

Jasjit S. Suri, Kecheng Liu, Sameer Singh, and Swamy Laxminarayan

CONTENTS

1.1 Introduction

Vascular diseases are one of the major sources of deaths in the United States. A report [1] states that "Aneurysm rupture is not a rare occurrence as evidenced by the fact that this event currently ranks thirteenth on the list for leading causes of death in the U.S.A." Also, this report [1] says that "Chronic venous insufficiency is a common problem in the U.S., affecting approximately 5% of the general population. It is estimated that half a million patients suffer from ulceration of the lower extremity as a result of longstanding venous disease." This report raises the importance of research needed in the area of angiography, the branch of medicine that deals with veins and arteries. In the field of cerebrovascular diseases [1], "Ischemic and hemorrhagic stroke account for one of the principal causes of death and disability in older aged population. In fact, stroke currently ranks third on the list of leading causes of death in the United States (see also [2–5]).

Each year, approximately 500,000 people suffer a new or recurrent stroke in the U.S., and approximately 150,000 die as a result of this process. In addition,

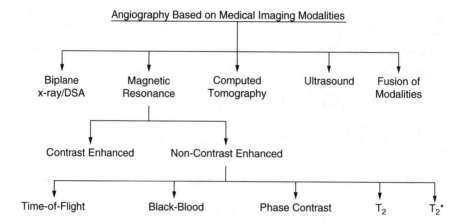

FIGURE 1.1

This chart shows the various ways angiography can be performed, based on the type of medical imaging modality used. Note that T_2 and T_2^* stand for T_2-weighted and T_2^*-weighted imaging.

more than one third of stroke survivors are left with permanent physical disability, which currently accounts for the leading cause of nursing home admissions in the U.S."

Having discussed the national concern on vascular diseases, we briefly present different imaging modalities that can perform angiography. Figure 1.1 shows the different ways angiography can be performed. The main modalities include biplane x-ray/digital subtraction angiography (DSA) (see [6–9]); MR angiography (MRA) (see [10–19]); CT angiography (CTA) (see [20–25]); ultrasound angiography[1] (see [26–32]); and angiography as a fusion of different medical imaging modalities (see [33–35]). From the clinical point of view, DSA[2] is considered the most reliable and accurate method for vascular imaging, a subset of x-ray. On the contrary, this method lacks three-dimensional information,[3] which is easily available via MR and CT techniques. The MR and CT techniques, however, lack the ability to locate tiny vessels and the morphological estimation of stenoses and aneurysms.

With advancements in MR technology and MR acquisition techniques,[4] the burden on vascular segmentation has certainly been reduced. But due to the complexity of the body vasculature, occlusions, small diameters of the vessels, and other factors, the segmentation problem has not been fully solved. Researchers are aggressively attempting to segment the vessels (arteries and veins) from the human body using computer vision, graphics, and image

---

[1]Most of the research done in ultrasound has been in the area of cardiovascular coronary arteries.
[2]Subtraction of the x-ray images without contrast material from x-ray angiograms.
[3]One can still achieve the 3-D information by using the stereo reconstruction from x-ray angiograms with multiple viewpoints.
[4]Pulse sequence programming.

processing (CVGIP) techniques and recently there has been tremendous interest in using automated segmentation of vasculature from MRA data sets. The main motivations for performing vascular segmentation include:

1. *Neuro-surgical planning, interventional procedures and treatments.* The ability to perform segmentation of three-dimensional brain vessels is important for neurosurgeons because it aids in the visualization of "intracranial saccular aneurysms" in relation to the vessels (see [36–39]). This helps in planning the brain surgery and in performing angioplasty. The position of the tumor can be localized using the three-dimensional venous structures as landmarks or roadmaps before and during the surgery (see [37]). Similar examples can be seen in the abdomen, such as for abdominal aortic aneurysms (AAA). Segmentation also helps in real-time operating room decision making and post-operative monitoring. Segmentation of the vasculature can help in endovascular treatment for intracranial saccular aneurysms (see [40]).

2. *Time saving.* Automated or semi-automated vasculature segmentation helps surgeons, radiologists, and oncologists in many different ways. For example, it can save radiologists a significant amount of time required for manual segmentation and can facilitate further data analysis. Another example is the preoperative evaluation of patients scheduled for endovascular repair by performing the computation of the minimum and maximum diameters of the lumen. These measurements are acquired in the planes perpendicular to a previously determined central lumen line at certain intervals.

3. *Distinguishing between the veins and arteries.* Segmentation also helps the radiologists and physicians in separating and visualizing arteries and veins (bright[5] blood and dark[6] blood vessels) (see Figure 1.4 and Figure 1.5).

4. *Relative placement of the brain structures.* Segmenting brain areas and brain blood vessels helps surgeons in studying the growth process of the brain structures and their relationships to each other.

5. *Blood flow process and hemodynamics.* Research is currently active in studying the relationship of the blood flow[7] in the blood vessel structures (see Figure 1.7). This includes hemodynamics and wall shear stress in the development and progression of atherosclerosis and other vascular diseases (see [41–43]). Wall shear stress

---

[5]Sometimes also called white.

[6]Sometimes also called black.

[7]The status of blood circulation in a given patient is helpful in predicting the results of potential treatment procedures.

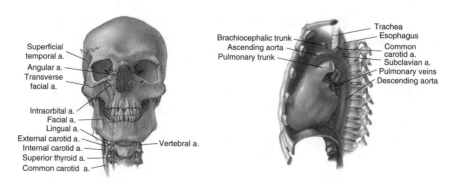

FIGURE 1.2 (See color insert.)

Vasculature system for the head and neck and the heart embedded in the skull and chest cavity, respectively. Left: Neck arteries entering the skull area. Right: Aorta seen in the chest cavity. (Courtesy of Professor Fishman, Johns Hopkins University, Baltimore, MD).

measurements in the abdominal aorta and other body parts need to be further researched (see [44]).

6. *Stenosis and aneurysm assessment/quantification.* Segmentation of vasculature is very useful for the detection and grading of stenoses and aneurysms and for assessment (see [45–49]), especially in the areas of brain, bronchial trees, and bile ducts. This is particularly helpful in the clinical evaluation of atherosclerosis. The shape, size, and location of aneurysms are critical in the embolization procedure.[8]

7. *Disease monitoring/remission.* Having an accurate description of vessel structures is important for monitoring disease progress or remission.

8. *Quantification of vascular structures.* Since the centerline vessel axis can serve as a basis for the description of quantitative diagnosis, vessel quantification is necessary (see [38]).

Having discussed the applications and sources of motivations for performing vascular segmentation, we now present the major difficulties in performing segmentation of the vasculature in MR data sets. The following are the main reasons contributing to the complexity in vasculature segmentation from MRA data sets (see [18]):

1. *Vessel shape complexity and variability.* The vessels are curvey, twisted (tortuous), and sometimes occluded,[9] or there could be superposition of structures/vessels (see Figures 1.2, 1.3, 1.4, 1.5, and 1.6

---

[8]Accurate delivery of anti-embolic material to avoid stroke.

[9]Overlap of vessels with one another.

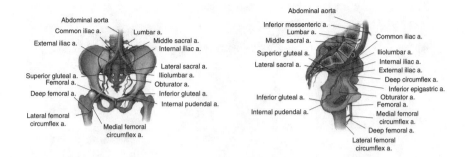

FIGURE 1.3 (See color insert.)
Vasculature system for pelvis region. Left: Pelvis frontal view. Right: Pelvis lateral view. (Courtesy of Professor Fishman, Johns Hopkins University, Baltimore, MD).

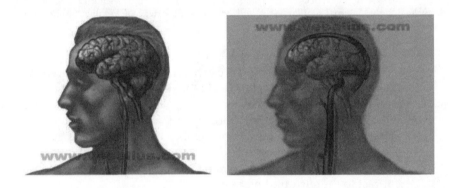

FIGURE 1.4 (See color insert.)
Right: The brain and its carotid artery supply. Left: The brain and its major venous drainage. (Courtesy of Vesalius Studios; www.vesalius.com/).

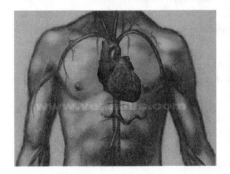
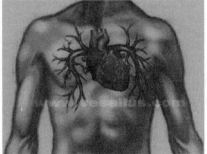

FIGURE 1.5 (See color insert.)
Vasculature system in the chest region. Left: Heart and aorta with major upper body branches. Right: The heart and pulmonary arteries. (Courtesy of Vesalius Studios; www.vesalius.com/.)

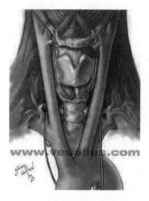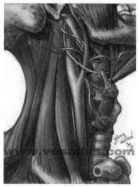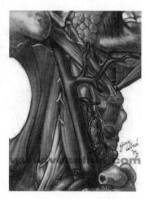

FIGURE 1.6 (See color insert.)
Vasculature system in the neck. Left: Anterior view of carotid arteries. Middle: Carotid artery branches. Right: Internal jugular veins and branches. (Courtesy of Vesalius Studios; www. vesalius.com/.)

corresponding to the vasculature in head, heart, pelvis, brain, chest, and neck areas, respectively). The branching of the vessels also contributes to the complexity in performing vasculature segmentation. Due to the topology and morphology of the vasculature, the vessel shapes and sizes may vary considerably, especially in the case of stenoses and aneurysms. In addition, the vessels are embedded in tissues with similar projection characteristics, permitting only a low contrast to the surrounding tissues.

2. *Vessel density and Diameter of small vessels.* The complexity of the segmentation increases with density and reduction of the diameter of vessels (see Figure 1.7, 7th image from top left corner). MRA has low resolution and contrast, especially with regard to the visibility of small vessels. The spatial continuity is poor along narrow, elongated objects such as thinner blood vessels, which are sometimes as thin as 1 to 2 mm.

3. *Noise and gaps in vessels.* The MRA acquisition process brings in gaps in the vessels, and the resulting data sets could be noisy. This poses difficulty in tracking the vessels.

4. *Dynamic range of intensities.* Many structures in the human body show high intensity values similar to vessel intensity values. The dynamic range of intensities is small between vessels and other structures. This is particularly seen in computer tomography angiography (CTA) data sets, where the intensity values of the vessels and bone are the same. Thus, the extraction of vessels becomes a challenging task to perform in CTA data sets. In the case of

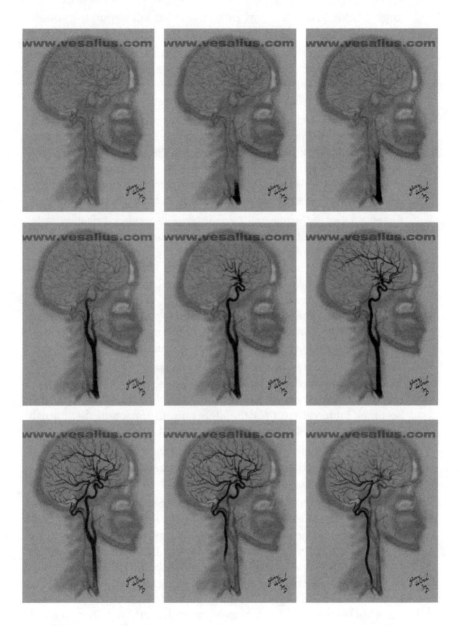

FIGURE 1.7 (See color insert.)
Lateral view of a carotid angiogram (arterial to venous). Top to bottom and left to right: shown are only limited angiogram frames: arterial (1–6) and venous (7–9) phases. Also, the density of the vessels and bifurcation can be appreciated. (Courtesy of Vesalius Studios; www.vesalius.com/.)

time-of-flight (TOF) MRA data sets, the variation in intensities is large. This is due to the flow properties of blood within the vessels (see [19]).

5. *Partial volume averaging.* Due to partial volume averaging (PVA), a voxel could have a combination of intensities from vessels and background. Particular difficulties occur at vessel bifurcations/branching due to PVA and calcification (which is common at bifurcations).

6. *White blood and black blood issues.* In the case of segmenting "white blood vessels," imaging conditions can cause some background areas to be as bright as other vessel areas; therefore, thresholding alone cannot be used. In the case of segmenting "dark-blood[10] vessels," imaging conditions can cause some background areas to be as dark as black blood vessels, making detection between them difficult.

7. *Characteristics of the imaging modality and motion/blood flow artifacts.* The resolution and clarity of the images play a critical role in vascular segmentation. This data acquisition process plays an equally critical role in the accuracy and robustness of the vascular segmentation process. For example, artifacts in MR imaging could be due to several kinds (for details, see [21] and [23]). In MRA, we can have ringing artifacts (see [24]) or artifacts due to patient motion or blood flow. This contributes to the intensity nonhomogeneity in the vessel, which makes the segmentation process difficult to perform.

8. *The ability to distinguish between arteries and veins.* Due to the similarity in the enhancement characteristics of the vessels and the proximity of arteries and veins, in addition being thin and curvey, it becomes more difficult for the algorithm to track and distinguish between these vessels (see Figures 1.4 and 1.5).

9. *Hemodynamics.* Due to imperfect timing of the arrival of the contrast agent and the partial volume effect, vessel detection and separation of the vein and the artery become very difficult.

10. *Scanning limitation.* In vascular image processing, for tracking the vessels, we find the imaging plane perpendicular to the vessel central axis. This plane is mathematically computed. Had the scanning system provided this imaging plane, the tracking of the vessels would have been very easy. Thus, one of the limitations in vascular tracking is the weakness of the scanning system for its inability to provide the orthogonal imaging planes to the central axis of the vessel. Also the vessels are curved, tortuous, and it is therefore not possible for the current MRA technology to scan the vascular structures in this manner. Because of this scanning limitation, we tailor

---

[10] Also called black blood vessels.

the image processing algorithms to perform the three-dimensional segmentation.

Having discussed the motivations and difficulties in vasculature segmentation, we next discuss the taxonomy of the vasculature[11] segmentation techniques (see Figure 1.8). The vasculature segmentation techniques are further divided into two types: *indirect or skeleton based*, and *direct or non-skeleton based*. Skeleton-based techniques are those that segment and reconstruct the vessels by first computing the skeleton of the vessels from the two-dimensional slices. These are also called indirect methods because the vessels are reconstructed by computing the vessel cross sections. Non-skeleton-based techniques are those that compute the vessels in three-dimensional directly. Here, the vessel reconstruction is done without estimating the vessel cross sections. Both of these broad techniques can be computed using one of two types: with multi-scale or without multi-scale.[12] Skeleton or indirect-based techniques are classified into three broad classes:

1. Skeleton with vessel cross-section estimation using edge-based techniques
2. Skeleton with vessel cross-section estimation using parametric-based models
3. Skeleton with vessel cross-section estimation using geometric-based models.

The difference between these three is in the way the cross section of the vessels is estimated, given the skeleton center line of the vessels. Non-skeleton or direct-based techniques are classified into eight different types:

1. Threshold based
2. Fitting based
3. Mathematical morphology based
4. Fuzzy connectivity based
5. Deformable model based
6. Scale-space line filter based
7. Pixel-classification in scale-space based
8. Differential geometry based.

In threshold-based techniques, one estimates the threshold to separate the vasculature from nonvasculature structures. The threshold estimation method

---

[11]See also the work by Coatrieux et al. [6].

[12]We will deal with the multi-scale concept later, but for now, think of multi-scale as a technique that can adjust the detection process of varying thickness by adjusting its scale-space (see [57–81]).

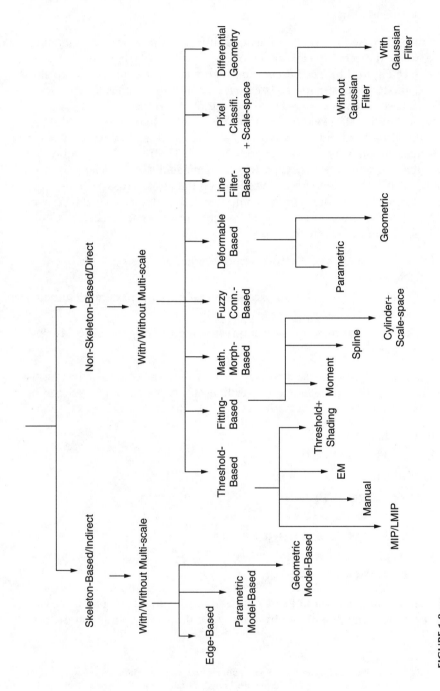

FIGURE 1.8
This chart shows vasculature segmentation techniques.

could be manual, semi-automatic, or automated. The threshold-based technique is divided into four types, depending on the method for computing the threshold:

1. MIP/local MIP
2. Manual
3. Expectation-maximization (EM) based (see [118])
4. Threshold followed by shading

The fitting-based method uses the method of fitting the cylindrical or elliptical models for vessels (see [120]). The main idea is to fit the piece-wise cylinders to the vessels. The fitting-based method is of three types:

1. Moment based
2. Spline based
3. Cylindrical plus scale-space based

The moment-based method uses three-dimensional moment rules for computation of orientations of the vasculature model. The spline-based method fits the spline with a certain degree of basis functions. The cylindrical scale-space-based method uses the cylindrical model to start with and then uses the scale-space for detection. The mathematical morphology-based technique uses the nonlinear mathematical operators along with connectivity for vascular segmentation (see [132]). The Fuzzy connectivity-based technique uses the the Fuzzy method for segmenting the vessels from the three-dimensional MRA volume (see [133, 134, 136, 137]). The deformable-based technique is divided into two types: (1) parametric and (2) geometric deformable models for segmenting the vessels from the MRA volume (see [145, 146]). The scale-space three-dimensional line filter method uses three-dimensional Hessian computation in scale-space for three-dimensional vascular segmentation (see [30, 150–152]). Pixel-classification in scale-space uses Markov Random Field (MRF) with Mean Field (MF) in scale-space for two-dimensional vessel extraction maximum intensity projection[13] images. Differential geometry is divided into two types: (1) with and (2) without Gaussian-based techniques, which use partial derivatives of the image volumes for computing the directions of the vessel.

Before we discuss the goals of this chapter, we will briefly discuss the differences between this chapter and previous review papers, such as [38, 107]. In [107], the role of MR physics in relation to vascular segmentation was discussed. Also discussed in detail were data acquisition techniques, followed

---

[13]We will discuss MIP in Subsection 1.3.1.1.

by a brief overview on the vascular segmentation techniques using magnetic resonance angiographic data sets. This article provides a detailed version of the vascular segmentation techniques applied to imaging modalities such as MR, CT, x-ray, and DSA. The following are the key differences between this Chapter and the article by Suri et al. [107]:

1. Reference [107] paper discusses in detail the vascular segmentation techniques and the comparative details among the other modalities.
2. Reference [107] paper gives a detailed classification division of two- and three-dimensional vascular segmentation techniques.
3. Reference [107] paper further highlights the pros and cons in detail on the different techniques and their implementations.
4. Reference [107] paper describes more about the practical issues related to vascular segmentation when dealing with different imaging modalities.

Having discussed the importance, motivations, difficulties, and the taxonomy of the vasculature segmentation, we will now define the goals of this chapter:

1. To learn about the fast expanding classification taxonomy of vascular segmentation techniques and the links between these core classes. Further, to establish the relationships between low-level computer vision and fast differential geometric techniques for a variety of vasculature applications.
2. To survey the state-of-the-art literature in:
   a. Region-based two- and three-dimensional vascular segmentation
   b. Boundary/surface-based two- and three-dimensional vascular segmentation
   c. The fusion of boundary/surface-based with region-based for two- and three-dimensional MRA vascular segmentation techniques.

   This will also involve discussing the pros and cons of the vascular segmentation techniques (especially from INRIA,[14] ISI-UU,[15]

---

[14]Institut National de Recherche en Informatique et Automatique, Sophia-Antipolis, France.
[15]Image Science Institute, Utrecht University, Utrecht, The Netherlands.

IMDM,[16] MIT,[17] NIH,[18] MMS,[19] UI,[20] UNO,[21] OU,[22] UPenn[23]) and the salient features. Special emphasis will be given on the success of scale-space vision and how the fusion of regional forces is incorporated into the topology driven snakes/surfaces in the level set framework using partial differential equations (PDEs).

3. To discuss the validation of vascular segmentation techniques, challenges in vasculature segmentation, and the future of vasculature segmentation.

4. To provide a comprehensive ready-reference for readers pursuing advanced vessel-imaging research covering the latest state-of-the-art literature and techniques, which solves the complex problem of two- and three-dimensional vasculature segmentation. Note that we will not discuss the work of segmentation used in endoscopy, although this branch is seeming to emerge rapidly. This is out of the scope of this chapter.

The remainder of this chapter is organized as follows. Section 1.3 presents the non-skeleton-based techniques and in Section 1.4, we present the skeleton-based segmentation techniques. Section 1.5 presents the discussions on non-skeleton and skeleton-based segmentation techniques.

1.2 A Brief Note on MRA Data Acquisition and Prefiltering

A brief understanding of MRA data acquisition is necessary to appreciate the vascular segmentation. Before we discuss the data acquisition, we first discuss the five kinds of surface receive coils used for collecting the MRA data sets. Figure 1.9 shows five types of radio-frequency (RF) surface receive coils used for collecting time-of-flight (TOF) MRA data sets. The Head Coil (top row middle), Anterior Neck Coil (top row right) and Posterior Neck Coil (bottom row left), and Integrated Spine Array (ISA) (bottom row right) Coils shown are manufactured by Marconi Medical Systems, Inc., Cleveland, OH. The Head Coil is a single channel receive-only design, used for imaging the head and its associated vasculature. The Anterior and Posterior Neck Coils

---

[16]Institute of Math. and Computer Science in Medicine, University Hospital Eppendorf, Hamburg, Germany.

[17]Massachusetts Institute of Technology, Cambridge, MA.

[18]National Institutes of Health, Bethesda, MD.

[19]Marconi Medical Systems, Inc., Cleveland, OH.

[20]University of Iowa, Ames, IA.

[21]University of North Carolina, Chapel Hill, NC.

[22]Osaka University, Osaka, Japan.

[23]University of Pennsylvania, Philadelphia, PA.

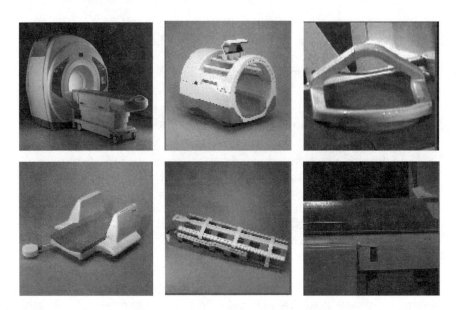

FIGURE 1.9

MRI system and the radio-frequency (RF) surface receive coils used for collecting the MR vasculature data sets. Top Left: MRI system (1.5 Tesla *Infinion^{TM}*). Top Middle: Head coil. Top Right:
Anterior neck coil. Bottom Left: Posterior neck coil. Bottom Middle: Peripheral vascular array
(PVA) coil. Bottom Right: Integrated spine array (ISA) coil. (Courtesy of Marconi Medical Systems, Inc., Cleveland, OH, and USAI, Aurora, OH.)

are each of single-channel, receive-only design, used to image the neck and its
associated vasculature in conjunction with the ISA Coil. The PVA (Peripheral
Vascular Array) Coil is a multi-channel receive-only design, manufactured by
USA Instruments, Inc., Aurora, OH. This coil covers the patient's body from
the heart to the ankle region and is used for run-off studies. The couch moves
in a multi-station fashion during the scan to follow the course of contrast
agent moving through the vasculature in the area covered by this coil.

Having discussed the hardware used for data acquisition, we now discuss the data acquisition process for MRA. This consists of two methods
(see Figure 1.1): (1) a non-contrast method and (2) a contrast method. In the
first case, no contrast agent is injected intraveneously, while in the second
method, Gadolinium-Dithylene-Triamine-Penta-Acetate (Gd-DPTA)[24] is injected. Both methods can be acquired as a two- or three-dimensional acquisition. The fundamental difference between two- and three-dimensional is that
in the two-dimensional case, images are acquired slice by slice using only *one
phase encoding* direction. In three-dimensional case, images are acquired in a
volume using *two phase encoding* directions. The signal-to-noise ratio (SNR) of

---

[24]*Magnevist^{TM}*, manufactured by Schering, Germany.

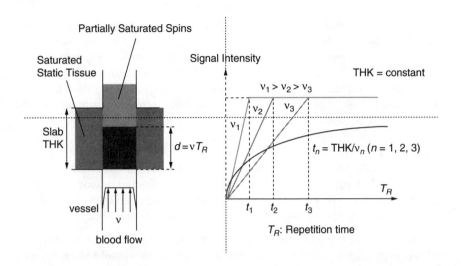

FIGURE 1.10 (See color insert.)
TOF technique: v_i is the velocity of blood flow, THK is the slice or slab thickness, T_R is the repetition time. Note $d = vT_R$ in the figure is same as $v \times T_R$. (Courtesy of Marconi Medical Systems, Inc.)

the three-dimensional acquisition is superior to that of the two-dimensional acquisition, while the acquisition time for three-dimensional MRA is longer than for two-dimensional MRA.

The following methods are currently widely used in practice with the non-contrast technique: (1) time-of-flight (TOF) MRA; (2) phase-contrast MR angiography (PC-MRA); (3) black-blood MRA; (4) T_2-weighted MRA; (5) T_2^*-weighted MRA. These methods can be used in combination along with different gating strategies (synchronizing with the cardiac cycle or respiratory motion) such as cardiac gating (ECG) or respiratory gating. Gating techniques improve the accuracy of blood flow information (blood flow varies in the systolic and diastolic phases) at the expense of extended imaging time.

1.2.1 Time-of-Flight (TOF) MR Angiography

TOF[25] utilizes the so-called *in-flow* effect (see [84–89]). Using a very short repetition time during data acquisition, the static surrounding tissue becomes saturated, resulting in low signal intensity in the acquired images. In contrast, the replenished flowing spins are less saturated, providing stronger signals and thus are able to be differentiated from the surrounding tissues. This is illustrated in Figure 1.10. As seen in this figure, the signal intensity from flowing spins depends on several parameters, including slice or slab thickness (THK), repetition time (T_R), flip angle, velocity vector (v) of blood

---

[25]From now on, whenever we use TOF, we mean TOF-MRA.

flow (magnitude and directions), and d, the displacement of flowing spins with a velocity of v for a given time period T_R. In other words, the replenishment of the flowing spins occurs within a known T_R. This exponential curve represents the spins from static tissue (surrounding tissue) recovering to their original state. As the graph shows, the shorter the repetition time, the smaller the signal, that is, the stronger the static tissue is suppressed. At a given time point, the difference between the exponential curve and the horizontal curve is the contrast between the blood signal and the surrounding tissue. As discussed above, $d = v \times T_R$. The larger the velocity v, the larger the displacement. In the case where $d = v \times T_R$ is greater than the slab thickness THK, the blood signal is completely replenished. Therefore, for a fixed T_R, when the velocity v is larger than a certain value, the signal intensity from the blood signal will stay a constant, as shown by the horizontal curve.

Pros and Cons of the TOF Technique: It should be pointed out that the TOF technique provides blood flow images instead of true vessel lumen images. The major *advantage* of TOF is that it is readily available because of its simplicity for the data acquisition and display. The major *disadvantages* of TOF include:

1. TOF technique is not robust under complicated flow conditions, including slowly flowing blood flow, turbulent blood flow, recirculated and swirling blood flow, which is usually present in tortuous vessels. Under such cases, signal void can appear, falsifying stenoses or occlusions.

2. Depending on the sequence parameters used and flow condition (oblique flow), TOF suffers from the phase shift effect, which causes misregistration between vessel lumen and blood flow, resulting in distortion (the flow images are not identical to the vessel lumen).

3. Another problem related to TOF includes slab boundary artifact due to imperfect radio-frequency (RF) pulse profiles in the multi-slab three-dimensional acquisition. This is particularly a nontrivial issue in three-dimensional acquisitions when it comes to imaging time, inflow enhancement, and complicated flow conditions. Recently, Liu et al. [33] proposed the SLINKY (SLiding INterleaved k_Y) method, which greatly reduces such artifacts, as shown in Figure 1.11.

The SLINKY technique, which uses an interleaved k_Y data acquisition strategy, equalizes flow-related signal intensity weighting across the entire slab dimension. This technique demodulates signal intensity changes along the slab direction and can essentially eliminate the slab boundary artifacts while retaining the same or better imaging time efficiency as that of conventional multi-slab three-dimensional TOF, providing robustness to complicated flow patterns and thereby resulting in a more accurate depiction of vascular morphology. In addition, this technique does not require specialized reconstruction and extra computation.

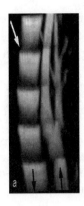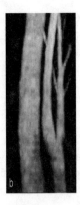

FIGURE 1.11
Carotid MRA maximum intensity projection (MIP) acquired without a superior flow presaturation RF pulse. Left: Three-dimensional multi-slab TOF technique with ramped RF pulse. White
arrow points to slab boundary artifact, black arrows show flow direction. Upward is arterial and
downward is venous. Right: SLINKY technique. The slab boundary artifacts are substantially
reduced in the SLINKY MIP. (Courtesy of Kecheng Liu (see Liu et al. [33]).)

Figure 1.11 illustrates a comparison study of carotid MRA from a healthy
volunteer. Neither superior nor inferior presaturation slab was applied.
On the left is shown the data acquired using conventional multi-slab three-
dimensional TOF with ramped RF pulses to compensate for the signal loss
of arterial flow. As theoretically indicated, ramped RF pulses render the flow
signal in one direction at the cost of exaggerating the slab boundary artifact
for the reversed flow (venous flow). On the right is shown the SLINKY technique without using ramped RF pulses. Slab boundary artifacts are nearly
absent despite the different flow direction, demonstrating the robustness of
the technique.

In clinical application, to improve vessel contrast and visualization, several
preparation RF pulses are recommended. Typically, proximal or distal pre-
saturations are used to selectively screen arteries or veins. MT (magnetization
transfer) pulses can also be used to improve the contrast. As an alternative,
fat saturation pulses are mostly used in body TOF MRA to suppress bright
signals from fat, which has a relatively short T_1.

1.2.2 Phase Contrast MR Angiography (PC-MRA)

Phase contrast MR angiography is based on the fact that for a given magnetic
gradient field, the flowing spins will experience phase shifts ϕ while the
static surrounding tissue will not (see [91–94]). This phase shift ϕ at the peak
of magnetization in the laboratory frame can be generally written as:

$$\phi = \int_0^{T_E} \gamma \overrightarrow{r}(t) \overrightarrow{G}(t) dt \qquad (1.1)$$

where $\vec{G}(t) = [G_x(t), G_y(t), G_z(t)]$ is the gradient vector, γ is the gyromagnetic ratio, T_E is the echo time, and $\vec{r}(t)$ is a time-varying spatial position function, which can be expressed using a Taylor's series as:

$$\vec{r}(t) = \vec{r}_0(t) + \vec{v}\,t + \frac{1}{2}\vec{a}\,t^2 + \cdots = \sum_{n=0}^{\infty} \frac{1}{n!} \frac{d^{(n)}\vec{r}}{dt^n} t^n \qquad (1.2)$$

where $\vec{r}_0(t)$ is the zero-order velocity, $\vec{v}$ is the first order velocity, $\vec{a}$ is the second-order acceleration, and $\vec{v}\,t$ is the product of first-order velocity and second-order acceleration. Considering the first-order velocity term and taking $n = 1$, the flow-related phase shift (Equation 1.1) can be expressed by the following equation:

$$\phi = \int_0^{T_E} \gamma(\vec{r}_0 + \vec{v}\,t)\,\vec{G}(t)dt = \phi_0 + \phi_v \qquad (1.3)$$

where $\phi_0 = \int_0^{T_E} \gamma \vec{r}_0 \vec{G}(t)dt$ is the phase shift of stationary tissue and $\phi_v = \int_0^{T_E} \gamma \vec{v}\,t\,\vec{G}(t)\,dt$ is the phase shift of first-order moving spins. Flow-related phase encoding is usually performed by applying a bipolar gradient, which has no effect on static signal. An example of PCA MIPs from the renal system is shown in Figure 1.12.

Pros and Cons of PCA: The major *advantages* of PCA include: (**1**) PCA is less sensitive to slowly flowing spins and is therefore able to provide more accurate vessel lumen. (**2**) PCA is able to provide flow velocity information, which is useful to study cardiac function and hemofluid dynamics. The major *disadvantage* of PCA is the long acquisition time. This is because at least four acquisitions are needed, which come from the three velocity components $[v_x, v_y, v_z]$. Thus, to measure these velocity components, at least three scans are acquired in three orthogonal directions plus one as a reference. Two conventional applications of PCA are Q-Flow (quantitative flow measurement) and MCA (magnitude contrast angiography). In the Q-Flow application, phase images are

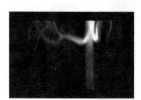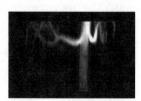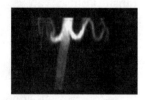

FIGURE 1.12
MIPs created from data acquired at various angles in the coronal to sagittal plane using the PCA technique for the renal system. Left: projection 2. Middle: projection 5. Right: projection 15. Image parameters used: $T_E = 6.3$ ms, $T_R = 85$ ms, FOV $= 24$ cm, matrix size $= 128 \times 256$, NSA $= 1$, flip angle $= 30°$, slice thickness $= 1.5$ mm, gap $= 0$ mm. (Courtesy of Marconi Medical Systems, Inc.)

acquired using the relationship: $\phi = \frac{Im(image)}{Re(image)}$, where Im and Re are the imaginary and real components of the image, respectively. The phase is proportional to one of the velocity components, depending on the encoding relationship. Thus, velocity images, $v = f(x, y, z, t)$, can be obtained. MCA is a specific case of PCA in which one image is acquired with a refocused phase shift while another image is acquired with a spoiled phase shift, presenting flow-related signal as a void. In the subtracted images, only blood "flow" is presented.

1.2.3 Black-Blood Angiography (BBA)

In contrast to TOF MRA, which attempts to maximize flow-related signal, black-blood-based MRA aims at minimizing flow-related signal, producing flow signal voids (see [53, 54, 95]). Thus, vessel lumens appear as dark areas. Therefore, black-blood MRA could truly delineate with the vasculature. Technically, black-blood MRA can be performed in different ways. A gradient recalled sequence can be used in combination, either with large bipolar gradients or presaturation RF pulses. Spin-echo (SE) style sequences utilize wash-out effects. This means a flowing spin will hardly experience an excitation and refocus RF pulses, contributing little or no signal to the final images. Therefore, SE style sequences are considered a self-disruptive technique for which neither large bipolar gradient nor presaturation RF pulses are necessary. Figure 1.13 (right) shows a black-blood MRA image of the knee acquired using T_2-weighted three-dimensional fast spin echo (FSE).

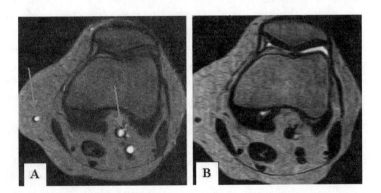

FIGURE 1.13
Axial images from a knee MRA. Left: The bright blood (**A**) and two-dimensional TOF, acquired in the axial plane. Right: The black-blood (**B**) and T_2-weighted three-dimensional FSE, acquired in the sagittal plane, reformatted here in the axial plane. The imaging time for three-dimensional FSE was comparable with two-dimensional TOF but covered a larger volume. In **A**, the arrows (flow images) point to vessels but they also have some black neighborhood around it. In **B**, the black-blood image shows perfect vessel capture. Thus, the left image has a weakness due to its acquisition methodology. (Courtesy of Kecheng Liu, Marconi Medical Systems, Inc.)

Pros and Cons of Black-Blood MRA Technique: The *advantages* of black-blood MRA include: (1) it is less sensitive to slowly flowing spins and complicated flow patterns, which would be problematic in TOF; (2) this presents an accurate depiction of true vessel lumen, instead of a blood flow image; and (3) it is also free from the phase shift effect, presenting no spatial misregistration or distortion. Therefore, black-blood MRA is more accurate than TOF images. The *disadvantages* of black-blood MRA is the difficulty in its image segmentation. This is because (1) two vascular systems are always presented together, causing complexity for radiologists in reading images; (2) there are other dark or black areas, such as tracts, sphenoid sinus, and dark muscles, which essentially hamper the use of minimum-intensity projection.

1.2.4   Contrast Enhanced MR Angiography (CE-MRA)

The process of acquiring CE-MRA consists of the following steps (see [99, 100]):

1. Injection of a contrast agent, such as Gd-DTPA dimelumine (Magnevistp^{TM}, Shering, Germany) into the vein, which is an intravascular but extracellular substance, and that substantially reduces the T_1 value of the blood. The injection procedure is not trivial. First, the injection rate (how fast the contrast agent is injected into the body) affects the arterial phase and venous phase, and therefore the shape of the curve. A power injector is recommended over manual injection to improve reliability and for consistency. Second, to guarantee detection of the bolus arrival, after injection of the contrast agent, the injector is switched to inject a certain amount of saline into the vein. In recent years, programmable power injectors with embedded microchips have been provided by several vendors.

2. Measurement of the timing of the bolus arrival. This can be achieved either by a test bolus method or real-time bolus tracking. The test bolus requires an extra injection. The first injection uses only a small amount (dose) of contrast agent, which measures the timing of the contrast agent arrival, as well as the *arterial phase* (arteries are filled with contrast agent) and *venous phase* (veins are filled with contrast agent). Those parameters are passed to the MR system and used when a full dose of the contrast agent is injected into the patient. Real-time bolus tracking can be performed either by monitoring k-space signal intensity changes (Smart-Prep^{TM}) or directly visualizing fluoroscopic images acquired at a rate of about 1 second/frame. As soon as the bolus arrival has been detected, the data acquisition is immediately switched into the three-dimensional acquisition in conjunction with so-called *centric elliptical phase encoding*. The greatest advantage of real-time bolus tracking is that it uses a single injection of contrast agent. This method, however, requires

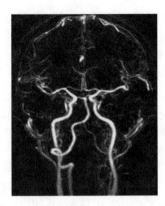 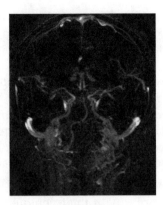

FIGURE 1.14
Coronal maximum intensity projections for CE-MRA acquisition: (**A**) first pass and (**B**) second pass. As this figure shows, the first pass (on the left) captured the arterial phase fairly well (venous flow almost absent), while the timing for the second pass (on the right) was a little too late (both arteries and veins are present with faded intensity). Imaging protocol used a single injection with fluoroscopic detection. (Courtesy of Marconi Medical Systems, Inc.)

higher system performance, such as faster acquisition and instant acquisition switching, etc. Timing in contrast-enhanced MRA plays a key role in the success of the data acquisition. Improper timing means using an incorrect acquisition time window, resulting in artifacts and degraded image quality (see Figure 1.14 where the imaging parameters used were: T_R/T_E = 4.6/2.1 ms, BW = 83.3 kHz, matrix = 192 × 220 (384 × 440), FOV = 270 mm, THK = 1.2 mm, 50 slices, 40 seconds/frame, two frames acquired in the coronal imaging plane).

3. Fast three-dimensional data acquisition. This is usually acquired in the coronal plane in order to cover a larger volume in a shorter period of time. In recent years, several state-of-the-art ultrafast MR techniques (see [102, 103]) have become popular for this purpose, such as SMASH™ and SENSE™, which can speed data acquisition.

Pros and Cons of CE-MRA: The following are the *advantages* of the CE-MRA technique:

1. Efficiency of data acquisition. Because the contrast-enhanced agent significantly reduces the T_1 value of blood, a very short repetition time can be used without penalties of SNR or CNR loss. Data can be collected in a very short time with superior SNR.

2. The method is virtually independent of flow behavior, such as velocity or flow pattern. Therefore, it results in more accurate description of the morphology and pathology, such as stenosis and occlusions, than the TOF method, which depends on the magnitude of velocity.

3. The method can provide not only morphological information but also physiological information, reflecting the functioning of the circulatory system.

The following are the major *disadvantages* of CE-MRA:

1. Requirements needed on specific hardware to guarantee certain performance, especially data acquisition speed. These include a programmable power injector for bolus (contrast agent) injection, and also specific computation capability for fast image reconstruction.

2. Cost per examination. It costs extra for the contrast agent.

3. Complexity of the technique. The entire data acquisition needs a highly synchronized operation (timing). Any mistake could result in deteriorated image quality, which could be inferior to non-contrast images. In some circumstances, a trade-off between temporal and spatial resolution has to be made.

Having discussed the different kinds of data acquisition techniques, their pros and cons, the limitations on two- and three-dimensional acquisitions, we will next discuss the segmentation techniques for extracting vessels in two- and three dimensions using MRA. Note that we did not discuss the T_2 and T_2^* techniques as they can be found in any book on basic MRI (for details, see [98]). Also note that we will not discuss the filtering or image enhancement algorithms for MRA here. Interested readers can look at [25, 31, 34–36].

1.3   Non-Skeleton (Direct) Vascular Segmentation Techniques

Segmentation in medical imaging modalities has been in existence for more than 40 years, but computer-assisted segmentation only began in the past 20 years. Good survey articles on segmentation have been written. Interested readers are referred to the latest book and survey articles by Suri et al. [21–23] and Valev et al. [55]. These articles cite more than ten good survey papers in the area of medical imaging. The discussion of those articles is out of the scope of this chapter. Segmentation in angiography has been active since 1985 when digital subtraction angiography (DSA) began (see [13, 14]).

The layout of this section is as follows. First, Section 1.3.1 presents the thresholding-based techniques. The fitting-based techniques are presented in Section 1.3.2. Techniques based on Fuzzy connectedness for vasculature segmentation are presented in Section 1.3.3. Vasculature segmentation using geometric deformable models is presented in Section 1.3.4. Segmentation techniques using mathematical morphology are presented in Section 1.3.5. Segmentation based on three-dimensional multi-scale line filter is presented

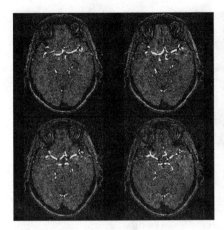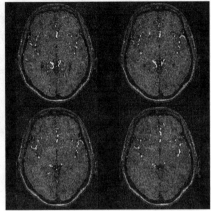

FIGURE 1.15
Images showing arterial flow (bright blood) in the brain. Imaging parameters used: volume (three-dimensional) TOF SLINKY technique acquired in the axial plane with a superior walking presat, $T_E = 6.7$ ms, $T_R = 27$ ms, FoV $= 20$ cm, matrix size $= 384 \times 512$, NSA $= 1$, flip angle $= 35°$, thickness $= 1$ mm, gap $= 0$ mm. (Courtesy of Marconi Medical Systems, Inc., Cleveland, OH.)

in Section 1.3.6. The multi-scale technique for vasculature segmentation is presented in Section 1.3.7.

1.3.1 Threshold-Based Segmentation Techniques: Manual and Automatic

Threshold-based techniques for vasculature segmentation are those using manual, semi-automatic, and automatic thresholding methods. This subsection has the following parts: In Subsection 1.3.1.1, we briefly present the Maximum Intensity Projection (MIP) and local MIP. Subsection 1.3.1.2 presents the manual thresholding for vascular segmentation techniques. Subsection 1.3.1.3 presents the thresholding method along with the shading techniques for vessel display. Automatic thresholding based on Expectation Maximization (EM) is discussed in Subsection 1.3.1.4.

1.3.1.1 Maximum Intensity Projection and Local Maximum Intensity Projection

MIP: Figure 1.15 shows a set of MRA images in the brain generated using the three-dimensional TOF technique. The MIP was generated by selecting the maximum value along an optical ray that corresponds to each pixel of the two-dimensional MIP image. The MIP results in three orthogonal planes are shown in Figure 1.16.[26] The display shows reasonably good presentation of the densitometry of vessels (compare Figure 1.16 and Figure 1.7).

---

[26]Note that the corresponding images and MIPs can also be displayed for the venous flow. For details on MIP, see [104, 105, 112, 113].

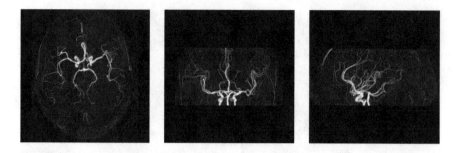

FIGURE 1.16
Orthogonal projections using the MIP algorithm for bright blood arterial images from Figure 1.15. Left: Transverse. Middle: Coronal. Right: Sagittal. Imaging parameters used: volume TOF technique, $T_E = 6.7$ ms, $T_R = 27$ ms, FoV $= 20$ cm, matrix size $= 384 \times 512$, thickness $= 1$ mm, gap $= 0$ mm, NSA $= 1$, flip angle $= 35°$. (Courtesy of Marconi Medical Systems, Inc., Cleveland, OH.)

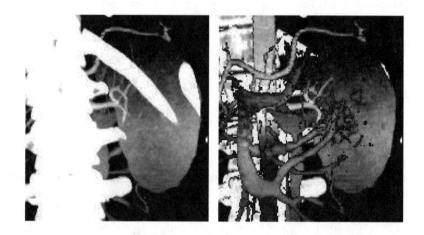

FIGURE 1.17
Comparison of MIP vs. Local MIP of CT renal volume. Left: MIP algorithm. Right: Local MIP (LMIP) algorithm. (Courtesy of Professor Sato, Osaka University, Osaka, Japan.)

Pros and Cons of MIP: The major *advantages* of MIP included: (1) easy design; (2) fast way for visualization of angiography data; and (3) MIP can be obtained irrespective of any direction of transverse, that is, front to back or back to front. The major *disadvantages* of MIP included: (1) loses the three-dimensional information, and (2) not helpful for finding stenosis.

Local MIP: The Local MIP (LMIP) was recently developed by Sato et al. [106], which showed improvements over MIP. The basic principle was to create an image by tracing an optical ray traversing three-dimensional data from the view points in the viewing direction, and then selecting the first local maximum value encountered that is larger than the preselected threshold value (see Figure 1.17), showing the renal system. For details, see Sato [106].

Pros and Cons of LMIP: The major *advantages* of LMIP included: (1) simple design, and (2) better performance compared to MIP. The major *disadvantages* of LMIP included: (1) sensitive to direction; (2) user selective threshold was used for LMIP generation; and (3) no three-dimensional information was produced. One way to improve upon this would be to use manual segmentation per slice to reconstruct the three-dimensional vasculature, which is discussed next. Another recent approach was by Mroz et al. [108]. Interested readers can research this algorithm.

1.3.1.2 Manual Thresholding for Vascular Segmentation

Manual and semi-automatic methods are used for vascular visualization and segmentation (see [109, 110]). Sample results on manual segmentation are shown in Figure 1.18. On the left in this figure is the manually selected threshold for TOF data for a single slice image, with the result of this seen on the right. The process is repeated for the entire volume on a slice-by-slice basis. The output results are displayed in three dimensions (see Figure 1.18, right).

Pros and Cons of Manual Vasculature Segmentation: The major *advantage* of using the manual segmentation method was: (1) traced manual methods

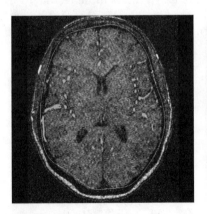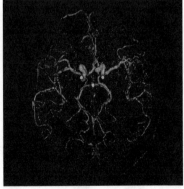

FIGURE 1.18
Manual segmentation results. Left: Manual segmentation of a slice from Figure 1.15 of a bright blood volume MRA TOF SLINKY image using manual thresholding. Right: Results of stacking of all the slices after manual segmentation on a slice-by-slice basis of the MRA images. Imaging parameters used: volume TOF technique, $T_E = 6.7$ ms, $T_R = 27$ ms, FoV = 20 cm, NSA = 1, flip angle = 35°, thickness = 1 mm, gap = 0 mm, matrix size = 384 × 512. (Courtesy of Marconi Medical Systems, Inc., Cleveland, OH.)

are considered the ground truth. The major *disadvantages* of using manual methods included:

1. They were tedious to use, as the data sets were very large.
2. This was a slow process, as it took a long time to perform the tracing.
3. Intra-observer errors were observed due to fatigue.
4. The threshold was adjusted manually for every desired vessel, for every slice, and for every view (axial, sagittal, and coronal), which was an enormous task to perform.
5. It was very difficult to track the tiny vessels due to their size and branching.
6. The quantification process for stenoses and aneurysms was cumbersome.
7. This was a repetitive process.
8. This was a machine-expensive, time-consuming process.

1.3.1.3 Computerized Thresholding and Shading

The surface rendering-based technique for vessel thresholding and display has been done by several authors (see [23, 111–114]). The basic principle was thresholding the volumetric data set and obtaining the binary image slices with the vessels identified or detected. Finally, surface shading was performed based on gradient methods (see Figure 1.19, right). Sample results for renal images can be seen in Figure 1.19. Others [38, 99, 111, 115, 116] have done thresholding on CT data and then surface shaded display (SSD).

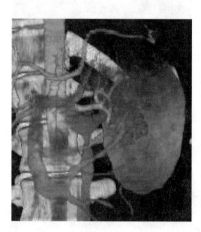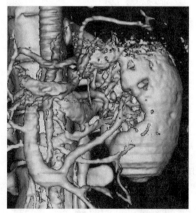

FIGURE 1.19

Comparison of surface shading vs. volume shading of the CT renal volume. Left: Volume rendering using Visual Tool Kit (VTK). Right: Surface rendering using surface shaded display (SSD) algorithm. (Courtesy of Dr. Sato, Osaka University, Osaka, Japan.)

Pros and Cons of Segmentation by Computerized Thresholding and Shading: The major *advantage* was: if the threshold was estimated correctly for applying the marching cube algorithm for surface rendering, then the shaded surface of the blood vessels was visually acceptable. The major *disadvantages* included: (1) It was very difficult to adjust the threshold for running the marching cubes algorithm. As a result, the thin vessels were missed. (2) The occlusion problem was not solved. We will see ahead that some of the drawbacks will be removed by automatic thresholding techniques.

1.3.1.4 *EM-Based Automatic Thresholding for Vascular Segmentation*

Nobel and co-worker (see [117, 118]) developed a technique for segmenting the arteries from the MRA volume by automatically thresholding the MRA volume based on the Expectation-Maximization (EM) algorithm (see [154]). The algorithm consisted of the following steps:

1. *Mixture modeling.* This consisted of modeling the mixture as the tissues of the brain MRA data set, which consisted of two tissue types: artery class (class 0) and two Gaussian distributions (classes 1 and 2). The model presented by Wilson et al. was:

$$p(x) = \underbrace{\frac{w_0}{I_{max}}}_{uniform} + \underbrace{\sum_{k=1}^{2} w_k \frac{1}{\sqrt{2\pi\sigma_k^2}} exp\left[-\frac{1}{2}\left(\frac{x-\mu_k}{\sigma_k}\right)^2\right]}_{Gaussian} \quad (1.4)$$

where μ_k and σ_k were the mean and standard deviation of the Gaussian distribution, respectively. Index k represented the two Gaussian distributions. w_k was the weight of each class k in the mixture.

2. *EM algorithm.* This step consisted of solving the iterative EM algorithm to estimate the mean, variance and weight. We will only present the updating values for the parameters μ_k^{new}, σ_k^{new} and w_k^{new}. For details on the EM algorithm, readers are referred to [81].

$$\mu_k^{new} = \frac{\sum_{i=1}^{i=N} p^{old}(k|x_i)\,x_i}{\sum_{i=1}^{i=N} p^{old}(k|x_i)} \quad (1.5)$$

$$\sigma_k^{new} = \frac{\sum_{i=1}^{i=N} p^{old}(k|x_i)\,\left(x_i - \mu_k^{new}\right)^2}{\sum_{i=1}^{i=N} p^{old}(k|x_i)} \quad (1.6)$$

$$w_k^{new} = \frac{1}{N}\sum_{i=1}^{i=N} p^{old}(k|x_i) \quad (1.7)$$

Note here that N was the total number of voxels being considered and x_i was the intensity of the voxel i, while the function $p^{old}(k|x_i)$

was the conditional probability of voxel i that belonged to class k at the current iteration and was defined as: $p^{old}(k|x_i) = \frac{w_k p^{old}(k|x_i)}{\sum_{j=0}^{M-1} p^{old}(x_i|j)}$.

3. *Threshold computation.* The threshold computed using the EM algorithm was based on the condition that the conditional probability of coming from the uniform class was *greater than* the conditional probability of coming from the other two Gaussian distributions; that is, $w_0 p(x_i|0) > w_k p(x_i|k)$, where k took the values 1 and 2. Following this condition, we obtained the threshold for the voxel x_i belonging to the artery class if and only if x_i was greater than $\left(\mu_k + \sigma_k \sqrt{2 \log \left(\frac{w_k}{w_0} \frac{1}{\sigma_k \sqrt{2\pi}} \right)} \right)$.

Pros and Cons of EM-Based Thresholding Algorithm: The major *advantage* of this technique was its simplicity and straightforwardness in use. The major *disadvantages* of this technique included: (1) it was computationally expensive; (2) the algorithm presented in the article did not show any validation scheme; and (3) the algorithm was applied to healthy volunteers only. There was no discussion on the data sets, except that the data set was TOF type.

1.3.2 Fitting-Based Segmentation Techniques: Moments and Spline Models

This class of indirect method consisted of estimating the vessel contours perpendicular to the vessel axis. These vessel contours were represented by generalized cylinders, B-splines, or triangulated surfaces (see [122–124, 147, 148]).

1.3.2.1 Moment-Based Approach for Vascular Segmentation

Coatrieux and co-workers (see [119–121]) developed an algorithm for blood vessel detection and quantification in MRA data sets. The algorithm consisted of the following steps:

1. Initial seed placement for tracking the three-dimensional vasculature.

2. Correction of the values by computing the orientation (α_0, β_0), which the projected axes of the cylinder made with the x-axis and z-axis, respectively. These values were computed based on the moments and were: $\alpha_0 = \tan^{-1}(\frac{2\mu_{110}}{\mu_{200} - \mu_{020}}) + k\frac{\pi}{2}$ and $\beta_0 = \tan^{-1}[(\frac{2\mu_{101}}{\cos}(\alpha_0) + \mu_{011} \sin(\alpha_0))(\mu_{002} - \mu_{200} \cos^2(\alpha_0) - \mu_{200} \sin^2(\alpha_0) - \mu_{110} \sin 2\alpha_0)^{-1}] + k\frac{\pi}{2}$, where μ's are moments about the axes and k was a constant. The μ's were given as: $\mu_{110} = \frac{(M_{110} - M_{110} M_{010})}{M_{000}}$, $\mu_{200} = M_{200} - \frac{(M_{100})^2}{M_{000}}$,

$\mu_{020} = M_{020} - \frac{(M_{010})^2}{M_{000}}$ and $\mu_{002} = M_{002} - \frac{(M_{001})^2}{M_{000}}$, where M_{prq} was defined as:

$$M_{pqr} = \sum_{i=-\frac{n}{2}}^{\frac{n}{2}} \sum_{j=-\frac{n}{2}}^{\frac{n}{2}} \sum_{k=-\frac{n}{2}}^{\frac{n}{2}} C(i, j, k) f_d(i, j, k) \qquad (1.8)$$

where

$$C(i, j, k) = \sum_{i=-\frac{m}{2}}^{\frac{m}{2}} \sum_{j=-\frac{m}{2}}^{\frac{m}{2}} \sum_{k=-\frac{m}{2}}^{\frac{m}{2}} (i')^p (j')^q (k')^r X(i', j', k'), \text{ and } X(i', j', k')$$

was the binary indicator which had a value of 1 inside the sphere and 0 outside the sphere. f_d was the density function given as:

$$f_d(i, j, k) = \int_{i-\frac{1}{2}}^{i+\frac{1}{2}} \int_{j-\frac{1}{2}}^{j+\frac{1}{2}} \int_{k-\frac{1}{2}}^{k+\frac{1}{2}} f(x, y, z) \, dx \, dy \, dz.$$

3. The diameter of the vessel was computed using the following expression:

$$d = n \left[1 - \left(\frac{\mu_{000} \frac{3}{4\pi} - I_c}{I_b - I_c} \right)^{\frac{2}{3}} \right]^{\frac{1}{2}}$$

where n was the size of the window, I_c was the vessel intensity and I_b was the background intensity.

4. The next step consisted of finding if the next voxel belonged to the vessel. The test was made using the thresholding procedure, if the intensity I was greater than or less than the threshold t, where t was given as:

$$t = \left[I_b \left(1 - \left(\frac{d_{min}}{2} \right)^2 \right)^{\frac{3}{2}} + I_c \left(1 - \left(1 - \left(\frac{d_{min}}{2} \right)^2 \right) \right)^{\frac{3}{2}} \right], \qquad (1.9)$$

where d_{min} was the minimum value of the diameter that has to be detected.

Pros and Cons of the Moment-Based Technique: The major *advantages* of the system included:

1. The method presented a technique to detect the vascular network in MRA data sets.

2. The method provided the local parameters characterizing the normal or abnormal morphology of a vessel based on a cylinder-shaped model.

3. The algorithm was independent of the window size.

The major *disadvantages* of the system included:

1. The model was not capable of understanding the forking or bifurcation behavior of the vessels. Thus, it was very difficult to design all the possible three-dimensional configurations, at least the detection of these deviations from the model and the re-initialization of the tracking procedure along these branches.
2. The window must be adaptive in size and only one vessel should be observed during the tracking procedure.
3. The fundamental assumption in the model was that the tissues consisted of only two classes: background and foreground. Thus, the methodology did not work for more than a two-class problem and usually in abnormal pathology, there are more than two classes.

1.3.2.2 *Vessel Segmentation Using Spline-Based Models*

Recently, Frangi et al. [70–73] developed a fitting model-based method for segmentation of vessels from TOF MRA data sets. The method was called "fitting model-based" because it used an energy minimization model for fitting the "initial spline" toward the "goal spline" for vessel segmentation. The initial spline was the raw spline that the user placed by selecting a few points in three-dimensional space. The goal spline was the spline that was estimated after fitting and consisted of a state of minimum energy. The algorithm consisted of the following steps. The first step consisted of finding the central vessel axis (CVA). This was modeled as: $\mathbf{C}(v) = \sum_{i=0}^{s} N_{in}(v)\mathbf{P}_i$, where $\mathbf{C}(v)$ was the representation for B-spline curve of degree n with $s+1$ control points, $\mathbf{P}_i$ were the control points, $N_{in}(v)$ was the i-th B-spline basis function of order n and $v \in [0, 1]$. This snake model was deformed toward the center of the vessel (goal state) by minimization of the energy function $\mathcal{E}^c$, which was mathematically[27] defined as: $\mathcal{E}^c = \mathcal{E}^c_{internal} + \mathcal{E}^c_{external}$, where $\mathcal{E}^c_{internal}$ was the internal energy of the spline which was the combination of stretching and bending given as: $\mathcal{E}^c_{internal} = \gamma^c_{stretch}\mathcal{E}^c_{stretch} + \gamma^c_{bend}\mathcal{E}^c_{bend}$. Note that $\gamma^c_{stretch}$ and γ^c_{bend} were the stretching and bending constants. The stretching and bending terms were standard due to Kass et al. [142] as the first and second partial derivatives of the central vessel axis contour $\mathbf{C}$. This was mathematically expressed as:

$$\mathcal{E}^c_{stretch} = \frac{1}{l}\int_0^1 \|\mathbf{C}_v(v)\|^2\|\mathbf{C}_v(v)\|dv \quad \text{and}$$

$$\mathcal{E}^c_{bend} = \frac{1}{l}\int_0^1 \|\mathbf{C}_{vv}(v)\|^2\|\mathbf{C}_{vv}(v)\|dv$$

---

[27] c represents the energy due to the central vessel axis fitting.

where $l = \frac{1}{l}\int_0^1 \|\mathbf{C}_v(v)\| dv$. The external energy term, $\mathcal{E}^c_{external}$ was defined mathematically as:

$$\mathcal{E}^c_{external} = -\frac{1}{l}\int_0^1 \underbrace{V(\mathbf{C}(v))}_{potential-energy} \|\mathbf{C}_v(v)\| dv$$

where $V(\mathbf{x}) = \max_{\sigma_{min} \leq \sigma \leq \sigma_{max}} v(\mathbf{x}, \sigma)$ and v was the discriminant function, which depended upon the cross-sectional geometry of the vessel. This discriminant function was actually developed by Frangi et al. [73] and was mathematically expressed as:

$$v(\mathbf{x}, \sigma) = \left[1 - exp\left(-\frac{\mathcal{R}_A^\epsilon}{2\alpha^2}\right) exp\left(-\frac{\mathcal{R}_B^\epsilon}{2\beta^2}\right)\right]\left[1 - exp\left(\frac{S^2}{2c^2}\right)\right]$$

where

$$\mathcal{R}_A = \frac{|\lambda_2|}{|\lambda_3|}$$

$$\mathcal{R}_B = \frac{|\lambda_1|}{\sqrt{|\lambda_2\lambda_3|}}$$

and

$$S = \|\mathcal{H}_\sigma\|_F = \sqrt{\sum_j \lambda_j^2}$$

Pros and Cons of the Spline-Based Methods: The major *advantage* of the system was its simplicity in implementation. The major *disadvantages* of the system included: (**1**) the method was susceptible to errors due to the energy constants; (**2**) the basis function needed to be carefully selected; and (**3**) the accuracy of the system depended on the external energy term due to the image intensities and was susceptible to errors for noisy data.

1.3.3 Scale-Space Fuzzy Connectedness Technique for Vascular Segmentation

Recently, Udupa and co-workers (see [137]) developed an algorithm for segmentation of vessels in three-dimensional based on scale-space Fuzzy connectedness (see the literatue on Fuzzy connectedness by Udupa and co-workers applied to medical image segmentation [133–137]). The algorithm for three-dimensional vessel segmentation consisted of the following steps:

1. κ-Affinity image generation.
2. C_κ-connectivity scene generation. This consisted of first, computation of the scale. This was done by solving the following equation:

$$FO_k(c) = \frac{\sum_{d \in B_k(c)} W_{\psi_s}(|f(c) - f(d)|)}{|B_k(c) - B_{k-1}(c)|} \qquad (1.10)$$

where $|B_k(c) - B_{k-1}(c)|$ was the number of pixels in $B_k(c) - B_{k-1}(c)$ and W_{ψ_s} was the homogeneity function used for defining ψ. This meant that while $FO_k(c)$ was greater than or equal to t_s, keep incrementing k. The scale was thus the last value of k. The connectivity scene generation consisted of the following: set all the elements of the scene to be 0 while the object was set to 1. Push all the elements $c \in C$ such that $\mu_\kappa(o, c) > 0$ to Q. Now the loop was run while Q was not empty. During this loop, f_{max} was computed. If f_{max} was greater than $f_{K_o(c)}$, $f_{K_o(c)}$ was assigned the value f_{max} and the pixels e were loaded in the queue, where $\mu_\kappa(c, e) > 0$.

3. Surface rendering using the shell-rendering technique (see [138]). Figure 1.20 shows the results of running the Fuzzy connectedness algorithm on MRA data sets. As can be seen in this figure, the scale-space method (right column) performed better than the non-scale-space (left column) method.

Pros and Cons of Scale-Space Fuzzy Technique: The major *advantages* of scale-space Fuzzy connectivity technique included:

1. The technique demonstrated that the scale-space method performed better than the non-scale-space-based method.
2. This technique was utilized for separating arteries from veins.
3. The method had been run on over 1500 patient studies for different applications such as brain white matter (WM) segmentation and fibroglandular tissue segmentation in breast x-ray digitized mammograms.

The major *disadvantages* of scale-space Fuzzy connectivity technique included:

1. The fuzzy connectivity was used only for CE-MRA data sets.
2. User interactiveness was needed for parameter estimation.
3. The Fuzzy connectedness technique needed a user-selected threshold for computing the connected scene. Recently, Kobashi et al. [83] came up with a Fuzzy approach to blood vessel segmentation.

1.3.4   Geometric Deformable Models for Vasculature Segmentation

Recently, Lorigo et al. [145] presented an algorithm for brain vessel reconstruction based on curve evolution in three dimensions, also known as "co-dimension two" in geodesic active contours (see [144]). This method used two components: (1) mean curvature flow (MCF) and (2) the directionality of vessels. The mean curvature flow component was used to derive the Eulerian representation of the level set equation. If ϕ was the signed distance transform

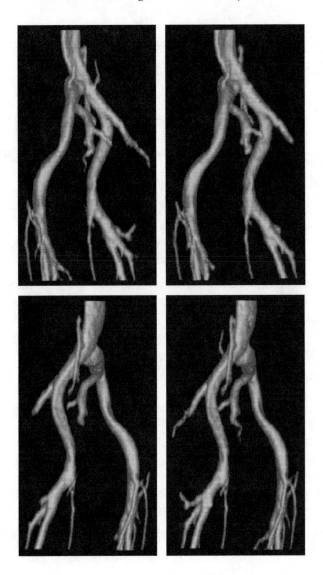

FIGURE 1.20
Three-dimensional vascular segmentation using non-scale (left column) and scale (right column) Fuzzy techniques for two views (top row and bottom row). Top left: Non-scale-based Fuzzy vessel extraction (view-1). Top right: Scale-based Fuzzy vessel extraction (view-1). Bottom left: Non-scale-based Fuzzy vessel extraction (view-2). Bottom right: Scale-based Fuzzy vessel extraction (view-2). (Courtesy of Dr. Udupa, University of Pennsylvania, Philadelphia, PA [136].)

(SDT) and $\lambda(\nabla\phi(\mathbf{x}, t), \nabla^2\phi(\mathbf{x}, t))$ was the eigenvalues of the projection operator: $\mathcal{P}_{\nabla\phi}\nabla^2\phi P_{\nabla\phi}$, where $\mathcal{P} = I - \frac{qq^T}{|q|^2}$ and q was a non-zero vector, then using these eigenvalues, the Eulerian representation of the curve evolution was given by Lorigo et al. as: $\frac{\partial\phi}{\partial t} = \lambda(\nabla\phi(\mathbf{x}, t), \nabla^2\phi(\mathbf{x}, t))$. The second component

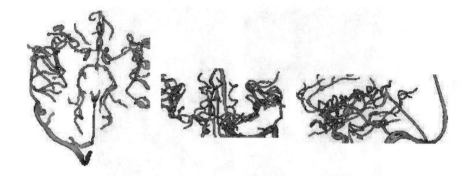

FIGURE 1.21
Segmentation results using Lorigo et al.'s technique [145, 146]. Left: Axial results. Middle: Coronal results. Right: Sagittal results. (Courtesy of Professor Grimson, MIT, Cambridge, MA.)

was the normal of these vessels projected onto the plane and was given as the product of $\nabla\phi$ with the projection vector d. This projection vector was computed using the Hessian of the intensity image I and was given as: $\frac{g'}{g}(H\frac{\nabla I}{|\nabla I|})$, where g was the edge detector operator. Adding these two components, the complete level set equation was:

$$\frac{\partial\phi}{\partial t} = \underbrace{\lambda(\nabla\,\phi(\mathbf{x},t),\nabla^2\phi(\mathbf{x},t))}_{mean-curvature-force} + \underbrace{D \times S \times \frac{g'}{g}\left(H\frac{\nabla I}{|\nabla I|}\right)}_{angular-balloon-force}, \quad (1.11)$$

where D was the directionality term, which was the dot product of $\nabla\phi$ and ∇I, which was the angle between these two vectors. S was the scale term. Note that the second term was like an angular balloon force that navigated the deformation process. The results of running the above algorithm can be seen in Figure 1.21, which shows the axial, coronal, and sagittal results, respectively.

Pros and Cons of Geometric Deformable Model Technique: The major *advantages* of this technique included:

1. The method successfully demonstrated the segmentation of vessels of the brain.
2. The method used the directional component in the level set framework, which was necessary for segmenting twisted, convoluted, and occluded vessels.
3. The technique was used to compute vessel radii, a clinically useful measurement.

The *disadvantages* of geometric deformable model based on the level set framework included:

1. Not much discussion was available on the computation of the scale factor S.

2. The method has yet to show the analytical model because the output of the system showed relatively thinner vessels compared to Maximum Intensity Projection (MIP)[28] and thresholding schemes.

3. There was no comparison made between segmented results and the ground truth; hence, this has not been validated. We will discuss the advantages and disadvantages of the geometric models in level set framework in Section 1.5.

1.3.5 Mathematical Morphology Approach for Vessel Segmentation

Masutani et al. [131] and then Cline [132] presented the algorithm based on mathematical morphology for estimation of the blood vessels from MRA data sets. This was based on the following four fundamental equations of mathematical morphology: dilation (ORing), erosion (ANDing), closing, and opening, expressed as: $M \oplus S = \bigcup_{x \in S} M_{+x}$; $M \ominus S = \bigcup_{x \in S} M_{+x}$; $M \bullet S = (M \oplus S) \ominus S$; and $M \circ S = (M \ominus S) \oplus S$. Figure 1.22 shows the algorithmic steps used for segmentation of the three-dimensional vessels from MRA data sets. The algorithm is self-explanatory; however, the steps are discussed briefly:

1. *Thresholding process.* This step consisted of binarization of the input gray-scale volume based on user threshold.

2. *Morphological smoothing.* This step consisted of eroding the binary volume using the structuring element like a sphere, followed by dilating the resulting volume with the same structuring element.

3. *Mask generation.* This step consisted of mask generation, which consisted of dilating the smoothed volume (computed from the previous step).

4. *Subtraction.* This step consisted of volume subtraction, where the smoothed volume was subtracted from the masked volume.

5. *Intersection.* This step consisted of computing the intersection of the subtracted volume with the original volume.

6. *Connectivity and display.* This step consisted of running the connectivity algorithm over the intersected volume and finally displaying the MIP of this volume for the three-dimensional vessel display.

Pros and Cons of Mathematical Morphology-Based Method: The mathematical morphology method had the following *advantage*: its simplicity and straightforwardness to you. The mathematical morphology method had the

---

[28]The MIP algorithm is a very popular technique. An example can be seen in [112].

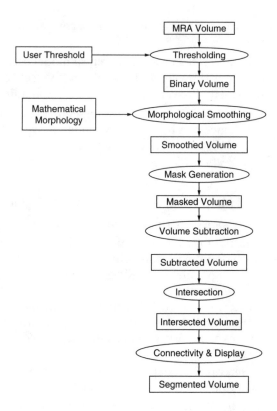

FIGURE 1.22

Cline's [132] method for segmentation of vessels based on three-dimensional mathematical morphology. The ellipses represent the process and the rectangles represent the objects or input/output. As seen in this figure, the main steps are: (1) thresholding, (2) morphological smoothing, (3) mask generation, (4) volume subtraction, (5) intersection estimation, and (6) connectivity and display.

following *disadvantages*: (1) initial stages needed user interaction; (2) no research had been done on the size of the structuring elements; and (3) there was no description on the validation of the algorithm.

1.3.6 Vasculature Segmentation Using Multi-scale Three-Dimensional Line Filter

Recently, Sato et al. [30, 150–152] presented work in the area of three-dimensional segmentation of curvilinear structures. The algorithm was applied to the MR and CT data sets for vessel segmentation. The steps of the algorithm were as follows:

1. *Isotropic volume generation.* This process consisted of changing the gray-scale volume to an isotropic volume where each size of each voxel was *unit cube*.

2. *Thresholding.* Thresholding the interpolated volume to generate the binary volume. This is done slice-by-slice and each image slice was thresholded based on the user-selected threshold.

3. *Connected component analysis for mask generation.* Extract the volume-of-interest (VOI) using connected components to obtain the mask or largest connected component. This step will be used ahead.

4. *Convolution using line filtering.* Take the same interpolated volume (from Step 1) and perform the line filtering by convolving the derivative of the Gaussian filter in three dimensions. This is given as:

$$I_{x^i y^j z^k}(\mathbf{x}, \sigma_f) = \frac{d^i}{d\mathbf{x}^i} G(\mathbf{x}, \sigma_f) \otimes \left\{ \frac{d^j}{d\mathbf{y}^j} G(\mathbf{y}, \sigma_f) \otimes \left\{ \underbrace{\frac{d^k}{d\mathbf{z}^k} G(\mathbf{z}, \sigma_f) \otimes I(\mathbf{x})}_{convolution-1} \right\} \right\},$$

$$\underbrace{\qquad\qquad\qquad\qquad\qquad\qquad}_{convolution-2}$$

$$\underbrace{\qquad\qquad\qquad\qquad\qquad\qquad\qquad\qquad}_{convolution-3}$$

(1.12)

where $I(\mathbf{x})$ was the interpolated gray scale volume, i, j, and k are the non-negative integers satisfying $i + j + k = 2$, and 3σ was used as the radius of the kernel. G was the Gaussian kernel in the x, y, and z directions. $\frac{d^k}{dz^k} G(\mathbf{z}, \sigma_f) \otimes I(\mathbf{x})$ was the convolution of the Gaussian kernel with standard deviation of σ_f. Note that three sets of convolutions are done to obtain the scale-space representation of the gray-scale volume rather than one convolution in three dimensions. This optimizes the speed from n^3 to $3n$ operations. This generates the Hessian matrix $H(x, y, z)$, which is the second derivative of the image volume ($\nabla^2 I$).

5. *Maximization of the multi-scale response (segmentation).* The above process was repeated for, say, n number of iterations and normalized by the scale-space factor σ_i; thus, the maximum scale-space representation was chosen by solving $M(\mathbf{x}) = \max_{1 \leq i \leq n}\{\sigma_i^2 \lambda_{123}(\mathbf{x}, \sigma_i)\}$, where σ_i was the normalization factor.

6. *Multi-scale response and scale-space optimization in the masked region.* Multiply the mask generated from Step 3 with the multi-scale line filter output (5). This will result in the segmented output in the region of interest. The process is optimized for the best σ.

7. *Cleaning using thresholding.* The final cleaning was done on the above segmented output by thresholding, and all voxel regions that have a size larger than ten voxels were removed.

8. *Display using surface rendering.* This step consisted of the final display of the vessel by surface rendering the above output. The results of the input and output of the system can be seen in Figure 1.23.

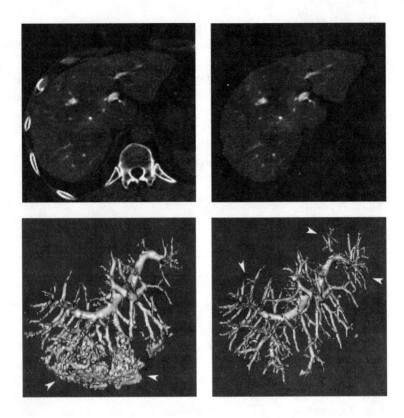

FIGURE 1.23

Surface rendering: Top: Input to the segmentation system. Bottom: Three-dimensional segmentation results using Sato et al.'s technique. (Courtesy of Dr. Sato, Osaka University. Reproduced with permission from Elsevier Science, *Medical Image Analysis*, Vol. 2. No. 2, pp. 143–168, 1998.)

Pros and Cons of the Multi-scale Line Filter: The major *advantages* of the above technique included:

1. The system was able to handle the variation of the curvilinear structures in embedded volumes.
2. The system was well validated using the synthetic model with vessel cross section of circular type and elliptical type.
3. The design of the line filtering was done using the decomposition in three directions, as shown in Equation. 4.26. This optimized the speed from n^3 to $3n$ operations.
4. The system was also parallelized using thread programming.

The major *disadvantage* of the above technique was that the user had to select the threshold for the masking procedure, which was susceptible to errors.

1.3.7 Skeleton-Based with Multi-scale Vessel Model

Krissian et al. [128–130] recently developed a three-dimensional segmentation method for brain vessel segmentation using MRA. The algorithm can be classified as a model-based technique using the scale-space framework. The algorithm consisted of the following steps:

1. *Framing initial model.* This model used was a cylinder with the axis of the cylinder along the z-axis with the cross section being a Gaussian function. This was represented using the following equation:

$$I_0(x, y, z) = CG_{\sigma_0}(x, y) = \frac{C}{2\pi\sigma_0^2}e^{\frac{-(x^2+y^2)}{2\sigma_0^2}} \qquad (1.13)$$

where C was a constant which depended upon choosing the size and location of the vessel and $\frac{C}{2\pi\sigma_0^2}$ represented the intensity at the center of the vessel. The reason for choosing this model was that when this model convolved with the Gaussian kernel of standard deviation s, the resulting image was another vessel that matched this model with a different radius.

2. *Multi-scale response computation.* This step had two parts: part one consisted of the preselection of the candidates using the eigenvalues of the Hessian matrix $H = \frac{I_0}{\sigma_0^4} H_0$. Part two consisted of computation of the scale-space response at one scale s and was given as:

$$R_\sigma(x) = \frac{1}{N} \sum_{i=0}^{N-1} -\nabla_\sigma I(x + \sigma \overrightarrow{v}_\alpha).\overrightarrow{v}_\alpha, \qquad (1.14)$$

where $\overrightarrow{v}_\alpha = cos(\alpha) \overrightarrow{v}_1 + sin(\alpha) \overrightarrow{v}_2$. α ranges from 0 to 2π.

3. *Local extrema computation.* This step consisted of finding the multi-scale response $R_{multi}(x)$ and was given as:

$$R_{multi}(x) = \max_s R_s(x), s \in [s_l, s_h], \qquad (1.15)$$

where $R_s(x)$ was the scale-space response at a scale s and the range of the scale was from s_l to s_h. $R_s(x)$ was computed as:

$$R_s(x) = \min\{|\nabla I_s(x + s \overrightarrow{v}) \cdot \overrightarrow{v}|, \quad \overrightarrow{v} \in \{\pm\overrightarrow{v}_1, \pm\overrightarrow{v}_2\}\}, \qquad (1.16)$$

where $\overrightarrow{v}_1$ and $\overrightarrow{v}_2$ were the eigenvectors of the Hessian matrix.

4. *Skeletonization and visualization.* This step consisted of skeletonization of the vessels.

Pros and Cons of Multi-scale with Vessel Model: The major *advantages* of using this method were: (1) the algorithm used the multi-scale approach for vascular segmentation; and (2) the algorithm showed good behavior on junctions and tangent vessels. The major *disadvantages* of multi-scale with vessel model included (1) the initial model taken was a cylinder, which was too simple for the complex vascular nature of the network; and (2) there was no discussion on the validation.

Although direct techniques are robust, accurate, and very attractive, there lies a major weakness with these techniques, that is, they are computationally very expensive and thus are slow when it comes to real-time data analysis. Thus, researchers are aggressively working on developing indirect methods, which have proved to be faster. We will discuss these techniques ahead.

1.4   Skeleton (Indirect) Vascular Segmentation Techniques

Skeleton or indirect-based techniques utilize the principle of building the skeleton of the vessels (see [182–192]). Section 1.4.1 presents the skeleton-based technique, which uses edge-based fusion for vessel cross-section estimation. Section 1.4.2 presents the skeleton-based technique, which uses deformable model for vessel cross-section estimation. Section 1.4.3 presents the wave propagation algorithm similar to the level set approach for segmentation of two-dimensional angiograms, and finally, this section concludes with segmentation techniques based on differential geometry in Section 1.4.4.

1.4.1   Skeleton-Based with Scale-Space Edge-Based Fusion

Recently, Viergever and co-workers (see [24, 180, 181]) developed a fast delineation technique for vessel reconstruction from different modalities such as computerized tomography angiography (CTA), phase contrast (PC)-MRA, and contrast enhanced (CE)-MRA. The algorithms consisted of the following steps:

1. *Manual initialization.* This step consisted of manually introducing the start and end points of the central vessel axis.

2. Computation of the next *candidate point* along the vessel.

3. *Estimation of the plane perpendicular to this candidate point.* In this step, the step vector was first computed, which consisted of the product of $\alpha \times d_{min}$, where α was a predetermined constant and d_{min} was the minimum diameter estimated of the vessel. The step vector was extended in the direction of the vector that joined the previous vessel center to the current vessel center. The perpendicular to this extended step vector was the perpendicular plane in which the search region s was defined.

4. *Estimating the vessel center in a search region in this perpendicular plane.* The vessel center was computed by finding the center likelihood measure, which was defined as:

$$CLm = \frac{1}{n} \sum_{i=1}^{n} \frac{min(|r_{1l_i}|, |r_{2l_i}|)}{min(|r_{1l_i}|, |r_{2l_i}|)} \tag{1.17}$$

where CLm was the center likelihood measure, n was the total number of rays or lines in the search region, $|r_{1l_i}|$ and $|r_{2l_i}|$ were the absolute value of the rays that originate from the center toward the border of the vessel along the lines l_i, which corresponded for the line i. The rays $|r_{1l_i}|$ and $|r_{2l_i}|$ were computed in opposite directions using the gradient change of the gray-scale intensity. The rays originated from the point source in radial directions. An average of $n = 12$ lines were drawn from the likelihood central point. The gradient component was computed as $\frac{\partial L}{\partial r} = \frac{r \nabla L}{r}$, where $\frac{\partial L}{\partial r}$ was the rate of change of image intensity along the radial direction and $\frac{r \nabla L}{r}$ was the product of the radial vector $\mathbf{r}$ and the gradient of the image intensity ∇L. Note that the gradient of the original image I was computed using Lindeberg's method [86, 87], which was mathematically given as $\nabla L = I \otimes \sigma^\gamma \nabla G$, where γ was the scale factor and G was the Gaussian smoothing function. Thus, given the CLm at all the points in the search region s, the location where CLm was at a maximum gave the vessel center location.

5. *Check of termination conditions.* Here one checks for the adaptation toward the central vessel axis and checking toward the termination conditions. If they were met, then the system exited, or else the process was repeated.

Pros and Cons of the Scale-Space Edge-Based Fusion Method: The major *advantages* of the system included:

1. The system was fast, because it found the central vessel axis in around 10 seconds.

2. One of the important aspects about this algorithm was the introduction of the smoothness constraint, which was responsible for tracking the sudden curvatures of the vessels. So basically, the direction of the tracking process was controlled by the new step vector, $\mathbf{b}_{new}$ (called the smoothed step vector), and was given as $\mathbf{b}_{new} = \frac{\gamma \mathbf{a} + (1-\gamma) \mathbf{c}_{new}}{|\gamma \mathbf{a} + (1-\gamma) \mathbf{c}_{new}|} |\mathbf{b}|$, where γ was the scale factor and had a range from 0 to 1. The larger the values of γ, the more robust the tracking process was to the abrupt changes in the direction of the central vessel axis. On the other hand, the smaller the values of γ, the algorithm prevented the tracking of highly curved vessels.

3. Wink et al. [24] also suggested a more robust method for computing the way to the vessel center in the search region. This was based on the *search tree* method, which explored different extensions to the current central vessel axis simultaneously and at a larger depth. This meant that for every position in this search tree, the *CLm* was computed. The tracking process now proceeded in the direction leading to the highest sum of center likelihoods along the tree. Although this method was more efficient, it was computationally expensive.

The major *disadvantages* of the system included:

1. There were too many parameters to adjust. They were α, the parameter that controlled the vector step; β, a constant that premultiplied the vector step to find the search region s; smoothness constraint γ, and n, the total number of rays that originated from the likelihood vessel center.

2. The system did not take into consideration any *a priori* knowledge for segmentation of the vessels.

3. The system did not show how the vessels were classified.

4. The computation time was linearly proportional to the number of rays originating from the vessel center in the search region.

5. It would have been better if the result showed the effect of the scale parameter γ, because it played a critical role in the tracking process.

6. There was no experimental comparison made between Wink et al.'s method and the indirect methods or other direct methods.

1.4.2 Skeleton-Based with Parametric-Based Model Fusion

Although deformable models[29] have been in existence since 1988, most of the applications were done in segmenting internal brain structures, or isolated structures. Not much was done in this area as applied to vasculature segmentation. Authors who did research in this application included Stein et al. [139] and Bulpitt and Efford [140]. Stein et al. [139] developed a technique to segment Nervus Alveolaris Inferior (NAI) present in the jaw–neck area. This algorithm consisted of the following steps:

1. *ROI reduction.* This step consisted of running the mathematical morphology operation to preprocess the CT images to reduce the search region where the nerve was to be segmented.

---

[29]The three major advantages of deformable models are: (1) ability to fuse regularizers; (2) ability to model the constraint in the imagery; and (3) ability to extend two-dimensional models to three and four dimensions.

2. *Minimum path estimation (guidewire estimation).* This step consisted of finding the most favorable path (called guide wire) between the starting and ending nodes or points. They used Dijkstra's algorithm for this purpose.

3. *Balloon inflation.* The last step consisted of applying the balloon force over the guidewire to inflate the guidewire to estimate the nerve structure.

Pros and Cons of Skeleton with Parametric-Based Fusion Method: The major *advantages* of the system included:

1. The system logically used the correct steps for estimation of the nerves: ROI reduction, guidewire estimation, and balloon inflation.

2. The system was fast because the region of process was reduced, based on mathematical morphology.

3. The system took advantage of interpolation because the data was tilted.

4. The concept of the soft classification was used, unlike hard classification. This gave the advantage that a path could go through small regions that showed a low probability of containing a nerve based on their own gray level.

The major *disadvantages* of the system included:

1. There was no discussion on the mathematical morphology operations. It was not clear what the size was of the structuring elements.

2. There was no discussion on the snake algorithm as to what the values were of the constants used in the minimization of the energy.

Bulpitt and Berry [141] recently used the deformable model to segment the branching vessels in abdominal aortic aneurysms (AAA).

1.4.3 Two-Dimensional Vessel Boundary Tracking Using Deformable Models

Recently, Quek and Kirbas [198] introduced a technique for segmentation of vessels in x-ray angiograms. This technique was similar to the concept of the propagation of the zero-level set contours in the level set framework. For complete details on level sets, see the review article by Suri et al. [231], but the sample results of Quek's method can be seen in Figure 1.24.

1.4.4 Skeleton-Based Approach Using Differential Geometry

A series of articles have appeared written by Deriche and co-workers from France (see [199–221]; see also [224–226]). These articles are based on the concept of differential geometry (see [222, 223]). The algorithm used was based

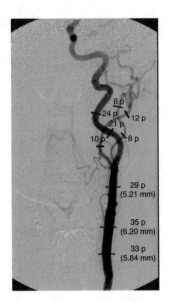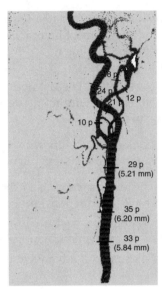

FIGURE 1.24

Wavefront propagation input and output. Left: Input image. Right: Output image. (Courtesy of F. K. H. Quek, Wright University, OH.)

on computing the principal curvatures and finding the ridge lines. Principal direction is defined as the direction of the vessel where the curvature change was at a minimum. The principal direction was estimated using the Weingarten matrix, which was the product of $F_1^{-1}F_2$, where F_1 and F_2 were given as the 3×3 matrix. F_1 was given as $[1 + I_x^2\ I_x I_y\ I_x I_z; I_x I_y\ 1 + I_y^2\ I_y I_z; I_x I_z\ I_y$ $I_z\ 1 + I_z^2]$ and F_2 was given as $[I_{xx}\ I_x I_y\ I_x I_z; I_x I_y\ I_{yy}\ I_y I_z; I_x I_z\ I_y I_z\ I_{zz}]$. Once W was computed, the eigenvalues and eigen directions were computed. This W was computed for each voxel position in the volume. An identification stage of k_{max}, k_{med}, and k_{min} was computed to determine the directional derivatives of the maximum and medium principal curvatures (DMC, DmC), which were given as $DMC = \nabla k_{max} \cdot t_{max}$ and $DmC = \nabla k_{med} \cdot t_{med}$. The zero crossing of the above equations defines the two surfaces in three dimensions and their intersections as a three-dimensional thin network. This zero-crossing was then computed as $em = (\nabla k_{max} \cdot t_{max}) \cdot (\nabla k_{med} \cdot t_{med})$. The method was actually run over the volume, which was obtained by the convolution of the decomposed higher-order derivatives, as originally developed by Deriche.

Pros and Cons of the Differential Geometry-Based Technique: The major *advantages* and *disadvantages* of the system included: The system was fast, and used the higher-order derivatives in terms of sine and cosines; the drawback was that the minimum direction was not estimated at the center of the vessel; and the technique was not very robust toward handling different diameters of vessels. This method did not use the scale-space concept.

1.4.5   Skeleton-Based Approach Using Training Models

Very recently, Toledo et al. [194, 195] developed a technique for segmenting the coronary vessels in angiograms. This technique used deformable models (for details on deformable models, see the extensive review in [196]), where the external energy was computed based on the training data set. The energy minimization was done using the following classical equation:

$$-\frac{\partial}{\partial s}(\alpha \mathbf{v}_s) + \frac{\partial^2}{\partial s^2}(\alpha \mathbf{v}_{ss}) + (cos\phi, sin\phi)\frac{\partial D}{\partial e_1} = 0 \qquad (1.18)$$

where the first and second terms are the smoothing and stretching energies. The third term is the external energy term composed from the training data matrix D. The way D is computed is as follows: first the higher-order Gaussian derivatives are computed to preserve the edges, ridges, and valleys, which are then convolved to give the scale-space representation. Then, the tensor is computed for the direction computation. This is similar to computing the Hessian of the scale-space represented image (see [72] or [197]). Then the eigenvalues are computed from this tensor matrix, which gives the directions of the vessels. Now the $D(m \times n)$ is built for all the points (m-index) at all the scales (n-index). $\frac{\partial D}{\partial e_1}$ is computed using the Mahanabolis distance in the e_1 direction which becomes an attractive force for the initial vessel contour. Thus, Equation 1.18 is optimized to yield the new contour points of the vessels.

Pros and Cons of Training-Based Skeleton Models: This technique is a novel concept of bringing together the training model with the deformable model and thus the external energy term computation. The main weakness of this method is that it is computationally very expensive because it has to undergo training data collection, D computation, tensor computation, and then the iterative optimization for the final contour position estimation. In addition to the above weakness, the training data is sensitive to the points collected for the vessels.

1.5   Discussions of Skeleton-Based vs. Non-Skeleton-Based Methods

We have seen that the taxonomy of vascular segmentation is highly dominated by non-skeleton (direct)- and skeleton (indirect)-based methods. In the non-skeleton (direct)-based methods, the scale-space methods as stand-alone, scale-space methods with Fuzzy connectivity, and geometric deformable model based on PDE and level set framework were the most widely used frameworks. In this section, we first discuss the advantages and disadvantages of the geometric framework using PDE and level sets for vascular segmentation, followed by a discussion on the implementation issues in the vascular segmentation algorithms.

1.5.1 Discussion of the PDE-Based Methods for Vascular Segmentation Algorithms

Geometric methods have started to dominate the segmentation area in a large way: (see the work by Faugeras[30] and Suri et al. [227–233]).[31] We will attempt to summarize the advantages and disadvantages of the geometric framework using level sets and PDEs for vascular segmentation. The *advantages* are as follows:

1. *Capture range.* The greatest advantage of this technique is that this algorithm increases the capture range of the "field flow," which increases the robustness of the initial contour placement.

2. *No need of elasticity coefficients.* These techniques are not controlled by the elasticity coefficients, unlike the classical parametric contour methods. There is no need to fit the tangents to the curves and compute the normals at each vertex. In this system, the normals are embedded in the system using the divergence of the field flow. These methods have the ability to model the incremental deformations in the shape.

3. *Suitability for medical image segmentation.* These techniques are very suitable for medical organ segmentation because they can handle any of the cavities, concavities, convolutedness, splitting, or merging.

4. *Finding the local and global minima.* There is no problem finding the local minima or global minima issues, unlike the optimization techniques of parametric snakes.

5. *Normal computation.* These techniques are less prone to the normal computational error, which is very easily incorporated in the "classical balloon force" snakes for segmentation.

6. *Automaticity.* It is very easy to extend this model from semi-automatic to completely automatic because the region is determined on the basis of prior information.

7. *Integration of regional statistics.* These techniques are based on the propagation of curves (just like the propagation of ripples in the tank or propagation of the fire flames) utilizing the region statistics.

8. *Flexible topology.* These techniques adjust to the topological changes of the given shape, such as joining and breaking of the curves.

9. *Wide applications.* This technique can be applied to unimodal, bimodal, and multi-modal imagery, which means it can have

---

[30]http://www-sop.inria.fr/robotvis/personnel/faugeras/faugeras-eng.html.
[31]We particularly refer readers to the extensive review article on level sets by Suri et al. [231], which compares research among more than ten research groups on level sets.

multiple gray-scale values in it. These PDE/level set-based methods have a wide range of applications in three-dimensional surface modeling.

10. *Speed of the system.* These techniques can be implemented using the fast marching methods in the narrow band and thus can be easily optimized.

11. *Extension.* This technique is an easy extension from two to three dimensions.

12. *Incorporation of regularizing terms.* This can easily incorporate other features for controlling the speed of the curve. This is done by adding an extra term to the region, gradient, and curvature speed terms.

13. *Handling corners.* The system takes care of the corners easily, unlike the classical parametric curves, where it needs special handling at the corners of the boundary.

14. *Resolution changes.* This technique is extendable to multi-scale resolutions, which means that at lower resolutions, one can compute regional segmentations. These segmented results can then be used for higher resolutions.

15. *Multi-phase processing.* These techniques are extendable to multi-phase, which means that if there are multiple level set functions, then they automatically merge and split during the course of the segmentation process.

16. *Surface tracking.* Tracking surfaces are implemented using level sets very smoothly.

17. *Quantification of three-dimensional structures.* Geometrical computations can be done in a natural way; for example, one can compute the curvature of three-dimensional surfaces directly while performing normal computations.

18. *Integration of regularization terms.* Allows easy integration of vision models for shape recovery such as Fuzzy clustering, Gibbs' model, Markov Random Fields, and Bayesian models (see [235]). This makes the system very powerful, robust, and accurate for medical shape recovery. One can segment any part of the brain, depending upon the membership function of the brain image. So, depending on the number of classes estimated, one can segment any shape in two or three dimensions.

19. *Concise descriptions.* One can give concise descriptions of differential structures using level set methods. This is because of the background mesh resolution controls.

20. *Hierarchical representations.* The level set offers a natural scale-space for hierarchical representations.

21. *Reparameterization.* There is no need for reparameterization for curve/ surface estimation during the propagation, unlike in the classical snakes model.

22. *Modeling in a continuous domain.* One can model the segmentation process in a continuous domain using PDEs. Thus, the formalism process is greatly simplified and is grid independent and isotropic.

23. *Stability issues.* With the help of research in numerical analysis, one can achieve highly stable segmentation algorithms using PDEs.

24. *Existence and uniqueness.* Using PDEs, one can derive not only successful algorithms but also useful theoretical results such as existence and uniqueness of solutions (see [236]).

1.5.2 Disadvantages of the Geometric Approaches

The major *disadvantages* of the geometric methods for vascular segmentation include:

1. *Convergence issue.* Although the edges will not be blurry when one performs the diffusion imaging, the issue of convergence always remains a challenge. In diffusion imaging, if the step size is small, then it takes longer to converge.

2. *Design of the constant force.* The design of the constant force in the PDE is another challenge. This involves computation of regional statistics in the region of the moving contour. There is a trade-off between the robustness of the regional design, computational time for the operation, and the accuracy of the segmentation. The design of the model plays a critical role in segmentation accuracy and remains a challenge. Another challenge occurs if the design force is internal or external (for details, see [231]).

3. *Stability issues.* The stability issues in PDEs are also important during the front propagation. The ratio of $\frac{\Delta t}{\Delta x}$, called the CFL number[32], is another factor that needs to be carefully designed.

4. *Initial placement of the contour.* One of the major drawbacks of the parametric active contours was its initial placement. This does not have either enough capture range or enough power to grab the topology of the shapes. Both of these drawbacks were removed by level sets, provided the initial contour was placed symmetrically with respect to the boundaries of interest. This ensures that the level sets reached object boundaries almost at the same time. On the contrary, if the initial contour was much closer to the first portion of the object boundary compared to the second portion, then the evolving contour crosses over the first portion of the object boundary. This is

---

[32]Courant number, named after the author Courant et al. [237].

because the stop function does not turn out to be zero. One of the controlling factors for the stop function is the gradient of the image. The relationship of the stop function to the gradient is its inverse and also depends on the index power m in the ratio $\frac{1}{1+|\nabla G_\sigma * I(x,y)|^m}$. For stopping the propagation, the denominator should be large, which means the image forces due to the gradient should be high. This means index m should be high. In other words, if m is high, then the gradient is high, which means the weak boundaries are not detected well and will be easily crossed over by the evolving curve. If m is low (low threshold), then the level set will stop at noisy or at isolated edges.

5. *Embedding of the object.* If some objects (e.g., the inner objects) are embedded in another object (the outer object), then the level set will not capture all the objects of interest. This is especially true if the embedded objects are asymmetrically situated. Under such conditions, one needs multiple initializations of the active contours. This means there can be only one active contour per object.

6. *Gaps in the objects.* This is one of the serious drawbacks of the level set method and has been pointed out by Siddiqi et al. [238]. Due to the gaps in the object, the evolving contour simply leaks through the gaps. As a result, the objects represented by incomplete contours are not captured correctly and fully. This is especially prominent in realistic images, such as in ultrasound and in multi-class MR and CT images.

7. *Problems due to shocks.* Shocks are among the most common problems in level sets. Kimia and co-workers [239–241] developed such a framework by representing shape as the set of singularities (called shocks) that arise in a rich space of shape deformations as classified into the following four types: (a) first-order shocks are orientation discontinuities (corners) and arise from protrusions and indentations; (b) second-order shocks are formed when a shape breaks into two parts during a deformation; (c) third-order shocks represent bends; and (d) fourth-order shocks are the seeds for each component of a shape. These shocks arise in level sets and can sometimes cause serious problems.

8. *Challenge in segmentation.* Although the level set segmentation method succeeds in the object and motion segmentation, it has weakness in segmenting many other kinds of images. These images mostly do not have a homogeneous background; instead, they are composed of many different regions, such as in natural scenery images (containing streets, mountains, trees, cars, and people). The method based on curve evolution will not produce the correct regions as desired. Such a segmentation problem is a challenge yet to be overcome.

In direct methods, the scale-space methods as stand-alone, scale-space methods with deformable models were used for segmentation. We will, however, discuss some of the key factors that affect the performance of the MRF during the vascular segmentation. They include:

1. *Image size.* The convergence time is directly proportional to the image size. The larger the image size, the longer it takes for the MRF-MF to compute the convergence.

2. *Multi-resolution.* The convergence time for the MRF-MF would be better controlled if the multi-resolution technique was adapted.

3. *Number of classes.* The convergence time is directly proportional to the number of classes used in the MRF-MF method.

4. *Boundary error.* The convergence time was also affected by the boundary error used for the convergence. If the boundary error was too small, then it would take a long time to converge.

1.5.3 Discussion of the Scale-Space Issues on Vascular Filtering and Segmentation

Although we present here some factors that affect the scale-space issues, this will be discussed in greater detail in Chapter 2.

1. *Vessel thickness sizes.* It is important to know to what level the largest scale should be chosen. If the vessels are very thick, then to filter out the largest thickness of vessels one needs scales on the order of 10. In such cases, it may be better to skip some scales and one can compute the intermediate or alternate volumes that can then be used for scale optimization.

2. *Gaussian kernel size.* The width of the Gaussian kernel is given as $W = 1 + 2.0 \times ceil(F \times \sigma)$, where F is the Gaussian fall constant. In our experiments of real and synthetic tests, we took the set of values 1.5 and 2.5. If the vessels were very thick, using a small value was better justified. For thicker vessels, we took $F = 2.5$.

3. *Separable vs. non-separable.* Three-dimensional Gaussian convolution was done using separable Gaussian kernels. This means the convolution was implemented in three different directions independently. This brought a significant speed improvement and reduced the order of complexity from k^3 to $3k$.

4. *ROI computation.* Most of the time, the processing was done in an ROI chosen in the volume. This was done by specifying the starting and ending coordinate positions in all three different directions. This saves much on computation time, as the eigenvalue and eigen directions were computed for each voxel position.

5. *Effect of large scales.* When the scales were large, there was little blurring of the thin vessels due to the large Gaussian window convolution. As a result, the intensities around the vessels increased and the vessel tends to be broader. On optimization, these blurred intensities show up and remove the crispness of the thin vessels. Thus, the thin vessels seem to be a little (say, one pixel) broader than expected.

6. *Quality speed trade-off.* Ellipsoidal filtering is a very powerful technique for segmentation of tubular structures. The results are very refined and the CNR ratio is very high when run on original MR data sets. But because ellipsoidal filtering requires volume generation at multiple scales, this may take huge computer runtime memory and space. It can be more troublesome if the volumetric data sets are very large. On an average, a data set can take up to 7.5 Gigabytes. Five to six volumes can take around 40 Gigabytes and can almost freeze the running machine. To avoid this problem, one has to down-sample the data size to have half the image size. This might bring some artifacts that are removed using Gaussian smoothing. This could bring blurring to these vessels and the second-order operation can make this more noisy and complicated.

7. *Eigenvalue/direction computations.* The eigenvalue and directions should be very carefully computed and all should be estimated to three to four decimal places. We used the computer vision library of Intel (freeware) but we also verified our computer program using Numerical Recipes in C (see [31]).

8. *Three-dimensional interpolation.* We followed a simple three-dimensional, trilinear interpolation for interpolating the three-dimensional angiographic volume. This was straightforward. Interested readers can look at the following research papers on voxel shift and sinc interpolation techniques (see [91–95]; see zero filled interpolation articles [96–99]. In this chapter we will not discuss the interpolation merits and demerits, as they will be discussed elsewhere.

1.6   Challenges, the Future, and Summary: Vascular Segmentation

The state-of-the-art vasculature segmentation techniques are filled with scale-space framework,[33] Fuzzy connectivity, classification, geometric frameworks, and skeletonization of the tubular structures. Although we are able to succeed to a large extent on the segmentation of the vessels, there still lie ahead greater

---

[33]We could not cover the cardiac application and tracking in this chapter. There has been a recent attempt [143] to track the aorta and articles on tracking and search heuristics (see [245–250]).

challenges and unresolved issues in vascular segmentation. This section has three parts: the challenges in the current data acquisition and vascular segmentation issues, some of the future issues in vascular segmentation, and a summary of this chapter.

1.6.1   Challenges in Data Acquisition and Segmentation Techniques

Some of the challenges in MRA data acquisition lie in: (1) the ability to automatically distinguish between the arteries and veins (see [234]); (2) the ability to automatically segment the arteries and veins simultaneously from the black-blood MRA; and (3) the ability to automatically achieve two steps independent of anatomy. Some of the challenges in vasculature segmentation techniques include: (1) the ability to integrate the Fuzzy connectivity or regularizers in the geometric framework for robust vasculature segmentation; (2) the ability to track the vessels to the second and third layers of branching; (3) the ability to distinguish arteries and veins from the TOF data; and (4) the development of methods that can incorporate the local object size in defining the connectedness, object material inhomogeneity, noise, blurring, and background variations.

1.6.2   The Future

Although the application of geometric techniques such as level sets and PDEs have gone well in the fields of medical imaging and biomedicine, we are still far away from achieving stable three-dimensional volumes and a standard segmentation in real-time. By standard, we mean that which can segment the three-dimensional volume with a wide variation in pulse sequence parameters. We will see in the near future the modeling of front propagation that takes into account the physical constraints of the problem, for example, minimization of variation geodesic distances, rather than simple distance transforms. We will also see more incorporation of likelihood functions and adaptive Fuzzy models to prevent leaking of the curves/surfaces. A good example of integration of the low-level processes into the evolution process would be given as: $\frac{\partial \phi}{\partial t} = L(x, y) (\beta_0 - \beta_1 \kappa) |\nabla \phi|$, where $L(x, y) = 1 - max(S_1, S_2, S_i, \ldots, S_n)$, where S_i is the low-level process from edge detection, optical flow, stereo disparity, texture, etc. The better the $S(x, y)$, the more robust would be the level set segmentation process. We also hope to see more articles on level sets where the segmentation step does require a reinitialization stage (see [242, 243]). It would also, however, be helpful if we can incorporate a faster triangulation algorithm for isosurface extraction in three-dimensional segmentation methods. Another issue in the future lies in the user interactiveness of the system design. No matter what computer algorithm is presented, user interaction is always a help in improving the accuracy of the system. The interpretation of the results are thus very essential. An attempt was made by Quek et al. [244] who designed an architecture, called the attentionally based interpretation model (AIM) for interpretation of the neurovascular system. We need such kinds of vascular interpretation systems to help provide better patient care.

1.6.3 Summary

The first part of the chapter introduced the importance of angiography, the motivation for performing MRA/CTA, and the major difficulties in vascular segmentation. The chapter then introduced five different sets of receive coils we used with the MRI system for MRA data acquisition. The chapter next presented the state-of-the-art vascular segmentation taxonomy, which consisted of primarily two broad classes: (1) *skeleton or indirect-based* and (2) *non-skeleton or direct-based*. We then presented three different *skeleton or indirect* techniques, along with their mathematical foundations, algorithms, and their pros and cons. Following this was the presentation of eight different techniques in the class of *non-skeleton or direct* methods. Extensive discussion was given on geometric and Fuzzy frameworks for vascular segmentation. Finally, the chapter concluded with the current challenges and the future of vascular segmentation techniques.

Acknowledgments

Thanks are due to Dr. Elaine Keeler from Marconi Medical Systems, Inc., Cleveland, OH, and Professor Linda Shapiro, University of Washington, Seattle, WA, for their motivation. Thanks also go to Dr. Larry Kasuboski, Marconi Medical Systems, Inc., for his encouragment during the course of this project. Thanks go to Professor Grimson, MIT, Medical Laboratories, and Professor Udupa, University of Pennsylvania, Department of Radiology, for the useful discussions on Fuzzy connectivity and images. Thanks go to Academic and IEEE Press for permissions to reproduce the necessary figures. Special thanks go also to Marconi Medical Systems, Inc., for the MR data sets.

References

1. http://www.med.jhu.edu/vascsurg/AAA1A1.html-Anchor-11481/.
2. North American Symptomatic Carotid Endarterectomy Trial (NASCET), *Stroke*, Vol. 22, No. 6, pp. 711–720, 1991.
3. European Carotid Surgery Trialists Collaborative Group, Randomised trial of endarterectomy for recently symptomatic carotid stenosis: final results of the

MRC European Carotid Surgery (ECST), *Lancet*, Vol. 351, No. 9113, pp. 1379–1387, 1998.

4. Wiebers, D. O., Torner, J. C., and Meissner, I., Impact of unruptured intracranial aneurysms on public health in the United States, *Stroke*, Vol. 23, No. 10, pp. 1416–1419, Oct. 1992.

5. ECRI, Health Technology Assessment Information Service, Magnetic resonance angiography (MRA) of the head and neck, Plymouth Meeting, PA, No. 66, p. 14, 1998.

6. Coatrieux, J. L., Garreau, M., Collorec, R., and Roux, C., Computer vision approaches for the three dimensional reconstruction of coronary arteries: review and prospects, *Crit. Rev. Biomed. Eng.*, Vol. 22, No. 1, pp. 1–38, Jan. 1994.

7. Higgins, W. E., Spyra, W. J. T., Karwoski, R. A., and Ritman, E. L., System for analyzing high-resolution three dimensional coronary angiograms, *IEEE Trans. Med. Imag.*, Vol. 15, No. 3, pp. 377–385, 1996.

8. Chan, R. C., Karl, W. C., and Lees, R. S., A new model-based technique for enhanced small-vessel measurements in x-ray cine-angiograms, *IEEE Trans. Med. Imag.*, Vol. 19, No. 3, pp. 243–255, 2000.

9. Herment, A., Sureda, F., Pellot, C., and Bloch, L., 3D Reconstruction of Blood Vessels by Multi-Modality Data Fusion Using Fuzzy and Markovian Modelling, *Lecture Notes in Computer Science*, Vol. 905, pp. 392–398, 1995, in Ayache, N., Ed., *Computer Vision, Virtual Reality and Robotics in Medicine*, First International Conference, CVRMed '95, Nice, France, 3–6 Apr., 1995, *Proceedings*, pp. 3–12; ISBN 3-540-59120-6, Berlin, Springer-Verlag, 1995.

10. Nishimura, Dwight et al., Magnetic resonance angiography, *IEEE Trans. Med. Imag.*, Vol. 5, No. 3, pp. 140–151, Sept. 1986.

11. Edelman, R. R., Mattle, H. P., Atkinson, D. J., and Hoogewould, H. M., MR angiography, *Am. J. Roentgenol.*, Vol. 154, No. 5, pp. 937–946, 1990.

12. Dumoulin, C. L. and Hart, H. R., MR angiography, *Radiology*, Vol. 161, No. 3, pp. 717–720, 1986.

13. Ritman, E. L., Robb, R. A., and Harris, L. D., *Imaging Physiological Functions: Experience with the Dynamic Spatial Reconstructor*, Praeger, New York, 1985.

14. Gerig, G., Kikinis, R., and Jolesz, F. A., Image processing of routine spin-echo MR images to enhance vascular structures: comparison with MR angiography, in Höhne, K. H., Fuchs, H., and Pizer, S. M., Eds., *3-D Imaging in Medicine*, NATO, ASI Series, F 60, pp. 121–132, 1990.

15. Potchen, E. J., Haacke, E. M., Siebert, J. E., and Gottschalk, A., *Magnetic Resonance Angiography: Concepts and Applications*, Mosby-Year Book, Inc., 1993.

16. Anderson, C. M., Edelman, R. R., and Turski, P. A., *Clinical Magnetic Resonance Angiography*, Lippincott-Raven Publishers, New York, 1993.

17. Johnson, D. B. S., Prince, M. R., and Chenevert, T. L., Magnetic resonance angiography: a review, *Acad. Radiol.*, Vol. 5, No. 4, pp. 289–305, Apr. 1998.

18. Vanninen, R. L., Manninen, H. I., Partamen, P. K., Tulla, H., and Vainio, P. A., How should we estimate carotid stenosis using MRA, *Neuroradiology*, Vol. 38, No. 4, pp. 299–305, 1996.

19. Debatin, J. F. and Hany, T. F., MR-based assessment of vascular morphology and functions, *Eur. Radiol.*, Vol. 8, No. 4, pp. 528–539, 1998.

20. Robin, G. D., Paik, D. S., Johnston, P. C., and Napel, S., Measurements of the aorta and its branches with helical CT, *Radiology*, Vol. 206, No. 3, pp. 823–829, 1999.

21. Kawata, Y., Niki, N., and Kumazaki, T., Computer-assisted analysis and 3-D visualization of blood vessels based on cone-beam CT images, in *Image Analysis Applications and Computer Graphics, Series Lecture Notes in Computer Science*, No. 1024, Chin, R., Ip, H., Naiman, A., and Pong, T. C., Eds., Springer-Verlag, Berlin, pp. 355–362, 1995.

22. Beier, J., Siekmann, R., Müller, F., Tröger, H., Schedel, H., Biamino, G., Fleck, E., and Felix, R., Planning and control of aortic stent implantations using 3-D reconstruction based on computer tomography (CT), in *Computer Assisted Radiology*, Lemeke, H. U., Vannier, M. W., and Inamura, K., Eds., Elsevier, Amsterdam, The Netherlands, pp. 716–720, 1996.

23. Marks, M. P., Napel, S., Jordan, J. E., and Enzmann, D. R., Diagnosis of Carotid Artery Disease: Preliminary Experience with MIP Spiral CT Angiography, *Am. J. Radiol.*, Vol. 160, No. 6, pp. 1267–1271, 1993.

24. Schwartz, R. B., Jones, K. M., Chernoff, D. M., Mukherji, S. K., Khorasani, R., Tice, H. M., Kikinis, R., Hooton, S. M., Stieg, P. E., and Polak, J. F., Common Carotid Artery Bifurcation: Evaluation with Spiral CT, *Radiology*, Vol. 185, No. 2, pp. 513–519, 1992.

25. Liang, C.-C., Singh, A., Chiu, M.-Y., Ezrielev, J., Fisler, R., and Hentschel, D., Method and Apparatus for Editing Abdominal CT Angiographic Images for Blood Vessel Visualization, U.S. Patent No.: 5,570,404, Oct. 29, 1996.

26. Rosenfield, K., Kaufman, J., and Pieczek, A. M., Human coronary and peripheral arteries: on-line three-dimensional reconstruction from 2-D intravascular US scans: Work in progress, *Radiology*, Vol. 184, No. 3, pp. 823–832, 1992.

27. Maurincomme, E., Magnin, I. E., Finct, G., and Goutte, R., Methodology for three-dimensional reconstruction of intravascular ultrasound images, *Proc. of SPIE - The International Society for Optical Engineering*, Vol. 1653, pp. 26–34, 1992.

28. Li, W., Gussenhoven, E. J., Zhong, Y., The, S. H., Pieterman, H., van Urk, H., and Bom, K., Temporal averaging for quantification of lumen dimensions in intravascular ultrasound images, *Ultrasound Med. Biol.*, Vol. 20, No. 2, pp. 117–122, 1994.

29. Thrust, A. J., Bonnett, D. E., Elliott, M. R., Kubob, S. S., and Evans, D. H., An evaluation of the potential and limitations of three-dimensional reconstructions from intravascular ultrasound images, Ultrasound, *Med. Biol.*, Vol. 23, No. 3, pp. 437–445, 1997.

30. Meier, D. S., Cotheren, R. M., Vince, D. G., and Cornhill, J. F., Automated morphometry of coronary arteries with digital image analysis of intravascular ultrasound, *Am. Heart J.*, Vol. 133, No. 6, pp. 681–690, 1997.

31. Shekhar, R., Cothren, R. M., Vince, D. G., Chandra, S., Thomas, J. D., and Cornhill, J. F., Three dimensional segmentation of luminal and adventitial borders in serial intravascular ultrasound images, *Computerized Medical Imaging and Graphics*, Vol. 23, No. 6, pp. 299–309, Nov. 1999.

32. Gill, J. D., Ladak, H. M., Steinman, D. A., and Fenster, A., Accuracy and variability assessment of a semiautomatic technique for segmentation of the carotid arteries from three-dimensional ultrasound images, *Med. Phys.*, Vol. 27, No. 6, pp. 1333–1342, June 2000.

33. Cothren, R. M., Shekhar, R., Tuzcu, E. M., Nissen, S. E., Cornhill, J. F., and Vince, D. G., Three dimensional reconstruction of the coronary artery wall by image fusion of intravascular ultrasound and bi-plane angiography, *Int. J. Card. Imaging*, Vol. 16, No. 2, pp. 69–85, 2000.

34. Borrello, J. A., MR Angiography versus conventional x-ray angiography in the lower extremities: everyone wins, *Radiology,* Vol. 187, No. 3, pp. 615–617, June 1993.

35. Anderson, C. M., Saloner, D., Lee, R. E., Griswold, V. J., Shapeero, L. G., Rapp, J. H., Nagarkar, S., Pan, X., and Gooding, G. A., Assessment of carotid artery stenosis by MR angiography: comparison with x-ray angiography and color-coded Doppler ultrasound, *Am. J. Neuroradiol.,* Vol. 13, No. 3, pp. 989–1003, 1992.

36. Nakajima, S., Atsumi, H., Kikinis, R., Moriarty, T. M., Metcalf, D. C., Jolesz, F. A., and Black, P. M., Use of cortical surface vessel registration for image-guided neurosurgery, *Neurosurgery,* Vol. 40, No. 6, pp. 1201–1210, 1997.

37. Kikinis, R., Gleason, P. L., Moriarty, T. M., Moore, M. R., Alexander, E., Stieg, P. E., Matsumae, M., Lorensen, W. E., Cline, H. E., Black, P. M., and Jolesz, F. A., Computer-assisted interactive three dimensional planning for neurosurgical procedures, *Neurosurgery,* Vol. 38, No. 4, pp. 640–651, 1996.

38. Broeders, I. A. J. M., Blankensteijn, J. D., Olree, M., Mali, W. P. Th. M., and Eikelboom, B. C., Preoperative sizing of grafts for transfemoral endovascular aneurysm management: a prospective comparative study of spiral CT angiography, arteriography and conventional CT imaging, *J. Endovasc. Surg.,* Vol. 4, No. 3, pp. 252–261, 1997.

39. Lanzino, G., Kaptain, G., Kallmes, D. F., Dix, J. E., and Kassell, N. F., Intracranial dissecting aneurysm causing subarachnoid hemorrhage: the role of computerized tomographic angiography and magnetic resonance angiography, *Surg. Neurol.,* Vol. 48, No. 5, pp. 477–481, 1997.

40. Guglielmi, F., Vinuela, I., Septka, I., and Macellar, V., Electrothromobrosis of saccular aneurysms via endovascular approach: electrochemical basis, technique and experimental, *J. Neurosurg.,* Vol. 75, No. 1, pp. 1–7, 1991.

41. Milner, J. S., Moore, J. A., Rutt, B. K., and Steinman, D. A., Hemodynamics of human artery bifurcations: computational studies with models reconstructed from MRI of normal subjects, *J. Vasc. Surg.,* Vol. 28, No. 1, pp. 143–156, 1998.

42. Moore, J. A., Steinman, D. A., and Holdsworth, D. W., Accuracy of computational hemodynamics in complex arterial geometries reconstructed from MRI, *Ann. Biomed. Eng.,* Vol. 27, No. 1, pp. 32–41, 1999.

43. Charbel, F., Shi, J., Quek, F., and Misra, M., Neurovascular flow simulation review, *Neurological Res.,* Vol. 20, No. 2, pp. 107-115, 1998.

44. Oshinski, J. N., Ku, D. N., Mukundan, S. J., Loth, F., and Pettigrew, R. I., Determination of wall shear stress in aorta with the use of MR phase velocity mapping, *J. Magn. Reson. Imag.,* Vol. 5, No. 6, pp. 640–647, 1995.

45. Masutani, Y., Kurihara, T., Suzuki, M., and Dohi, T., Quantitative Vascular Shape Analysis for 3-D MR- Angiography Using Mathematical Morphology, in Ayache, N., Ed., *Computer Vision, Virtual Reality and Robotics in Medicine,* Berlin, pp. 449–459, 1995.

46. Anderson, C. M., Lee, R. E., Levin, D. L., de la Torre Alonso, S., and Saloner, D., Measurement of internal carotid artery stenosis from source MR angiograms, *Radiology,* Vol. 193, No. 1, pp. 219–226, 1994.

47. Yim, P. J., Mullick, R., Summers, R. M., Marcos, H., Cebral, J. R., Lohner, R., and Choyke, Peter L., Measurement of stenosis from magnetic resonance angiography using vessel skeletons, *Proc. of SPIE - The International Society for Optical Engineering,* Vol. 3978, pp. 245–255, 1993.

48. Hoogeveen, C., Bakker, J. G., and Viergever, M. A., Limits to the accuracy of vessel diameter measurement in MR angiography, *J. Magn. Reson. Med.*, Vol. 8, No. 6, pp. 1228–1235, 1998.

49. Hoogeveen, C., Bakker, J. G., and Viergever, M. A., MR phase-constrast flow measurement with limited spatial resolution in small vessels: value of model-based image analysis, *Magn. Reson. Med.*, Vol. 41, No. 3, pp. 520–528, March 1999.

50. Patel, M. R., Klufas, R. A., Kim, D., Edelman, R. R., and Kent, K. C., MR angiography of the carotid bifurcation: artifacts and limitations, *Am. J. Roentgenol.*, Vol. 162, No. 6, pp. 1431–1437, 1994.

51. Yucel, E. K., *Magnetic Resonance Angiography: A Practical Approach*, McGraw-Hill, New York, 1995.

52. Suri, J. S., Singh, S., and Reden, L., computer vision and pattern recognition techniques for 2-D and 3-D MR cerebral cortical segmentation (Part-I): a state-of-the-art review, to appear in *Int. J. Pattern Anal. Appl.*, Vol. 4, No. 3, Sept. 2001.

53. Suri, J. S., Singh, S., and Reden, L., Fusion of region and boundary/surface-based computer vision & pattern recognition techniques for 2-D and 3-D MR cerebral cortical segmentation (Part-II): a state-of-the-art review, to appear in *Int. J. Patt. Anal. Appl.*, Vol. 4, No. 4, Dec. 2001.

54. Suri, J. S., Setarehdan, S. K., and Singh, S., *Advanced Algorithmic Approaches to Medical Image Segmentation: State-of-the-Art Applications in Cardiology, Neurology, Mammography and Pathology*, 1st ed., in press, 2001.

55. Valev, V., Wang, G., and Vannier, M. W., Techniques of CT colonography (virtual colonoscopy), *Crit. Rev. Biomed. Eng.*, Vol. 27, No. 1–2, pp. 1–25, 1999.

56. Wink, O., Niessen, W. J., and Viergever, M. A., Fast delineation and visualization of vessels in 3-D angiographic images, *IEEE Trans. Med. Imag.*, Vol. 19, No. 4, pp. 337–346, 2000.

57. Rosenfeld, A. and Thurston, M., Edge and curve detection for visual scene analysis, *IEEE Trans. Computer*, Vol. 20, No. 5, pp. 562–569, 1971.

58. Vandarbrug, S. J., Semilinear line detectors, *Comput. Graphics Image Processing*, Vol. 4, pp. 287–293, 1975.

59. Fischler, M. A., Tenenbaum, J. M., and Wolf, H. C., Detection of roads and linear structures in low-resolution aerial imagery using a multi-source knowledge integration, *Comput. Graphics and Image Process (CGIP)*, Vol. 15, No. 3, pp. 201–223, 1981.

60. Haralick, R. M., Watson, L. T., and Laffey, T. J., The topographic primal sketch, *Int. J. Robotic Res.*, Vol. 2, No. 1, pp. 50–72, 1983.

61. Lindeberg, T., Scale-space for discrete signals, *IEEE Patt. Anal. Mach. Intell.*, Vol. 12, No. 3, pp. 234–254, 1990.

62. Lindeberg, T., On scale selection for differential operators, *Proc. 8th Scandinavian Conf. Image Analysis (SCIA)*, pp. 857–866, 1993.

63. Lindeberg, T., Detecting salient blob-like image structures and their scales with a scale-space primal sketch: a method for focus of attention, *Int. J. Computer Vision*, Vol. 11, No. 3, pp. 283–318, 1993.

64. Lindeberg, T., Edge detection and ridge detection with automatic scale selection, in *Proc. of Computer Vision and Pattern Recognition*, pp. 465–470, 1996.

65. Lindeberg, T., Feature detection with automatic scale-space selection, *Int. J. Computer Vision*, Vol. 30, No. 2, pp. 79–116, 1998.

66. Lindeberg, T., *Scale-space Theory in Computer Vision*, Kluwer Academic Publishers, 1994.

67. Lindeberg, T., Discrete derivative approximations with scale-space properties: a basis for low-level feature extraction, *J. Mathematical Imaging and Vision*, Vol. 3, No. 4, pp. 349–376, 1993.

68. Witkin, A. P., Scale-space filtering, *Proc. of 8th Int. J. Artificial Intelligence*, Karlsruhe, West Germany, Vol. 2, pp. 1019–1022, 1983.

69. Koenderink, J. J., The structure of images, *Biol. Cyb.*, Vol. 50, pp. 363–370, 1984.

70. Koller, T. M., Gerig, G., Székely, G., and Dettwiler, D., Multiscale detection of curvilinear structures in 2-D and 3-D image data, *IEEE Int. Conference on Computer Vision (ICCV)*, pp. 864–869, 1995.

71. Koller, T. M., From Data to Information: Segmentation, Description and Analysis of the Cerebral Vascularity, Ph.D. thesis, Swiss Federal Institute of Technology, Zürich, 1995.

72. Gerig, G., Koller, M. Th., Székely, Brechbuhler, C., and Kubler, O., Symbolic description of 3-D structures applied to cerebral vessel tree obtained from MR angiography volume data, in *Proceedings of IPMI, Series Lecture Notes in Computer Science*, No. 687, Barett, H. H. and Gmitro, A. F., Eds., Springer-Verlag, Berlin, pp. 94–111, 1993.

73. Thirion, J. P. and Gourdon, A., The 3-D marching lines algorithm, *Graphics Models Image Processing*, Vol. 58, No. 6, pp. 503–509, 1996.

74. Lorenz, C., Carlsen, I.-C., Buzug, T. M., Fassnacht, C., and Wesse, J., Multi-scale line segmentation with automatic estimation of width, contrast and tangential direction in 2-D and 3-D medical images, *Proc. Joint Conf. CVRMed and MRCAS*, pp. 233–242, 1997.

75. Fidrich, M., Following features lines across scale, in *Proc. of Scale-Space Theory in Computer Vision, Series Lectures Notes in Computer Science*, No. 1252, ter Haar Romeny, B., Florack, L., Loeenderink, J. and Viergever, M., Eds., Springer-Verlag, Berlin, pp. 140–151, 1997.

76. Prinet, V., Monga, O., and Rocchisani, J. M., Vessel Representation in 2D and 3D Angiograms, *International Congress Series (ICS)*, ISSN: 0531-5131, Vol. 1134, pp. 240–245, 1998.

77. Prinet, V., Monga, O., Ge, C., Loa, X. S., and Ma, S., Thin network extraction in 3-D images: application of medical angiograms, *Int. Conf. Patt. Recog.*, Aug. 1996.

78. Griffin, L., Colchester, A., and Robinson, G., Scale and segmentation of images using maximum gradient paths, *Image and Vision Computing*, Vol. 10, No. 6, pp. 389–402, 1992.

79. Koenderink, J. and van Doorn, A., Local features of smooth shapes: ridges and course, *SPIE Proc. Geometric Methods in Computer Vision-II*, Vol. 2031, pp. 2–13, 1993.

80. Koenderink, J. and van Doorn, A., Two-plus-one-dimensional differential geometry, *Patt. Recog. Lett.*, Vol. 15, No. 5, pp. 439–444, 1994.

81. Majer, P., A Statistical Approach to Feature Detection and Scale Selection in Images, Ph.D. thesis, University of Göttingen, Gesellschaft für wissenschaftliche Datenverarbeitung mbH Göttingen, Germany, July 2000.

82. Koenderink, J. J., *Solid Shapes*, MIT Press, Cambridge, MA, 1990.

83. Kobashi, S., Kamiura, N., Hata, Y., and Miyawaki, F., Fuzzy Information Granulation on Blood Vessel Extraction from 3D TOF MRA Image, Vol. 14, No. 4, pp. 409–425, 2000.

84. Laub, G. A., and Kaiser, W. A., MR Angiography with gradient motion refocussing, *J. Comput. Assist. Tomogr.*, Vol. 12, No. 3, pp. 377–382, 1988.

85. Laub, G. A., Time-of-flight method of MR angiography, *Magn. Reson. Imag. Clin. North Am.*, Vol. 3, No. 3, pp. 391–398, 1995.

86. Lewin, J. S., Laub, G., and Hausmann, R., Three-dimensional time-of-flight MR angiography: application in the abdomen and thorax, *Radiology*, Vol. 179, No. 1, pp. 261–264, 1992.

87. Atkinson, D., Brant-Zawadzki, M., and Laub, G., Improved MR angiography: magnetization transfer suppression with variable flip angle excitation and increased resolution, *Radiology*, Vol. 190, No. 3, pp. 890–894, 1994.

88. Wehrli, F. W., Shimakawa, A., Gullnerg, G. T., and MacFall, J. R., Time-of-flight MR flow imaging: selective saturation recovery with gradient refocussing, *Radiology*, Vol. 160, No. 3, pp. 781–785, 1986.

89. Parker, D. L., Yuan, C., and Blatter, D. D., MR angiography by multiple thin slab 3-D acquisition (MOTSA), *Magn. Reson. Med.*, Vol. 17, No. 2, pp. 434–451, 1991.

90. Liu, K., and Rutt, B. K., Sliding Interleaved kY (SLINKY) Acquisition: A Novel 3-D TOF MRA Technique with Suppressed Slab Boundary Artifact, *J. Magn. Reson. Imag.*, Vol. 8, No. 4, pp. 905–911, 1998.

91. Dumoulin, C. L., Phase contrast MR angiography techniques, *Magn. Reson. Imag. Clin. North Am.*, Vol. 3, pp. 399–411, 1995.

92. Dumoulin, C. L., Souza, S. P., and Walker, M. F., Three-dimensional phase contrast angiography, *Magn. Reson. Med.*, Vol. 9, No. 1, pp. 139–149, 1989.

93. Hausmann, R., Lwein, J. S., and Laub, G., Phase-contrast MR angiography with reduced acquisition time: new concepts in sequence design, *J. Magn. Reson. Imag.*, Vol. 1, No. 4, pp. 415–422, 1991.

94. Pelc, N. J., Bernstein, M. A., Shimakawa, A., and Glover, G. H., Encoding strategies for three-direction phase-contrast MR imaging of flow, *J. Magn. Reson. Imag.*, Vol. 1, No. 4, pp. 405–413, 1991.

95. Edelman, R. R., Mattle, H. P., Wallner, B., Bajkian, R., Kleefied, J., Kent, C., Skillman, J. J., Mendel, J. B., and Atkinson, D. J., Extracranial Carotid arteries: evaluation with "black blood" MR angiography, *Radiology*, Vol. 177, No. 1, pp. 45–50, 1990.

96. Chien, D., Goldmann, A., and Edelman, R. R., High speed black blood imaging of vessel stenosis in the presence of pulsatile flow, *J. Magn. Reson. Imag.*, Vol. 2, No. 4, pp. 437–441, 1992.

97. Edelman, R. R., Chien, D., and Kim, D., Fast selective black blood MR imaging, *Radiology*, Vol. 181, No. 3, pp. 655–660, 1991.

98. Reichenbach, J. R., Essig, M., Haacke, E. M., Lee, B. C. P. , Przetak, C., Kaiser, W. A., and Schad, L. R., High-resolution venography of the brain using magnetic resonance imaging, *Magn. Reson. Mater. Biol. Phys. Med.*, Vol. 6, No. 1, pp. 62–69, 1998.

99. Prince, M. R., Yucel, E., Kaufman, J., Harrison, D. C., and Geller, S. C., Dynamic gadolinium-enhanced three-dimensional abdominal MR arteriography, *J. Magn. Reson. Imag.*, Vol. 3, No. 6, pp. 877–881, 1993.

100. Prince, M. R., Narashmham, D. L., Stanley, J. C., Chenevert, T. L., Williams, D. M., Marx, M. V., and Cho, K. J., Breath-hold gadolinium-enhanced MR angiography of the abdominal aorta and its major branches, *Radiology*, Vol. 197, No. 3, pp. 785–792, 1995.

101. Prince, M. R., Body MR angiography with gadolinium contrast agents, *Magn. Reson. Imag. Clin. North. Am.*, Vol. 4, No. 1, pp. 11–24, 1996.

102. Sodickson, D. K. and Manning, W. J., Simultaneous acquisition of spatial harmonics (SMASH): Fast imaging with radiofrequency coil arrays, *Magn. Reson. Med.*, Vol. 35, No. 4, pp. 591–603, 1997.

103. Pruessmann, K. P., Weiger, M., Scheidegger, M. B., Markus, B., and Boesiger, P., SENSE: Sensitivity encoding for fast MRI, *Magn. Reson. Med.*, Vol. 42, No. 5, pp. 952–962, 1999.

104. Rossnick, S., Kennedy, D., Laub, G., Braeckle, G., Bachus, R., Kennedy, D., Nelson, A., Dzik, S., and Starewicz, P., Three dimensional display of blood vessels in MRI, *IEEE Computers in Cardiology*, pp. 193–196, 1986.

105. Laub, G. A. and Kaiser, W. A., MR angiography with gradient motion refocusing, *J. Comput. Assist. Tomogr.*, Vol. 12, No. 3, pp. 377–382, 1988.

106. Sato, Y., Shiraga, N., Nakajima, S., Tamura, S., and Kikinis, R., Local maximum intensity projection: a new rendering method for vascular visualization, *J. Comput. Assist. Tomogr.*, Vol. 22, No. 6, pp. 912–917, Dec. 1998.

107. Suri, J. S., Liu, K., Reden, L., and Laxminarayan, S., A state-of-the-art review of vascular segmentation algorithms from magnetic resonance angiography data, submitted 2001.

108. Mroz, L., Hauser, H., and Groller, E., Interactive high-quality maximum intensity projection, *Computer Graphics Forum*, Vol. 19, No. 3, pp. 341–350, 2000.

109. Ney, D. R. and Fishman, E. K., Editing tools for 3-D medical imaging, *IEEE Computer Graphics and Applications*, Vol. 11, No. 6, pp. 63–71, Nov. 1991.

110. Shiffman, S., Rubin, G., and Napel, S., Semi-automated editing of computed tomography sections for visualization of vasculature, Vol. 2707, pp. 140–151, 1996.

111. Cline, H. E., Lorensen, W. E., Souza, S. P., Jolesz, F. A., Kikinis, R., Gerig, G., and Kennedy, T. E., 3-D surface rendered MR images of the brain and its vasculature, *J. Comput. Assist. Tomogr.*, Vol. 15, No. 2, pp. 344–351, 1991.

112. Suri, J. S. and Bernstein, R., 2-D and 3-D display of aneurysms from magnetic resonance angiographic data, *6th Int. Conf. Computer Assisted Radiology*, pp. 666–672, 1992.

113. Suri, J. S., Kathuria, C., and Bernstein, R., Segmentation of aneurysms and its 3-D display from MRA data sets, *Proceedings of SPIE–The International Society for Optical Engineering*, Vol. 1771, pp. 58–66, 1992.

114. Okuda, S., Kikinis, R., Geva, T., Chung, T., Dumanil, H., and Powell, A. J., 3D-shaded surface rendering of gadolinium-enhanced MR angiography in congenital heart disease, *Pediatr. Radiol.*, Vol. 30, No. 8, pp. 540–545, Aug. 2000.

115. Halpern, E. J., Wechsler, R. J., and DiCampli, D., Threshold selection for CT angiography shaded surface display of the renal arteries, *J. Digital Imag.*, Vol. 8, No. 3, pp. 142–147, 1995.

116. Cline, H. E., Dumoulin, C. L., Lorensen, W. E., Souza, S. P., and Adams, W. J., Volume rendering and connectivity algorithms for MR angiography, *J. Magn. Reson. Med.*, Vol. 18, No. 2, pp. 384–394, 1991.

117. Wilson, D. L. and Nobel, J. A., Segmentation of cerebral vessels and aneurysms for MR angiography data, *Proc. of Image Processing in Medical Imaging (IPMI)*, *Lecture Notes in Computer Science*, Vol. 1230, pp. 423–428, 1997.

118. Wilson, D. L. and Noble, J. A., An adaptive segmentation algorithm for extracting arteries and aneurysms from time-of-flight MRA data, *IEEE Trans. Med. Imag.*, Vol. 18, No. 10, pp. 938–945, Oct. 1999.

119. Luo, L. M., Hamitouche, C., Dillenseger, J. L., and Coatrieux, J. L., A moment based three dimensional edge operator, *IEEE Trans. Biomed. Eng.*, Vol. 40, No. 3, pp. 693–703, 1993.

120. Reuze, P., Coatrieux, J. L., Luo, L. M., and Dillenseger, J. L., A 3-D moment based approach for blood vessel detection and quantification in MRA, *Technol. Health Care*, Vol. 1, No. 2, pp. 181–188, 1993.

121. Prokop, R. J. and Reeves, A. P., A survey of moment-based techniques for unoccluded object representation and recognition, *Computer Vision, Graphics and Image Processing*, Vol. 54, No. 5, pp. 438–460, 1992.

122. Verdonck, B., Bloch, I., Maitre, H., Vandermeulen, D., Suetens, P., and Marchal, G., Blood vessel segmentation and visualization in 3-D MR and spiral CT angiography, in *Computer Assisted Radiology (CAR)*, Lemke, H. U., Inamaura, K., Jaffe, C. C., and Vannier, M. W., Eds., Springer-Verlag, Berlin, pp. 177–182, 1995.

123. Verdonck, B., Bloch, H., Maitre, H., Vandermeulen, D., Suetens, P., and Marchal, G., Accurate segmentation of blood vessels from 3-D medical images, *Proc. IEEE Int. Conf. Img. Proc.*, Vol. 3, pp. 311–314, 1996.

124. O'Donnel, T., Gupta, A., and Boult, T., A new model for the recovery of cylindrical structures from medical image data, in *Proc. of CVRMed and MRCAS*, *Ser. Lecture Notes in Computer Science*, Troccaz, J., Grimson, E., and Mösgez, R., Eds., Springer-Verlag, Berlin, No. 1205, pp. 223–232, 1997.

125. Frangi, A. F., Niessen, W. J., Hoogeveen, R. M., van Walsum, Th., and Viergever, M. A., Model-based quantification of 3-D magnetic resonance angiographic images, *IEEE Trans. Med. Imag.*, Vol. 18, No. 10, pp. 946–956, Oct. 1999.

126. Frangi, A. F., Niessen, W. J., Nederkoorn, P. J., Elgersma, O. E. H., and Viergever, M. A., Three-dimensional model-based stenosis quantification of the carotid arteries from contrast-enhance MR angiography, in *IEEE Workshop of Mathematical Methods in Biomedical Image Analysis (MMBIA)*, pp. 110–118, 2000.

127. Frangi, A. F., Niessen, W. J., Hoogeveen, R. M., van Walsum, Th., and Viergever, M. A., Quantitation of vessel morphology from 3D MRA, in *Medical Image Computing and Computer-Assisted Intervention - MICCAI'99*, Taylor, C. and Colchester, A., Eds., *Lecture Notes in Computer Science*, Springer-Verlag, Berlin, Vol. 1679, pp. 358–367, 1999.

128. Krissian, K., Malandain, G., Ayache, N., Vaillant, R., and Trousset, Y., Model based detection of tubular structures in 3D images *Computer Vision and Image Understanding*, Vol. 80, No. 2, pp. 130–171, Nov. 2000.

129. Krissian, K., Malandain, G., Ayache, N., Vaillant, R., and Trousset, Y., Model based multiscale detection of 3D vessels, in *Proc. Computer Vision and Pattern Recognition*, pp. 722–727, 1998.

130. Krissian, K., Malandain, G., Ayache, N., Vaillant, R., and Trousset, Y., Model based multiscale detection of 3D vessels, in *Workshop on Biomedical Image Analysis (WBIA)*, pp. 202–208, 1998.

131. Masutani, Y., Kurihara, T., and Suzuki, M., Quantitative vascular shape analysis for 3D MR-angiography using mathematical morphology, *Int. Conference on Computer Vision, Virtual Reality and Robotics in Medicine (ICCVVRRM)*, pp. 449–454, April 1995.

132. Cline, H. E., Enhanced Visualization of Weak Image Sources in the Vicinity of Dominant Sources, U.S. Patent No. 6,058,218, May 2, 2000.

133. Udupa, J. K., Odhner, D., Tian, J., Holland, G., and Axel, L., Automatic clutter free volume rendering for MR angiography using fuzzy connectedness, *SPIE Proc.*, Vol. 3034, pp. 114–119, 1997.

134. Udupa, J. K. and Samarasekera, S., Fuzzy connectedness and object delineation: theory, algorithm, and applications in image segmentation, *Graphical Models and Image Processing*, Vol. 58, No. 3, pp. 246–261, 1996.

135. Lei, T., Udupa, J. K., Saha, P. K., and Odhner, D., MR angiographic visualization and artery-vein separation, *Proc. of SPIE—The International Society for Optical Engineering*, Vol. 3658, pp. 58–66, 1999.

136. Saha, P. K. and Udupa, J. K., Scale-based fuzzy connectivity: a novel image segmentation methodology and its validation, *Proceedings of the SPIE Conference on Medical Imaging*, Vol. 3661, pp. 246–257, 1999.

137. Saha, P. K., Udupa, J. K., and Odhner, D., Scale-based fuzzy connected image segmentation: theory, algorithm, and validation, *Computer Vision and Image Understanding*, Vol. 77, No. 2, pp. 145–174, 2000.

138. Udupa, J. K. and Odhner, D., Shell rendering, *IEEE Comp. Graph. Appl.*, Vol. 13, No. 6, pp. 58–67, 1993.

139. Stein, W., Hassfeld, S., and Muhling, J., Tracing of thin tubular structures in computer tomographic data, *Comput. Aided Surg.*, Vol. 3, No. 2, pp. 83–88, 1998.

140. Bulpitt, A. J. and Efford, N. D., An efficient 3-D deformable model with a self-optimizing mesh, *Image and Vision Computing*, Vol. 14, No. 8, pp. 573–580, 1996.

141. Bulpitt, A. J. and Berry, E., Spiral CT of abdominal aneurysms: comparison of segmentation with an automatic 3D deformable model and iterative segmentation, *Proc. SPIE, Medical Imaging*, Vol. 3338, pp. 938–946, 1998.

142. Kass, M., Witkin, A., and Terzopoulos, D., Snakes: active contour models, *Int. J. Computer Vision*, Vol. 1, No. 4, pp. 321–331, 1988.

143. Rueckert, D., Burger, P., Forbat, S. M., Mohiaddin, R. D., and Yang, G. Z., Automatic tracking of the aorta in cardiovascular MR images using deformable models, *IEEE Trans. Med. Imag.*, Vol. 16, No. 5, pp. 581–590, Oct. 1997.

144. Ambrosio, L. and Soner, H. M., Level set approach to mean curvature flow in arbitrary co-dimension, *J. Different. Geom.*, Vol. 43, No. 4, pp. 693–737, 1996.

145. Lorigo, L. M., Faugeras, O., Grimson, W. E. L., Keriven, R., Kikinis, R., and Westin, Carl-Fredrik, Co-dimension 2 geodesic active contours for MRA segmentation, in *Proc. 16th Int. Conf. Information Processing in Medical Imaging*, Visegrad, Hungary, *Lecture Notes in Computer Science*, Volume 1613, pp. 126–139, June/July 1999.

146. Lorigo, L. M., Grimson, W. Eric L., Faugeras, O., Keriven, R., Kikinis, R., Nabavi, A., and Westin, Carl-Fredrick, Two Geodesic Active Contours for the Segmentation of Tubular Structures, in *Proc. Computer Vision and Pattern Recognition (CVPR)*, pp. 444–451, June 2000.

147. Terzopoulos, D., Witkin, A., and Kass, M., Constraints on deformable models: recovering 3-D shape and nonrigid motion, *Artificial Intell.*, Vol. 36, No. 1, pp. 91–123, 1988.

148. Sequeira, J., Ebel, R., and Schmitt, F., 3-D modeling of tree-like anatomical structures, *Computerized Med. Imag. Graph.*, Vol. 17, No. 4/5, pp. 333–337, 1993.

149. Sato, Y., Nakajima, S., Shiraga, N., Atsumi, H., Yoshida, S., Koller, T., Gerig, G., and Kikinis, R., Three-dimensional multi-scale line filter for segmentation and visualization of curvilinear structures in medical images (see Web site: http://www.spl.harvard.edu:8000/pages/papers/yoshi/cr.html), *Med. Image Anal. (MIA)*, Vol. 2, No. 2, pp. 143–168, 1998.

150. Sato, Y., Chen, J., Harada, N., Tamura, S., and Shiga, T., Automatic extraction and measurements of leukocyte motion in microvessels using spatiotemporal image analysis, *IEEE Trans. Biomed. Eng.*, Vol. 44, No. 4, pp. 225–236, 1997.

151. Sato, Y., Nakajima, S., Atsumi, H., Koller, T., Gerig, G, Yoshida, S., and Kikinis, R., 3-D multi-scale line filter for segmentation and visualization of curvilinear structures in medical images, in *Proc. on CVRMed and MRCAS (CVRMed/MRCAS)*, pp. 213–222, 1997.

152. Sato, Y., Araki, T., Hanayama, M., Naito, H., and Tamura, S., A viewpoint determination system for stenosis diagnosis and quantification in coronary angiographic image acquisition, *IEEE Trans. Med. Imag.*, Vol. 17, No. 1, pp. 121–137, 1998.

153. Sato, Y., Westin, C.-F., Bhalerao, A., Nakajima, S., Tamura, S., and Kikinis, R., Tissue classification based on 3-D local intensity structures for volume rendering, *IEEE Trans. on Visualization and Computer Graphics*, Vol. 8, No. 2, pp. 160–180, April-June, 2000.

154. Geman, S. and Geman, D., Stochastic relaxation, Gibbs distribution and the Bayesian restoration of images, *IEEE Trans. on Pattern Analysis and Machine Intelligence*, Vol. 6, pp. 721–741, 1984.

155. Dempster, A. D., Laird, N. M., and Rubin, D. B., Maximum likelihood from incomplete data via the EM algorithm, *J. R. Stat. Soc.*, Vol. 39, pp. 1–37, 1977.

156. Suri, J. S. and Gao, J., Bi-directional regional forces for level set propagation: an application to static and motion imagery, to appear in *Proceedings of the International Conference on Signal and Image Processing (SIP2001)*, Hawaii, Aug. 13–16, 2001.

157. Suri, J. S. and Liu, K., Level set regularizers for shape recovery in medical images, to appear in the *Proceedings of the 14th Int. Symposium on Computer-Based Medical Systems (CBMS)*, National Library of Medicine, National Institutes of Health, Bethesda, MD, July 2001.

158. Suri, J. S., White matter/gray matter boundary segmentation using geometric snakes: a fuzzy deformable model, *Proc. International Conference on Advances in Pattern Recognition, Lecture Notes in Computer Science (LNCS)*, Singh, S., Murshed, N., and Kropatsch, W., Eds., Springer-Verlag, Rio de Janeiro, Brazil (11-14 March), No. 2013, pp. 331–338, 2001.

159. Suri, J. S., Two dimensional fast MR brain segmentation using a region-based level set approach, to appear in *International Journal of Engineering in Medicine and Biology (EMBS)*, May 2001.

160. Suri, J. S., Singh, S., Laxminarayan, S., Zeng, X., Liu, K., and Reden, L., Shape recovery algorithms using level sets in 2-D/3-D medical imagery: a state-of-the-art review, to appear in *IEEE Trans. in Information Technology in Biomedicine (ITB)*, Vol. 4, Dec. 2001.

161. Suri, J. S., Modeling segmentation via geometric deformable regularizers, PDE and level sets in still/motion imagery: a revisit, submitted 2001.

162. Suri, J. S., Advanced segmentation tools and techniques for medical imaging, submitted, 2002.

163. Simonetti, O. P., Display of 3-D MRA Images in which Arteries can be Distinguished from Veins, U.S. Patent No. 6,073,042, June 6, 2000.

164. Paragios, N. and Deriche, R., Coupled geodesic active regions for image segmentation: a level set approach, in the *Sixth European Conference on Computer Vision (ECCV)*, Trinity College, Dublin, Ireland, Vol. II, pp. 224–240, 26th June-1st July, 2000.

165. Alvarez, L., Fuichard, F., Lions, P.-L., and Morel, J. M., Axioms and fundamental equations on image processing, *Arch. Ration. Mech.*, Vol. 123, No. 3, pp. 199–257, 1993.

166. Courant, R., Friedrichs, K. O., and Lewy, H., On the partial difference equations of mathematical physics, *IBM J.*, Vol. 11, pp. 215–235, 1967.

167. Siddiqi, K., Lauriere, Y. B., Tannenbaum, A., and Zucker, S. W., Area and length minimizing flows for shape segmentation, *IEEE Trans. Image Processing*, Vol. 7, pp. 433–443, 1998.

168. Kimia, B. B., Tannenbaum, A. R., and Zucker, S. W., Shapes, shocks and deformations. I. The components of shape and the reaction-diffusion space, *Int. J. Computer Vision (IJCV)*, Vol. 15, No. 3, pp. 189–224, 1995.

169. Siddiqi, K., Tresness, K. J., and Kimia, B. B., Parts of visual form: ecological and psychophysical aspects, *Perception*, Vol. 25, No. 4, pp. 399–424, 1996.

170. Stoll, P., Tek, H., and Kimia, B. B., Shocks from images: propagation of orientation elements, in *Proceedings of Computer Vision and Pattern Recognition (CVPR)*, Puerto Rico, IEEE Computer Society Press, pp. 839–845, June 15-16, 1997.

171. Zhao, H. K., Chan, T., Merriman, B., and Osher, S., A variational level set approach to multiphase motion, *J. Computational Phys.*, Vol. 127, No. 1, pp. 179–195, 1996.

172. Evans, L. C. and Spruck, J., Motion of level sets by mean curvature: I, *J. Differential Geom.*, Vol. 33, pp. 635–681, 1991.

173. Quek, F. K. H., Kirbas, C., and Charbel, F. T., AIM: attentionally-based interaction model for the interpretation on vascular angiography, *IEEE Trans. Information Technology in Biomedicine*, Vol. 3, No. 2, pp. 151–157, 1999.

174. Villasenor, J. and Vincent, A., An algorithm for space recognition and time tracking of vorticy tubes in turbulence, *Computer Vision, Graphics, Image Processing and Image Understanding*, Vol. 55, No. 1, pp. 27–35, Jan. 1992.

175. Noordmas, H. J. and Smeulders, A. W. M., High accuracy tracking of 2-D/3-D curved line-structures by consecutive cross-section matching, *Patt. Recog. Lett.*, *(PRL)*, Vol. 19, No. 5, pp. 97–111, 1998.

176. Kwa, J. B. H., An admissible bidirectional staged heuristic search algorithm, *Artificial Intelligence*, Vol. 38, pp. 95–109, 1989.

177. Cherkassky, V. B., Goldberg, A. V., and Radzik, T., Shortest paths algorithms: theory and experimental evaluation, *Mathematical Programming*, Vol. 73, pp. 129–174, 1996.

178. Hartmann, E., On the curvature of curves and surfaces defined by normal forms, *Computer Aided Geometric Design*, Vol. 16, No. 5, pp. 355–376, 1999. ISSN 0167-8396.

179. Press, W. H., Flannery, B. P., Teukolsky, S. A., and Vetterling, W. T., *Numerical Recipes in C*, Cambridge University Press, 1988.

180. Wink, O., Niessen, W. J., and Viergever, M. A., Fast quantification of abdominal aortic aneurysms from CTA volumes, in *Proc. Medical Image Computing and Computer Assisted Intervention*, pp. 138–145, Oct. 1998.

181. Niessen, W. J., Montauban van Swijndregt, A. D., Elsman, B. H. P., Wink, O., Mali, W. P. Th. M., and Viergever, M. A., Improved artery visualization in blood pool MRA of the peripheral vasculature, in *Proc. Computer Assisted Radiology and Surgery (CARS)*, pp. 119–123, 1999.

182. Bulpitt, E., Liu, A., Aylward, S., Solys, M., Rosenman, J., and Pizer, S. M., Methods for displaying intracerebral vascular anatomy, *Am. J. Neuro Radiol.*, Vol. 18, pp. 417–420, 1997.

183. Aylward, S., Bulpitt, E., Pizer, S., and Eberly, D., Intensity ridge and widths for tubular object segmentation and description, *Proceedings of the Workshop on Mathematical Methods in Biomedical Image Analysis*, Amini, A. A., Brookstein, F. L., Wilson D. C., et al., Eds., pp. 131–138, 21–22 June, 1996.

184. Nystrom, I., Skeletonization applied to magnetic resonance angiography images, *Proc. SPIE*, Vol. 3338, pp. 693–701, 1998.

185. Lee, T.-C., Kashyap, R. L., and Chu, C. N., Building skeleton models via 3-D medial surface/axis thinning algorithms, *CVGIP: Graphical Models and Image Processing*, Vol. 56, No. 6, pp. 462–478, 1994.

186. Lam, L., Lee, W. S., and Suen, C. Y., Thinning methodologies-A comprehensive survey, *IEEE Trans. Patt. Anal. Mach. Intell.*, Vol. 14, No. 9, pp. 869–885, Sept. 1992.

187. Lopez, A., Toledo, R., Serrat, J., and Villanueva, J., Extraction of vessel centerlines from 2-D coronary angiographies, *8th Spanish Conf. on Pattern Recognition and Image Analysis*, Vol. 1, pp. 489–496, 1999.

188. Morse, B. S., Pizer, S. M., and Liu, A., Multiscale medial analysis of medical images, *Proc. of the Information Processing in Medical Imaging (IPMI)*, in *Lecture Notes in Computer Science*, Barret, H. H. and Gmitro, A. F., Eds., Springer-Verlag, Vol. 687, pp. 112–131, 1993.

189. Morse, B. S., Computation of Object Cores from Grey Level Images, Ph.D. dissertation, University of North Carolina, Chapel Hill, NC, 1994.

190. Pizer, S. M., Eberly, D., Morse, B. S., and Fritsch, D. S., Zoom-invariant vision of figural shape: the mathematics of cores, *Computer Vision and Image Understanding*, Vol. 69, No. 1, pp. 55–71, 1996.

191. Szekely, G., Koller, T., Kikinis, R., and Gerig, G., Structural description and combined 3-D display for superior analysis of cerebral vascularity from MRA, *SPIE*, pp. 272–281, 1994.

192. Fritsch, D. S., Pizer, S. M., Morse, B. S., Eberly, D. H., and Liu, A., The multiscale medial axis and its applications in image registration, *Patt. Recog. Lett.*, Vol. 15, No. 5, pp. 445–452, 1994.

193. Eberly, D., Gardner, R., Morse, B., Pizer, S., and Scharlach, C., Ridges for image analysis, *J. Math. Imag., Vision*, Vol. 4, No. 4, pp. 351–371, 1994.

194. Toledo, R., Orriols, X., Radeva, P., Vitria, J., Canero, C., and Villanueva, J. J., Eigensnakes for vessel segmentation in angiography, *Proc. Int. Conf. in Pattern Recog.*, pp. 340–343, Sept. 2000.

195. Toledo, R., Radeva, P., von Land, C., and Villanueva, J., 3-D dynamic model of the coronary tree, *Computers in Cardiology*, pp. 777–780, 1998.

196. Suri, J. S., Liu, K., Singh, S., Laxminarayana, S., and Reden, L., Shape recovery algorithms using level sets in 2-D/3-D medical imagery: a state-of-the-art review, accepted for publication in *Int. J. IEEE Trans. Information Technology in Biomedicine*, 2001.

197. Suri, J. S., Liu, K., Reden, L., and Laxminarayana, S., White and Black Blood Volumetric Angiographic Filtering: Ellipsoidal Scale-Space Approach, submitted 2001.

198. Quek, F. K. H. and Kirbas, C., Vessel Extraction in Medical Images by Wave-Propagation and Traceback, *IEEE Trans. Med. Imag.*, Vol. 20, No. 2, pp. 117–131, Feb. 2001.

199. Deriche, R., Using Canny's Criteria to Derive a Recursively Implemented Optimal Edge Detector, *Int. J. Computer Vision*, Vol. 1, No. 2, pp. 167–187, 1987.

200. Deriche, R., Optimal edge detection using recursive filtering, *Proc. First Int. Conf. Computer Vision,* London, pp. 501–505, 1987.
201. Monga, O., Deriche, R., Malandain G., and Cocquerez, J. P., Recursive filtering and edge tracking: two primary tools for 3-D edge detection, *Image and Vision Computing (IVC),* Vol. 4, No. 9, pp. 203–214, Aug. 1991.
202. Deriche, R., Implementing the Gaussian and its derivatives, *Int. Conf. Image Processing,* pp. 263–267, Sept. 1992.
203. Monga, O., Lengagne, R., and Deriche, R., Extraction of the zero-crossing of the curvature in volumetric 3-D medical images: a multi-scale approach, *IEEE Conf. Computer Vision and Pattern Recog.,* (CVPR), 1994.
204. Monga, O., Ayache, N., and Sander, P., From voxel to curvature, *IEEE Conf. Computer Vision and Pattern Recog.,* pp. 644–649, 1991.
205. Monga, O., Benayoun, S., and Faugeras, O. D., From partial derivatives of 3-D density images to ridge lines, *IEEE Conf. Computer Vision and Pattern Recog.,* pp. 354–359, Urbana-Champaign, IL, June 1992.
206. Monga, O., Benayoun, S., and Faugeras, O. D., Using the third order derivatives to extract ridge lines in 3d images, *IEEE Conf. Computer Vision and Pattern Recog.,* Urbana-Champaign, IL, June 1992.
207. Monga, O., Benayoun, S., and Faugeras, O., Using differential geometry in r^4 to extract typical surface features, *IEEE Conf. Computer Vision and Pattern Recog.,* pp. 684–685, June 1993.
208. Monga, O., Lengagne, R., Deriche, R., and Ma, S. D., A Multi-Scale Approach for Crest Line Extraction in 3-D Medical Images, International Workshop on Machine Vision and Applications (IWMVA), Kawasaki, Japan, Dec. 1994.
209. Prinet, V., Monga, O., and Ma, S. D., Extraction of Vascular Network in 3-D Images, *Int. Conf. Image Processing,* (ICIP), Lausanne, Switz., Sept. 1996.
210. Monga, O. and Benayoun, S., Using partial derivatives of 3-D images to extract typical features, *CVGIP: or Computer Vision and Image Understanding (CVIU),* Vol. 61, No. 2, pp. 171–189, 1995 (also the INRIA internal report, 1992).
211. Prinet, V. and Monga, O., Crest-lines for vessels detection in angiograms, *Asian Conference on Computer Vision (ACCV),* Singapore, Dec. 1995.
212. Armande, N., Monga, O., and Montesinos, P., Using crest lines to extract thin networks in images: application to roads and blood vessels, in *XIVth International Conference on Information Processing in Medical Imaging (IPMI), Lecture Notes in Computer Science,* Springer-Verlag, France, June 1995.
213. Prinet, V., Monga, O., and Rocchisani, J. M., Multi-Dimensional Vessels Extraction Using Crest-Lines, *IEEE Engineering in Medicine and Biology Conference,* Montreal, Canada, Sept. 1995.
214. Armande, N., Montesinos, P., and Monga, O., A 3-D thin nets extraction method for medical imaging, *13th Int. Conf. on Pattern Recog.,* (ICPR), Vienna, Austria, Vol. 1, pp. 642–646, 1996.
215. Prinet, V., Monga, O., Ge, C., and Ma, S. D., Thin network extraction in 3D images: application to medical angiograms, *Int. Conf. Pattern Recog.,* (ICPR), Vienna, Austria, Vol. 3, pp. 386–390, Aug. 1996.
216. Prinet, V., Rocchisani, J. M., and Monga, O., Vessels representation in 2-D and 3-D angiograms, *Computer Assisted Radiology,* Berlin, Germany, pp. 240–245, July 1997.
217. Monga, O., Armande, N., and Montesinos, P., Using crest lines to extract thin networks in images: application to roads and blood vessels, *CVGIP: Image Understanding,* Vol. 66, No. 1, pp. 248–257, July 1997.

218. Monga, O., Armande, N., and Montesinos, P., Thin nets and crest lines: application to satellite data and medical images, *Computer Vision and Image Understanding*, Vol. 67, No. 3, pp. 285–295, Sept. 1997.

219. Armande, N., Monga, O., and Montesinos, P., Extraction of Thin Nets in Grey-level Images Application: Roads and Blood Vessels, *Proc. SCIA, 9th Scandinavian Conf. Image Analysis*, pp. 287–295, June 1995.

220. Bricault, I. and Monga, O., From volume medical images to quadratic surface patches, *CVGIP: or Computer Vision and Image Understanding (CVIU)*, Vol. 67, No. 1, pp. 24–38, July 1997.

221. Armande, N., Montesinos, P., Monga, O., and Vaysseix, G., Thin Nets Extraction Using a Multi-scale Approach, *CVGIP: Image Understanding*, Vol. 73, No. 2, pp. 248–257, Feb. 1999.

222. de Carmo, M. P., *Differential Forms and Applications*, Springer-Verlag, Berlin, 1994.

223. Carmo, M. D., *Differential Geometry of Curves and Surfaces*, Prentice Hall, New York, 1976.

224. Romeny, B. H., Florack, L., Salden, A., and Viergever, M., Higher order differential structure of images, in Barrett, H. H. and Gmitor A. F. Eds., in *Proc. of Information Processing in Medical Imaging*, pp. 77–93, June 1993.

225. Sander, P. T. and Zucker, S. W., Inferring surface trace and differential structures from 3-D images, *IEEE Trans. Patt. Anal. Mach. Intell.*, Vol. 12, No. 9, pp. 833–854, Sept. 1990.

226. Leung, A., *Modelling and Reconstruction of Vascular Trees in Medical Images*, Ecole Polytechnique-France, 1996.

227. Suri, J. S. and Gao, J., Bi-directional regional forces for level set propagation: an application to static and motion imagery, to appear in *Proc. Int. Conf. Signal and Image Processing (SIP2001)*, Hawaii, Aug. 13–16, 2001.

228. Suri, J. S. and Liu, K., Level set regularizers for shape recovery in medical images, to appear in the *Proc. 14th Int. Symp. Computer-Based Medical Systems (CBMS)*, National Library of Medicine, National Institutes of Health, Bethesda, MD, July 2001.

229. Suri, J. S., White Matter/Gray Matter Boundary Segmentation Using Geometric Snakes: A Fuzzy Deformable Model, *Proc. Int. Conf. Advances in Pattern Recognition, Lecture Notes in Computer Science (LNCS)*, Singh, S., Murshed, N., and Kropatsch, W., Eds., Springer-Verlag, Rio de Janeiro, Brazil (11–14 March), No. 2013, pp. 331–338, 2001.

230. Suri, J. S., Two dimensional fast MR brain segmentation using a region-based level set approach, to appear in *Int. J. Engineering in Medicine and Biology (EMBS)*, May 2001.

231. Suri, J. S., Singh, S., Laxminarayan, S., Zeng, X., Liu, K., and Reden, L., Shape recovery algorithms using level sets in 2-D/3-D medical imagery: a state-of-the-art review, to appear in *IEEE Trans. Information Technology in Biomedicine (ITB)*, Vol. 4, Dec. 2001.

232. Suri, J. S., Modeling segmentation via geometric deformable regularizers, PDE and level sets in still/motion imagery: a revisit, submitted 2001.

233. Suri, J. S., Advanced segmentation tools and techniques for medical imaging, submitted 2002.

234. Simonetti, O. P., Display of 3-D MRA Images in which Arteries Can Be Distinguished from Veins, U.S. Patent No. 6,073,042, June 6, 2000.

235. Paragios, N. and Deriche, R., Coupled geodesic active regions for image segmentation: a level set approach, in *Sixth European Conf. Computer Vision (ECCV)*, Trinity College, Dublin, Ireland, Vol. II, pp. 224–240, 26th June–1st July, 2000.

236. Alvarez, L., Fuichard, F., Lions, P.-L., and Morel, J. M., Axioms and fundamental equations on image processing, *Arch. Ration. Mech.*, Vol. 123, No. 3, pp. 199–257, 1993.

237. Courant, R., Friedrichs, K. O., and Lewy, H., On the partial difference equations of mathematical physics, *IBM J.*, Vol. 11, pp. 215–235, 1967.

238. Siddiqi, K., Lauriere, Y. B., Tannenbaum, A., and Zucker, S. W., Area and length minimizing flows for shape segmentation, *IEEE Trans. Image Processing*, Vol. 7, pp. 433–443, 1998.

239. Kimia, B. B., Tannenbaum, A. R., and Zucker, S. W., Shapes, shocks and deformations. I. The components of shape and the reaction-diffusion space, *Int. J. Computer Vision (IJCV)*, Vol. 15, No. 3, pp. 189–224, 1995.

240. Siddiqi, K., Tresness, K. J., and Kimia, B. B., Parts of visual form: ecological and psychophysical aspects, *Perception*, Vol. 25, No. 4, pp. 399–424, 1996.

241. Stoll, P., Tek, H., and Kimia, B. B., Shocks from images: propagation of orientation elements, in *Proc. Computer Vision and Pattern Recognition (CVPR)*, Puerto Rico, IEEE Computer Society Press, pp. 839–845, June 15–16, 1997.

242. Zhao, H. K., Chan, T., Merriman, B., and Osher, S., A variational level set approach to multiphase motion, *J. Computational Phys.*, Vol. 127, No. 1, pp. 179–195, 1996.

243. Evans, L. C. and Spruck, J., Motion of level sets by mean curvature. I, *J. Differential Geom.*, Vol. 33, pp. 635–681, 1991.

244. Quek, F. K. H., Kirbas, C., and Charbel, F. T., AIM: attentionally-based interaction model for the interpretation on vascular angiography, *IEEE Trans. Information Technology in Biomedicine*, Vol. 3, No. 2, pp. 151–157, 1999.

245. Villasenor, J. and Vincent, A., An algorithm for space recognition and time tracking of vorticy tubes in turbulence, *Computer Vision, Graphics, Image Processing and Image Understanding*, Vol. 55, No. 1, pp. 27–35, Jan. 1992.

246. Noordmas, H. J. and Smeulders, A. W. M., High accuracy tracking of 2-D/3-D curved line-structures by consecutive cross-section matching, *Patt. Recog. Lett., (PRL)*, Vol. 19, No. 5, pp. 97–111, 1998.

247. Kwa, J. B. H., An admissible bidirectional staged heuristic search algorithm, *Artificial Intelligence*, Vol. 38, pp. 95–109, 1989.

248. Cherkassky, V. B., Goldberg, A. V., and Radzik, T., Shortest paths algorithms: theory and experimental evaluation, *Mathematical Programming*, Vol. 73, pp. 129–174, 1996.

249. Yim, P. J., Choyke, P. L., and Summers, R. M., Gray-scale skeletonization of small vessels in magnetic resonance angiography, *IEEE Trans. Med. Imag.*, Vol. 19, No. 6, pp. 568–576, June 2000.

250. Yim, P. J., Kim, D., and Summers, R. M., A path-wise definition of the watershed line and a watershed-like skeltonization, submitted 2001.

2

Scale-Space 3-D Ellipsoidal Filtering for White and Black Blood MRA

Jasjit S. Suri, Kecheng Liu, Sameer Singh, and Swamy Laxminarayan

CONTENTS

2.1 Introduction

Vascular diseases are one of the major sources of deaths in the U.S. A report [1] states that "Aneurysm rupture is not a rare occurrence as evidenced by the fact that this event currently ranks thirteenth on the list for leading causes of death in the U.S.A." Also, this report [1] says that "Chronic venous insufficiency is a common problem in the U.S., affecting approximately 5% of the general population. It is estimated that half a million patients suffer from ulceration of the lower extremity as a result of longstanding venous disease." This report raises the importance of research needed in the area of angiography, the branch of medicine which deals with veins and arteries. In the field of cerebrovascular diseases [1], "Ischemic and hemorrhagic stroke account for one of the principal causes of death and disability in older aged population. In fact, stroke currently ranks third on the list of leading causes of death in the United States (see also trial reports from North America (NASCET) [2] and Europe (ECST) [3], and Wiebers et al. [4]). Each year approximately 500,000 people suffer a new or recurrent stroke in the U.S., and approximately 150,000 die as a result of this process. In addition, more than one third of stroke survivors are left with permanent physical disability which currently accounts for the leading cause of nursing home admissions in the U.S."

The branch of medicine that deals with studies of the arteries and veins or vasculature is angiography. The different ways angiography can be performed are: bi-plane x-ray/digital subtraction angiography (DSA), MR angiography (MRA), CT angiography (CTA), and ultrasound angiography. From the clinical point of view, DSA[1] is considered the most reliable and accurate method for vascular imaging, a subset of x-rays. On the contrary, this method lacks three-dimensional information,[2] which is easily available via MR and CT techniques. The MR and CT techniques lack the ability to locate tiny vessels and the morphological estimation of stenoses and aneurysms. One of the main reasons MR and CT techniques are not as successful in detection as DSA is due to the presence of nonvascular structures and background noise.

This chapter focuses on white-blood angiography (WBA) and black-blood angiography (BBA) using MR, and more importantly, on the prefiltering of the MR data sets for removal of nonvascular tissues and background noise suppression. The main motivation for performing vascular filtering is for three-dimensional segmentation, which in turn helps in the following areas:

1. Neurosurgical planning, interventional procedures, and treatments
2. Time saving for performing three-dimensional segmentation
3. Distinguishing between the veins and arteries
4. Relative placement of the anatomical structures with respect to vasculature
5. Blood flow process and hemodynamics
6. Stenosis and aneurysm assessment/quantification
7. Disease monitoring/remission, and
8. Quantification of vascular structures

Having discussed some of the sources of motivations for performing *vascular image processing* (VIP), we now present the major difficulties in performing filtering of the vasculature in MR data sets. The following include the main reasons that contribute to the complexity in vasculature filtering from MRA data sets (see [18–20]):

1. *Vessel shape complexity and variability.* The vessels are curvey, twisted (tortuous), and sometimes occluded,[3] or there could be superposition of structures/vessels corresponding to the vasculature in various areas of the body, such as in the head, heart, and neck.
2. *Vessel density and diameter of small vessels.* The complexity of the filtering increases with density and reduction of the diameter of vessels (see Figure 2.1).

---

[1]Subtraction of the x-ray images without contrast material from x-ray angiograms.
[2]One can still achieve the three-dimensional information using the stereo reconstruction from x-ray angiograms with multiple viewpoints.
[3]Overlap of vessels with one another.

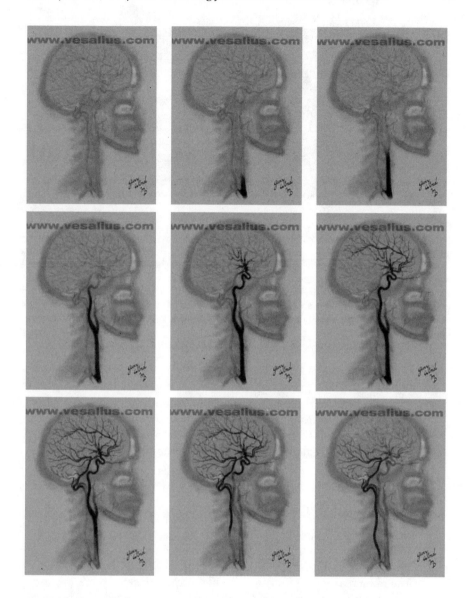

FIGURE 2.1 (See color insert.)
Lateral view of a carotid angiogram (arterial to venous). Top to bottom and left to right: shown are only limited angiogram frames: arterial (frames 1–6) and venous (frames 7–9) phases. Also, the density of the vessels and bifurcation can be appreciated. (Courtesy of Vesalius; www.vesalius.com/.)

3. *Noise and gaps in vessels.* The MRA acquisition process brings in gaps in the vessels, and the resulting data sets could be noisy.

4. *Dynamic range of intensities.* Many structures in the human body show high intensity values similar to vessel intensity values. The

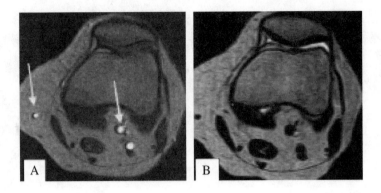

FIGURE 2.2
Axial images from a knee MRA. Left: The bright blood (A) two-dimensional TOF, acquired in the axial plane. Right: The black-blood (B) T_2-weighted three-dimensional FSE, acquired in the sagittal plane, reformatted here in the axial plane. The imaging time for three-dimensional FSE was comparable with two-dimensional TOF but covered a larger volume. In (A), the arrows (flow images) point to vessels but they also have some black neighborhood around them. In (B), the black-blood image shows perfect vessel capture. Thus, the left image has a weakness due to its acquisition methodology. (MR data, Courtesy of Philips Medical Systems, Inc., Cleveland, OH.)

dynamic range of intensities is small between vessels and other objects.

5. *Partial volume averaging.* Due to partial volume averaging (PVA), a voxel could have a combination of intensities from vessels and background. Particular difficulties occur at vessel bifurcations/branching due to PVA and calcification (which is common at bifurcations).

6. *White blood and black blood issues.* In the case of segmenting "white-blood vessels," imaging conditions can cause some background areas to be as bright as other vessel areas; therefore, thresholding alone cannot be used. In the case of "black-blood vessels," imaging conditions can cause some background areas to be as dark as black-blood vessels, making detection between them difficult. From the image processing perspective, BBA is more complicated than WBA. The main reasons for this problem include (a) muscles, bone, air, and vessels show as black in intensity; (b) two neighboring bones can touch each other, thereby making the black region thicker (if they do not touch each other, then they can have gray-level tissue in between); (c) air or muscle pockets are irregular shapes which can very large, or very small. The very large ones can be longitudinal or circular in nature (see Figure 2.2, right); (d) the blood vessels are black and sometimes of the same size as that of air pockets or small bony structures, causing great difficulty in distinguishing between the blood vessels and small air pockets, or small bone circular structures; and (e) the bone lining (cartilage) and the vessels are equally

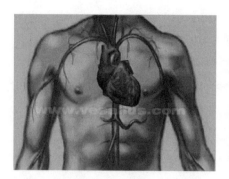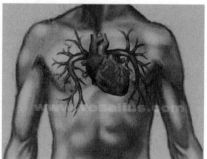

FIGURE 2.3 (See color insert.)
Vasculature system in the chest region. Left: Heart and aorta with major upper body branches. Right: The heart and pulmonary arteries. (Courtesy of Vesalius Studios; www.vesalius.com/.)

thin in diameter (see Figure 2.2, right). Using median filtering with subtraction will remove both the thin vessels and the thin lining. Similarly, using Gaussian blurring along with subtraction will also remove both the thin lining and the thin vessels. Consequently, we have to carefully select filter sizes for thin vessel detection. We will discuss this in detail in Section 2.3.

7. *Characteristics of the imaging modality and motion/blood flow artifacts.* The resolution and clarity of the images play a critical role in *vascular image processing*. This data acquisition process plays an equally critical role in the accuracy and robustness of the vascular segmentation process. For example, artifacts in MR imaging could be due to several kinds (for details, see [21–23]). In MRA, we can have ringing artifacts (see [24]), or artifacts due to patient motion or blood flow. This contributes to the intensity nonhomogeneity in the vessel, which makes the segmentation process difficult to perform.

8. *Ability to distinguish between arteries and veins.* Due to the similarity in the enhancement characteristics of the vessels and close proximity of arteries and veins, it becomes more difficult for the tracking algorithms to distinguish between the arteries and veins (see Figure 2.3 and Figure 2.4).

9. *Hemodynamics.* Because of imperfect timing of the arrival of the contrast agent and the partial volume effect, vessel detection and separation of the vein and the artery become very problematic.

10. *Scanning limitation.* In vascular image processing, for tracking the vessels, we find the imaging plane perpendicular to the vessel's central axis. This plane is mathematically computed. Had the scanning system provided this imaging plane, tracking of the vessels would have been very easy. Therefore, one of the limitations in vascular

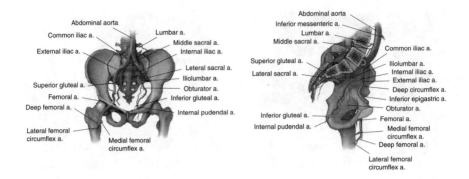

FIGURE 2.4 (See color insert.)
Vasculature system for pelvis region. Left: Pelvis frontal view. Right: Pelvis lateral view. (Courtesy of Professor Fishman, Johns Hopkins University, Baltimore, MD.)

> tracking is the weakness of the scanning system for its inability to provide the orthogonal imaging planes to the central axis of the vessel. In addition, the vessels are curved, tortuous, and it is therefore not possible for current MRA technology to scan the vascular structures in this manner. Because of this scanning limitation, we tailor the image processing algorithms to perform the three-dimensional segmentation.

Having discussed the difficulties of performing vascular image processing, we will very briefly list some of the work from previous authors who attempted to perform prefiltering on MRA data sets. One of the active groups is Parker and co-workers (see [25–27]). Some of the earlier VIP techniques are from: Vandermeulen et al. [31], Lin et al. [34], Chen et al. [35, 36], Gerig et al. [79], Orkisz et al. [38], and Chen et al. [39]. These techniques do not exploit any kind of image processing to remove the nonvascular structures and background suppression of noise. They mostly use data acquisition techniques to improve the signal-to-noise (SNR) or contrast-to-noise ratio (CNR).

The latest trend has been developed by Frangi et al. [73]. This chapter is in the spirit of Frangi et al.'s approach, but as applied to both WBA and BBA. The goals of this chapter are to devise:

1. A generic MRA prefiltering algorithm that can remove the nonvascular structures, and suppress noise and background variations

2. An automatic vascular imaging processing system that can detect thin and thick vessels simultaneously

3. A system that is insensitive to different MR acquisition techniques and parameters, such as phase contrast, contrast-enhanced, time-of-flight, white-blood angiography and black-blood angiography

4. A vascular image processing system that can then be used with other advanced image processing segmentation tools such as pixel/voxel classifiers.

Note that this chapter is limited to angiography filtering and, henceforth, we will limit our discussions to filtering[4] MR angiographic data sets only, for WBA or BBA. The layout of this chapter is as follows. A brief theory on ellipsoidal filtering is discussed in Section 2.2. The same section presents the results on ellipsoidal filtering over several data sets. Section 2.3 shows the comparison between different filtering algorithms. A discussion on the implementation issues involved with filtering algorithms is presented in Section 2.4. The chapter concludes by presenting the conclusions, challenges, and the future on MRA filtering algorithms in Section 2.5.

2.2 Theory and Algorithm of Ellipsoidal Filtering

Consider an image I and its Taylor expansion in the neighborhood of a point $\mathbf{x}_0$ as:

$$I(\mathbf{x}_0 + \delta\mathbf{x}_0, \sigma) = \underbrace{I(\mathbf{x}_0, \sigma)}_{0^{th}\text{-order}} + \underbrace{\delta\mathbf{x}_0^T \nabla_{0,\sigma}}_{1^{st}\text{-order}} + \underbrace{\delta\mathbf{x}_0^T \mathcal{H}_{0,\sigma} \delta\mathbf{x}_0}_{2^{nd}\text{-order}} + \cdots \qquad (2.1)$$

This expansion approximates the structure of the image up to the second order. $\nabla_{0,\sigma}$ and $\mathcal{H}_{0,\sigma}$ are the gradient vector and Hessian matrix of the image computed at $\mathbf{x}_0$ at scale σ. To calculate the differential operators I, the scale-space framework is adapted. In this framework, the differentiation is defined as a convolution with Derivative of Gaussian (DoG). This is given as:

$$\frac{\partial}{\partial \mathbf{x}} L(\mathbf{x}, \sigma) = \sigma^\gamma I(\mathbf{x}) \otimes \frac{\partial G}{\partial \mathbf{x}}(\mathbf{x}, \sigma) \qquad (2.2)$$

where $G(\mathbf{x}, \sigma)$ is the three-dimensional Gaussian kernel defined as:

$$G(\mathbf{x}, \sigma) = \frac{1}{(2\pi\sigma^2)^{\frac{D}{2}}} e^{\frac{\|\mathbf{x}\|^2}{2\sigma^2}} \qquad (2.3)$$

where $D = 3$, due to three-dimensional processing. The parameter γ was introduced by Lindeberg[5] (see [83–89]). This was used to define a family of normalized derivatives. This normalization was particularly important for a fair comparison of the response of differential operators at multiple scales. With no scales used, $LC = 1.0$. The second-order information (called Hessian)

---

[4]From now on, whenever we use "filtering," we mean "MRA filtering."
[5]Known as the Lindeberg constant (LC).

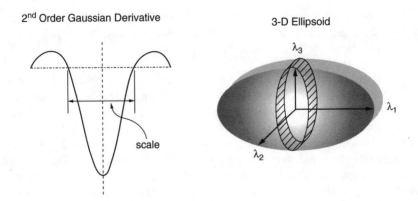

FIGURE 2.5
Concept of second-order Gaussian derivative for edge estimation and ellipsoidal concept for direction estimation. Left: Second-order Gaussian derivative. Right: Three-dimensional ellipsoid.

has an intuitive justification in the context of the tubular structure detection. The second derivative of a Gaussian kernel at scale σ generates a probe kernel that measures the contrast between the regions inside and outside the range $(-\sigma, \sigma)$. This can be seen in Figure 2.5 (left), shown below. The third term in Equation 2.1 gives the second-order directional derivative:

$$\delta \mathbf{x}_0{}^T \mathcal{H}_{0,\sigma} \, \delta \mathbf{x}_0 = \left(\frac{\partial}{\partial \delta \mathbf{x}_0}\right) \left(\frac{\partial}{\partial \delta \mathbf{x}_0}\right) I(\mathbf{x}_0, \sigma) \qquad (2.4)$$

The main concept behind the eigenvalue of the Hessian is to extract the principal directions in which the local second-order structure of the image can be decomposed. Because this directly gives the direction of the smallest curvature (along the direction of the vessel), application of several filters in multiple orientations is avoided. This latter approach is computationally more expensive and requires a discretization of the orientation space. If $\lambda_{\sigma,k}$ is the eigenvalue corresponding to the kth normalized eigenvector $\mathbf{u}_{\sigma,k}$ of the Hessian $\mathcal{H}_{0,\sigma}$ computed at scale σ, then from the definition of the eigenvalues:

$$\mathcal{H}_{0,\sigma} \, \hat{\mathbf{u}}_{\sigma,k} = \lambda_{\sigma,k} \hat{\mathbf{u}}_{\sigma,k} \qquad (2.5)$$

The above equation has the following geometric interpretation. The eigenvalue decomposition extracts three orthonormal directions that are invariant up to a scaling factor when mapped by the Hessian matrix. In particular, a spherical neighborhood centered at $\mathbf{x}_0$ and having a radius of unity will be mapped by $\mathcal{H}_0$ onto an ellipsoid whose axes are along the directions given by the eigenvectors of the Hessian and the corresponding axis semi-lengths are the magnitudes of the respective eigenvalues. This ellipsoid locally describes the second-order structure of the image (see Figure 2.5, right). Thus, the problem comes down to the estimation of the eigenvalues and eigenvectors at

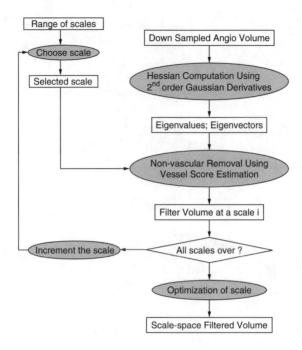

FIGURE 2.6
Algorithm pipeline for the three-dimensional ellipsoidal filter.

each voxel location in the three-dimensional volume. The algorithm for filtering is framed in Section 2.2.1.

2.2.1   Algorithmic Steps for Ellipsoidal Filtering

The algorithm consists of the following steps and is in the spirit of Frangi et al.'s approach [73]. The algorithmic pipeline is shown in Figure 2.6, whose steps are discussed below:

1. *Preprocessing of the MRA data sets.* This consists of changing the anisotropic voxels to isotropic voxels. We used trilinear interpolation for this conversion. The second step in this preprocessing is the image resizing, primarily for speed concerns. We used the standard wavelet transform method to down-sample the volume to preserve the high-frequency components of the lumen edges.

2. *Edge volume generation.* Here, the convolution is performed between the image volume with the higher-order Gaussian derivative operators. The computation of the second derivatives of Gaussian in the Hessian matrix is implemented using three separate convolutions

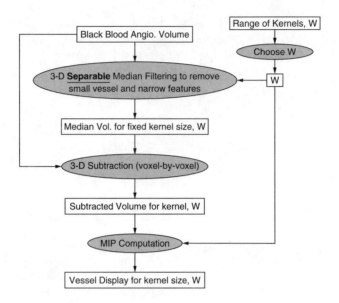

FIGURE 2.7
Object process diagram of three-dimensional median filtering algorithm for black-blood angiography (BBA) (see Alexander et al.'s [27] algorithm).

with one-dimensional kernels, given as:

$$I_{x^i y^j z^k}(\mathbf{x}, \sigma_f) = \frac{d^i}{d\mathbf{x}^i} G(\mathbf{x}, \sigma_f) \otimes \left\{ \frac{d^j}{d\mathbf{y}^j} G(\mathbf{y}, \sigma_f) \otimes \left\{ \underbrace{\frac{d^k}{d\mathbf{z}^k} G(\mathbf{z}, \sigma_f) \otimes I(\mathbf{x})}_{\text{convolution-1}} \right\} \right\}$$

$$\text{convolution-2}$$

$$\text{convolution-3}$$

(2.6)

where $I(\mathbf{x})$ is the interpolated gray scale volume; i, j, and k are the nonnegative integers satisfying $i + j + k = 2$; and 3σ was used as the radius of the kernel. G is the Gaussian kernel in the x, y, and z directions. $\frac{d^k}{d\mathbf{z}^k} G(\mathbf{z}, \sigma_f) \otimes I(\mathbf{x})$ is the convolution of the Gaussian kernel with a standard deviation of σ_f. Note that three sets of convolutions are done to obtain the scale-space representation of the gray-scale volume rather than one convolution in three dimensions. A similar example of three-dimensional convolution in MRA can be seen in [30].

3. *Hessian analysis.* Running the directional processor for computing the eigenvalues, which is computed using Jacobi's method (see [31]).

4. *Nonvascular removal.* Here, the computation of the vessel score is performed to distinguish between the vessels from non-vessels using

the eigenvalues based on connectivity, scale, and contrast. This can be computed using the combination of components that are computed using the geometry of the shape, which in turn is a function of the eigenvalues, λ_1, λ_2, and λ_3,

$$\mathcal{V}(\sigma, \gamma) = \begin{cases} 0 \text{ if } |\lambda_2| > 0 \text{ or } |\lambda_3| > 0 \\ \left(1 - exp\left(-\dfrac{\mathcal{R}_A^2}{2\alpha^2}\right)\right) exp\left(-\dfrac{\mathcal{R}_B^2}{2\beta^2}\right)\left(1 - exp\left(-\dfrac{\mathcal{S}^2}{2\epsilon^2}\right)\right) \end{cases} \quad (2.7)$$

where γ is the Lindeberg constant and α, β, and ϵ are the thresholds that control the sensitivity of the filter for the measurements of features of the image such as area, blobness, and distinguishing property given by notations $\mathcal{R}_A^2$, $\mathcal{R}_B^2$, and $\mathcal{S}^2$. The first two geometric ratios are gray-level invariants. This means they remain constant under intensity rescaling. The geometrical meaning of $\mathcal{R}_B^2$ is the derivation from a blob-like structure but cannot distinguish between a line and a plate-like pattern. The $\mathcal{R}_B^2$ is computed as the ratio of the volume of the ellipsoid to the largest cross-sectional area, which came out to be a fraction $\frac{|\lambda_1|}{\sqrt{|\lambda_2 \lambda_3|}}$. The "blob-term" is at a maximum for a blob-like structure and is close to zero if λ_1, or λ_1 and λ_2, tend to vanish. $\mathcal{R}_A^2$ referred to the largest area of the cross section of the ellipsoid in the plane, which was perpendicular to the vessel direction (the least eigenvalue direction). It is computed as the ratio of the two largest second-order derivatives. This ratio is basically distinguishing between the plate and line-like structures. Mathematically, it is given as $\frac{|\lambda_2|}{|\lambda_3|}$. The third term helps in distinguishing the vessel and non-vessel structures. This term is computed as the magnitude of the derivatives, which is the magnitude of the eigenvalues. It is computed using the norm of the Hessian. Frobenius matrix norm[6] was used because it was straightforward in terms of the three eigenvalues and was given as:

$$\mathcal{S} = \sqrt{\lambda_1^2 + \lambda_2^2, \lambda_3^2}$$

5. *Iteration for all scales.* Repeating Steps 2, 3, and 4 from the starting scale, σ_{min}, to the ending scale, σ_{max}.

6. *Compositing volumes.* Scale optimization to remove the nonvascular and background structures. The filter optimization was done by finding the best scale σ. This is computed as:

$$\mathcal{V}(\gamma) = \max_{\sigma_{min} \leq \sigma \leq \sigma_{max}} \mathcal{V}(\sigma, \gamma)$$

The volume corresponding to the best scale σ_{opt} is the filtered volume.

---

[6]The Frobenius matrix of a given matrix, say $\mathbf{A}$, is the rational canonical form of $\mathbf{A}$ and is mathematically equivalent to $\mathbf{Q}^{-1}\mathbf{AQ}$, where $\mathbf{Q}$ is the transformation matrix.

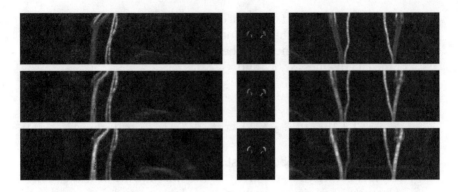

FIGURE 2.8
Effect of increasing the scale value over the scale-space ellipsoidal filtering over the MRA carotid data set. Left column: Sagittal view. Middle column: Transverse view. Right column: Coronal view. The scale (σ) increases from top to bottom. Top row: $\sigma = 1.0$. Middle row: $\sigma = 2.0$. Bottom row: $\sigma = 3.0$. Data size: $256 \times 256 \times 150$. Note the capture of thin vessels at small scale and thick vessels at large scale.

2.2.2 Experimental Protocol for WBA/BBA Filtering

This subsection briefly discusses the results of the WBA and BBA using the ellipsoidal filtering protocol.

1. *Increasing scale experiment.* In the first set of experiments, we observed the behavior of changing the scale σ from 1.0 to 5.0 in increments of 1.0. The results can be seen in Figure 2.8. The first column shows the sagittal view, the second column shows the transverse view, and the third column shows the coronal view of the carotid area. Note that as we go from lower scales (say 1.0) to higher scales (3.0), we find that the thick vessels are captured by the vessel filter. We took the Lindeberg constant as 0.7, α and β were both taken as 0.5, and ϵ was taken as 0.25 times the I_{max}. We took another data set of the knee, shown in Figure 2.9. The increasing scale experiment in this example was run and the results can be seen in Figure 2.10. This projection clearly captures the figure of "N", which corresponds to three different vessels (see Figure 2.9 showing three white circular dots, seen starting from the left edge of the images).

2. *Vessel score optimization experiment.* In the second set of experiments, we ran the complete cycle by optimization of the vessel score. Here, we computed the optimized vessel score using the equation: $\mathcal{V}(\gamma) = \max\limits_{\sigma_{min} \leq \sigma \leq \sigma_{max}} \mathcal{V}(\sigma, \gamma)$. The results can be seen in Figures 2.11, 2.12 and 2.13. The right column in each of these figures shows the optimized results. Also seen in Figures 2.12 and 2.13 are the MIP of the mean (middle row) and variance (bottom row) images. The composite volume results have high CNRs and SNRs.

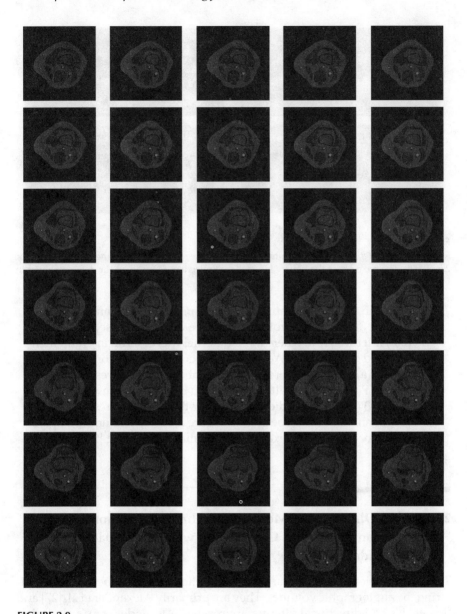

FIGURE 2.9
White blood transverse slices of the knee MR data. Note the three cross-sectional vessels when moving from the left edge of the image to right edge of the image. This will make a figure "N" in the MIP when seen in the coronal projection.

3. *MIP comparison between raw, median filter, and scale-space ellipsoidal filtering.* In the third set of experiments, we compared the results of the ellipsoidal filter with the raw MIP and median filtering MIP in the carotids. The MIP from the raw data set was straightforward.

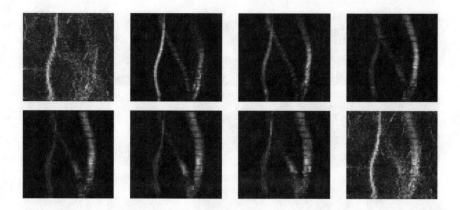

FIGURE 2.10

MIPs obtained after filtering the volume with scale-space-ellipsoidal filtering (data size: 256 × 256 × 150). The recovery of the figure "N" in these projections is based on the data set shown in Figure 2.9.

The MIP was also computed after running the median filtering of size $3 \times 3 \times 3$. In this protocol, the three-dimensional separable median filter was run, where the 1-D kernel was first run in x, and then in y and z-directions. We took two sets of data sets for this experiment: (a) carotids, (b) renal, and (c) abdomen. The results for the raw MIP and median filtering MIP can be seen in Figures 2.11, 2.12 and 2.13 (left and middle columns) for the neck. The results for the abdomen data set can be seen in Figure 2.14. We will now compare our algorithm with Alexander et al.'s median filtering [27] on BBA.

2.3   Three-Dimensional Median and Three-Dimensional Directional Filtering: Comparison with Scale-Space Ellipsoidal Filtering

This section briefly presents the previous methods that have been used for filtering the angiographic volumes. They are primarily Alexander et al. [27] and Sun et al.'s [26] directional filtering approaches. Alexander et al.'s algorithm is discussed using the Object process diagram (OPD) shown in Figure 2.7.

2.3.1   Alexander et al.'s Three-Dimensional Separable Median BBA Filtering Algorithm

Alexander et al.'s method exploited the fact that most intracranial vessels are narrower than other structures that appear dark in the image (called black-blood angiography). Keeping the characteristics of BBA in mind, as discussed

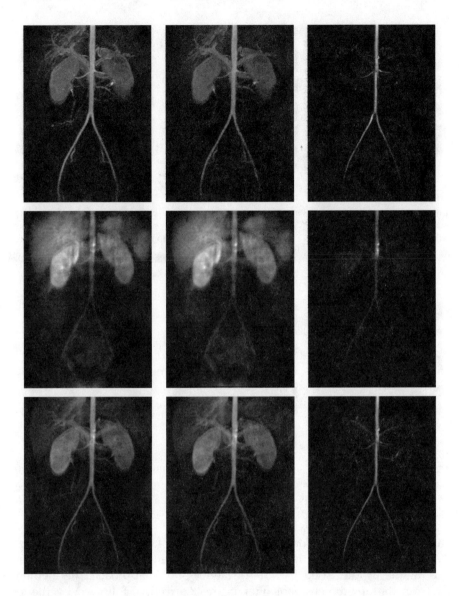

FIGURE 2.11
Raw vs. median vs. ellipsoidal filtering for the carotid arteries in the transverse plane (data size: 256 × 256 × 130). Top row: MIP of raw vs. median filter vs. ellipsoidal filter. Middle row: MIP of mean of raw vs. median filter vs. ellipsoidal filter. Bottom row: MIP of variance of raw vs. median filter vs. ellipsoidal filter.

in Section 2.1, we here present Alexander et al.'s algorithm along with the results. The algorithm consisted of finding the median value of the voxels that constitute the cube region. Alexander et al. implemented this by applying one-dimensional median filters in three orthogonal directions to the original

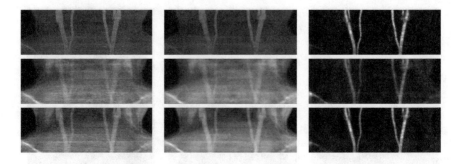

FIGURE 2.12
Raw vs. median filter vs. ellipsoidal filtering for the carotid arteries in the coronal plane (data size: $256 \times 256 \times 130$). Top row: MIP of raw vs. median filter vs. ellipsoidal filter. Middle row: MIP of mean of raw vs. median filter vs. ellipsoidal filter. Bottom row: MIP of variance of raw vs. median filter vs. ellipsoidal filter.

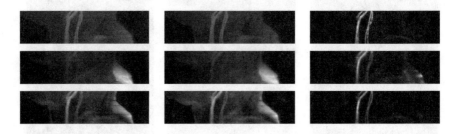

FIGURE 2.13
Raw vs. median vs. ellipsoidal filtering for the carotid arteries in the sagittal plane. Data size: $256 \times 256 \times 130$. Top row: MIP of raw vs. median filter vs. ellipsoidal filter. Middle row: MIP of mean of raw vs. median filter vs. ellipsoidal filter. Bottom row: MIP of variance of raw vs. median filter vs. ellipsoidal filter.

three-dimensional MRA data set. A median filter kernel (whose width was W) operated by sorting the W values and selecting the value that was in the middle of the sorted list. In Alexander et al.'s approach, the method first ran the one-dimensional filter in the z-direction, followed by the x- and y-directions. This was done to remove vessels and narrow structures. This process generated the *masked volume*. Because air and bone in the brain were also dark (in BBA), the above mask would preserve the signal contrast of the brain parenchyma and the boundaries between regions of tissues, bone, and air. Thus, the original volume was subtracted from the masked volume to generate the subtracted volume, which had the vessels in it. The algorithm is shown in Figure 2.7, right. Note that the method needs a kernel whose width is $3W$. Alexander et al. used a kernel size of $9 \times 9 \times 7$ in three different directions.

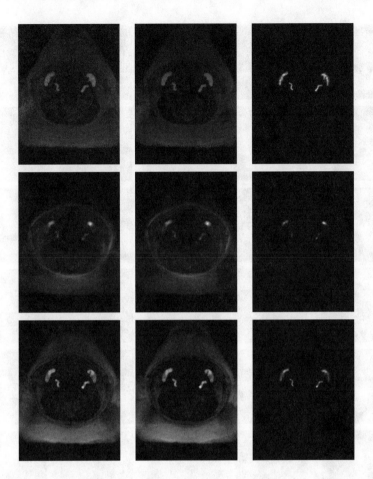

FIGURE 2.14
Raw vs. median filter vs. ellipsoidal filtering for the abdomen data set. Data size: $256 \times 256 \times 130$. Top row: MIP of raw vs. median filter vs. ellipsoidal filter. Middle row: MIP of mean of raw vs. median filter vs. ellipsoidal filter. Bottom row: MIP of variance of raw vs. median filter vs. ellipsoidal filter.

2.3.2 Results on Alexander et al.'s Technique and Their Pros and Cons

Our protocol consisted of taking the BBA of the knee data set of $256 \times 256 \times 147$. Sample slices are shown in Figure 4.33. After performing median filtering and subtraction, the resultant slices can be seen in Figure 4.34. Finally, the MIP of the subtracted results can be seen in Figure 4.35. We have shown this protocol using different kernel sizes, W.

The major *advantage* of the system is that the three-dimensional median filter is implemented in a separable mode to improve the speed. The major *disadvantages* of the system include that the method: (1) was too sensitive to the kernel size W; (2) used a slow sorting method such as heap sort (see the

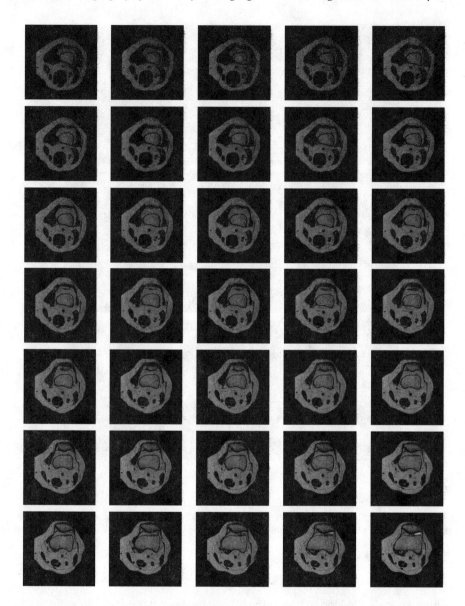

FIGURE 2.15
Transverse slices acquired for black-blood angiography (BBA) data set of the knee.

recent paper by Suri [44], on heap sorting using back pointer technique); (3) was only demonstrated for brain BBA and there were no experiments on vasculature in other areas of the body; (4) did not show any timing issues for a comparison between the separable vs. nonseparable three-dimensional median filter; (5) did not remove the background and nonvasculature

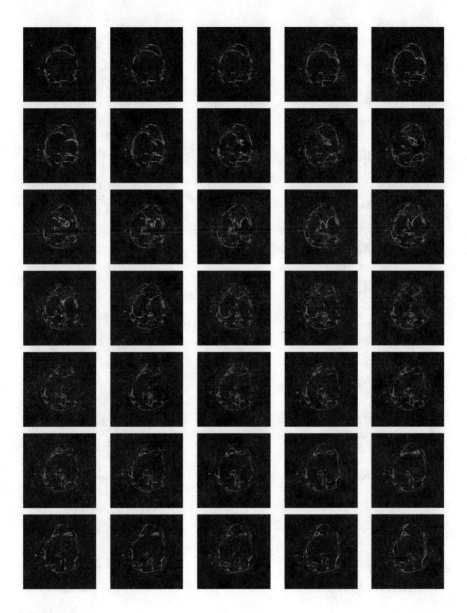

FIGURE 2.16
Protocol for black-blood angiography (BBA) for three-dimensional FSE MR knee data set. Implementation of Alexander and Parker et al.'s algorithm. Subtracted results of the three-dimensional data set, kernel size of $9 \times 9 \times 9$ separable median filter from the raw data set. Only nonoverlapping vessels are unidentified.

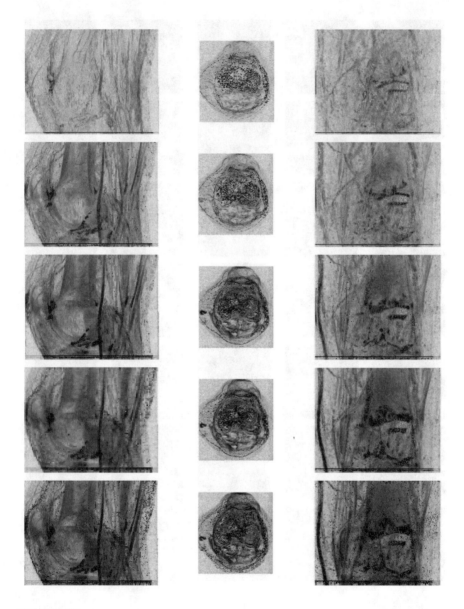

FIGURE 2.17
Effect of kernel size on median filtering for the knee data set shown in Figure 4.33. Top row to bottom row, kernel size one-dimensional window, $W = 5, 7, 9, 11$, and 13. Left column: Sagittal MIP views. Middle column: Transverse MIP views. Right column: Coronal MIP views.

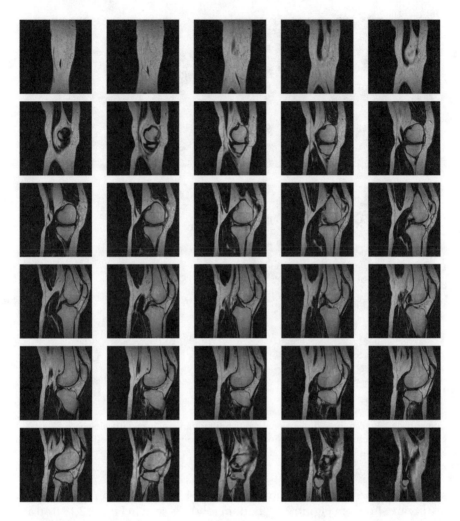

FIGURE 2.18
Sagittal slices acquired for black-blood angiography (BBA) data set of the knee. Slice positions shown are in increments of five, starting from slice number 25.

structures; and (6) the article did not show any performance evaluation of the technique.

Figure 2.19 shows the comparison between the three-dimensional median filter and the three-dimensional ellipsoidal filter presented here for the BBA of the knee images. Two orientations were acquired for this experiment, transverse and sagittal. Figure 4.33 shows the transverse slices acquired of the BBA knee data set. The median filter vs. ellipsoidal results are shown in Figure 2.19 (top row). In the second experiment, we acquired the sagittal data set from the

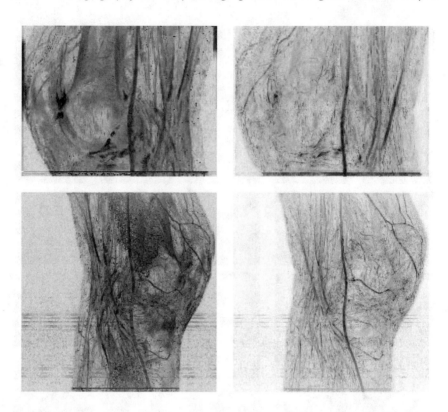

FIGURE 2.19
Comparison between three-dimensional median filtering vs. ellipsoidal scale-space filtering algorithm. Left column: Three-dimensional median filtering. Right column: Three-dimensional ellipsoidal filtering.

same knee. These slices are shown in Figure 4.36. The median vs. ellipsoidal results are shown in Figure 2.19 (bottom row). As seen in Figure 2.19 (top and bottom rows), the background noise was greatly suppressed in the Ellipsoidal Scale-Space Filter (ESSF) for both the views (right column). Also, the black vessels were more accurately detected with the ellipsoidal filtering method. The greatest advantage of ESSF was the removal of the non-vascular structures, such as the air pockets and bone, which has not been done in previous research papers.

2.3.3   Sun et al.'s Local Maximum Mean Filtering Algorithm

Sun et al. [26] recently presented the directional filtering approach for filtering the MRA white-blood angiographic volume. At each voxel of interest in the original data, Sun et al. considered $k \times k \times k$ (where k was an odd integer)

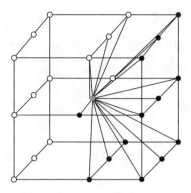

FIGURE 2.20
Thirteen directions shown with filled-in circles.

cube centered at the voxel of interest. If $k = 3$, then there are a total of $M = 13$ line segments in the $3 \times 3 \times 3$ cube, as shown in Figure 2.20. Sun et al.'s local maximum mean processing algorithm consisted of finding the local maximum mean (LMM) in the cube and was defined as the maximum of the M local means, where M are the directions. Suppose a cube centered at a vessel voxel S contained a voxel-wide straight line vessel going through the voxel S; and if there were M k-voxel line segments in the cube, then Sun et al. assumed that the Mth line segment was the vessel that consisted of k vessel voxels S, S_1, S_2, ... S_{k-1}. The local mean was given as: $\bar{S}^i = \frac{\Sigma_i^k S_i}{k}$. The LMM in this cube was $\hat{S} = max\{\bar{S}^i, \ldots, \bar{S}^M\}$. We implemented Sun et al.'s algorithm to compare with our results for WBA data sets. We found a very slight improvement in Sun et al.'s method when compared to the raw MIP; but when compared to ellipsoidal filtering, the CNR and SNR were still high.

Pros and Cons of Sun et al.'s Filtering: The major *advantages* of the system are that: (1) the technique took advantage of both the local and global characteristics of the image volume. This means both thin and thick blood vessels could be captured; and (2) the article presented a very good performance evaluation technique for measuring the performance of the prefilter. The major *disadvantages* of the system are that the method: (1) was not robust enough to remove the nonvascular and background structures; (2) was demonstrated only for a kernel size of $3 \times 3 \times 3$, although theoretically it was shown how many line segments would be necessary for the filtering operation; (3) showed the results only for WBA. No experiments were done on BBA; and previously, (4) was only demonstrated on cerebral images.

Having discussed ellipsoidal filtering in Section 2.2, median and directional filtering in Section 2.3, we will now discuss the implementation issues.

2.4   MR Angiography Filtering: Implementation Issues

The following are the main issues related to ellipsoidal filtering:

1. *Vessel thickness sizes.* It is important to know the maximum scale width σ_{max}. If the vessels are very thick, then to filter out the largest thickness of vessels one needs scales on the order of 10. In such cases, it may be better to skip some scales and one can compute the intermediate or alternate volumes that can then be used for scale optimization.

2. *Gaussian kernel size.* The width of the Gaussian kernel was given as $W = 1 + 2.0 \times ceil(F \times \sigma)$, where F is the Gaussian fall constant. In our experiments of real and synthetic tests, we took the set of values of 1.5 and 2.5. If the vessels were very thick, using a small F value was better justified. For thicker vessels, we took $F = 2.5$.

3. *Separable vs. nonseparable.* Three-dimensional Gaussian convolution was done using separable Gaussian kernels. This means the convolution was implemented in three different directions independently. This brought significant speed improvement and reduced the order of complexity from k^3 to $3k$.

4. *ROI computation.* Most of the time, the processing was done in an ROI chosen in the volume. This was done by specifying the starting and ending coordinate positions in all three directions. This saves much computation time as the eigenvalues and eigen directions were computed for each voxel position.

5. *Effect of large scales.* When the scales were large, there was little blurring of the thin vessels due to the large Gaussian window convolution. As a result, the intensities around the vessels increased and the vessels tended to be broader. On optimization, these blurred intensities show up and remove the crispness of the thin vessels, causing the thin vessels seem to be a little broader than expected (approximately one pixel).

6. *Quality speed trade-off.* Ellipsoidal filtering is a very powerful technique for segmentation of tubular structures. The results are very refined and the CNR ratio is very high when run on original MRA data sets. Because ellipsoidal filtering requires volume generation at multiple scales, this may take huge computer runtime, memory, and space. It can be more troublesome if the volumetric data sets are very large. On average, a data set can take up to 7.5 Gigabytes. Five to six volumes can take around 40 Gigabytes and can almost freeze the running machine. To avoid this problem, one has to downsample the data size to half the image size. This might bring in some artifacts, which are removed using Gaussian smoothing. However,

blurring to vessels and the second-order operation can make this more noisy and complicated.

7. *Effect of Lindeberg constants.* It is necessary to keep the constants in mind and their respective ranges. In all our experiments, we kept the Lindeberg constant at 0.7. A good range can be from 0.4 to 0.8, depending on the noise in the data sets. The constants α, β, and ϵ are the thresholds that control the sensitivity of the filter for the measurements of features of the image such as area and blobness. In all our experiments we fixed α and β at 0.5. These two constants did not play a very critical role for our data sets. An important factor, ϵ, was taken as a product of $\sigma \times I_{max}$, where σ was the scale factor and I_{max} was the maximum intensity level in the image volume.

8. *Eigenvalue/Direction Computations.* The eigenvalues and directions should be very carefully computed and should be estimated at three to four decimal places. We used the computer vision library of Intel (freeware), but we also verified our computer program using Numerical Recipes in C (see Press et al. [31]).

9. *Three-dimensional interpolation.* We followed a simple three-dimensional trilinear interpolation for interpolating the three-dimensional angiographic volume. This method was found to be very straightforward. Interested readers can look at the following research articles on voxel shift and sinc interpolation techniques: see [90–95]; see zero filled interpolation [96–99]. The interpolation merits and demerits are too lengthy to be discussed in this chapter; however, they will be addressed elsewhere.

2.5 Conclusions, Challenges, and the Future: Angiographic Filtering

2.5.1 Conclusions

The first part of this chapter introduced the importance of vascular image processing and prefiltering. The major part of this chapter focused on the scale-space ellipsoidal filtering. We presented several experiments and demonstrated that the SNR and CNR for the filtered MIP were far superior to the raw MIPs. Our results were compared with three-dimensional median filtering. We also presented the experiments on BBA and compared our algorithm with Alexander et al. and Sun et al.'s algorithms (recently published). A full discussion was presented on the implementation issues of scale-space ellipsoidal filtering.

2.5.2 Challenges

Some of the challenges in vasculature filtering techniques include the ability: (1) to distinguish between the air and bone pockets in comparison to blood vessels in black-blood angiography; (2) to integrate the regularizers in the geometric framework for robust vasculature filteration; (3) to distinguish arteries and veins during the filteration process; and (4) to develop methods that can incorporate the local object size in defining the connectedness, object material inhomogeneity, noise, blurring, and background variations.

2.5.3 The Future

We demonstrated the ellipsoidal scale-space filtering algorithm for white and black blood MR angiography. Although the method was successfully demonstrated on more than 20 patient studies and was also compared with existing start-of-the-art filtering algorithms, the method needs further improvements in the computation of the vessel score for each voxel position in the three-dimensional volume. Such methods are called regularizers and make the system more robust, accurate, and insensitive to variation in the parameters used in the MR data acquisition methods. Terms like Fuzzy connectivity, classification, geometric frameworks, and skeletonization of the tubular structures must be brought into the scale-space framework for better filtration. Another topic to explore would be to understand the filtering quality–speed trade-off. We do the convolution in separable mode, which is very fast, but sometimes this can be longer if the kernel size is very large. The authors are working aggressively toward new and improved methods keeping the above issues in mind (see [20–22, 43]).

Acknowledgments

Thanks are due to Dr. Elaine Keeler and Dr. Larry Kasuboski from Philips[7] Medical Systems, Inc., Cleveland, OH; and Professor Linda Shapiro, University of Washington, Seattle, WA, for their encouragment during the course of this project. We thank Alejandro F. Frangi, Universidad de Zaragoza, Spain, and Dr. Sato, Osaka University, Japan, for useful discussions. We are also grateful to Philips Medical Systems, Inc., Cleveland, OH, for the MR data sets. Special thanks to IEEE Press for allowing us to reproduce this journal paper of IEEE *Transactions in Information Technology in Biomedicine*.

---

[7]Formerly known as Marconi Medical Systems, Inc.

References

1. Suri, J. S., Setarehdan, S. K., and Singh, S., *Advanced Algorithmic Approaches to Medical Image Segmentation: State-of-the-Art Applications in Cardiology, Neurology, Mammography and Pathology*, ISBN 1-85233-389-8, Springer-Verlag, Dec. 2001.

2. Alexander, A. L., Champman, B. E., Tsuruda, J. S., and Parker, D. L., A Median Filter for 3-D Fast Spin Echo Black Blood Images of Cerebral Vessel, *Magn. Reson. Med.*, Vol. 43, No. 2, pp. 310–313, 2000.

3. Sun, Y. and Parker, D. L., Performance analysis of maximum intensity projection algorithm for display of MRA images, *IEEE Trans. Med. Imag.*, Vol. 18, No. 12, pp. 1154–1169, Dec. 1999.

4. http://www.med.jhu.edu/vascsurg/AAA1A1.html-Anchor-11481/.

5. North American Symptomatic Carotid Endarterectomy Trial (NASCET), *Stroke*, Vol. 22, No. 6, pp. 711–720, 1991.

6. European Carotid Surgery Trialists Collaborative Group, Randomised trial of endarterectomy for recently symptomatic carotid stenosis: Final results of the MRC European Carotid Surgery (ECST), *Lancet*, Vol. 351, No. 9113, pp. 1379–1387, 1998.

7. Wiebers, D. O., Torner, J. C., and Meissner, I., Impact of unruptured intracranial aneurysms on public health in the United States, *Stroke*, Vol. 23, No. 10, pp. 1416–1419, Oct. 1992.

8. Patel, M. R., Klufas, R. A., Kim, D., Edelman, R. R., and Kent, K. C., MR angiography of the carotid bifurcation: artifacts and limitations, *Am. J. Roentgenol.*, Vol. 162, No. 6, pp. 1431–1437, 1994.

9. Yucel, E. K., *Magnetic Resonance Angiography: A Practical Approach*, McGraw-Hill, New York, 1995.

10. Suri, J. S., Liu, K., Reden, L., and Laxminarayan, S., A state-of-the-art review of vascular segmentation algorithms from magnetic resonance angiography data, submitted 2002.

11. Suri, J. S., Singh, S., and Reden, L., Computer vision and pattern recognition techniques for 2-D and 3-D MR cerebral cortical segmentation. I. A state-of-the-art review, to appear in *Int. J. Pattern Analysis and Applications*, Vol. 4, No. 3, Sept. 2001.

12. Suri, J. S., Singh, S., and Reden, L., Fusion of region and boundary/surface-based computer vision & pattern recognition techniques for 2-D and 3-D MR cerebral cortical segmentation. II. A state-of-the-art review, to appear in *Int. J. Pattern Analysis and Applications*, Vol. 4, No. 4, Dec. 2001.

13. Wink, O., Niessen, W. J., and Viergever, M. A., Fast delineation and visualization of vessels in 3-D angiographic images, *IEEE Trans. Med. Imag.*, Vol. 19, No. 4, pp. 337–346, 2000.

14. Du, Y. P. and Parker, D. L., Vessel enhancement filtering in three dimensional angiograms using long range signal correlation, *J. Magn. Reson. Imag.*, Vol. 7, No. 2, pp. 447–450, 1997.

15. Vandermeulen, D., Delaere, D., Suetens, P., Bosmans, H., and Marchal, G., Local filtering and global optimization methods for 3-D MRA image enhancement, in *Proc. Visualization in Biomedical Computing*, pp. 274–288, 1992.

16. Lin, W., Haacke, E. M., Masaryk, T. J., and Smith, A. S., Automated local maximum-intensity projection with three dimensional vessel tracking, *J. Magn. Reson. Imag.*, Vol. 2, No. 5, pp. 519–526, 1992.

17. Chen, H. and Hale, J., An algorithm for MR angiography image enhancement, *J. Magn. Reson. Imag.*, Vol. 33, No. 4, pp. 534–540, 1995.

18. Chen, H., Li, A., Kaufman, L., and Hale, J., A fast filtering algorithm for image enhancement, *IEEE Trans. Med. Imag.*, Vol. 13, No. 3, pp. 557–564, Sept. 1994.

19. Gerig, G., Kubler, O., and Jolesz, F. A., Nonlinear anisotropic filtering of MRI data, *IEEE Trans. Med. Imag.*, Vol. 11, No. 2, pp. 221–232, 1992.

20. Orkisz, M. M., Bresson, C., Magnin, I. E., Champin, O., and Douek, P. C., Improved vessel visualization in MR angiography by nonlinear anisotropic filtering, *J. Magn. Reson. Med.*, Vol. 37, No. 6, pp. 914–919, 1997.

21. Chen, H. and Hale, J., An algorithm for MR angiography image enhancement, *Magn. Reson. Med.*, Vol. 33, No. 4, pp. 534–540, 1995.

22. Frangi, A. F., Niessen, W. J., Vincken, K. L., and Viergever, M. A., Multiscale vessel enhancement filtering, in *Proc. Medical Image Computing and Computer-Assisted Intervention (MICCAI)*, Vol. 1496, pp. 130–137, 1998.

23. Lindeberg, T., Scale-space for discrete signals, *IEEE Pattern Analysis and Machine Intelligence*, Vol. 12, No. 3, pp. 234–254, 1990.

24. Lindeberg, T., On scale selection for differential operators, *Proc. 8th Scandinavian Conf. Image Analysis (SCIA)*, pp. 857–866, 1993.

25. Lindeberg, T., Detecting salient blob-like image structures and their scales with a scale-space primal sketch: a method for focus of attention, *Int. J. Computer Vision*, Vol. 11, No. 3, pp. 283–318, 1993.

26. Lindeberg, T., Edge detection and ridge detection with automatic scale selection, in *Proc. Computer Vision and Pattern Recognition*, pp. 465–470, 1996.

27. Lindeberg, T., Feature detection with automatic scale-space selection, *Int. J. Computer Vision*, Vol. 30, No. 2, pp. 79–116, 1998.

28. Lindeberg, T., *Scale-Space Theory in Computer Vision*, Kluwer Academic Publishers, 1994.

29. Lindeberg, T., Discrete derivative approximations with scale-space properties: a basis for low-level feature extraction, *J. Mathematical Imaging and Vision*, Vol. 3, No. 4, pp. 349–376, 1993.

30. Sato, Y., Nakajima, S., Shiraga, N., Atsumi, H., Yoshida, S., Koller, T., Gerig, G., and Kikinis, R., Three-dimensional multi-scale line filter for segmentation and visualization of curvilinear structures in medical images (see Web site: http://www.spl.harvard.edu:8000/pages/papers/yoshi/cr.html), *Med. Image Anal. (MIA)*, Vol. 2, No. 2, pp. 143–168, 1998.

31. Press, W. H., Flannery, B. P., Teukolsky, S. A., and Vetterling, W. T., *Numerical Recipes in C*, Cambridge University Press, 1988.

32. Suri, J. S., Two Dimensional Fast MR Brain Segmentation Using a Region-Based Level Set Approach, *IEEE J. Eng. in Medicine and Biology (EMBS)*, Vol. 20, No. 4, pp. 84–95, July/Aug. 2001.

33. Schanze, T., Sinc interpolation of discrete periodic signals, *IEEE Trans. Signal Processing*, Vol. 43, No. 6, pp. 1502–1503, June 1995.

34. Yaroslavsky, L. P., Signal sinc-interpolation: a fast computer algorithm, *Bioimaging*, Vol. 4, pp. 225–231, 1996.

35. Yaroslavsky, L. P., Efficient algorithm for discrete sinc-interpolation, *Applied Optics*, Vol. 36, No. 2, pp. 460–463, Jan. 1997.

36. Candocia F. M. and Principe, J. C., Comments on sinc interpolation of discrete periodic signals, *IEEE Trans. Signal Processing*, Vol. 46, No. 7, pp. 2044–2047, July 1998.
37. Sato, Y., Westin, C.-F., Bhalerao, A., Nakajima, S., Tamura, S., and Kikinis, R., Tissue classification based on 3-D local intensity structures for volume rendering, *IEEE Trans. Visualization and Computer Graphics*, Vol. 8, No. 2, pp. 160–180, April–June, 2000.
38. Kober, V., Unser, M. and Yaroslavsky, L. P., Spline and sinc signal interpolations in image geometrical transforms, *Proc. SPIE Fifth International Workshop on Digital Image Processing and Computer Graphics (DIP'94)*, Samara, Russia, Vol. 2363, pp. 152–156, August 23–26, 1994.
39. Parker, J. A., Kenyon, R. V., and Troxel, D. E., Comparison of interpolating methods for image resampling, *IEEE Trans. Med. Imag.*, Vol. 2, No. 1, pp. 31–39, March 1983.
40. Hylton, N. M., Simovsky, I., Li, A. J., and Hale, J. D., Impact of section doubling on MR angiography, *Radiology*, Vol. 185, No. 3, pp. 899–902, Dec. 1992.
41. Du, Y. P., Parker, D. L., Davis, W. L., and Cao, G., Reduction of partial-volume artifacts using zero-filled interpolation in three-dimensional MR angiography, *J. Magn. Reson. Imag.*, Vol. 4, No. 5, pp. 733–741, 1994.
42. Chapman, B. E., Goodrick, K. C., Alexander, A. L., Blatter, D. D., and Parker, D. L., Two alternative forced choice evaluations of vessel visibility increases due to zero-filled interpolation in MR angiography, in *Proc. 15th Int. Conf. Information Processing in Medical Imaging, (LNCS)*, Springer-Verlag, Berlin, Vol. 1230, pp. 543–548, 1997.
43. Suri, J. S., Liu, K., Reden, L., and Laxminarayan, S., Detectability of black blood vessels in magnetic resonance angiography volumes: a review, submitted, 2001.

3

Three-Dimensional Interactive Vascular Postprocessing Techniques: Industrial Perspective

James Williams, Huseyin Tek, Dorin Comaniciu, and Brian Avants

CONTENTS

3.1   Introduction

3.1.1   Problem Domain

The focus of this chapter is on the design and construction of interactive software to aid in the task of detection, diagnosis, and quantification of vascular pathology from three-dimensional imaging modalities (currently CT, MR, and rotational angiography). We do not expect or attempt to achieve a fully automated diagnostic process. Instead, the role of the software system is to augment human capabilities. There is an implicit guideline for the division of tasks: target the software at those tasks for which automation is best suited.

3.1.2 Chapter Structure

We begin the chapter with a discussion of the clinical problem domains characterized by the body region involved. After these problems are laid out, we continue with a section outlining the platform and environment of the software application we have created and the design choices we have made regarding visualization and segmentation methods. Visualization methods are then covered, with particular focus on the suitability and limitations of these techniques with regard to clinical vascular postprocessing. Following visualization, a survey of segmentation methods is given before launching into the detailed discussion of the techniques we have created and deployed to support clinical workflow in our medical workstation environment.

3.2 Clinical Problem Domains

The requirements of a vascular postprocessing system vary, depending on the body region being imaged (see Figure 3.1). This section provides an overview of the major domains and the particular needs of each type.

3.2.1 Abdominal

Abdominal vascular imaging is one of the most challenging body areas for postprocessing. In addition to basic diagnostic inspection and quantification, surgical planning is needed. The placement of stents using noninvasive intravascular surgery requires detailed geometric information prior to the procedure and similarly detailed evaluation during follow-up examinations. Consider the placement of a stent in the aorta. A number of facts must be obtained prior to the procedure including:

1. What diameter and length of stent should be used?
2. Is the aneurysm far enough below the renal arteries to allow a standard stent, or must a stent with renal branches be used?
3. Which approach (right or left) is less tortuous and allows more room for the surgeon to maneuver? Will the stent fit through this approach path?
4. How far from the entry point should the stent be deployed?
5. What is the thickness of thrombus inside the aneurysm?

Answering these questions requires making precise measurements of the vascular structures and is a primary guideline for the design of the suite of measurement tools inside the application.

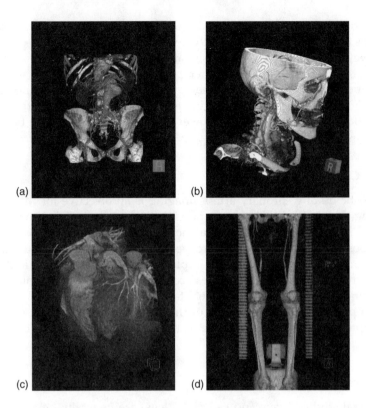

(a) (b) (c) (d)

FIGURE 3.1 (See color insert.)
Angio studies: (a) abdominal, (b) carotid, (c) cardiac, and (d) peripheral.

3.2.2 Head and Neck

The analysis of carotid pathology, particularly stenosis (narrowing) of the carotid artery has relied on projective x-ray angiography as a gold standard. There are strong arguments that three-dimensional modalities (MR, CT) may provide more accurate quantification of pathology. A basic tenet of this belief is simple geometry. X-ray only shows one of a possible 360 degrees of rotated views. It is possible that the chosen projection either exaggerates or hides pathology—in a three-dimensional modality, the true geometry of the vessel is available for measurement.

For intercranial studies, aneurysm detection and measurement is probably the most common goal. For interventions, however, the three-dimensional study is just a precursor and the dynamic fluoro images are used for the detailed inspection. Recently, three-dimensional rotational angiography has become more common in the interventional suite. In this imaging protocol, contrast is injected into the vasculature of interest and the x-ray gantry is rotated around the axis of the patient, producing between 50 and 200 projections. A three-dimensional volume is then reconstructed through back projection.

An exciting aspect of three-dimensional-angio is that the isotropic voxel resolutions can be 0.2 mm or less for the reconstructions.

However, because three-dimensional-angio is an interventional imaging medium, it requires an even faster processing loop than the diagnostic modalities and does not fit into the application workflow described in this chapter. The algorithmic and imaging techniques still apply, but the level of user guidance available is much lower and response times must be significantly faster in the interventional suite.

3.2.3   Cardiac

Diagnostic quality coronary artery imaging is an objective for MR and CT imaging that is finally becoming possible, especially in CT. New gantries with 0.5 second or less rotational latency, coupled with multi-row detectors, make possible prospective and retrospectively gated cardiac reconstructions with minimal motion artifacts and in-plane resolutions of 0.5 mm and better. In current images, calcified plaques are clearly visible and soft plaques are beginning to become resolvable. Qualitative and quantitative analysis of soft arterial plaque is likely to be one of the most active fields of research and development for both diagnostic and healthy-patient screening during the next decade.

3.2.4   Peripheral

Peripheral studies (arms and especially legs) are generally detection problems with some moderate amount of associated quantification, usually to give direction for a surgical intervention. However, as resolution increases, peripheral studies will become important to whole-patient screening procedures.

3.3   An Application for Vascular Postprocessing

3.3.1   Vessel View

The many vascular diagnosis problems share a common archetype. First there is the problem of pathology detection, which is primarily a qualitative visual task. Once pathology has been detected and localized, further enhanced visualization of the target area and measurement are the key. The software package that embodies the algorithms and methods described in this chapter is Vessel View. Vessel View was developed for Siemens postprocessing workstations for use on both MR and CT data. It is integrated into a suite of applications available on a medical imaging workstation platform. The workstation software runs on commodity (x86 and Alpha) hardware and is layered on top of a commercial WIN32 operating system.

A high level of three-dimensional graphics performance is required on these workstations and current high-end OpenGL accelerated graphics cards support fast visualization at a commodity price. Allowable memory overhead for a single application should not exceed the 1-GB level, even for the largest of data sets. These assets, coupled with the design concept of interactive processing have guided the design and selection of the visualization and segmentation components of the system. An important design consideration was to what extent vessel detection was required, if at all.

3.3.2 Vessel Detection vs. Segmentation

There is a clear distinction between the problems of detection and segmentation of the vasculature. In our system, the detection of vessels and localization of pathologies is a user task supported by high-speed interactive visualization. The problem of vessel detection is not approached for a practical reason. The diagnostic process is an interactive one that requires a human operator in the loop for safety concerns. Generally, the operator is a radiological technician (RT) or, in some practices, the reading radiologist. In either case, the operator is a skilled expert. Given the availability of this resource, it makes sense to make maximal use of operator skill at junctures where it would streamline the workflow and speed up the end-to-end processing time. Vessel detection in a three-dimensional rendering is an easy task for such a user. Also, the user has a host of background information on the task, such as body region, the reason for the scan, and the conditions of the acquisition that may have affected the images. Human flexibility is an asset of which we seek to take full advantage.

3.4 Visualization

Visualization (see Figure 3.2) and segmentation are tightly coupled in the postprocessing workflow. The earliest and most prevalent visualization technique for MR and CT angio studies has been the maximum intensity projection (MIP). MIP visualization projects the entire volume along a single direction vector onto a plane. The intensity value of a pixel in the projected image is the maximum intensity value of all voxels that project to that particular two-dimensional point. MIP is an excellent tool for vascular visualization but it lacks depth information. The impression of three dimensions is conveyed through interactive rotation of the view, but it is difficult for the user to discern when vessels pass in front of or behind one another. It is also difficult to see surface features of vessels (for example, the small bump of a nascent aneurysm) because surface information is lost in the projection.

Surface shaded display (SSD) is a technique in which the volume is initially thresholded so that all pixels above a certain intensity value are labeled as

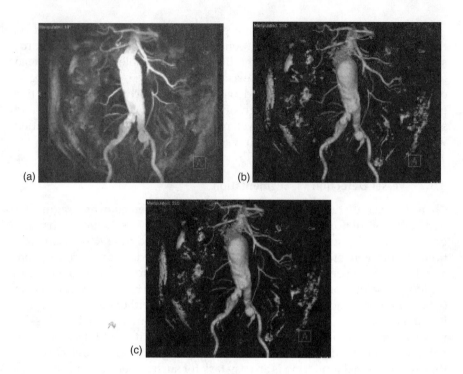

FIGURE 3.2
Three types of visualization techniques: (a) MIP, (b) VRT, and (c) SSD.

belonging to the object(s) to be visualized. Object voxels are considered completely opacified and are rendered using lighting and local surface normal computations to reveal details through shading and specular highlights. The highlights provide strong visual clues to surface irregularities such as bumps and depressions. Because only those voxels on the surface of the object are visible to the user, SSD can be easily optimized to operate at real-time speed without the need for special hardware acceleration. SSD is very effective for visualizing CT vascular data, which can be reliably thresholded. For MR, however, inhomogeneities in the signal due to coil proximity artifacts and gain irregularities make SSD unreliable in moderate to low quality MR studies.

The primary visualization mode we use is the alpha-composited volume rendering technique (VRT) [29]. In the past 5 years, improved CPU and graphics accelerator technology driven by the consumer PC market have made volume rendering visualization possible on low-cost platforms. Previously, interactive volume rendering was possible only on expensive specialized hardware.

VRT visualization is dependent on a transfer function. A transfer function maps voxel intensity values to (R, G, B, α) tuples. In these color tuples, α is an opacity value ranging from 0 (transparent) to 1 (completely opacified). The volume is projected along rays onto an image plane. Blending is performed starting at the voxels most distant from the projection plane and finishing with those most proximal to the plane. Along each ray, the blending equation is applied on a voxel-by-voxel basis.

Given a ray with current color C and opacity α, and a new voxel with color C_1 and alpha α_1, the resulting new alpha (A_{new}) and color (C_{new}) are:

$$C_{new} = C(1 - \alpha_1) + C_1 * \alpha_1 \qquad (3.1)$$

$$A_{new} = 1 - (1 - \alpha) * (1 - \alpha_1) \qquad (3.2)$$

Through interactive adjustment of the transfer function, a wide range of appearances can be generated for the data. With the increased versatility also comes added user complexity. Helper tools for the selection of transfer functions are required to make VRT a practical medium. Most applications provide for this need by supplying transfer function galleries and/or transfer function generation heuristics targeted at the types of evaluation to be performed.

3.4.1 Integrating Visualization and Segmentation

The volume-rendered view of the data is not a passive visualization. It is an interactive, selectable part of the UI. The opacified volume can be selected by pointing and clicking. When selected, a ray is cast back through the volume to determine the front-most opacified point. A target pointer is then drawn at this location (see Figure 3.3). This feature lets the user set seed points and select vessels directly in the three-dimensional visualization. The placement of seed points and region selection are vital to the initialization and guidance of the segmentation algorithms, which will be described later in this chapter.

Visualization, in turn, benefits from the segmentations when they are created. Given a segmentation of the vessel in three-dimensions, it is possible to automatically generate a range of targeted visualizations. The simplest is to use the segmentation as a volume mask for MIP or volume rendering. Removal of the background tissues allows more detailed review of the vessels. Anatomical context is, however, important so the application gives the user a dimming control for the portions of the volume that have been masked away. This fader control changes the opacity of the background voxels as they are piped into the volume-rendering engine.

Other types of targeted visualization are possible only if a central axis path is available for a vessel. Two-dimensional multi-planar reformat (MPR) views can be constructed orthogonal to the vessel to provide reference images for making accurate vessel diameter and area measurements.

In addition, given the central axis curve, a curved planar reformat of the vessel can be produced. This is a two-dimensional image produced by

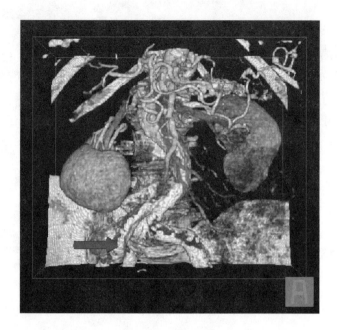

FIGURE 3.3 (See color insert.)
Volume-rendered image of contrast-enhanced abdominal CT data.

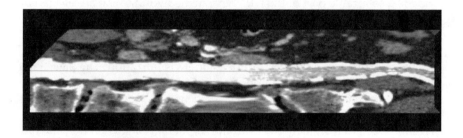

FIGURE 3.4
Curved planar reformat of an aorta from CT.

sweeping a line segment along the path in an orientation orthogonal to the tangent direction (see Figure 3.4).

Given an arc-length parameterized curve $\vec{C}(t)$, and the tangent function of this curve $\vec{T}(t) = \frac{\vec{C}'(t)}{\|\vec{C}'(t)\|}$, let $V(x, y, z)$ be the intensity function of the volume. The curved reformat image $I(u, v)$ is defined to be:

$$I(u, v) = V(\vec{C}(u) + \vec{N}(u) * (v - .5)) \tag{3.3}$$

where u, v in $[0..1]$ and $\vec{N}(u)$ is a continuous normal function that is orthogonal to $\vec{T}(t)$.

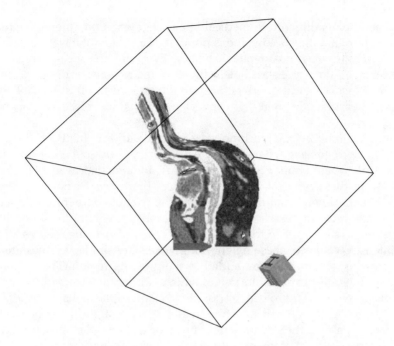

FIGURE 3.5
Curved planar reformat depicted in three-dimensional view before flattening.

We choose the normal function $\vec{N}(u)$, which minimizes the integral of torsion of the local frame $(\vec{T}(t), \vec{N}(t), \vec{T}(t) \times \vec{N}(t))$ over the length of C. An example of this curved visualization is shown in Figure 3.5.

3.5 Related Work in Vascular Segmentation

Segmentation is a required precursor to semi-automatic or automatic quantification. The vessel segmentation problem for MRA and CTA images has been the subject of a broad variety of investigations. These techniques have ranged from simple thresholding and region growing to complex differential-geometry-based filtering schemes. This section provides a partial overview of these techniques grouped into an informal taxonomy.

3.5.1 Statistical Methods

One of the simplest statistical segmentation techniques is global thresholding, where pixels are classified based on their intensity values. However, choosing the right intensity threshold, which typically varies from one data set to another, is difficult. In medical image segmentation, interactive manual selection of a threshold value is popular, but finding the right threshold value can be tedious and operator sensitive. Even with the optimal threshold, final segmentation can create holes, disconnected regions, or merge adjacent regions. Morphological filters [43, 75] are often used to fill in the holes via closing operations or break the connected regions into pieces via opening operations.

One of the most popular techniques for segmentation of medical structures is *seeded region growing* where initialized seeds grow by collecting "similar" pixels, and where similarity is often defined by a statistical test [2, 11, 37, 45, 104]. In these types of algorithms, a user first selects a point or region from a three-dimensional image which is the part of a structure of interest (e.g., bright areas of vessels in CE-MRA). Second, a region filling algorithm recursively is then applied to voxels in the vicinity of growing regions. When the intensity values of these neighboring voxels are similar to the statistics of a growing region, they are added to the growing region. The similarity measure includes a threshold value, which is often determined by a user and plays an important role in the quality of results. Like global thresholding algorithms, segmentation results from region growing algorithms can contain holes, miss parts of the structure of interest, or include other structures, due to the inhomogeneity of image data. Again, morphological operators [43, 75] are often used to correct these errors.

More advanced statistical methods try to automatically determine the intensity threshold by fitting a mixture of Gaussian distributions to the intensity values, and estimating the distribution parameters using the expectation maximization (EM) algorithm [26, 72]. Once the parameters are estimated, classical Bayesian decision theory [33] is used to find the decision boundaries. Specifically, Wilson and Noble [97] and Chung and Noble [19] used the expectation maximization algorithm (EM) to find an appropriate threshold value for separating vessels from background.

3.5.2   Deformable Contour and Surfaces for Medical Image Segmentation

Deformable model-based segmentation algorithms can be divided into explicit methods and implicit methods, based on how the deformable surface is represented. In this section we briefly review the "deformable models" literature as is pertinent to this chapter. A more detailed review of deformable models for medical image segmentation can be found in [63, 100].

3.5.2.1   Active Contours and Surfaces: Explicit Methods

Active contours, or snakes [48], are deformable models based on energy minimization of controlled-continuity splines. When placed near the boundary of objects, they will lock onto salient image features under the guidance of internal and external forces. Formally, let $C(s) = (x(s), y(s))$ be the coordinates of a point on the snake, where s is the length parameter. The energy functional of a snake is defined as:

$$E(\mathcal{C}) = \int_0^1 [E_{int}(\mathcal{C}(s)) + E_{image}(\mathcal{C}(s)) + E_{con}(\mathcal{C}(s))]\,ds \qquad (3.4)$$

where E_{int} represents the internal energy of the spline due to bending, E_{image} represents image forces, and E_{con} are the external constraint forces. First, the internal energy, $E_{int} = w_1|\mathcal{C}'(s)|^2 + w_2|\mathcal{C}''(s)|^2$, imposes regularity on the curve, and w_1 and w_2 correspond to elasticity and rigidity, respectively. Second, the image forces are responsible for pushing the snake toward salient image features. E_{con} corresponds to the user-specified constraints.

Snakes perform well when they are placed close to the desired shapes. However, snakes heavily rely on a proper initialization close to the boundary, multiple initializations, one per object of interest. To overcome some of the initialization difficulties with snakes, Cohen and Cohen [20] introduced a deformable model based on the snakes idea. This model resembles a "balloon" that is inflated by an additional force [90] which pushes the active contour to object boundaries, even when it is initialized far from the initial boundary. Numerous papers have been published in last decade for improving these models see, for example, [5, 21, 25, 42, 55, 101].

Hernandez-Hoyos et al. [44] presented a snake model with a single point initialization for segmenting vessel boundaries in the planes orthogonal to the vessel centerline. The centerline of vessels is detected via an expansible skeleton method based on a tracking strategy. Specifically, the user initializes a point within a vessel and then the algorithm iteratively estimates the consecutive axis points. Once the centerline is detected, the cross-sectional vessel boundaries are detected via an efficient and fast snake method.

Wink et al. [98] used ray propagation for fast segmentation of vessels and detection of their centerline. In this approach, Wink et al. used the intensity gradients to stop the propagation of rays. However, this approach faces difficulties when the vessel boundaries are not sharp, that is, due to partial volume effects, and also when vessels contain isolated noises (e.g., calcifications in CT images).

Traditionally, snakes or balloons cannot handle *topological changes*, that is, merging and splitting. McInerney and Terzopoulos [62, 65] presented the topologically adaptable snakes for semi-automatic segmentation of medical images in two dimensions. Specifically, they used the affine cell image decomposition (ACID) framework for enabling topological flexibility. They have illustrated that this algorithm, which is computationally efficient in two dimensions, can be used to segment complex-shaped biological structures from medical images (e.g., blood vessel in a retinal angiogram). This two-dimensional approach was then extended to three dimension [64] for volume segmentation.

3.5.2.2 Level Set Evolution: Implicit Methods

The most popular approach for the solution of the topological problems of snakes is the use of the level set evolution proposed by Osher and Sethian for flame propagation [69], introduced to computer vision for shape representation [51] and first applied to active contours in [14, 61].

The level set approach considers a curve C as the zero level set of a surface, $\phi(x, y) = 0$. Caselles et al. [14, 61] proposed that the zero level set of the function ϕ, $\{x \in R^2 : \phi(t, x) = 0\}$, evolves in the normal direction according to

$$\phi_t = S(x, y)(\beta_0 - \beta_1 \kappa(x, y))|\nabla \phi| \tag{3.5}$$

where β_0, and β_1 are constants, $\kappa(x, y)$ is the curvature of level sets, $\nabla \phi$ is the normal to the level set, and $S(x, y)$ is the image-based speed function defined as $S(x, y) = \frac{1}{1 + |\nabla G_\sigma * I(x, y)|}$. ϕ_0 is the initial surface which is often chosen to be a signed distance transform of the initial curve C_0. Several interesting relevant approaches [15, 16, 49, 74, 78, 80, 102] have been proposed since the original work of Caselles et al. [14] and Malladi et al. [61]. Unlike snakes, this active contour model can handle topological changes such as merging and splitting without any computational difficulty.

Tek and Kimia [84–86] proposed a reaction-diffusion bubble technique for segmenting three-dimensional medical images such as carotid arteries in MRA images (Figure 3.6). In this approach, bubbles, small deformable models, are randomly initialized in either uniform areas of image or structure of interests which then grow, shrink, merge, split, and disappear, and in general deform unless influenced by image information to confirm or invalidate the existence of an object and its parts, leading to a segmentation of images. In addition, a particular mean-Gauss curvature deformation [67] is used to serve as the diffusion process, leading to the following reaction-diffusion evolution,

$$\frac{\partial \Psi}{\partial t} = S(x, y, z)(\beta_0 - \beta_1 sign(H)\sqrt{G + |G|})|\nabla \Psi| \tag{3.6}$$

where Ψ is the four-dimensional evolving surface whose zero level set represents the deformable model. $|\nabla \Psi|$ is the normal to the level set. H is the

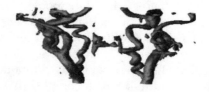

FIGURE 3.6 (See color insert.)
This figure illustrates the quality of reconstruction of the vascular structure from MRA images via three-dimensional bubbles [85, 86].

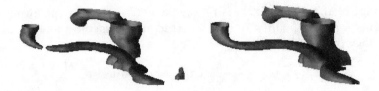

FIGURE 3.7 (See color insert.)
This figure illustrates the importance of diffusion process in the three-dimensional bubbles technique. In the reaction process, bubbles cross over the small weak boundary segments, finally causing the vessels to split into pieces. However, in the diffusion process, bubbles do not enter these regions; thus, they reconstruct smooth shapes [86].

mean curvature and G is the Gaussian curvature. Similarly, $S(x, y, z)$ is the speed function derived from three-dimensional image information. The three-dimensional reaction-diffusion bubbles are intrinsic, can deal with a variety of gaps, and place captured surfaces in a hierarchy of scale. For example, consider Figure 3.7, which is a small volume cropped from a large MRA image. Observe that a small area located at the bent part of the long vascular structure surface lacks edge evidence. Thereby, three-dimensional reaction bubbles fail to fully capture the vascular area. In contrast, the addition of diffusion regularizes the evolving bubble surface to capture this structure.

Siddiqi and Vasilevskiy [81] proposed a three-dimensional level sets method based on maximizing the rate of an auxiliary vector field through a curve for segmentation of blood vessels in computational rotational angiography (CRA). Specifically, for a compact embedded surface S, they proposed:

$$S_t = div(\mathcal{V})\mathcal{N} \qquad (3.7)$$

where $\mathcal{N}$ is the normal vector and $\mathcal{V}$ is chosen to be the gradient ∇I of the original intensity image I. Similar to three-dimensional bubbles [86], several small spheres are automatically placed in regions of high flux (bright regions), which then follow the direction of blood flow to reconstruct blood vessels.

Lorigo et al. [58, 59] proposed a level set method for segmentation of blood vessels that specifically aims to recover low-contrast thin vessels as well as large ones. Traditionally, level sets methods use the mean curvature to regularize the geometric flow in three dimensions [16, 49, 61]. However, the mean curvature-based flows tend to annihilate thin structures. Lorigo et al. then proposed to use the curvature of a three-dimensional curve. Specifically, they used the elegant theoretical results of Ambrosio and Soner [4], who developed level sets theory for mean curvature flows in arbitrary co-dimension. These theoretical results suggest a nice solution for the problem of three-dimensional curve evolution via its curvature. In fact, Lorigo et al. developed the implementation of these theoretical results and illustrated that three-dimensional curves represented by a tubular structure can be smoothed without creating self-intersections. However, the main contribution of Lorigo et al. is the extension of these theoretical results to geodesic active contours for segmentation of tubular structures in medical images. Specifically, they proposed

$$\Psi_t = \lambda(\nabla\Psi, \nabla^2\Psi) + \rho(\nabla\Psi \cdot \nabla I)\frac{g'}{g}\nabla\Psi \cdot H\frac{\nabla I}{||\nabla I||} \qquad (3.8)$$

where Ψ is, again, the embedded surface whose zero level is the evolving three-dimensional curve C. Specifically, they suggested ϵ-level set representation for the numerical simulations. $\lambda(\nabla\Psi, \nabla^2\Psi)$ is the smaller non-zero eigenvalue of a certain matrix defined in [4]. Intuitively, the smaller eigenvalue corresponds to the larger principal curvature, which is related to the geometry of curve C. I is the image and the function g is an image-dependent decreasing function such as $g(r) = exp(-r)$. H is the Hessian of the intensity function. Lorigo et al. illustrated several examples where the proposed evolution successfully segments blood vessels in several primary phase contrast MRA (PC-MRA) data sets and an aorta MRA data set.

A key disadvantage of the level set method is their high computational complexity, due to the additional embedding dimensional, even when the computation is restricted to a narrow band around the curve. To overcome the computational complexity, narrowband level set evolutions have been proposed [1, 61, 95]. Similarly, Sethian [77] proposed fast marching methods for simulating the monotonically advancing front. This method does not require any additional surface, but it is limited to simulate one-directional flows (i.e., no curvature smoothing). Deschamps and Cohen [27, 28] developed a technique based on the fast marching method for determining the paths of tubular structures in medical images. Specifically, they first extended the minimal path planing technique of Cohen and Kimmel [22] to three-dimensional images. Second, they adapted this technique to detect tubular anatomical structures in medical images such as vessels and the colon.

3.5.3   Graph Algorithms

Graph algorithms are powerful tools for image segmentation and clustering. The data is represented by a weighted graph, composed of a set of vertices representing the data points, a set of edges connecting them, and a weight assigning function that measures the affinity between adjacent data points. Depending on the method, the graph may or may not be complete. The term "adjacency graph" is used when the data represents image pixels.

In one of the earliest works on clustering based on graph theory, Zahn [103] used the minimum spanning tree of the graph to select large edges for breaking the clusters. Urquhart [91] introduced the idea of edge normalization based on region information. Wu [99] transformed first the graph into an equivalent tree, and then used the tree to successively remove edges and optimally divide the image into K parts. More recently, Felzenszwalb and Huttenlocher [36] introduced a region comparison function and provided an efficient segmentation algorithm that is closely related to Kruskal's minimum spanning tree.

Using the graph-theoretic framework, problems that were first analyzed in network flow theory find direct application in image data analysis. For segmentation, one is interested in finding the maximum flow from one vertex to another, or the maximum flow between every pair of vertices. The Ford–Fulkerson theorem [38] makes the link between maximum flow from one vertex to another and the minimum cut separating the two vertices. See [41] for a discussion of polynomial-time maximum flow algorithms. Karger and Stein [47] developed a randomized, strongly polynomial algorithm that finds the minimum cut in an undirected graph with high probability. The algorithm was applied by Gdalyahu et al. [40] to stochastic clustering and image segmentation. In a different approach, Jermyn and Ishikawa [46] employed a minimum mean weight cycle algorithm to determine the global optima of an energy functional used in image segmentation.

To capture nonlocal properties of the image, Shi and Malik [79] introduced a normalization of the graph cut. The resulting segmentation captures salient parts of an image. However, because the resulting optimization is still NP-hard, they solved the problem using an approximation based on generalized eigenvectors. Weiss [94] discussed in detail segmentation methods relying on eigenvectors.

Boykov and Jolly [12] presented a technique for interactive segmentation with graph cuts based on hard constraints (i.e., user-selected seeds representing the foreground vs. background). An efficient maximum flow algorithm assures close to real-time user interaction with the algorithm. The globally optimal solution is updated when the user adds or removes any hard constraints. The method allows the introduction of soft constraints in terms of region and boundary properties. It extends easily to volumetric data, such as kidney segmentation in three-dimensional MRI angiography.

A different class of techniques relies on shortest path algorithms [30]. Jolly and Gupta [32] developed a method for tracking deformable templates using Dijkstra's shortest path algorithm. They used the method to track and motion-compensate coronary arteries in x-ray angiography. Concepts such as *live wire* and *live lane* [35] and *intelligent scissors* [66] are also based on the minimal cost path algorithm. They provide fast user interaction by interactively presenting the boundary segments between the user-defined starting point and the current position of the cursor.

3.5.4 Differential Geometry-Based Filtering Approaches

Koller et al. [52] presented a nonlinear filtering method for the detection of curvilinear structures in two- and three-dimensional images such as vessels in MRA data. This filtering technique combines responses from across scale-space to detect the various sizes of curvilinear structures. In addition, it uses the eigenvalues of the Hessian matrix to determine the orientation of filters in three dimensions. Specifically, the Hessian matrix of image I is given by:

$$H(x, y, z) = \begin{bmatrix} I_{xx} & I_{xy} & I_{xz} \\ I_{yx} & I_{yy} & I_{yz} \\ I_{zx} & I_{zy} & I_{zz} \end{bmatrix} \qquad (3.9)$$

and describes the local intensity variations of a voxel in a three-dimensional image. The eigenvalues of a Hessian matrix were also used in [39, 54, 57, 73] to determine the local shape of structure in the image. Specifically, the three-dimensional images are smoothed via the three-dimensional line (or vessel) filters, which are designed from the detailed analysis of eigenvectors of the Hessian matrix. Because vessels in three-dimensional images can be in different sizes, images are convolved with multi-scale filters and maximum response over all scales is stored in each voxel. However, for a fair comparison of the responses at multiple scales, a normalization parameter [56] is added to the definition of the line filters. This scale information stored in each voxel is then used to determine the size of vessels. These multi-scale filtered images can then be used in direct visualization or segmentation. Specifically, Sato et al. [73] illustrated the threshold segmented vessels in MRA images and the quality of volume rendering visualization after multi-scale filtering. Frangi et al. [39] showed that MIP visualizations of these filtered images are much better than the original images. Lorenz et al. [57] and Krissian et al. [53, 54] used these results for detection of centerlines of vessels in medical images.

Another interesting set of approaches tried to detect vessel centerlines directly from three-dimensional medical images. Specifically, Aylward et al. [8] and Bullit et al. [13] detected the ridges of images as the centerlines of vessels. Like the approaches in [57, 73], the width of vessels is then determined from the multi-scale response of a medialness function. Similarly, Prinet et al. [71] considered a three-dimensional image as a four-dimensional hyper-surface, that is, a volume image I is represented by $(x, y, z, I(x, y, z))$. They proposed that the crest-lines of this hyper-surface correspond to the centerline of tubular structures. They then proposed a mathematical model for detecting these crest-lines that is based on the three principle curvatures of this hyper-surface.

3.6 Workflow Constraints

Segmentation of vessels is essential to support quantification. However, one must take into consideration the data domain and clinical workflow before choosing a segmentation algorithm. One of the primary constraints, and a strong argument for using interactive methods for vessel detection, is that data sizes, especially of CT images, are generally too large for efficient application of global detection or preprocessing techniques. Current state-of-the art scanners can easily generate data series of 1000 512×512 slices for body angio and peripheral runoff cases. Given the 12-bit intensity resolution, such studies reach 0.5 GB in their raw form.

Consider also that most segmentation techniques will require additional data stored on a per-voxel basis to maintain state information during the execution of the algorithm. Memory overhead multipliers of 2X, 3X, etc. are not feasible when dealing with volumes of this scale. Given these constraints, we use only algorithms that have memory overhead multipliers which are dependent on the size of the segmented region. Vascular structures, as a rule of thumb, will rarely occupy more than 5 to 10% of the image volume.

The approach that we take relies on two stages of segmentation. The first step is a voxel-based three-dimensional segmentation that relies on the user to place seed points at the extrema of vessels. This first step segments the vessels at the resolution of the voxel grid and produces central axis curves. The second stage automatically segments two-dimensional orthogonal cross sections of the vessels at sub-voxel resolution. This level of precision is required to make accurate measurements of the cross-sectional area and min/max vessel diameter.

3.7 Three-Dimensional Vessel Segmentation

The initial three-dimensional segmentation is a learning procedure that provides both a metric and bounds for an explicit vessel centerline search. Vessel axes encode the vessel tree more sparsely. Our method makes the extraction of such abstractions sufficiently fast to make axis creation and manipulation part of a real-time, interactive clinical workflow. No preprocessing of the images is required and we demonstrate that the algorithm is parsimonious in its search of the volume—examining primarily those voxels needed to segment and delineate the vessels without appreciable wasted analysis of background regions.

3.7.1 Seeded Vessel Segmentation

The three-dimensional vessel segmentation algorithm relies on the user to place seed points at extremal points of the vessels of interest. This placement is supported by the "touchable" volume-rendered view and also by an additional enhancement. When the user clicks during seed point placement, the selection point is not placed on the surface of the foremost opacified object. Instead, the ray cast to find the nearest opaque voxels is continued until it re-enters translucent or empty space, and the seed is placed halfway in the middle of the opacified region, bringing it closer to the true center of the vessel.

A max-probability front propagation algorithm then makes a dynamic segmentation of the vessels containing the seeds. Front propagation in this case indicates that there is always a layer of "candidate" voxels that are added to the segmented volume sequentially, depending on a membership probability that adjusts dynamically as the segmentation expands. The initial segmentation step provides data that is then used to help determine parameters for the subsequent minimal path calculation used to approximate the vessel centerlines. The distribution of intensity values inside the segmented region is also useful for later processing or subsequent segmentations. In MR images, spatial variation in the distribution of grey values inside the segmented vessel region can be used as input for intensity inhomogeneity correction.

3.7.1.1   Graph-Based Approach

In our application, we view the image volume as a k-regular graph (where "k" denotes the number of edges at each node/voxel) through which we would like to compute a small set of the minimal connectivity. The user contributes the location of nodes to be connected through the image volume. The algorithm then consists of two parts: a volume search and a path search. The first part searches for the subset of the full image graph that is most likely to contain the paths between the user's seed points. The associated volumes are also given a statistical characterization. The edge cost function for the second phase is determined from the statistical distribution of the voxels explored during the first phase. The second phase computes the minimal connectivity of the selected vessel tree points according to parameters set by the partial segmentation results. The constraint of the minimal path computation to only those regions that contain the objects to be connected is an important part of the efficiency and correctness of the algorithm if it is to operate on volumetric data. If unnecessary (non-object) regions of the image are searched, not only does the execution time rapidly increase (as the algorithm is $O(N \log N)$), but the chance that the path will mistakenly cross an object boundary increases. It is imperative, then, to restrain the search to only those regions in which it is probable to have a true path.

3.7.1.2   Surface Expansion

Our approach to the segmentation aspect of this problem is motivated by Sethian's fast marching method. He observes [77] that the fast marching method, which is a level set surface propagation tool, is fundamentally the same as Dijkstra's algorithm in a regular graph. The former, however, computes velocities (inversely proportional to edge costs) incrementally according to the local solution to the Eikonal partial differential equation (pde). The latter is defined, usually, over a simple network with fixed edge costs. Sethian describes his method as producing a gradient field for the arrival time of the front such that:

$$|\nabla T| = \frac{1}{F} \tag{3.10}$$

In his application of the fast marching method on medical images [60], the velocity function is given by:

$$F = e^{-\alpha|\nabla GI|}, \quad \alpha > 0 \tag{3.11}$$

where ∇GI is the gradient of the image pre-processed with a Gaussian filter and α is a constant governing the global expansion rate. Time is zero at all initialized source points and arrival time is calculated such that $T > 0$ at all successive iterations. The proof of the algorithm's correctness is given in [76].

We incorporate a similar approach to Sethian's but do not focus entirely on segmentation. The surface propagation is simultaneously used to learn an appropriate data-based cost function for calculating the minimal path. Also, in our case, the velocity model is probabilistic and nonviscous, thereby allowing velocity to be determined by data at a particular voxel rather than the voxel's neighborhood. This probabilistic model effectively learns the intensity distribution of the segmented region and is subsequently used to generate a data-based closed form for the edge cost function. We redefine the speed function such that we are examining the probability of the local data being included in a known set. Then, the speed function for each node is determined by maximizing the probability of advancement in each possible direction of new exploration. We sample the data locally according to Dijkstra's method (analogous to the Eikonal model of front advancement if connectivity is k-regular) and then define speed to be:

$$F_{ijk} = vP(\text{data included in known set}) \tag{3.12}$$

If $v = 1$ (expansive), then F_{ijk} can be written:

$$F_{ijk} = 1 - P(\text{data } not \text{ included in known set}) \tag{3.13}$$

and we see the parallel between this and Sethian's purely geometric method. The change in time is then given by:

$$|\nabla T| = \frac{1}{max(F_{ijk}(P))} \tag{3.14}$$

Initially, the front will expand most rapidly in the most probable directions. After long times, however, lower probability regions can be explored. This fits with the intuitive notion that probable events occur often and improbable ones occur only at large intervals. If the probability calculation varies only according to data at each voxel, the exploration will execute in $O(N \log N)$. If the probability changes according to the delivery from the min-heap, the entire boundary should be recomputed (as it must be with pure level set methods.) This guarantees the maximum probability exploration, given the elapse of time, but reduces efficiency with a worst-case bound of N^2. Instead, we use a bounded-error approach where recomputation is performed only when the potential maximum error exceeds a given threshold. This generates an error-bounded approximation of the maximum probability exploration with relatively little loss in efficiency.

3.7.1.3 Edge Cost/Velocity Model

The probability model given for the data determines our speed function. In vessel path finding for CTA/CE-MRA, we are interested in quickly connecting vessel-like regions without crossing neighboring non-vessel regions. Stated another way, we are interested in discrimination between energy levels, with vessel membership being analogous to a particular energy level. Therefore, we want rapid propagation through regions of similar energy and slow movement elsewhere.

3.7.1.4 Partitioning Distributions

We formulate the vessel search in terms of a thermodynamic partitioning problem. Sections of the image are allowed two possibilities: vessel and non-vessel, where the existence of one state excludes the other. Each image region, whether it is a single voxel or collection of voxels, is then treated as a canonical ensemble. The comparison of two regions is performed with the partition function [6] given by:

$$Q = \sum_{\text{all states}} e^{\frac{E_i}{\kappa T}} \tag{3.15}$$

where each state is described by its energy E and all states share the constants κT.

Equilibrium requires that, given a system, we have a time-independent minimum of information to describe it. That information for equilibrium systems (and our image) is given by N, the number of particles (proportional to the number of voxels), volume V (the sum of voxel volumes), and temperature T, which we can set. We assume that, from the macroscopic perspective, we can also measure the system's average energy.

3.7.1.5 The Fermi-Dirac Distribution

These assumptions lead directly to the Fermi-Dirac probability function for two states [6]:

$$P_{FD} = \frac{1}{1 + e^{\left(\frac{E_1 - E_0}{\kappa T}\right)}} \tag{3.16}$$

P_{FD} is a step function with slope determined by the size of κT. The inflection point occurs where E_1 (the ensemble temperature) equals E_0, beyond which probability approaches one. Therefore, the κT term determines the parsimony in the allocation of probability. Increasing κT makes the slope gentle, supplying slowly changing probabilities to a broad range of energies about E_1. As the temperature approaches absolute zero, the function approaches zero slope. Higher temperatures result in steep vertical slopes.

3.7.1.6 Implementation

In our framework, given fixed temperature, we can examine the change of an equilibrium system surrounded by a narrow border of ensembles that may or not contain the vessel. We choose a low temperature (generally such that κT is within an order of magnitude of unity) to make propagation through high probability energy regions fast, and low probability regions slow. Initialization occurs when the user selects seeds. Each seed is considered a vessel containing system for which we have N, the system size, V, the volume, the time T, and the energy of the ensemble,

$$E_1 = \frac{1}{N} \sum_{\text{ensemble}} E_i(I) \tag{3.17}$$

which is the standard averaging procedure, where $N = 1$ and $E_i(I)$ is the intensity. These points are treated as ensembles, as stated above. For each source, surrounding regions are explored and compared point-by-point to the expanding ensemble E with which they are in contact. The border point with the highest probability of being vessel tissue will have the smallest arrival time. That voxel is added to its source ensemble such that the latter becomes a system of size $N + 1$. E_1 is then re-measured and the process repeats.

3.7.1.7 Approximation Methods

We could simplify our calculation by weighting the source points with large N values and giving all border systems $N = 1$ such that adding a new voxel won't appreciably change E_1, the mean of the ensemble values. However, for calculating the average and standard deviation of the vessel intensity (needed for the path finding parameters), we would like more exact discrimination. We therefore may be forced to recompute border probabilities when we re-measure E_1. This increases the order by a factor of N. However, we can use the monotonicity of the p.d.f. as well as the relative stability of E_1 over time to limit the frequency of recomputation. The derivative of P_{FD} is:

$$\frac{d}{dE} P_{FD} = \frac{-m}{(m + e^{(E_0 - E_1)})(m + e^{(E_0 - E_1)})} \tag{3.18}$$

where $m = \frac{1}{\kappa T}$. We first note that the derivative of our p.d.f. approaches the delta function if temperature decreases. As temperature increases, the derivative spreads and its magnitude decreases. Generally speaking, the error is only appreciable along the region of the p.d.f where there is a significant slope. For the low-temperature Fermi function, this region is narrow. We can illustrate the nature of the measurement error as follows:

$$P_{FD}(E_{+\epsilon}) = \frac{1}{1 + e^{(E_1(1+\epsilon) - E_0)}} \tag{3.19}$$

We see that our error can be thought of as occurring on the measurement of E_1. We can then limit our error concern to only those values of E_1 where

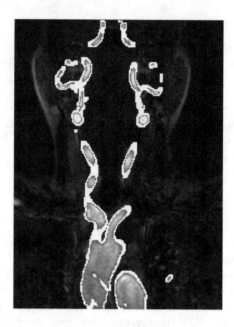

FIGURE 3.8

Slice from a segmented three-dimensional carotid CE-MRA data set illustrates the region explored and segmented by phase 1 of the algorithm. The explored region is highlighted by a white boundary.

the error might be appreciable. We expect to encounter three cases:

$$E_0 > (E_1 + |dE|), \text{ error rapidly diminishing as } E_0 \text{ increases} \quad (3.20)$$
$$(E_1 - |dE|) < E_0 < (E_1 + |dE|), \text{ error significant} \quad (3.21)$$
$$E_0 < (E_1 - |dE|), \text{ error rapidly diminishing as } E_0 \text{ decreases} \quad (3.22)$$

We store, for each E_0 probability computed, the value of E_1 against which it was compared. Then, at the time of delivery, we compute:

$$Error \approx P_{FD}(E_0|E_{1old}) - P_{FD}(E_0|E_{1new}) \quad (3.23)$$

If this value is greater than c, the error tolerance, then we recompute the probability and re-insert the voxel. This process is repeated for all delivered nodes with error greater than the tolerance. Generally, we apply a 5% rule to case 3.20 and 3.21 errors, and 10% to case 3.22 errors that could benefit from updating. Fortunately, not only is the range that we need to recompute small, but the value E_1 stabilizes over time. In practice, this means that the vast majority of border recomputations occur early in the expansion process when the boundaries contain relatively few nodes.

3.7.2 Path Finding

3.7.2.1 Speed Function

The speed function for the path finding derives naturally from our former statements. Here, we do not have to choose between two states. The only state we are concerned with is the vessel state.

Due to our surface exploration, then, we know the degeneracy (histogram) of energy levels in the vessel. So, we use that knowledge along with the canonical distribution to compute our speed function:

$$F_{ijk} = L W_j P_{canonical}(E_j) = L W_j e^{\left(\frac{-E_j}{\kappa T}\right)} \qquad (3.24)$$

where W_j is the degeneracy of energy E_j and L is a Euclidean term that gives inter-voxel distance in patient space. The advantage that we have here is that we already know the intensity distribution of the segmented region and can normalize the computation by the "known" natural temperature of the distribution. It is proportional to the standard deviation of the intensities in the region, which we measured in our surface propagation algorithm. This guarantees that we have a provably minimal path that will move through the vessel region with a very high probability. Even if there is error in the segmentation, the use of the canonical distribution for the speed function makes it highly unlikely that the actual minimal path will deviate into the erroneously segmented parts of the volume. This is because the canonical distribution peaks around E_1 due to the large degeneracy of that energy level [6].

The speed function is also modulated by a morphologically derived term. We compute the approximate Euclidean Distance Transform (EDT) of the segmented region. For each voxel in the segmented region, the distance to the closest background voxel is computed. The highest values of the EDT lie close to the centerlines of the vessels. The EDT value is used as a direct multiplier to the speed function to encourage propagation near the vessel centers.

3.7.2.2 Active Backtracking and System Equilibration

Although we instantiate a min-heap for each source, we compute the minimum over all heaps for the expansion of exploration. In this way, we have a virtual single min-heap. The movement of all surfaces, then, is governed by the interaction of the set of heaps. This, naturally, leads to surfaces in more homogeneous regions of the image propagating more rapidly and thus initiating meetings with other surfaces first.

Surface meetings occur when different surfaces share osculating border points. This is the condition for producing a path. We set the parameters for the path finding by measuring the degeneracy of the energy levels within each surface and computing the (approximate) standard deviation of the energies. An instance of Dijkstra's algorithm with the above speed function is then initiated from the osculating points backward into each surface, thus producing a minimal path as it goes. The stopping condition for this search is the discovery of either an original source or a minimal path computed at a previous meeting.

After the paths are computed, the two osculating regions then share statistical information and merge into a single heap. Then, the algorithm continues as before, but with one less surface. The final termination condition is that all surfaces have met and all paths connecting them have been computed. The data structures containing the vessel boundaries, paths, and sources are maintained. This allows subsequent sources to be added to the image volume.

The algorithm will then begin a new set of surface searches, and meetings will be handled in the same way as before, except that if the old surface is met, active backtracking is not symmetric. Instead, the new surface is allowed to find paths both backward into its volume and forward toward the paths computed in prior executions of the algorithm.

3.7.3   Vessel Tree Morphology

The path finding algorithm is versatile in that it is able to handle seeded segmentations of linear vessels and of complete vessel trees without resorting to ad-hoc methods. Simple guidance is given to the user that the best place to set seed points is at the extremal points and junctions of the vessels of interest. By following these instructions, the user provides exactly the information needed for correct topological separation of individual vessels.

This is easiest to explain by example. Consider the aorta and the two branching iliac arteries. Following the guideline, seed points are placed at the three extremal points and at the junction, and region expansion is initiated. The expansion of the region at the junction effectively "plugs" the junction so the expanding regions originating at the extrema will not be able to join directly to one another. The first expanding front to meet the junction will form a linear "leg" of the final tree and subsequent meetings will also form legs attached to the junction locus.

We include an additional topology check at the end of the segmentation to ensure that the axis tree produced truly has a tree topology and this serves as a safety fall-back. However, there is at least one vascular feature that does not fit neatly into the tree topology, the Circle of Willis. This is a rather unique anatomical structure that is a closed loop. However, in the vast majority of cases, the tree structure predominates.

3.7.4   Limitations

The unusual case of the Circle of Willis aside, there are other limitations to our three-dimensional segmentation method. First and foremost, in the case of total or nearly total occlusion of an artery, the algorithm's cost function will tend to explore every other healthy arterial path or even connect through other bright tissues (such as unsuppressed fat in MR or bone in CT) before jumping the dark occluded region. Because the expanding regions have only local

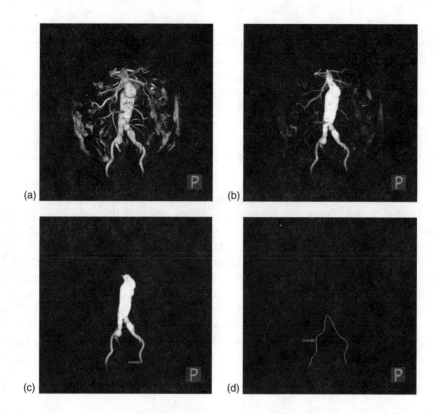

FIGURE 3.9
3-D segmentation stages: (a) presegmented data, (b) seeds set, (c) segmentation complete, and (d) generated paths.

knowledge of their segmented regions, there is no hint that the vessel should be continued across a complete gap. For the human operator, however, such failures are immediately obvious and can be corrected by manually bridging the gap using the path editing interface.

3.7.5 Performance

The performance of the three-dimensional segmentation is data dependent. Both the size of the region to be segmented and the intensity distribution affect the running time, as of course does the seeding pattern given by the user.

Putting those factors aside for the moment, we focus on the real-world performance of the application. The deployment platform is a 1.5-GHz Intel machine with 1 to 2 GB of RAM. The typical CT abdominal study contains 250 to 400 512 × 512 slices. Three-dimensional segmentation of the aorta from above the renal branch to below the iliac bifurcation generally requires less than 5 seconds; the additional path generation and visualization steps add an additional 5 to 10 seconds to the total execution time.

MR studies are faster because of the lower resolution. In CT, other narrow-vessel studies such as coronaries and peripherals require less time because the total volume of the segmented region is usually significantly smaller than that of the large aorta.

3.7.6 From Coarse Three-Dimensional to Fine Two-Dimensional Segmentations

Extraction of vessels in three dimensions using the algorithm described provides the user with a voxel-resolution segmentation of the vessel and a centerline that can be used to accurately position an orthogonal MPR plane. In this plane, the vessel diameter and cross-sectional area can be accurately measured. A goal of our implementation is to provide vessel cross-sectional area measurements automatically once the three-dimensional segmentation is completed. These measurements should be given with sub-voxel precision to support evaluation in cases where the vessel may only have a diameter of 2 or 3 voxels. To accomplish this goal, we use a two-dimensional ray propagation method in conjunction with a mean-shift-based noise modulation technique.

3.8 Cross-Sectional Vessel Boundary Detection by Two-Dimensional Ray Propagation

In this section, we describe a ray propagation technique for detecting vessel boundaries in the planes orthogonal to their centerlines [83].

Let the front be represented by a two-dimensional curve $C(s, t) = (x(s, t), y(s, t))$, where x and y are the Cartesian coordinates, s is the length parameter, and t is time. The evolution is then governed by [51]:

$$\begin{cases} \frac{\partial C(s,t)}{\partial t} = S(x, y)\vec{N} \\ C(s, 0) = C_0(s) \end{cases} \tag{3.25}$$

where $C_0(s) = (x(s, 0), y(s, 0))$ is the initial curve, $\vec{N}$ is the unit normal vector, and $S(x, y)$ is the speed of a ray at point (x, y).

The approach that we consider in this section is based on explicit front propagation via normal vectors. Specifically, the contour is sampled and the evolution of each sample is followed in time by rewriting the Eikonal equation [69] in vector form, namely:

$$\begin{cases} x_t(s, t) = S(x, y)\dfrac{y_s}{\sqrt{x_s^2 + y_s^2}} \\ y_t(s, t) = S(x, y)\dfrac{x_s}{\sqrt{x_s^2 + y_s^2}}. \end{cases} \tag{3.26}$$

The speed of rays, $S(x, y)$ depends on image information and shape priors, which is explained in the next sections.

This evolution is Lagrangian because the physical coordinate system moves with the propagating wavefront. However, the applications of ray propagation for curve evolution have been limited. This is because, when the normals to the wavefront collide (formation of shocks), this approach exhibits numerical instabilities due to an accumulated density of sample points, thus requiring special care, such as reparametrization of the wavefront. Also, topological changes are not handled naturally; that is, an external procedure is required.

Previously, ray propagation has been used to implement the *full-width at half-maximum* (FWHM) technique for quantification of two-dimensional airway geometry [31]. In the FWHM technique, the maximum and minimum intensity values along the rays are computed to determine the "half-maximum" intensity value, which is the half-intensity value between the maximum and minimum. However, stable computation of the maximum and minimum along the rays is quite difficult due to high signal variations. In addition, ray propagation was used by Wink et al. [98] for fast segmentation of vessels and detection of their centerline. In this approach, Wink et al. used the intensity gradients to stop the propagation of rays. However, this approach faces difficulties when the vessel boundaries are not sharp (due to partial volume effects) and also when vessels contain isolated noises (e.g., calcifications in CT images).

The main shortcomings of these approaches stem from the computation of image gradients that are not robust relative to the image noise. In this section, we propose to use *mean shift analysis* for detecting vessel boundaries efficiently and robustly. Comaniciu and Meer [23, 24] showed that the image discontinuities are robustly revealed by a mean-shift process that evolves in both the intensity and image space.

We first review nonlinear smoothing algorithms; second, describe the mean shift analysis; third, illustrate an approach where the mean shift procedure is applied to select discontinuities in one dimensional signal; and finally, present the mean-shift-based ray propagation approach for segmentation of medical structures (e.g., vessels).

3.8.1 PDE-Based Smoothing Methods

Often, smoothing is used to remove noise present in three-dimensional images without affecting the important features, such as vascular structures. Traditionally, images are smoothed via the Gaussian function. However, Gaussian smoothing is not an appropriate method for smoothing medical images containing vascular structures because it shrinks shapes and dislocates boundaries when moving from finer to coarser scales. Instead, nonlinear filters are proposed for removing the noise present in three-dimensional images while keeping the important geometrical structures.

Perona and Malik proposed a nonlinear diffusion filtering method that reduces smoothing at the edges to preserve the contrast information and the location of the object boundaries [70]. Specifically, they proposed that:

$$\begin{cases} u_t = div(f(|\nabla u|^2)\nabla u) \\ u(x, y, 0) = I(x, y) \end{cases} \tag{3.27}$$

where $I(x, y)$ is the image, $f(|\nabla u|^2) = \frac{1}{1+|\nabla u|^2/\lambda^2}$, and $\lambda \geq 0$. This method preserves the strong edges for a long time during the smoothing process by turning off the smoothing at high brightness gradient locations. Thus, this approach smooths regions of low brightness gradient while regions of high gradients are not smoothed. Catté et al. [17] suggest a slight modification in which the gradient in $f(|\nabla u|^2)$ is computed from the Gaussian smoothed image to account for the large noise in the image:

$$u_t = div(f(|\nabla(u * G_\sigma)|)\nabla u) \tag{3.28}$$

A similar scheme was proposed by Whitaker and Pizer [96].

However, these anisotropic diffusion approaches are contrast driven and smooth globally salient but low contrast image features [50]. Thus, geometry-driven diffusion techniques are proposed to deal with low-contrast structures. One particular approach is based on curvature-based smoothing of grey-level intensity images. The curvature deformation of surface $\phi(x, y, t)$, which is also known as the mean curvature flow,

$$\phi_t = div\left(\frac{\nabla\phi}{|\nabla\phi|}\right)|\nabla\phi| \tag{3.29}$$

was studied by Evans and Spruck [34] and by Chen et al. [18]. Kimia and Siddiqi [50] also used this evolution for image smoothing. Similarly, Alvarez et al. [3] studied a class of nonlinear parabolic differential equations defined by:

$$\begin{cases} \phi_t = g(|G * \nabla\phi)div\left(\frac{\nabla\phi}{|\nabla\phi|}\right)|\nabla\phi| \\ \phi(x, y, 0) = \phi_0(x, y) \end{cases} \tag{3.30}$$

where G is a smoothing kernel (e.g., the Gaussian). This is similar to Perona Malik's anisotropic smoothing in that curvature smoothing is turned off in the vicinity of a high brightness gradient. Osher and Rudin [68] proposed shock filters for image smoothing and enhancement. Other works on the nonlinear geometric diffusion can be found in [82, 88, 89]. Specifically, Weickert presented an excellent review of the related approaches in [93]. We now present mean-shift analysis, a robust way of measuring image discontinuities and smoothing images at the same time.

3.8.2 Mean-Shift Analysis

Given the set $\{x_i\}_{i=1,...,n}$ of d-dimensional points, the mean-shift vector computed at location x is given by [23, 24]:

$$M_h(\mathbf{x}) = \frac{\sum_{i=1}^{n} \mathbf{x} K\left(\frac{\mathbf{x} - \mathbf{x}_i}{h}\right)}{\sum_{i=1}^{n} K\left(\frac{\mathbf{x} - \mathbf{x}_i}{h}\right)} - \mathbf{x} \qquad (3.31)$$

where K represents a kernel with a monotonically decreasing profile and h is the bandwidth of the kernel.

It can be shown that (Equation 3.31) represents an estimate of the normalized density gradient computed at location x; that is, the mean shift vector always points toward the direction of the maximum increase in the density. As a result, the successive computation of expression (Equation 3.31), followed by the translation of the kernel K by $M_h(\mathbf{x})$, will define a path that converges to a local maximum of the underlying density. This algorithm is called the *mean shift procedure*, a simple and efficient statistical technique for mode detection.

The mean-shift procedure can be applied for the data points in the joint *spatial-range* domain [23, 24], where the space of the two-dimensional lattice represents the *spatial* domain and the space of intensity values constitutes the *range* domain. In this approach, a data point defined in the joint spatial range domain is assigned with a point of convergence that represents the local mode of the density in this space, e.g., a three-dimensional space for gray-level images. One can define the displacement vector in the spatial domain as the spatial difference between the convergence point and the original point.

When each pixel in the image is associated with the new range (intensity) information carried by the point of convergence, the algorithm produces discontinuity, preserving smoothing. Conceptually, this process is similar to anisotropic diffusion, nonlinear filtering, or bilateral filtering [9].

However, when the spatial information corresponding to the convergence point is also exploited, one can define a segmentation process based on the displacement vectors of each pixel. The convergence points sufficiently close in this joint domain are gathered together to form uniform regions for image segmentation [23, 24].

In this section, we will exploit the mean-shift-generated displacement vectors to guide active contour models. The robustness of the mean shift is thus combined with *a priori* information regarding the smoothness of the object contours. This processing is integrated into our computationally efficient framework based on ray propagation. The new algorithm allows real-time segmentation of medical structures.

3.8.3 Mean-Shift Filtering Along a Vector

Let us first illustrate the mean-shift procedure applied to a one-dimensional intensity profile obtained from a two-dimensional gray-level image. Specifically, let $\{x_i, I_i\}_{i=1,...,N}$ and $\{x^*_i, I^*_i\}_{i=1,...,N}$ be the two-dimensional original and filtered N image points in the spatial-range domain. In addition, the output of the mean-shift filter includes a displacement vector $\{d_i\}_{i=1,...,N}$ that measures the spatial movement of each spatial point. In our algorithm, each point in this spatial range domain is processed via the mean-shift operator until convergence. Specifically, the algorithm consists of three steps:

For each $i = 1, \ldots, N$:

1. Initialize $k = 1$ and $(x^{*k}_i, I^{*k}_i, d_i) = (x_i, I_i, 0)$
2. Compute

$$x^{*k+1}_i = \frac{\sum_{j=1}^{M} x_j e^{\frac{-(x^{*k}_i - x_j)^2}{2\sigma_x^2}} e^{\frac{-(I^{*k}_i - I_j)^2}{2\sigma_I^2}}}{\sum_{j=1}^{M} e^{\frac{-(x^{*k}_i - x_j)^2}{2\sigma_x^2}} e^{\frac{-(I^{*k}_i - I_j)^2}{2\sigma_I^2}}}$$

$$I^{*k+1}_i = \frac{\sum_{j=1}^{M} I_j e^{\frac{-(x^{*k}_i - x_j)^2}{2\sigma_x^2}} e^{\frac{-(I^{*k}_i - I_j)^2}{2\sigma_I^2}}}{\sum_{j=1}^{M} e^{\frac{-(x^{*k}_i - x_j)^2}{2\sigma_x^2}} e^{\frac{-(I^{*k}_i - I_j)^2}{2\sigma_I^2}}}$$

(3.32)

until the displacement of spatial points x_i are small (i.e., $|x^{*k+1}_i - x^{*k}_i| < \epsilon$) and where σ_x and σ_I determine the Gaussian spatial and range kernels size, respectively.

3. Assign $d_i = (x^{*k+1}_i - x_i)$
4. Assign $(x^*_i, I^*_i) = (x_i, I^*_i)$

Observe that in the last step of the procedure, the original spatial locations (namely, x_i's) are assigned with the smoothed intensity values. Figure 3.10a illustrates an example where 1-dimensional intensity data is obtained from a slice of a CT image. Figures 3.10b and c illustrate the original intensity profile and the smoothed intensity profile, respectively. Observe that the mean shift procedure smooths the intensity data while preserving and sharpening its discontinuities. Similarly, Figure 3.10d depicts the displacement vectors along this 1-D signal. Our boundary detection framework exploits the information contained in these displacement vectors.

3.8.4   Mean-Shift-Based Ray Propagation

Semi-automatic segmentation procedures are very well-accepted in medical image applications because of their fast execution times and their stability. In fact, active contours have been extensively used in medical image segmentation. In this section, we advocate ray propagation from a single point for vessel segmentation. Specifically, we assume that the vessels are orthogonal to the viewing plane and their boundaries are very similar to circular/elliptical objects [7]. Thus, ray propagation is very well suited to this problem for the following reasons. First, ray propagation is very fast. Second, no topological

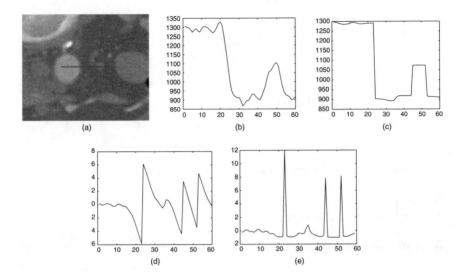

FIGURE 3.10
(a) A one-dimensional intensity profile is obtained along the line from a CT image containing the aorta. The left endpoint of the line is the beginning of data and right endpoint is the end of data. (b) Original intensity profile. (c) Intensity profile after mean shift filtering, with $\sigma_x = 3$ and $\sigma_I = 100$. (d) The displacement vectors of each spatial point and their first derivatives (e). (©2001 IEEE.)

changes are necessary and no shocks form during the propagation, because rays from a single source point do not collide with each other. Recall that level sets have been the choice of curve evolution problems [51] due to formation of shocks and topological changes that may happen during the evolution. However, based on our experiments, level set-based segmentation techniques e.g., [61, 80] are still slow for real-time image segmentation.

Now we are ready to define the speed term $S(x, y)$ of the ray propagation framework defined by the Equation 3.26. Specifically, we propose that:

$$S(x, y) = \alpha \frac{f(x, y)}{1.0 + |\nabla d(x, y)|^2} + \beta \kappa(x, y) \qquad (3.33)$$

where $d(x, y)$ is the displacement function computed by the mean-shift procedure, $\kappa(x, y)$ is the discrete curvature, α and β are constants, and $f(x, y)$ is given by:

$$f(x, y) = \begin{cases} -sign(d(x, y)) & if \ |\nabla d(x, y)| > 3\sigma_d \\ 1 & else \end{cases} \qquad (3.34)$$

Ideally, rays should propagate freely toward the object boundaries when they are away from them, and they should slow down in the vicinity of these object boundaries. If they cross over the boundaries, they should come back to the boundary. Observe that all these requirements are satisfied by the choice of speed function. The mean-shift-generated displacement vectors have high

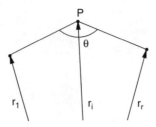

FIGURE 3.11
The curvature of a ray r_i at P is approximated by the angle θ at that vertex. (©2001 IEEE.)

gradient magnitude (Figure 3.10e) and diverge (Figure 3.10d) at the aorta boundary. Note that the high gradient magnitude results in low propagation speed, while the divergence property determines the direction of the propagation, that is, outward inside the aorta and inward outside the aorta.

Often, intensity values inside vessels are not smoothly changing. In fact, it is possible that there may be isolated noise that then creates severe problems for the propagation of rays. In addition, the object boundaries may be distorted at isolated locations due to interaction with nearby structures. Because of these irregularities inside vessels and on their boundaries, we believe that there must be some smoothness constraints on the evolving contour via rays. Thus, we add $\kappa(x, y)$ to the speed function of rays, which forces the front to be smooth during the propagation. We currently use $\kappa(x, y) = (1 - (\frac{\theta}{\pi})^2)$ as the curvature value of a ray at point (x, y) where θ is the angle between two contour segments (Figure 3.11). The ratio α/β controls the degree of desired smoothness.

Our speed function contains the σ_d parameter. This statistical parameter is the variation of the magnitude of displacement function in a region and is learned from the data. Specifically, first rays are initially propagated via constant speed in a small region (circular region). Second, first-order statistics — namely, mean, μ, and standard deviation σ_d of gradient displacement function — are computed from this sample. It is assumed that locations of the small gradients in a displacement function (less than $3\sigma_d$) should not be part of any object boundary.

3.8.5   Results

Figure 3.12 illustrates the mean-shift-based ray propagation for a CT (top) and an MR image (bottom). Specifically, we depict the displacement vectors obtained from mean-shift filtering in middle column to show the strength of the mean-shift filtering. In this figure, black color indicates a vector pointing toward the center and, similarly, white colors are the vectors pointing outward from the center of rays. Observe the divergence of the displacement vectors in the vicinity of aorta boundaries. This divergence of vectors are integrated via rays, which then leads to the segmentation of aorta.

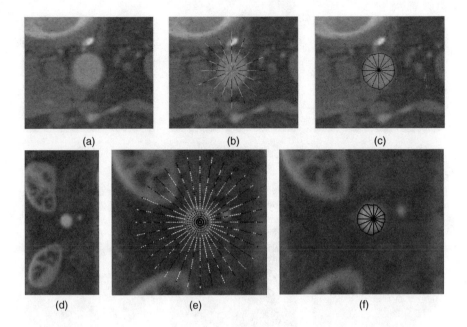

FIGURE 3.12

This figure illustrates the mean-shift-based ray propagation on a CT (top) and MR image aorta (bottom). Both images contain aorta. Right: Original image. Middle: The unit displacement vectors of mean-shift procedure are computed via propagating unit speed rays; that is, speed function is unity. The white indicates a vector pointing outward from the center and the black color indicates a vector pointing toward the center. Observe that our speed function in Equation 3.34 includes the negative sign of the displacement vectors. Thus initially, rays are pushed toward the vessel boundaries and, if they cross over them, they come back due to the sign change in the speed function. Right: The segmentation of vessel via mean-shift-based ray propagation. (©2001 IEEE.)

We have tested the stability of our algorithm on a variety of CT and MR images, as well as on CT phantom data (Figure 3.13). Further validation studies will be done by the experts.

Figure 3.14 illustrates the need for shape priors; for example, smoothness constraints in segmentation on an MR image and a CT image. Shape priors are necessary for two reasons: (1) Figure 3.14a depicts a case where renal arteries branch from the aorta. The segmentation of aorta for quantitative measurements via ray propagation without any smoothness constraint would result in large errors due to renal arteries (Figure 3.14b). The addition of a strong smoothness constraint results in better segmentation of the aorta for quantitative measurements, Figure 3.14c. This example illustrates that our algorithm is capable of incorporating simple shape priors. (2) The smoothness constraint is often needed for the stability of a segmentation process. Figure 3.14a illustrates a structure in a CT image that has diffused boundaries and a circular dark region in it. Observe that the ray passing over the circular dark region is stopped due to the high displacement vector (or high intensity gradient)

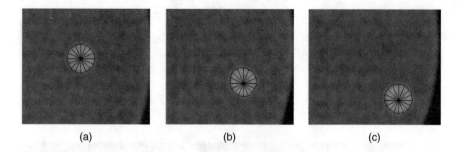

FIGURE 3.13
This example illustrates the stability of our results on CT phantom data depicting coronory arteries. The boundaries are detected by a single click inside the vessels. (©2001 IEEE.)

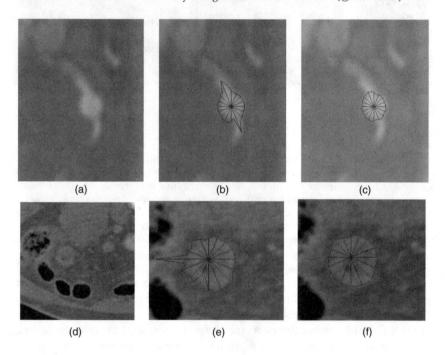

FIGURE 3.14
This figure illustrates the need for a smoothness constraint in segmentation on an MR image and a CT image. Left: Original image. Middle: Boundary detection by mean shift-based ray propagation without any shape priors. Right: Boundary detection by mean shift based ray propagation with smoothing constraints. Observe that (e) and (f) depict a zoomed area of the original image shown in (d). (©2001 IEEE.)

(Figure 3.14b). In addition, one ray did not stop at the correct boundary due to the very low gradient. Figure 3.14c illustrates that these isolated errors in the segmentation process can be corrected by the addition of smoothness constraints.

3.8.6 Observations

The two-dimensional ray propagation technique has proved for us to be an efficient and reliable tool for the quantification of vessel cross sections. However, in the evaluation of an aneurysm, volume is the critical statistic.

3.9 Three-Dimensional Ray Propagation

In this section, we propose that the two-dimensional ray propagation algorithm for detecting cross-sectional vessel boundaries can be extended to three-dimensions [87]. Specifically, we advocate ray propagation from a single point source for the segmentation of blob-like structures found in medical images, such as aneurysms and brain tumors. In fact, ray propagation is well suited for these problems because it is very fast, no topological changes are necessary, and no shocks form during the propagation, because rays from a single source point do not collide with each other.

Let the front be represented by a three-dimensional surface $\psi(\xi, \eta, t) = (x(\xi, \eta, t), y(\xi, \eta, t), z(\xi, \eta, t))$, where x, y, and z are the Cartesian coordinates; ξ, η parameterize the surface; and t is time. The front evolution is governed by:

$$\begin{cases} \frac{\partial \psi}{\partial t} = S(x, y, z)\vec{N} \\ \psi(\xi, \eta, 0) = \psi_0(\xi, \eta) \end{cases} \tag{3.35}$$

where $\psi_0(\xi, \eta) = (x(\xi, \eta, 0), y(\xi, \eta, 0), z(\xi, \eta, 0))$ is the initial surface, $\vec{N}$ is the unit normal vector, and $S(x, y, z)$ is the speed of the surface at point (x, y, z).

Like the two-dimensional case, the approach that we consider is based on explicit front propagation via normal vectors. The surface is sampled and the evolution of each sample is followed in time by rewriting the Eikonal equation [77] in vector form; namely:

$$\begin{cases} x_t = S(x, y, z)\frac{\vec{N_x}}{\|\vec{N}\|} \\ y_t = S(x, y, z)\frac{\vec{N_y}}{\|\vec{N}\|} \\ z_t = S(x, y, z)\frac{\vec{N_z}}{\|\vec{N}\|} \end{cases} \tag{3.36}$$

The speed function $S(x, y, z)$ plays an important role in the quality of the segmentation results. The speed of rays $S(x, y, z)$ depends on image information and shape priors. Specifically, we propose to use $S(x, y, z) = S_0(x, y, z) + \beta S_1(x, y, z)$, where $S_0(x, y, z)$ measures image discontinuities, $S_1(x, y, z)$ represents shape priors, and β balances these two terms.

The first part of the speed term can be now defined by $S_0(x, y, z) = \frac{f(x,y,z)}{1.0 + |\nabla d(x,y,z)|^2}$. The function $d(x, y, z)$ is obtained by summarizing the information provided by the displacement vectors described in Section 3.8.3.

For a given location along a ray, $d(x, y, z)$ is positive when the corresponding displacement vector is pointing outbound and is negative when the vector points toward the seed point. The term $f(x, y, z)$ is given by:

$$f(x, y, z) = \begin{cases} -sign(d(x, y, z)) & if \; |\nabla d(x, y, z)| > 3\sigma_d \\ 1 & else \end{cases} \tag{3.37}$$

In this formulation, rays propagate freely toward the object boundaries when they are away from them and slow down in the vicinity of boundaries. If a ray crosses over a boundary, it returns to the boundary. The estimation of the σ_d parameter is described in Section 3.8.

3.9.1   Smoothness Constraints

Problems related to missing data are common in the segmentation of medical structures. A solution to missing data is to exploit *a priori* knowledge by imposing smoothness constraints on the evolving surface. We use two types of smoothness constraints in this work: one on the speed of neighboring rays, the other on the local curvature of the front.

Thus, the speed function $S_0(x, y, z)$ of a ray is filtered by employing the speed information in a neighborhood. In addition, the speed term $S_1(x, y, z)$ imposes the smoothness of the front. Currently, we employ the mean curvature given by $S_1(x, y, z) = \frac{\kappa_1 + \kappa_2}{2}$, where κ_1 and κ_2 are the principal curvatures. However, other geometric smoothing techniques, such as the mean-Gaussian curvature [67], can be used.

3.9.2   Implementation

For the initialization of rays, we use an algorithm that provides an approximation to equidistant placement of points on a sphere by employing several subdivisions of an octahedron. The octahedron is initialized with the six points $(1, 0, 0)$, $(-1, 0, 0)$, $(0, 1, 0)$, $(0, -1, 0)$, $(0, 0, 1)$, and $(0, 0, -1)$, and connections between neighboring points give the first primitive triangulization of the unit sphere. In the subdivision process, each triangle is subdivided into four new ones by placing one new point on the middle of every edge, projecting it onto the unit sphere and connecting the neighboring points. Rays are then shot from the seed point along the direction given by this approximation of the unit sphere.

To estimate the surface curvature at the current position of a ray, we use the following algorithm [10, 92]: Compute the first matrix $\mathcal{S}$:

$$\mathcal{S} = \left(\frac{1}{2N} \sum_{i=1}^{N} \mathbf{n}_i \mathbf{n}_i^t \right) + \frac{1}{2} \mathbf{p} \mathbf{p}^t$$

where N is the number of neighbors, $\mathbf{n}_i$ denotes the vector to the current position of the ith neighbor, and $\mathbf{p}$ is the vector to the current position of the ray in question. The positive definite matrix S is called *structure tensor* or *scatter matrix*. A principle component analysis provides the eigenvalues $\sigma_1 \geq \sigma_2 \geq \sigma_3$ and eigenvectors $\mathbf{v}_1$, $\mathbf{v}_2$, $\mathbf{v}_3$ of S. The eigenvector $\mathbf{v}_1$ corresponding to the largest eigenvalue σ_1 is in normal tangential direction. The other two eigenvectors point in the directions of the principal curvatures. Although the corresponding eigenvalues σ_2 and σ_3 already give an estimate of the degree of curvature in these directions, they do not give information on their orientation, forcing us to include another step. Therefore, for every neighbor we also calculate the dot product of the neighbor vector and the principal curvature vector. This coefficient is then multiplied the difference of $\frac{\pi}{2}$ and the angle between the normal tangential vector $\mathbf{v}_1$ and the vector connecting $\mathbf{p}$ and the neighbor. The sum over this weighted angle difference is positive for convex areas and negative for concave areas. Hence, the final formulas for principal curvatures are:

$$
\begin{aligned}
\kappa_1 &= \sum_{i=1}^{N} \frac{|\mathbf{v}_2 \cdot \mathbf{n}_i|}{|\mathbf{v}_2||\mathbf{n}_i|} \left(\arccos \left(\frac{\mathbf{v}_1 \cdot (\mathbf{n}_i - \mathbf{p})}{|\mathbf{v}_1||\mathbf{n}_i - \mathbf{p}|} \right) - \frac{\pi}{2} \right) \\
\kappa_2 &= \sum_{i=1}^{N} \frac{|\mathbf{v}_3 \cdot \mathbf{n}_i|}{|\mathbf{v}_3||\mathbf{n}_i|} \left(\arccos \left(\frac{\mathbf{v}_1 \cdot (\mathbf{n}_i - \mathbf{p})}{|\mathbf{v}_1||\mathbf{n}_i - \mathbf{p}|} \right) - \frac{\pi}{2} \right)
\end{aligned}
\tag{3.38}
$$

3.9.3 Results

In this section, we have presented a user-friendly, three-dimensional volume segmentation algorithm. Figure 3.15 shows the segmentation of the inner boundary of an aneurysm on CE-CTA data [87]. This proposed algorithm is very fast due to ray propagation. Second, the analysis based on mean shift makes our algorithm robust to outliers inherent in CT and MR images. Third, the use of shape priors such as smoothness constraints implies a reduced sensitivity of the algorithm to missing data, that is, surfaces that are not well defined or missing. Fourth, our algorithm is user-friendly because one click inside the three-dimensional medical structure is often sufficient.

3.10 Conclusion: From Diagnosis to Screening

In this chapter we have described a set of vascular visualization and segmentation techniques that were chosen or designed as part of an interactive clinical application for MRA and CTA postprocessing. The purpose of this application is diagnostic: to find and quantify pathology in syptomatic patients.

However, the future of vascular postprocessing lies beyond diagnosis in the field of healthy patient screening. Dosage levels for CT studies are decreasing with every new generation of detectors, and MR resolution is continually increasing. Both modalities are approaching the goal of soft-plaque visualization.

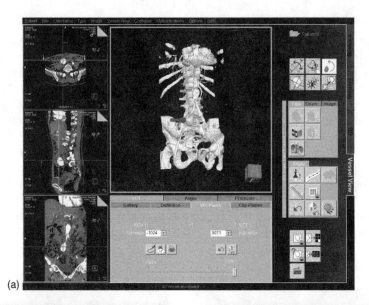

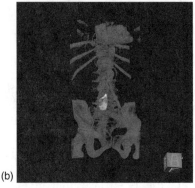
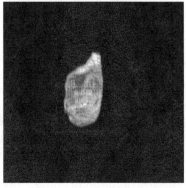

FIGURE 3.15

This figure summarizes the method described in this section. (a) Illustrates the original (CE-CTA) data in multi-planar reformats (MPRs) and volume rendering. This data set contains an aneurysm that is indicated by the arrow. In addition, MPRs (orthogonal views) are centered on this pathology. The system allows the radiologist to quickly detect pathologies from different visualizations. The next step is the quantification of these pathologies. The goal of this work is to provide a mechanism such that a user can quickly measure the volume of blob-like structures by simply clicking on them. In this example, the user clicks on a structure of interest and the three-dimensional ray propagation algorithm detects the boundary of the structure and computes its volume. (b) The detected aneurysm (lumen boundary) is blended with the original data. (c) Segmented aneurysm (lumen boundary). (©2002 Springer-Verlag.)

When the imaging of soft arterial plaque matures, plaque analysis will supplant current techniques such as cardiac calcium scoring as routine and reliable preventative medicine. The key to the success of plaque analysis will be efficient, robust postprocessing software.

References

1. D. Adalsteinsson and J. Sethian. A fast level set method for propagating interfaces. *J. Comput. Phys.*, 118:269–277, 1995.
2. R. Adams and L. Bischof. Seeded region growing. *IEEE Trans. Pattern Analysis and Machine Intelligence*, 16(6):641–647, 1994.
3. L. Alvarez, P.-L. Lions, and J.-M. Morel. Image selective smoothing and edge detection by nonlinear diffusion. II. *SIAM Journal of Numerical Analysis*, 29(3):845–866, June 1992.
4. L. Ambrosio and M. Soner. Level set approach to mean curvature flow in arbitrary codimension. *Journal of Differential Geometry*, 43:693–737, 1996.
5. A. A. Amini, T. Weymouth, and R. Jain. Using dynamic programming for solving variational problems in vision. *IEEE Trans. Patt. Anal. Mach. Intell.*, 12:855–867, 1990.
6. F. C. Andrews. *Equilibrium Statistical Mechanics, 2nd edition*, John Wiley & Sons, 1975.
7. B. B. Avants and J. P. Williams. An adaptive minimal path generation technique for vessel tracking in CTA/CE-MRA volume images. In *Medical Image Computing and Computer-Assisted Intervention MICCAI*, pages 707–716, 2000.
8. S. Aylward, S. Pizer, E. Bullitt, and D. Eberly. Intensity ridge and widths for 3d object segmentation and description. In *IEEE Proc. Workshop Mathematical Models Biomedical Image Analysis*, pages 131–138, 1996.
9. D. Barash. Bilateral Filtering and Anisotropic Diffusion: Towards a Unified Viewpoint. Technical Report HPL-2000-18(R.1), Hewlett-Packard, 2000.
10. J. Berkmann and T. Caelli. On the relationship between surface covariance and differential geometry. *Shape in Picture. Mathematical Description of Shape in Grey-Level Images*. Springer-Verlag, pages 343–352, 1994.
11. J. R. Beveridge, J. Griffith, R. R. Kohler, A. R. Hanson, and E. M. Riseman. Segmenting images using localized histograms and region merging. *Int. J. Computer Vision*, 2:311–347, 1989.
12. Y. Boykov and M. Jolly. Interactive graph cuts for optimal boundary and region segmentation of objects in N-D images. In *International Conference Computer Vision*, Volume I, pages 105–112, 2001.
13. E. Bullitt, S. Aylward, A. Liu, J. Stone, S. K. Mukherjee, C. Coey, G. Gerig, and S. M. Pizer. 3d graph description of the intracerebral vasculature from segmented MRA and tests of accuracy by comparison with x-ray angiograms. In *IPMI*, pages 308–321, 1999.
14. V. Caselles, F. Catte, T. Coll, and F. Dibos. A Geometric Model for Active Contours in Image Processing. Technical Report No 9210, CEREMADE, 1992.
15. V. Caselles, R. Kimmel, and G. Sapiro. Geodesic active contours. In *ICCV95*, pages 694–699, 1995.
16. V. Caselles, R. Kimmel, G. Sapiro, and C. Sbert. Minimal surfaces based object segmentation. *IEEE Trans. Patt. Anal. Mach. Intell.*, 19(4):394–398, 1997.
17. F. Catté, P.-L. Lions, J.-M. Morel, and T. Coll. Image selective smoothing and edge detection by nonlinear diffusion. *SIAM Journal of Numerical Analysis*, 29(1):182–193, February 1992.

18. Y. Chen, Y. Giga, and S. Goto. Uniqueness and existence of viscosity solutions of generalized mean curvature flow equations. *J. Differential Geom.*, 33:749–786, 1991.

19. A. Chung and J. A. Noble. Statistical 3D vessel segmentation using a Rician distribution. In *Medical Image Conference and Computer Assisted Interventions (MICCAI)*, pages 82–89, 1999.

20. L. D. Cohen. Note on active contour models and balloons. *CVGIP: Image Understanding*, 53(2):211–218, 1991.

21. L. D. Cohen and I. Cohen. Finite element methods for active contour models and balloons for 2D and 3D images. *IEEE Trans. Patt. Anal. Mach. Intell.*, 15(11):1131–1147, 1993.

22. L. D. Cohen and R. Kimmel. Global minimum for active contour models: A minimal path approach. *Int. J. Computer Vision*, 24(1):57–78, August 1997.

23. D. Comaniciu and P. Meer. Mean shift analysis and applications. In *IEEE International Conference on Computer Vision*, pages 1197–1203, 1999.

24. D. Comaniciu and P. Meer. Mean shift: a robust approach toward feature space analysis. *IEEE Trans. Patt. Anal. Mach. Intell.*, 24(5): 603–619, 2002.

25. D. DeCarlo and D. N. Metaxas. Blended deformable models. *IEEE Trans. Patt. Anal. Mach. Intell.*, 18(4):443–448, 1996.

26. A. Dempster, N. Laird, and D. Rubin. Maximum likelihood from incomplete data via the EM algorithm. *J. Roy. Statistical Soc., Series B*, 39:1–38, 1977.

27. T. Deschamps and L. Cohen. Minimal paths in 3d images and application to virtual endoscopy. In *Eur. Conf. Computer Vision*, 2000.

28. T. Deschamps and L. Cohen. Fast extraction of minimal paths in 3d images and applications to virtual endoscopy. *Med. Image Anal.*, 5(4):281–299, 2001.

29. R. A. Drebin, L. Carpenter, and P. Hanrahan. Volume rendering. *Computer Graphics (ACM Siggraph Proceedings)*, 22(4):65–74, 1988.

30. S. Dreyfus. An appraisal of some shortest path algorithms. *Oper. Res.*, 17:395–412, 1969.

31. N. D. D'Souza, J. M. Reinhardt, and E. A. Hoffman. ASAP: interactive quantification of 2d airway geometry. In *Meical Imaging 1996: Physiology and function from multidimensional images*, Eric A. Hoffman, Ed., *Proc. SPIE 2709*, pages 180–196, 1996.

32. M. Dubuisson-Jolly and A. Gupta. Tracking deformable templates using the shortest path algorithm. *Computer Vision and Image Understanding*, 81:26–45, 2001.

33. R. O. Duda and P. E. Hart. *Pattern Classification and Scene Analysis*. Wiley, 1973.

34. L. C. Evans and J. Spruck. Motion of level sets by mean curvature I. *J. Differential Geom.*, 33(3):635–681, May 1991.

35. A. Falcao, J. Udupa, S. Samarasekera, and S. Sharma. User-steered image segmentation paradigms: Live wire and live lane. *Graphical Models and Image Processing*, 60:233–260, 1998.

36. P. F. Felzenszwalb and D. P. Huttenlocher. Image segmentation using local variation. In *IEEE Conference on Computer Vision and Pattern Recognition*, Santa Barbara, CA, pages 98–103, June 1998.

37. N. Flasque, M. Desvignes, J.-M. Constans, and M. Revenu. System for analyzing highresolution three-dimensional coronary angiograms. *Med. Image Anal.*, 5:173–183, 2001.

38. L. Ford and E. Fulkerson. *Flows in Networks*. Princeton University Press, 1962.

39. A. F. Frangi, W. J. Niessen, K. L. Vincken, and M. A. Viergever. Multiscale vessel enhancement filtering. In *Medical Image Conference and Computer Assisted Interventions (MICCAI)*, pages 82–89, 1998.

40. Y. Gdalyahu, D. Weinshall, and M. Werman. Self-organization in vision: stochastic clustering for image segmentation, perceptual grouping, and image database organization. *IEEE Trans. Patt. Anal. Mach. Intell.*, 23(10):1053–1074, 2001.

41. A. Goldberg and R. Tarjan. A new approach to the maximum-flow problem. *J. ACM*, 35(4):921–940, 1988.

42. A. Gupta and R. Bajsy. Volumetric segmentation of range images of 3d objects using superquadric models. *CVGIP*, 58(3):302–326, November 1993.

43. R. M. Haralick, S. R. Sternberg, and X. Zhuang. Image analysis using mathematical morphology. *IEEE Trans. Pattern Anal. Machine Intell.*, 9(4):532–550, July 1987.

44. M. Hernandez-Hoyos, A. Anwander, M. Orkisz, J. P. Roux, and I. E. M. P. Doueck. A deformable vessel model with single point initialization for segmentation, quantification and visualization of blood vessesl in 3D MRA. In *MICCAI'00*, pages 735–745, 2000.

45. W. Higgins, W. Spyra, R. Karwoski, and E. Ritman. System for analyzing high resolution three-dimensional coronary angiograms. *IEEE Tran. Med. Imag.*, 15(3):377–385, 1996.

46. I. Jermyn and H. Ishikawa. Globally optimal regions and boundaries. In *Int. Conf. Computer Vision*, Volume II, pages 904–910, 1999.

47. D. Karger and C. Stein. A new approach to the minimum cut problem. *J. ACM*, 43:601–640, 1996.

48. M. Kass, A. Witkin, and D. Terzopoulos. Snakes: active contour models. *Int. J. Computer Vision*, 1(4):321–331, 1988.

49. S. Kichenassamy, A. Kumar, P. Olver, A. Tannenbaum, and A. Yezzi. Gradient flows and geometric active contour models. In *Fifth Int. Conf. Computer Vision*, pages 810–815, 1995.

50. B. B. Kimia and K. Siddiqi. Geometric heat equation and nonlinear diffusion of shapes and images. *Computer Vision Graphics and Image Processing: Image Understanding*, 64(3):305–322, November 1996.

51. B. B. Kimia, A. R. Tannenbaum, and S. W. Zucker. Shapes, shocks, and deformations. I. The components of shape and the reaction-diffusion space. *IJCV*, 15:189–224, 1995.

52. T. M. Koller, G. Gerig, and G. S. an D. Dettwiler. Multiscale detection of curvilinear structures in 2-d and 3-d image data. In *Int. Conf. Computer Vision*, pages 864–869, 1995.

53. K. Krissian, G. Malandain, and N. Ayache. Directional anisotropic diffusion applied to segmentation of vessels in 3d images. In *Int. Conf. Scale-Space*, pages 345–348, 1997.

54. K. Krissian, G. Malandain, N. Ayache, R. Vaillant, and Y. Trousset. Model based multiscale detection of 3d vessels. In *IEEE Conf. Comp. Vision and Pattern Recognition*, pages 722–727, 1998.

55. F. Leymarie and M. D. Levine. Tracking deformable objects in the plane using an active contour model. *IEEE Trans. Patt. Anal. Mach. Intell.*, 15(6):617–633, 1993.

56. T. Lindeberg. Edge detection with automatic scale selection. In *IEEE Computer Vision and Pattern Recognition*, pages 465–470, 1996.

57. C. Lorenz, I.-C. Carlsen, T. M. Buzug, C. Fassnacht, and J. Weese. Multi-scale line segmentation with automatic estimation of width, contrast and tangential direction in 2d and 3d medical images. In *CVRMed-MRCAS'97 (Lecture Notes in Computer Science)*, pages 233–242, 1997.

58. L. M. Lorigo, O. Faugeras, W. E. L. Grimson, R. Keriven, R. Kikinis, A. Nabavi, and C. Westin. Codimension-two geodesic active contours for the segmentation of tubular structures. In *IEEE Conference on Computer Vision and Pattern Recognition*, 2000.

59. L. M. Lorigo, O. Faugeras, W. E. L. Grimson, R. Keriven, R. Kikinis, A. Nabavi, and C. Westin. CURVES: Curve evolution for vessel segmentation. *Med. Image Anal.*, 5(3):195–206, 2001.

60. R. Malladi and J. A. Sethian. A real time algorithm for medical shape recovery. In *International Conference on Computer Vision*, pages 304–310, January 1998.

61. R. Malladi, J. A. Sethian, and B. C. Vemuri. Shape modelling with front propagation: a level set approach. *IEEE Trans. Patt. Anal. Mach. Intell.*, 17, 1995.

62. T. McInerney and D. Terzopoulos. Topologically adaptible snakes. In *IEEE Int. Conf. Computer Vision*, pages 840–845, 1995.

63. T. McInerney and D. Terzopoulos. Deformable models in medical images analysis: a survey. *Med. Image Anal.*, 1(2):91–108, 1996.

64. T. McInerney and D. Terzopoulos. Topology adaptive deformable surfaces for medical image volume segmentation. *IEEE Trans. Med. Imag.*, 18(10):840–850, 1999.

65. T. McInerney and D. Terzopoulos. Snakes: topology adaptive snakes. *Med. Image Anal.*, 4:73–91, 2000.

66. E. Mortensen and W. Barrett. Interactive segmentation with intelligent scissors. *Graphical Models and Image Processing*, 60:349–384, 1998.

67. P. Neskovic and B. B. Kimia. Three-Dimensional Shape Representation from Curvature-Dependent Deformations. Technical Report 128, LEMS, Brown University, November 1993.

68. S. Osher and L. I. Rudin. Feature-oriented image enhancement using shock filters. *SIAM J. Numerical Analysis*, 27(4):919–940, August 1990.

69. S. Osher and J. A. Sethian. Fronts propagating with curvature dependent speed: algorithms based on Hamilton-Jacobi formulations. *J. Computational Physics*, 79:12–49, 1988.

70. P. Perona and J. Malik. Scale-space and edge detection using ansiotropic diffusion. *IEEE Trans. Patt. Anal. Mach. Intell.*, 12(7):629–639, 1990.

71. V. Prinet, O. Monga, C. Ge, L. Sheng, and S. Ma. Thin network extraction in 3d images: application to medical angiograms. In *Int. Conf. Pattern Recognition*, Volume 3, pages 386–390, 1996.

72. R. A. Redner and H. F. Walker. Mixture densities, maximum likelihood and the EM algorithm. *SIAM Review*, 26(2):195–239, 1984.

73. Y. Sato, S. Nakajima, N. Shiraga, H. Atsumi, S. Yoshida, T. Koller, G. Gerig, and R. Kikinis. Three-dimensional multi-scale line filter for segmentation and visualisation of curvilinear structures in medical images. *Med. Image Anal.*, 2(2):143–168, 1998.

74. T. B. Sebastian, H. Tek, J. J. Crisco, S. W. Wolfe, and B. B. Kimia. Segmentation of carpal bones from 3d CT images using skeletally coupled deformable models. In *MICCAI*, pages 1184–1194, 1998.

75. J. Serra, editor. *Image Analysis and Mathematical Morphology*. Academic Press, 1982.
76. J. Sethian. A fast marching level set method for monotonically advancing fronts. *Proc. Nat. Acad. Sci.*, 93:1591–1595, 1996.
77. J. A. Sethian. *Level Set Methods and Fast Marching Methods*, 2nd edition, Cambridge University Press, New York, 1999.
78. J. Shah. A common framework for curve evolution, segmentation and anisotropic diffusion. In *IEEE Conference on Computer Vision and Pattern Recognition*, 1996.
79. J. Shi and J. Malik. Normalized cuts and image segmentation. *IEEE Trans. Patt. Anal. Mach. Intell.*, 22(8):888–905, 2000.
80. K. Siddiqi, A. Tannenbaum, and S. Zucker. Area and length minimizing flows for image segmentation. *IEEE Trans. Image Processing*, 7:433–444, 1998.
81. K. Siddiqi and A. Vasilevskiy. 3d flux maximizing flows. In *International Workshop on Energy Minimizing Methods in Computer Vision*, 2001.
82. N. A. Sochen, R. Kimmel, and A. M. Bruckstein. Diffusions and confusions in signal and image processing. *J. Math. Imaging Vision*, 14(3):195–209, 2001.
83. H. Tek, D. Comaniciu, and J. Williams. Vessel detection by mean shift based ray propagation. In *Workshop on Mathematical Models in Biomedical Image Analysis*, 2001.
84. H. Tek and B. B. Kimia. Image segmentation by reaction-diffusion bubbles. In *IEEE Int. Conf. Computer Vision*, pages 156–162, 1995.
85. H. Tek and B. B. Kimia. Volumetric segmentation of medical images by three-dimensional bubbles. In *Workshop on Physics-Based Modeling in Computer Vision*, pages 9–16, 1995.
86. H. Tek and B. B. Kimia. Volumetric segmentation of medical images by three-dimensional bubbles. *CVIU*, 64(2):246–258, February 1997.
87. H. Tek, M. Bergtholdt, D. Comaniciu, and J. Williams. Segmentation of 3D medical structures using robust ray propagation. *MICAA*, 572–579, September 2002.
88. B. M. ter Haar Romeny, Editor. *Geometry-Driven Diffusion in Computer Vision*. Kluwer, September 1994.
89. B. M. ter Haar Romeny, L. Florack, J. Koenderink, and M. Viergever, Editors. *Scale-Space Theory in Computer Vision*. Springer, July 1997.
90. D. Terzopoulos and A. Witkin. Constraints on deformable models: recovering shape and non-rigid motion. *Artificial Intelligence*, 36:91–123, 1988.
91. R. Urquhart. Graph theoretical clustering based on limited neighborhood sets. *Pattern Recognition*, 15:173–187, 1982.
92. B. Vemuri, A. Mitiche, and J. Aggarwal. Curvature-based representation of objects from range data. *Image and Vision Computing*, 4(2):107–114, 1986.
93. J. Weickert. Review of nonlinear diffusion filtering. In *First International Conference, Scale-Space*, pages 3–28, Utrecht, The Netherlands, 1997. Springer.
94. Y. Weiss. Segmentation suing eigenvectors: A unifying view. In *Int. Conf. Computer Vision*, pages 975–982, 1999.
95. R. Whitaker. Algorithms for implicit deformable models. In *Int. Conf. Computer Vision 1995*, pages 822–827, 1995.
96. R. T. Whitaker. Geometry-limited diffusion in the characterization of geometric patches in images. *CVGIP*, 57(1):111–120, January 1993.
97. D. Wilson and J. Noble. Segmentation of cerebral vessels and aneurysms from mr angiography data. In *IPMI*, pages 423–428, 1997.

98. O. Wink, W. Niessen, and M. A. Viergever. Fast delination and visualization of vessels in 3-D angiographic images. *IEEE Trans. Med. Imag.*, 19(4):337–345, 2000.

99. Z. Wu. An optimal graph theoretic approach to data clustering: theory and its application to image segmentation. *IEEE Trans. Patt. Anal. Mach. Intell.*, 15(11):1101–1113, 1993.

100. C. Xu, D. L. Pham, and J. L. Prince. Medical image segmentation using deformable models. In J. M. Fitzpatrick and M. Sonka, Editors, *Handbook of Medical Imaging. Volume 2: Medical Image Processing and Analysis*, pages 129–174. SPIE Press, May 2000.

101. C. Xu and J. Prince. Snakes, shapes, and gradient vector flow. *IEEE Trans. Image Proc.*, pages 359–369, 1998.

102. A. Yezzi, S. Kichenassamy, A. Kumar, P. Oliver, and A. Tannenbaum. A geometric snake model for segmentation of medical imagery. *IEEE Trans. Med. Imag.*, 16(2), 1997.

103. C. Zahn. Graph-theoretic methods for detecting and describing gestalt clusters. *IEEE Trans. Comput.*, 20:68–86, 1971.

104. S. C. Zhu and A. L. Yuille. Region competition: Unifying Snakes, Region growing, and Bayes/MDL for multiband Image Segmentation. *IEEE Trans. Patt. Anal. Mach. Intell.*, 18(9):884–900, 1996.

4

Masking Strategies for Black-Blood Angiography

Jasjit S. Suri, Kecheng Liu, Sameer Singh, and Swamy Laxminarayan

CONTENTS

4.1 Introduction

Vascular diseases are one of the major sources of deaths in the United States. A report [1] states that "Aneurysm rupture is not a rare occurrence as evidenced by the fact that this event currently ranks thirteenth on the list for leading causes of death in the U.S.A." This report [1] also says that "Chronic venous insufficiency is a common problem in the U.S., affecting approximately 5% of the general population. It is estimated that half a million patients suffer from ulceration of the lower extremity as a result of longstanding venous disease." This report raises the importance of research needed in the area of angiography, the branch of medicine that deals with veins and arteries. In the field of cerebrovascular diseases [1], "Ischemic and hemorrhagic stroke account for one of the principal causes of death and disability in older aged population. In fact, stroke currently ranks third on the list of leading causes of death in the United States (also see [2–4]). Each year approximately 500,000 people suffer a new or recurrent stroke in the U.S., and approximately 150,000 of them die as a result. In addition, more than one-third of stroke survivors

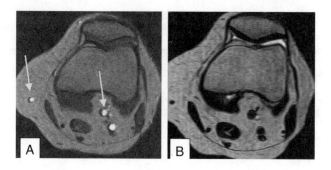

FIGURE 4.1

Axial images from a knee MRA: Left (A): The bright blood two-dimensional TOF, acquired in the axial plane. Right (B): The black blood T_2-weighted three-dimensional FSE, acquired in the sagittal plane, reformatted here in the axial plane. The imaging time for three-dimensional FSE was comparable with two-dimensional TOF but covered a larger volume. In (A), the arrows point to vessels but they also have some black neighborhood areas around them. In (B), the black-blood image shows perfect vessel capture. Thus, the WBA has a weakness compared to BBA due to its acquisition methodology. (Courtesy of Kecheng Liu, Philips Medical Systems, Inc., Cleveland, OH.)

are left with permanent physical disability, which currently accounts for the leading cause of nursing home admissions in the U.S."

The branch of medicine that deals with studies of the arteries and veins or vasculature is angiography. The different ways angiography can be performed are bi-plane x-ray/digital subtraction angiography (DSA), MR angiography (MRA), CT angiography (CTA), and ultrasound angiography. From the clinical point of view, DSA[1] is considered the most reliable and accurate method for vascular imaging, a subset of x-rays. On the contrary, this method lacks three-dimensional information,[2] which is easily available via magnetic resonance (MR) and computer tomography (CT) techniques. The MR and CT techniques lack the ability to locate tiny vessels and provide the morphological estimation of stenoses and aneurysms. The presence of nonvascular structures and background noise makes differentiation more challenging and is one of the main reasons MR and CT techniques are not as successful in the detection of vasculature as DSA.

Unlike most conventional angiography in MR and CT, black-blood magnetic resonance angiography[3] (BB-MRA) presents vascular morphology as a dark vasculature region with a gray background. Figure 4.1 illustrates the difference between conventional white-blood angiography (WBA) (left) and black-blood angiography (BBA) (right). Although the BBA images can be

---

[1]Subtraction of the x-ray images without using contrast material from x-ray angiograms.

[2]One can still achieve the three-dimensional information by using the stereo reconstruction from x-ray angiograms with multiple viewpoints.

[3]From now, when we say BBA, we mean BB-MRA.

converted to reversed gray scale, that is, black vessels in gray background into white vessels in gray background, the concept behind BB-MRA is that the signal from blood flow is nulled so that it appears as signal voids in the reconstructed images. We discuss the principles of BBA in the next section.

The importance of BBA has grown tremendously in recent years (see [5–8]). This chapter focuses on BBA using MR and, more importantly, on the prefiltering of the BBA data sets for removal of nonvascular structures and background noise suppression. The main motivation for performing BBA vascular filtering is for three-dimensional segmentation which, in turn, helps in the following areas:

1. Neurosurgical planning, interventional procedures, and treatments
2. Time saving for three-dimensional segmentation
3. Distinguishing between the veins and arteries
4. Studying relative placement of the structures
5. Blood flow process and hemodynamics
6. Stenosis and aneurysm assessment/quantification
7. Disease monitoring/remission
8. Quantification of vascular structures

Interested readers can explore the following articles to understand the importance of vascular image processing needs: [9–17].

Having discussed some of the sources of motivations for performing black-blood *vascular image processing* (BB-VIP), we now present the major difficulties in performing filtering of the BBA volumes. The following include the main reasons that contribute to the complexity in vasculature filtering from BBA data sets (see [18–20]):

1. *Vessel shape complexity and variability.* The vessels are curvey, twisted (tortuous), and sometimes occluded,[4] or there could be superposition of structures/vessels corresponding to the vasculature in various areas of the body, such as in the head, heart, and neck.

2. *Vessel density and diameter of small vessels.* The complexity of the filtering increases with density and reduction of the diameter of vessels (see Figure 4.2).

3. *Noise and gaps in vessels.* The MRA acquisition process brings in gaps in the vessels, and the resulting data sets could be noisy.

4. *Dynamic range of intensities.* Many structures in the human body show high intensity values similar to vessel intensity values. The dynamic range of intensities is small between vessels and other objects.

---

[4]Overlap of vessels with one another.

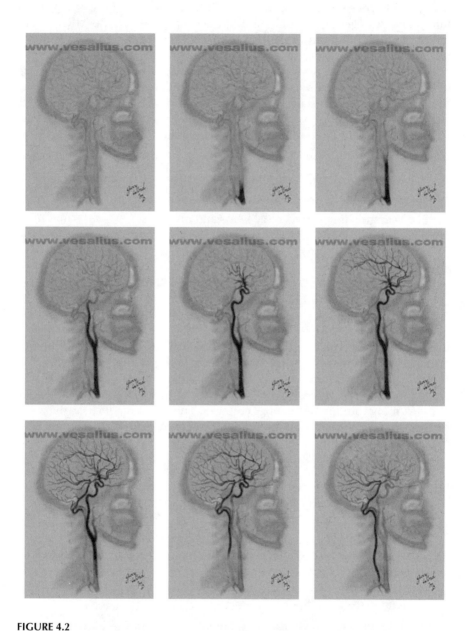

FIGURE 4.2
Lateral view of a carotid angiogram (arterial to venous). Top to bottom and left to right: shown are only limited angiogram frames: arterial (frames 1 to 6) and venous (frames 7 to 9) phases. Also, the density of the vessels and bifurcation can be appreciated. (Courtesy of Vesalius Studios, www.vesalius.com.)

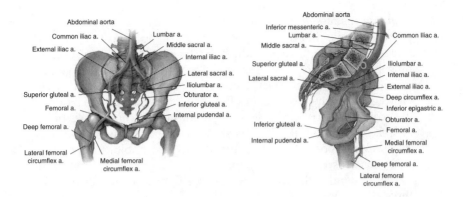

FIGURE 4.3
Vasculature system for pelvis region. Left: Pelvis frontal view. Right: Pelvis lateral view. (Courtesy of Professor Fishman, Johns Hopkins University, Baltimore, MD.)

5. *Partial volume averaging.* Due to partial volume averaging (PVA), a voxel could have a combination of intensities from vessels and background. Particular difficulties can occur at vessel bifurcations/branching due to PVA and calcification (which is common at bifurcations).

6. *White blood and black blood issues.* In the case of segmenting "white blood vessels," imaging conditions can cause some background areas to be as bright as other vessel areas; therefore, nonstatistical thresholding alone cannot be used. In the case of "black blood vessels," imaging conditions can cause some background areas to be as dark as black blood vessels, making detection between them difficult.

7. *Characteristics of the imaging modality and motion/blood flow artifacts.* The resolution and clarity of the images play a critical role in *vascular image processing*. This data acquisition process plays an equally critical role in the accuracy and robustness of the vascular segmentation process. For example, artifacts in MR imaging could be due to several kinds (for details, see [21–23]). In MRA, we might have ringing artifacts (see [24]), or artifacts due to patient motion or blood flow. This contributes to the intensity nonhomogeneity in the vessel, which makes the segmentation process difficult to perform.

8. *Ability to distinguish between arteries and veins.* Due to the similarity in the enhancement characteristics of the vessels and close proximity of arteries and veins, it becomes more difficult for the tracking algorithms to distinguish between the arteries and veins.

9. *Hemodynamics.* Due to imperfect timing of the arrival of the contrast agent and the partial volume effect, vessel detection and separating of the vein and the artery become very difficult.

10. *Scanning limitation.* When tracking the vessels in vascular image processing, we find the imaging plane perpendicular to the vessel central axis. This plane is mathematically computed. Had the scanning system provided this imaging plane, the tracking of the vessels would have been very easy. One of the major limitations in vascular tracking is the weakness of the scanning system in its inability to provide the orthogonal imaging planes to the central axis of the vessel. In addition, the vessels are curved and tortuous, and it is therefore not possible for the current MRA technology to scan the vascular structures in this manner. Because of this scanning limitation, we tailor the image processing algorithms to perform the three-dimensional segmentation.

Now that we have discussed the *motivation* for and *difficulties* in performing vascular image processing, we very briefly list some of the work from previous authors who attempted to perform prefiltering on MR data sets. We have seen that most techniques come from Parker and co-workers (see [25–27]). Some of the older techniques [31, 34–36, 38, 39, 79] do not exploit real image processing to remove the nonvascular structures and background suppression of noise. We have covered some of these in detail (see [42, 43]).

Historically, not many researchers have looked into BBA. Only recently has much attention been given to this method. Currently, the researchers actively pursuing this include Robarts Research Institute, University of Western Ontario, London, Canada; University of Washington, Seattle; and Philips Medical Systems, Cleveland, OH. Most of the work in BBA to date has been in two-dimensional black blood images. This requires extraction of the boundaries of the blood vessels in the two-dimensional slices of the BBA volume. The boundary extraction process uses a modified version of the classical snake model (see [14, 16, 17]). Although these articles do discuss the boundary estimation problems of vessel cross sections in two dimensions, they use classical snakes, which are very sensitive to noise, and important issues such as stability (see articles on boundary estimation based on level sets [44–49]).

The focus of this chapter is on three-dimensional BBA masking strategies, vessel detection, and nonvascular filtering. The latest trend was developed by Frangi et al. [73] and recently by Suri et al. [42] (see also [43]). This chapter is in the same spirit of Frangi/Suri et al.'s approaches as applied to BBA. Because BBA has other black structures present in the cross-sectional slices, it is not straightforward to implement these approaches to filter BBA volume. Moreover, the scale-space techniques are highly dependent on scale and on selecting and medium to large scales (see Chapter 2, and [50, 51]), can bring edge artifacts around these black structures. One of the major problems in black blood is that non-black-blood structures are irregular in shape and the cross-section behavior is of noncircular and nontubular type. Because plain scale-space approaches are based on higher-order derivatives of Gaussian models, it gives edges around these irregular shaped objects. Thus, there is a motivation to get rid of these nontubular cross sections in these BBA slices before one can take advantage of the scale-space approaches. To get rid of these irregular black objects in these BBA slices, one can develop a mask that shows just these irregular black objects. The masking strategy can differ in approach, depending on the body structure (e.g., if it is neuro or knee). We discuss these masking strategies in Section 4.3. Because we know that scale-space approaches work well on WBA volumes, to preserve that property, we need another step to convert the BBA volume to a volume closer to the WBA. Therefore, we have devised an approach that changes the black-blood volume to a pseudo-white-blood volume and then apply Frangi/Suri et al.'s approach. Because this volume very much resembles the white-blood volumes, we call it pseudo-white-blood volume. Our motivation is to remove the black nonvascular structures using the tissue characteristics in the neighborhood, and then generate the pseudo-WBA volumes, which are now ready for application using Frangi and Suri approaches.

Keeping this motivation in mind, the goals of this chapter are to:

1. Devise a generic BBA prefiltering algorithm that can remove the nonvascular structures, and suppress noise and background variations

2. Devise an automatic vascular imaging processing system that can detect thin and thick vessels simultaneously

3. Devise a system that is insensitive to different imaging parameters for the BBA

4. Design a vascular image processing system that can then be used with other advanced image processing segmentation tools such as pixel/voxel classifiers.

The layout of this chapter is as follows. Section 4.2 presents the image generation for BBA. Section 4.4 is the main body of this chapter and discusses the effect of the pixel-classification algorithm over scale-space filtering. We compare the three-dimensional median filtering algorithm with our system in Section 4.5. A discussion on the implementation issues involved with filtering algorithms is presented in Section 4.6. The chapter concludes by discussing the challenges and future of filtering algorithms in Section 4.7.

4.2 Physics of Black-Blood Angiography Image Generation

A brief understanding of the BBA data acquisition process is necessary to appreciate vascular segmentation. Before we discuss the BBA data acquisition process, we first discuss the hardware and the five kinds of surface receive coils used for collecting the BBA data sets. Figure 4.4 shows five

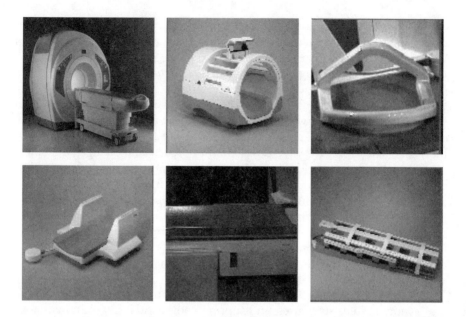

FIGURE 4.4

MRI system and the radio-frequency (RF) surface receive coils used for collecting the MR vasculature data sets. Top Row, Left: MRI system (1.5 Tesla Infinion™, Philips Medical Systems, Inc., Cleveland, OH). Top Row, Middle: Head coil. Top Row, Right: Anterior neck coil. Bottom Row, Left: Posterior neck coil. Bottom Row, Middle: Integrated spine array (ISA) coil. Bottom Row, Right: Peripheral vascular array (PVA) coil. (Courtesy of Philips Medical Systems, Inc., Cleveland, OH; and PVA coil, courtesy of USAI, Aurora, OH.)

types of radio-frequency (RF) surface receive coils used for collecting our BBA data sets, along with the MRI system (top row, left), the head coil (top row, middle), anterior neck coil (top row, right), and posterior neck coil (bottom row, left), integrated spine array (ISA) (bottom row, middle), and the peripheral vascular array (PVA) coil (bottom row, right). The first four coils shown are manufactured by Philips Medical Systems, Inc., Cleveland, OH. The head coil is of single-channel, receive-only design, and used for imaging the head and its associated vasculature. The anterior and posterior neck coils are each of single-channel, receive-only design, and used to image the neck and its associated vasculature in conjunction with the ISA coil. The PVA coil (bottom row, right) is a multi-channel, receive-only design, manufactured by USA Instruments, Inc., Aurora, OH. This coil covers the patient's body from the renal area to the ankle region and is used for run-off studies. The couch moves in a multi-station fashion during the scan to follow the course of the contrast agent (Gad) moving through the vasculature in the area covered by this coil. Principally, in contrast to time-of-flight (TOF) MRA, which attempts to maximize flow-related signal, black-blood-based MRA aims at minimizing flow-related signal, producing flow signal voids (see [52–54]). Thus, vessel lumen appear as dark areas. This technique is less sensitive to slowly flowing spins and complicated flow patterns, which can be troublesome in TOF. Second, BBA is more accurate than TOF because it depicts true lumen instead of only flow images. BBA is free from the phase shift effect, presenting no spatial misregistration and/or distortion. In general, black-blood MRA provides more information than white-blood MRA, such as background tissue and contrast. For this reason, black-blood MRA is more useful in studying vessel wall rupture and plaque formation (see [55–57, 64, 65]). Furthermore, there are different techniques in BBA that provide a depiction of the true vessel lumen and position of the vessel instead of just inner vessel lumen or flow images. These are discussed later in this section.

BBA can be acquired in different ways. A gradient recalled sequence can be used in combination either with large bipolar gradients or presaturation RF pulses. Spin echo (SE) style sequences utilize *washout* effects. This means a flowing spin will hardly experience both excitation and refocus RF pulses, contributing no signal to the final images. Therefore, SE style sequences are considered a self-disruptive technique for which neither large bipolar gradient nor presaturation RF pulses are necessary. Depending on the techniques used to acquire the data, the physical mechanisms of BBA can be principally divided into the two major categories: (1) blood-flow behavior independent and (2) blood-flow behavior dependent (see Figure 4.5). The third category is a combination of these two types, as mentioned above. Here, blood-flow behavior refers to blood hemodynamics: velocity, acceleration, flow pattern, viscosity, Reno's number, etc.

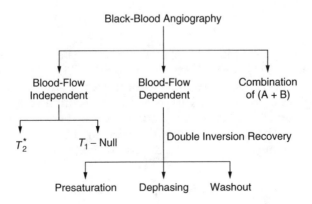

FIGURE 4.5
Black-blood data acquisition techniques.

4.2.1   Blood Flow Independent: T_2^*

This technique utilizes the effect of T_2 changes due to local magnetic field fluctuations, which is a function of any physiological activities, such as a change of oxygen partial pressure (see [66–69]). This is mathematically expressed as:

$$\frac{1}{T_2^*} = \frac{1}{T_2} + (\gamma \times \triangle B_0) \tag{4.1}$$

where T_2 is the spin-spin relaxation of a tissue, γ is the gyromagnetic ratio, and $\triangle B_0$ is the local field change. In angiographic imaging, B_0 depends on the oxygen level change, especially in small veins. This effect is similar to the blood oxygen level dependent (BOLD) technique. Technically, a long TE field echo (FE) sequence can also be used to detect such an effect. To avoid any possible motion and flow pulsatility, this technique is most suitable for intracranial veins. It should be noted that because this depends on oxygen level change, it may not give a complete depiction of vessel morphology.

4.2.2   Blood Flow Independent: T_1-Nulling

At a 1.5-Tesla magnetic field, the T_1 (spin-lattice) values for blood are about 1200 ms in arteries and 1000 ms in veins, respectively. Knowing these values, the blood signal can be selectively suppressed using proper spin preparations (see [53, 54]). A typical technique is to use an inversion recovery (IR) RF pulse for spin preparation, of which a 180° RF pulse is applied and, after a certain delay, the acquisition commences. The inversion time, TI, can be calculated from:

$$M_z = -M_0 \, e^{\frac{TI}{T_1}} + M_0 \left(1 - e^{\frac{TI}{T_1}} \right) = 0 \tag{4.2}$$

Thus, the inversion time, TI, can be determined by:

$$TI = T_1 \times ln2 \tag{4.3}$$

For a given T_1 value of blood (1200 ms), *TI* needs to be set to around 500 to 600 ms. When the *TI* is raised, this technique is called FLAIR (fluid attenuated inversion recovery) and is very suitable for use in the situation where blood flow is stagnant or very slow. This technique does bring some side effects, namely the contrast change of surrounding issues when T_1 values are close to that of blood. Therefore, to combat this problem, FLAIR can be combined with other techniques, which will be discussed ahead.

4.2.3   Blood-Flow Dependent Technique: Presaturation

Unlike TOF, the concept behind presaturation is to exclude the signal from flowing spins by setting the presaturating flowing spins. The presaturation technique uses additional RF pulses to excite regions adjacent to the imaging

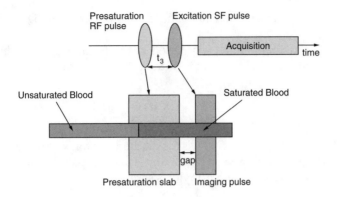

FIGURE 4.6
Scheme for presaturation preparation: a presaturation RF pulse is applied before conventional data acquisition. The flowing spins that experience the presaturation RF pulse have a very short time to recover and contribute less signal to the final images. The effectiveness of presaturation depends on flow behavior (the velocity) and imaging parameters, such as gap and time delay t_d.

region prior to data acquisition using a very short inversion time delay, usually a few milliseconds (see [52]). Following the excitation RF pulse, flowing spins will experience a very short recovery time, and therefore barely contribute signal to the final reconstructed images, as illustrated in Figure 4.6. Mathematically, this is expressed as:

$$I_{flow} = M_0 \left(1 - e^{\frac{TI}{T_1}}\right) = 0, \tag{4.4}$$

where $TI = t_d$ is the time delay between the presaturation RF pulse and excitation RF pulse, and T_1 is blood, about 1200 ms. TI is usually very small, about 1 to 4 ms. Therefore, flow-related signal I_{flow} is nearly zero. This technique is simple and widely used in clinical imaging. In practice, however, blood-flow patterns are rather complicated *in vivo*, such as in turbulent flow or disturbed flow with a wide range of velocities. Thus, the suppression of flow signal depends on many factors, such as slab thickness of presaturation, time delay between presaturation and excitation RF pulses, the gap between presaturation and the imaging slab, the phase of the cardiac cycle, etc. (see [57]). Specifically, in the case of very slow blood flow or a wide range of blood-flow velocity (from very fast to very slow flow), it becomes difficult to suppress all flowing spins.

4.2.4 Blood-Flow Dependent Technique: Phase Dispersion (Dephasing)

In this technique, the velocity of a flowing spin can be mapped into a phase shift using a proper gradient. When a large bipolar gradient is applied, flow spins possess a wide range of phase dispersion, resulting in signal cancellation, while the static spins remain unchanged (see patents [58, 59] and articles [60–63]).

This can be mathematically expressed in the following ways. In the laboratory framework, the phase shift at the echo top of magnetization can be written as:

$$\phi = \int_0^{T_E} \gamma \, \overrightarrow{r}(t) \, \overrightarrow{G}(t) \, dt \tag{4.5}$$

where $\overrightarrow{G}(t) = [G_x(t), G_y(t), G_z(t)]$ is the gradient vector, γ is the gyromagnetic ratio, T_E is the echo time, and $\overrightarrow{r}(t)$ is a time-varying spatial position function, which can be expressed using a Taylor's series as:

$$\overrightarrow{r}(t) = \overrightarrow{r_0}(t) + \overrightarrow{v} \, t + \frac{1}{2} \overrightarrow{a} \, t^2 + \cdots = \sum_{n=0}^{\infty} \frac{1}{n!} \frac{d^{(n)} \overrightarrow{r}}{dt^n} t^n \tag{4.6}$$

where $\overrightarrow{r_0}(t)$ is the zero-order component (the position), $\overrightarrow{v}$ is the first-order component (the velocity), and $\overrightarrow{a}$ is the second-order component (the acceleration). Considering the first-order velocity term and taking $n = 1$, the flow-related phase shift (Equation 4.6) can be expressed by the following equation:

$$\phi = \int_0^{T_E} \gamma \, (\overrightarrow{r_0} + \overrightarrow{v} \, t) \, \overrightarrow{G}(t) \, dt = \phi_0 + \phi_v \tag{4.7}$$

where $\phi_0 = \int_0^{T_E} \gamma \, \overrightarrow{r_0} \overrightarrow{G}(t) \, dt$ is the phase shift of *stationary* tissue and $\phi_v = \int_0^{T_E} \gamma \, \overrightarrow{v} \, t \, \overrightarrow{G}(t) \, dt$ is the phase shift of first-order *moving* spins. Flow-related phase encoding is usually performed by applying a bipolar gradient, which has no effect on static signal. Note that if $M_0 = \int G(t) \, dt$ and $M_1 = \int r G(t) \, dt$, then Equation 4.7 can be rewritten as: $\phi_0 = \gamma \times r_0 M_0$ and $\phi_v = \gamma \times v M_1$. By bipolar gradient, we mean $M_0 = 0$ and $M_1 \neq 0$.

Phase dispersion is of particular importance in the multi-echo acquisition technique. When spins are moving along the frequency (readout) or phase encoding direction, the phase dispersion will progressively increase, resulting in complete signal voids. For fast spin echo (FSE) type sequences, the discrepancy between spin echo and the stimulated echo will also become larger (see Figure 4.7).

4.2.5 Blood-Flow Dependent Technique: Washout Effect

In MRI, certain sequences, such as spin echo, fast spin echo, rapid acquisition refocused echo (RARE), and gradient recall acquisition spin echo (GRASE), signal can be formed only when spins completely experience a train of RF pulses, typically 90° to 180°, with n = 1 (see [28–30]). This is true for the spins that are static but is not true for the spins that are moving, such as blood flow. This phenomenon is called *washout*. Figure 4.8 illustrates such a situation.

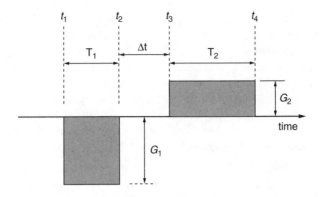

FIGURE 4.7
Phase dispersion is particularly important in the multi-echo acquisition technique. When spins are moving along the frequency (readout) or phase encoding direction, the phase dispersion will progressively increase, resulting in complete signal voids. For fast spin echo type sequences, the discrepancy between spin echo and stimulated echo will also become larger.

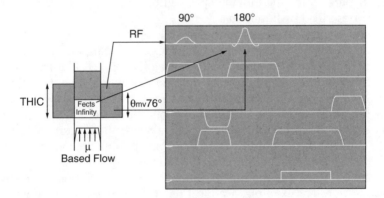

FIGURE 4.8
Left: Scheme of the *washout* effect. Right: Spin echo sequence diagram. Spin echo style sequences show the *washout* effect. The static spins can see both 90° and 180° pulses, while the flowing spins cannot see both the RF pulses. As a result, this contributes almost little or no signal.

For multi-echo sequences such as FSE, a RF pulse train is employed. Thus, if a later echo is placed into the center of k-space, to achieve, for example, T_2-weighting, the flowing spins can hardly experience the entire echo train, resulting in signal void. In such a case, the cut-off velocity, the slowest moving spins that can form signal, can be expressed as:

$$v > \frac{ST}{\frac{TE_{eff,\,n}}{2}} = 2\frac{ST}{n \times ESP} \tag{4.8}$$

where $n = 1, 2, \ldots n$, $TE_{eff, n}$ is the effective echo time as a function of the nth echo in the center of k-space, and ESP is the inter-echo spacing time. The equation shows that as the effective echo time $TE_{eff, n}$ increases, there is less possibility of forming signal, even in the case of slow or pulsatile flow. In a dual-contrast FSE sequence, the first echo is usually set in the center k-space for the PD-weighted and T_2-weighted images, while the later echo is located in the center of k-space for the T_2-weighted images. This explicitly elucidates why the T_2-weighted images are less sensitive to slow flow (smaller v) than the PD-weighted images (the first echo is in the center of k-space).

4.2.6   Clinically Applied Techniques and Examples: TOF vs. FSE

As mentioned above, in a FSE acquisition, a train of RF pulses will be used, usually $90° - n \times 180°$, with $n = 4, \ldots, 32$. The produced black-blood MRA is principally based on two effects: (**1**) *washout* effect for the moving spins perpendicular to the imaging plane, as described by Equation 4.8; and (**2**) phase dispersion for the moving spins within the imaging plane (in-plane flow), as described by Equation 4.7.

In comparison with the conventional TOF for the white-blood technique, a three-dimensional FSE shows its advantages of imaging time efficiency and flexibility of imaging parameter choices (see [32, 33]). TOF purely relies on the in-flow effect, which is largely determined by the repetition time, the flip angle and flow vector (direction and speed). Consequently, for a given larger flip angle and under a slow flow condition, the repetition time cannot be set too short, and the imaging plane needs to be positioned perpendicularly to the in-flow direction as much as possible. In contrast, the FSE-based black-blood angiogram is mainly affected by the effective echo time and therefore those constraints do not apply, thus permitting more efficient data collection. For example, a typical repetition time in three-dimensional TOF is 30 ms. while in a three-dimensional FSE technique, a typical inter-echo spacing ranges from 9 to 16 ms. Figure 4.9 illustrates such a situation of identical imaging parameters except for the flip angle, repetition time, and echo time. Within the comparable imaging time (11 min. 31 sec for the three-dimensional TOF vs. 9 min. 31 sec for the three-dimensional FSE), the dual-contrast three-dimensional FSE technique provides more information content than the three-dimensional TOF does. In addition, the angiographic information, the dual-contrast three-dimensional FSE also provides two types of images using complementary contrast. Conversely, the three-dimensional TOF acquisition can merely provide angiographic information with suppressed background. Therefore, for a given imaging time, spatial resolution and information content, a dual-contrast three-dimensional FSE acquisition can be considered more efficient than a three-dimensional TOF acquisition.

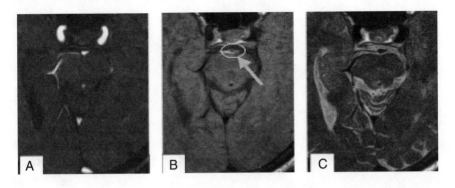

FIGURE 4.9

Axial source images of a healthy volunteer, acquired on a 1.5T MRI scanner (Philips, Cleveland, OH, Eclipse™). Left: A TOF image acquired with a three-dimensional SLiding INterleaved Ky space (SLINKY) sequence. Middle: Proton-density weighted image. Right: T_2-weighted image. Middle–Right were obtained with a dual contrast three-dimensional FSE. Common imaging parameters were: FOV = 220 mm, THK = 1.0 mm, 256 × 256 acquisition matrix, nine slabs with eight partitions, BW = 20.8 kHz, (512 × 512 × 16) × 9 reconstruction matrix. For the three-dimensional TOF (left), the parameters used were: $T_R = 30$ ms, $T_E = 6.9$ ms, flip angle = 30°, magnetization transfer contrast (MTC), with a total imaging time = 11 min. 31 sec. For the dual-contrast, three-dimensional FSE (middle and right, respectively), $T_R = 1843$ ms, effective $T_E = 12/120$ ms, flip angle (FA) = 90/120°, and total imaging time = 9 min. 31 sec (see [65]).

4.2.7 Combined Technique: Double IR Preparation

The double inversion recovery (IR) acquisition consists of two parts: a preparation part and a data acquisition part. In the preparation part, a selective 180° inversion RF pulse is transmitted to invert all spins, moving or static, within the imaging plane. Consequently, a nonselective 180° inversion RF pulse is transmitted to reverse all the static spins within the imaging plane, and reverse all the spins (static or moving) that are outside the imaging plane. Some of the slow-moving spins within the imaging plane can still experience both of these inversion pulses. The acquisition will commence after a specified delay as described by Equation 4.1, usually 500 ms. During that period, the slowly moving spins that were originally within the plane will move out, contributing nothing to the reconstructed images; while the flowing spins that originally were outside the imaging plane will be nulled. Therefore, double IR preparation utilizes *washout* and T_1 characteristics of blood flow to minimize the flow signal. For these reasons, this is a robust and reliable technique, less dependent upon imaging parameters, such as ECG gating and pre-saturation, etc. If a double IR preparation is combined with a FSE acquisition, minimizing the flow signal will be further enhanced. In particular, double-IR and dual-contrast FSE can be used to study plaque development and vessel wall ruptures. In addition, PD-weighted and T_2-weighted contrast can help to identify vessel wall calcifications and early stages of plaque development. Figure 4.10 shows a set of axial images of extracranial vasculature from a

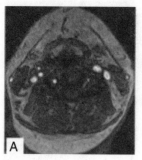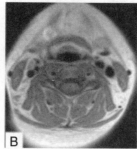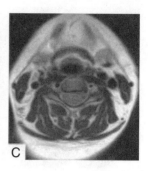

FIGURE 4.10

Axial images of neck vasculature from a healthy volunteer, acquired with: (A) Reference, three-dimensional TOF without any presaturation; (B) *PD*-weighted double-IR FSE; and (C) T_2-weighted double-IR FSE. Imaging parameters for B–C: dual-contrast FSE, ETL = 8, ESP = 8.0 ms, TR/TE1/TE2 = 800 ms/8 ms/64 ms, FOV = 240 mm, THK = 5.0 mm, 192 × 256, BW = 41.7 kHz, 1.0T Polaris™, Philips Medical Systems, Inc., Cleveland, volume-neck coil. No ECG gating was used for A–C (see [65]).

healthy volunteer, acquired with several sequences. Figure 4.10A is a reference image obtained with a three-dimensional TOF sequence. Figures 4.10B and 4.10C present the *PD*-weighted and T_2-weighted images from double-IR dual contrast FSE without ECG gating, respectively. The blood signal is completely nulled in both images, providing clear and sharper vasculature. The T_2-weighted-weighted image (Figure 4.10C) from the double-IR, dual-contrast FSE sequence also gave dark, sharp BB images of the vasculature. Double-IR BBA is less sensitive to ghosting artifacts due to pulsatile blood flow. Complementary contrast images may be useful to characterize plaque formation.

4.2.8   Pros and Cons of the Black-Blood MRA Technique

The *advantages* of BBA include:

1. It is less sensitive to slowly flowing spins and complicated flow patterns, which would be problematic in TOF.

2. BBA images present an accurate depiction of true vessel lumen, instead of just a blood flow image.

3. BBA is also free from the phase shift effect, presenting no spatial misregistration or distortion. Therefore, BBA images are more accurate than TOF images.

The *disadvantages* of BBA include the difficulty in its image segmentation. This is because two vascular systems are always presented together, causing complexity for radiologists in reading these images; and there are other dark, or black areas, such as tracts, sphenoid sinus, and dark muscles, which essentially hamper the use of minimum intensity projection.

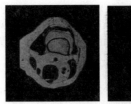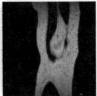

FIGURE 4.11
Left: Axial slice acquired for black-blood angiography (BBA) data set of the knee. Right: Sagittal slice acquired for black-blood angiography (BBA) data set of the knee.

4.3 Mask Generation Systems for Black-Blood Angiography

4.3.1 Mask Using Bayesian Techniques: An Application in Black-Blood Orthopedic Images

In Section 4.2 we presented the nature of the BBA volumetric data sets. Representative BBA slices for transverse and sagittal data set are shown in Figure 4.11. Seen in this figure are black blobs such as muscle pockets and air lining. Although not shown in the figure, areas of the air, muscles and bone are also seen as black in intensity in images. Thus, bone, air, and muscles are all black, in addition to the vessel themselves. The rest of the image consists of tissues that are gray in contrast. Also note that the shapes and sizes of the black nonvascular structures vary from area to area of the body. Some muscle shapes can be tapering, some can be blobby, and some can be as thin as a vessel. These shapes interfere in segmentation of the "black vessels." One way to handle the segmentation of the black vessels would be to remove these black muscle pockets using mathematical morphology on a slice-by-slice basis. One could use the gray-scale mathematical morphology to erode these shapes, but this would need a different set of structuring elements. Also, because the variability is so high, it would be very difficult to keep the vessels and remove the rest. Therefore, we have approached the black vessel segmentation as a pixel-classification problem in scale-space. It is known that the white-blood angiographic images can be successfully used in scale-space vessel segmentation (well established); we therefore try to create the pseudo-white-blood angiographic images from the black-blood angiographic image volumes. This pseudo-white-blood angiographic image volume can then be used in scale-space for blood vessel segmentation. Conversion from black blood to pseudo white blood can be done by assigning the gray tissue intensities to the black interfering objects, such as muscle or air masks. To perform the conversion, it is necessary to identify the black object regions in the image slices and then remove these using the gray-scale intensities of the tissues. However, the important aspect to keep in mind is not to lose the black-blood vessels. If they become lost, then the scale-space method will not be able to find the blood vessels in the image volume. To identify the black-blood blobby regions of black muscles and air pockets, this problem can be posed as a two-class problem: class 1 is the black regions and class 2 is the tissue regions. The two-class problem can be solved using the Bayesian classifier problem of maximization of the maximum *a posteriori* probability, given the Gaussian distribution of the probability in the image model.

Several researchers have used the application of Bayesian pixel classification in medical imaging (see [74–81]).

Having discussed the motivation for introducing the pixel classifier for classifying the black-blood pixels in comparision to the tissue pixels, we here propose a generic pipeline, called vessel detection and analysis system for black-blood angiography (VDAAS-BBA), for filtering the black-blood angiographic volumes. This system is shown in Figure 4.12. VDAAS-BBA consists of three major image processing components: (1) the pixel classification block, (2) the black-blood to pseudo-white-blood converter, and (3) the scale-space filtering block. The last stage is the vessel display system based on the classical maximum intensity projection algorithm. Note that our attempt is to show that this system as a pipeline works well for black-blood angiographic volumes that have large black structured geometric shapes in addition to the black-blood vessels. We are not by any means claiming the

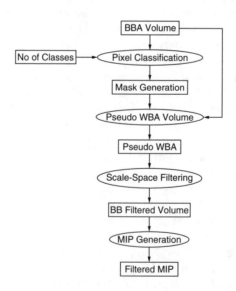

FIGURE 4.12
Vessel detection and analysis system for black-blood angiography (VDAAS-BBA). System shows three components: mask generation using pixel classifier, BBA to WBA converter for pseudo-WBA generation, and nonvascular tissue removal using scale-space filter.

novelty of each of these blocks, but rather presenting a system-based approach that can help in the detection of vessels in black-blood angiographic volumes.

In this approach, image segmentation is posed as a classification problem where each pixel is assigned to one of K image classes. Specifically, suppose the input image is $\mathbf{y} = \{\mathbf{y}_{i,j}, (i,j) \in \mathbf{L}\}$, where $\mathbf{y}_{i,j}$ is a pixel and $\mathbf{L}$ is a square lattice. Denote the segmentation as $\mathbf{z} = \{\mathbf{z}_{i,j}, (i,j) \in \mathbf{L}\}$. Here, $\mathbf{z}_{i,j}$ is a binary *indicator vector* of dimension K, with only one component being 1 and the others being 0. For example, when $K = 3$, $\mathbf{z}_{i,j} = [0,1,0]^T$ means we assign the pixel at (i,j) to class 2.

Using the notation introduced above, the segmentation problem can be formulated as the following MAP (maximum *a posteriori*) inference problem:

$$\hat{\mathbf{z}} = \arg\max_{\mathbf{z}}[p(\mathbf{y}|\mathbf{z}, \Phi)] \qquad (4.9)$$

where Φ is model parameters. In this work, we assume that the pixels in $\mathbf{y}$ are conditionally independent given $\mathbf{z}$; that is:

$$p(\mathbf{y}|\mathbf{z}, \Phi) = \Pi_{i,j}\, p(\mathbf{y}_{i,j}|\mathbf{z}_{i,j}, \Phi) \qquad (4.10)$$

Furthermore, we assume that conditioned on $\mathbf{z}_{i,j}$, the pixel $\mathbf{y}_{i,j}$ has a multivariate Gaussian density [77]; that is:

$$p(\mathbf{y}_{i,j}|\mathbf{z}_{i,j} = \mathbf{e}_k, \Phi) = \frac{1}{(2\pi)^{3/2}|\mathbf{C}_k|^{1/2}} e^{-\frac{1}{2}(\mathbf{y}_{i,j}-\mathbf{m}_k)^T \mathbf{C}_k^{-1}(\mathbf{y}_{i,j}-\mathbf{m}_k)}, \quad k = 1, 2, \ldots, K \qquad (4.11)$$

where $\mathbf{e}_k$ is a K-dimensional binary indicator vector with the kth component being 1. From this,

$$\Phi = \{\mathbf{m}_k, \mathbf{C}_k\}_{k=1}^K \qquad (4.12)$$

contains the mean vectors and covariance matrices for the K image classes.

Here is the scheme for updating the parameter estimates:

$$\pi_k^{(n)} = \frac{\sum_{i,j} \langle \mathbf{z}_{i,jk}^{(n-1)} \rangle}{\sum_{i,jk} \langle \mathbf{z}_{i,jk}^{(n-1)} \rangle}, \qquad (4.13)$$

$$\langle \mathbf{z}_{i,jk}^{(n)} \rangle = \frac{p^{(n)}(y_{i,j}|z_{i,j} = e_k, \Phi)\pi_k^{(n)}}{\sum_k p^{(n)}(y_{i,j}|z_{i,j} = e_k, \Phi)\pi_k^{(n)}}, \qquad (4.14)$$

$$\hat{\mathbf{m}}_k^{(n+1)} = \frac{\sum_{i,j} \langle z_{i,jk}^{(n)} \rangle \mathbf{y}_{i,j}}{\sum_{i,j} \langle z_{i,jk}^{(n)} \rangle}, \qquad (4.15)$$

$$\hat{\mathbf{C}}_k^{(n+1)} = \frac{\sum_{i,j} \langle z_{i,jk}^{(n)} \rangle [\mathbf{y}_{i,j} - \hat{\mathbf{m}}_k^{(n+1)}][\mathbf{y}_{i,j} - \hat{\mathbf{m}}_k^{(n+1)}]^T}{\sum_{i,j} \langle z_{i,jk}^{(n)} \rangle} \qquad (4.16)$$

where $k = 1, 2, \ldots, K$, z_{i,j_k} is the kth component of $\mathbf{z}_{i,j}$.

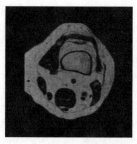
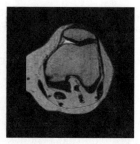

BBA slices of the axial knee

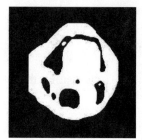
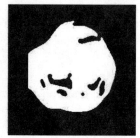

Bayesian followed by binary opening

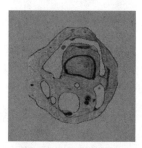
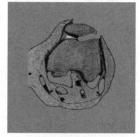

Mean intensity assigment using inverted mask

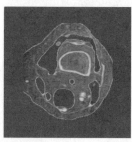
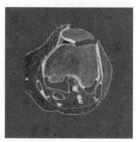

Pseudo-white-blood slices

FIGURE 4.13

Pseudo-white-blood volume generation. Left Column: Slice number 30. Right Column: Slice number 80. Topmost Row: Original BBA slices. 2nd Topmost Row: Bayesian masks. 3rd Topmost Row: Muscle and air removal. Bottommost Row: Pseudo-white-blood results. (MR data, courtesy of Philips Medical Systems, Inc., Cleveland, OH.)

These formulas, in addition to providing the estimate of Φ, also produce a segmentation. Specifically, at each iteration, $\langle z_{i,j_k}^{(n)} \rangle$ is interpreted as the probability that $\mathbf{y}_{i,j}$ should be assigned to class k. Hence, after a sufficient number of iterations, we can obtain the segmentation $\mathbf{z}$ by for each $(i, j) \in \mathbf{L}$:

$$\mathbf{z}_{i,j} = \mathbf{e}_{k_0}, \quad \text{if } k_0 = \arg\max_{1 \leq k \leq K} \langle z_{i,j_k} \rangle. \tag{4.17}$$

The results of the Bayesian classifier as a mask is shown in the Figure 4.13 (2nd topmost row, left and right). This binary raw mask volume undergoes binary mathematical morphology of erosion followed by dilation — so-called binary opening. This ensures that tiny circular vessels are removed, if any. This becomes the refined binary masked volume. Using this volume and the original gray-scale black-blood volume, we assign the mean intensity of the original gray-scale black-blood volume (obtained from the inverted binary masked volume) to the masked volume. Thus, the black regions are removed in the black-blood volume. This is then inverted to reflect the pseudo-white-blood volume for scale-space processing, as discussed in the next section.

4.3.2 Mask Using Fuzzy Techniques: An Application in Black-Blood Neuro Images

Mask generation becomes critical in cases of black-blood neuro images. This is because in BBA, the arteries and veins that are black in structure are embedded in the black neighborhood regions. This is particularly seen for venous flow, because the veins are at the edges of the brain and the region next to the veins is the CSF, which is also black (see Figure 4.14). As seen in the slice, the veins

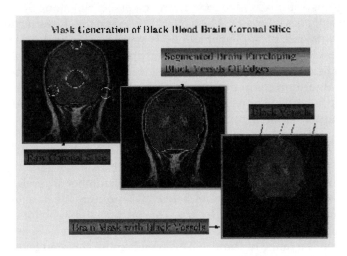

FIGURE 4.14
Figures showing the venous flow in the black-blood neuro image. (Courtesy of Philips Medical Systems, previously known as Marconi Medical Systems, Inc., Cleveland, OH.)

are almost half-embedded in the gray matter and half in the CSF region. One way to approach this problem is to find the region of the gray matter (GM) and make it as a mask, enlarge the mask in few directions, and then we can be very close to detecting the black veins. In this approach, we will thus need a mask of the gray matter, and thus the motivation for the mask generation process.

There are several ways the GM mask can be generated. We have developed an algorithm that is based on recursive connected component analysis and recursive mathematical morphology embedded in the Fuzzy framework. First the Fuzzy C mean algorithm is run over the BBA neuro images by detecting the three major classes: the vessels inside the WM area, the WM itself (along with some GM), and background. We can then choose the WM region because it is the largest region in the brain images. Because the region below the brain, such as neck, etc., may have intensities close to the WM region, they will also be selected. To detach these regions, we use the concept of recursive mathematical morphology and recursive connected component analysis. The connected component analysis is run in the run length mode. The mathematical morphology is binary in nature and consists of four major functions such as dilation, erosion, opening, and closing.

4.3.2.1   FCM Algorithm for Mask Generation in Black-Blood Neuro Images

In this step, we classified each pixel. Usually, the classification algorithm expects one to know how many classes (roughly) the image would have. The number of classes in the image would be the same as the number of tissue types. A pixel could belong to more than one class; therefore, we used the fuzzy membership function to associate with each pixel in the image. There are several algorithms used to compute membership functions, and one of the most efficient ones is Fuzzy C Mean (FCM), based on the clustering technique. Because of its ease of implementation for spectral data, it is preferred over other pixel classification techniques. Mathematically, we express the FCM algorithm below, but for complete details, readers are advised to see [40, 41]. The FCM algorithm computed the measure of membership termed the *fuzzy membership function*. Suppose the observed pixel intensities in a multi-spectral image at a pixel location j was given as:

$$\mathbf{y}_j = [y_{j1}\ y_{j2}\ \ldots,\ y_{jN}]^T \tag{4.18}$$

where j takes the pixel location, and N is the total number of pixels in the data set. In FCM, the algorithm iterates between computing the *fuzzy membership function* and the centroid of each class. This membership function is the pixel location for each class (tissue type), and the value of the membership function lies between the range of 0 and 1. This membership function actually represents the degree of similarity between the pixel vector at a pixel location and the centroid of the class (tissue type). For example, if the membership function has a value close to 1, then the pixel at the pixel location is close to the centroid of the pixel vector for that particular class. The algorithm can be presented in the following four steps. If $u_{jk}^{(p)}$ is the membership value at location j for class k at iteration p, then $\Sigma_{k=1}^{3} u_{jk} = 1$. As defined before, $\mathbf{y}_j$ is the observed pixel vector at location j and $\mathbf{v}_k^{(p)}$ is the centroid of class k at iteration p; thus, the FCM steps for computing the fuzzy membership values are:

1. Choose the number of classes (K) and the error threshold ϵ_{th}, and set the initial guess for the centroids $\mathbf{v}_k^{(0)}$ where the iteration number $p = 0$.

2. Compute the fuzzy membership function, given by the equation:

$$u_{jk}^{(p)} = \frac{\|\mathbf{y}_j - \mathbf{v}_k^{(p)}\|^{-2}}{\sum_{l=1}^{K} \|\mathbf{y}_j - \mathbf{v}^{(p)}\|^{-2}} \tag{4.19}$$

where $j = 1, \ldots, M$ and $k = 1, \ldots, K$.

3. Compute the new centroids using the equation:

$$\mathbf{v}^{(p+1)} = \frac{\sum_{j=1}^{N} \left(u_{jk}^{(p)}\right)^2 \mathbf{y}_j}{\sum_{j=1}^{N} \left(u_{jk}^{(p)}\right)^2} \tag{4.20}$$

4. Convergence was checked by computing the error between the previous and current centroids ($\|\mathbf{v}^{(p+1)} - \mathbf{v}^{(p)}\|$). If the algorithm had converged, an exit would be required; otherwise, one would increment p and go to Step 2 for computing the fuzzy membership function again.

We use this classified image to generate the mask discussed in next section.

4.3.2.2 Recursive Mathematical Morphology with Connected Component Analysis

Having classified the brain images into three classes, one then selects the class with the largest number of connected pixels. Obviously, this would be the white matter region. Such a conversion process is basically called binarization process. This binary volume (as binary slices) is run-length converted so as to run the connected component analysis. The idea is to choose the largest connected component in the above binary brain images. Because other regions below the brain might also have intensities that would be similar to the white matter region, we would like to disconnect that neck region from the brain region using the mathematical morphology erosion process. This eroded image is further run by connected component analysis and the largest connected components are framed, which is the same white matter. The process is repeated three to four times until the entire brain is obtained. In the last stage, we find that due to the binary mathematical morphology, there is a possibility of hole formation. We thus need a last stage of hole filling and the mask is ready. Figure 4.15 shows the raw brain images. The results of running the intermediate steps are shown in Figure 4.16 through Figure 4.29. The final results can then be taken as the mask.

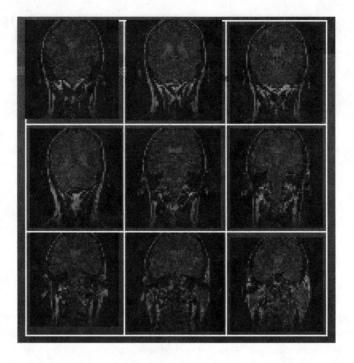

FIGURE 4.15

Step 1: raw MR black-blood neuro images. Note that slices are shown in the gap of ten slices each to give an idea of the other structures besides just the brain. (Courtesy of Philips Medical Systems, previously known as Marconi Medical Systems, Inc., Cleveland, OH.)

4.4 Black-Blood Angiographic Filtering System

4.4.1 Ellipsoidal Scale-Space Filtering for BBA Vascular Segmentation

Consider an image I and its Taylor expansion in the neighborhood of a point $\mathbf{x}_0$ and given as:

$$I(\mathbf{x}_0 + \delta\mathbf{x}_0, \sigma) = \underbrace{I(\mathbf{x}_0, \sigma)}_{0^{th}-order} + \underbrace{\delta\mathbf{x}_0^T \nabla_{0,\sigma}}_{1^{st}-order} + \underbrace{\delta\mathbf{x}_0^T \mathcal{H}_{0,\sigma} \delta\mathbf{x}_0}_{2^{nd}-order} + \cdots \qquad (4.21)$$

This expansion approximates the structure of the image up to the second order. $\nabla_{0,\sigma}$ and $\mathcal{H}_{0,\sigma}$ are the gradient vector and Hessian matrix of the image computed at $\mathbf{x}_0$ at scale σ, respectively. To calculate the differential operators I, the scale-space framework is adapted. In this framework, the differentiation is defined as a convolution with Derivative of Gaussian (DoG). This is given as:

$$\frac{\partial}{\partial x} L(\mathbf{x}, \sigma) = \sigma^\gamma I(\mathbf{x}) \otimes \frac{\partial G}{\partial \mathbf{x}}(\mathbf{x}, \sigma) \qquad (4.22)$$

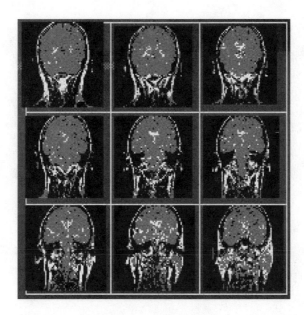

FIGURE 4.16
Step 2: running fuzzy connectivity algorithm by taking three classes into account. (Courtesy of Philips Medical Systems, previously known as Marconi Medical Systems, Inc., Cleveland, OH.)

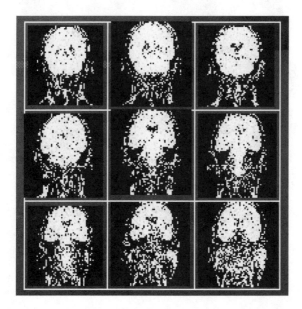

FIGURE 4.17
Step 3: binarization of the output of the Fuzzy connectivity algorithm. (Courtesy of Philips Medical Systems, previously known as Marconi Medical Systems, Inc., Cleveland, OH.)

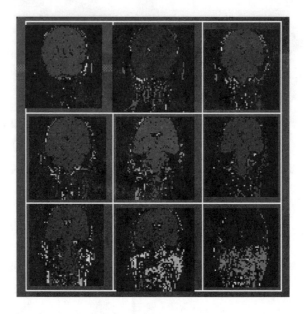

FIGURE 4.18
Step 4: labeling the different components of the binary images of the brain. (Courtesy of Philips Medical Systems, previously known as Marconi Medical Systems, Inc., Cleveland, OH.)

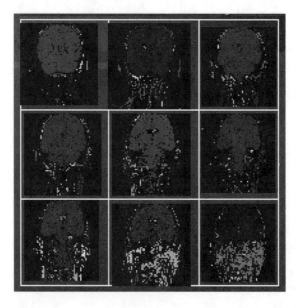

FIGURE 4.19
Step 5: Selecting the largest connected component of the brain. (Courtesy of Philips Medical Systems, previously known as Marconi Medical Systems, Inc., Cleveland, OH.)

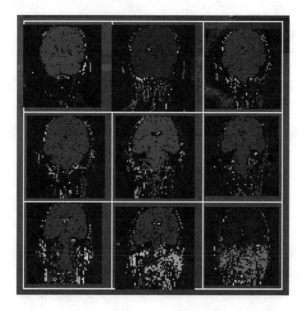

FIGURE 4.20
Step 6: running the connected component labeling algorithm in run-length representation. (Courtesy of Philips Medical Systems, previously known as Marconi Medical Systems, Inc., Cleveland, OH.)

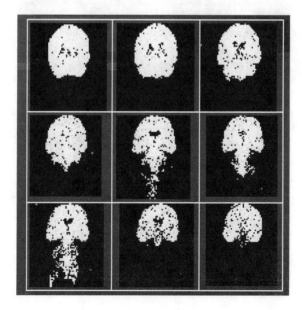

FIGURE 4.21
Step 7: selecting the largest connected component of the brain image again. (Courtesy of Philips Medical Systems, previously known as Marconi Medical Systems, Inc., Cleveland, OH.)

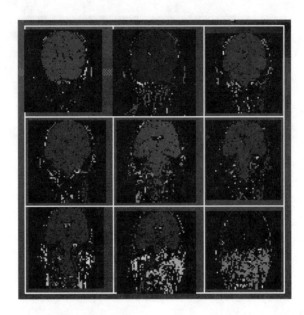

FIGURE 4.22
Step 8: labeling the different components of the brain. (Courtesy of Philips Medical Systems, previously known as Marconi Medical Systems, Inc., Cleveland, OH.)

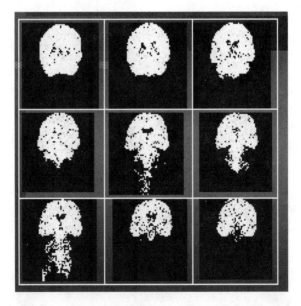

FIGURE 4.23
Step 9: labeling the different components of the brain. (Courtesy of Philips Medical Systems, previously known as Marconi Medical Systems, Inc., Cleveland, OH.)

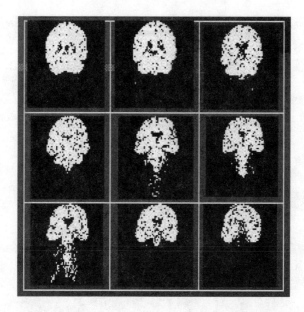

FIGURE 4.24
Step 10: running mathematical morphology such as binary erosion to remove the small islands. (Courtesy of Philips Medical Systems, previously known as Marconi Medical Systems, Inc., Cleveland, OH.)

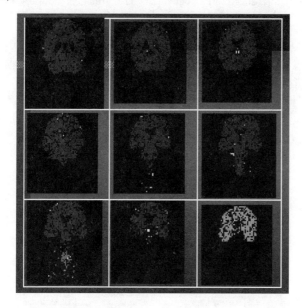

FIGURE 4.25
Step 11: running the connected components again to give labels to each of the regions. (Courtesy of Philips Medical Systems, previously known as Marconi Medical Systems, Inc., Cleveland, OH.)

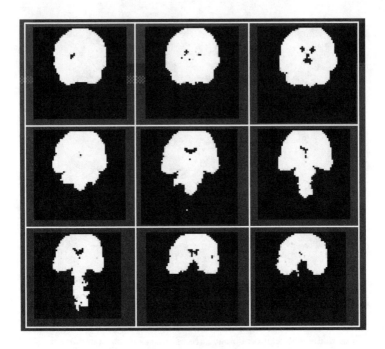

FIGURE 4.26
Step 12: running mathematical morphology such as binary dilation. (Courtesy of Philips Medical Systems, previously known as Marconi Medical Systems, Inc., Cleveland, OH.)

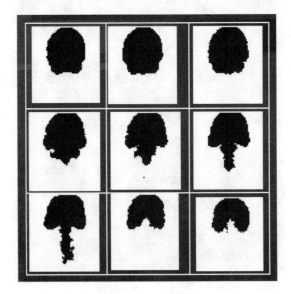

FIGURE 4.27
Step 13: hole filling and brain mask extraction. (Courtesy of Philips Medical Systems, previously known as Marconi Medical Systems, Inc., Cleveland, OH.)

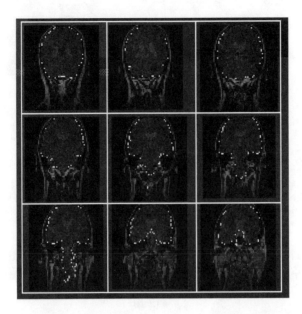

FIGURE 4.28
Step 14: superposition of the boundary of the mask over the original gray-scale images of brain. (Courtesy of Philips Medical Systems, previously known as Marconi Medical Systems, Inc., Cleveland, OH.)

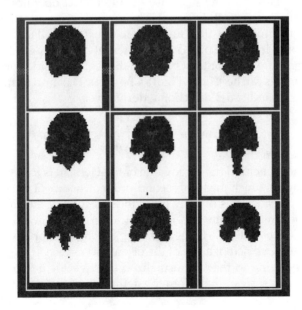

FIGURE 4.29
Step 15: gray-scale mask showing the segmented brain. (Courtesy of Philips Medical Systems, previously known as Marconi Medical Systems, Inc., Cleveland, OH.)

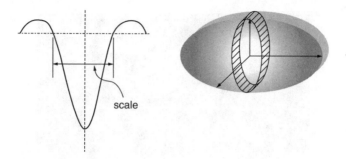

FIGURE 4.30
Concept of second-order Gaussian derivative for edge estimation and ellipsoidal concept for direction estimation. Left: Second-order Gaussian derivative. Right: Three-dimensional ellipsoid.

where $G(\mathbf{x}, \sigma)$ is the three-dimensional Gaussian kernel defined as:

$$G(\mathbf{x}, \sigma) = \frac{1}{(2\pi\sigma^2)^{\frac{D}{2}}} e^{\frac{\|\mathbf{x}\|^2}{2\sigma^2}} \qquad (4.23)$$

where $D = 3$, due to three-dimensional processing. The parameter γ was introduced by Lindeberg[5] (see [83–89]). This was used to define a family of normalized derivatives. This normalization was particularly important for a fair comparison of the response of differential operators at multiple scales. With no scales used, $LC = 1.0$. The second-order information (called Hessian) has an intuitive justification in the context of tubular structure detection. The second derivative of a Gaussian kernel at scale σ generates a probe kernel that measures the contrast between the regions inside and outside the range $(-\sigma, \sigma)$. This can be seen in Figure 4.30 (left). The third term in Equation 4.22 gives the second-order directional derivative:

$$\delta\mathbf{x}_0{}^T \mathcal{H}_{0,\sigma}\, \delta\mathbf{x}_0 = \left(\frac{\partial}{\partial\delta\mathbf{x}_0}\right)\left(\frac{\partial}{\partial\delta\mathbf{x}_0}\right) I(\mathbf{x}_0, \sigma). \qquad (4.24)$$

The main concept behind the eigenvalue of the Hessian is to extract the principal directions in which the local second-order structure of the image can be decomposed. Because this directly gives the direction of the smallest curvature (along the direction of the vessel), application of several filters in multiple orientations is avoided. This latter approach is computationally more expensive and requires a discretization of the orientation space. If $\lambda_{\sigma,k}$ is the eigenvalue corresponding to the kth normalized eigenvector $\hat{\mathbf{u}}_{\sigma,k}$ of the Hessian $\mathcal{H}_{0,\sigma}$ computed at scale σ, then from the definition of the eigenvalues:

$$\mathcal{H}_{0,\sigma}\, \hat{\mathbf{u}}_{\sigma,k} = \lambda_{\sigma,k}\hat{\mathbf{u}}_{\sigma,k} \qquad (4.25)$$

---

[5]Known as the Lindeberg Constant (LC).

The above equation has the following geometric interpretation. The eigen-value decomposition extracts three orthonormal directions that are invariant up to a scaling factor when mapped by the Hessian matrix. In particular, a spherical neighborhood centered at x_0 having a radius of unity will be mapped by $\mathcal{H}_0$ onto an ellipsoid whose axes are along the directions given by the eigenvectors of the Hessian, and the corresponding axis semi-lengths are the magnitudes of the respective eigenvalues. This ellipsoid locally describes the second-order structure of the image (see Figure 4.30, right). Thus, the problem comes down to an estimation of the eigenvalues and eigenvectors at each voxel location in the three-dimensional volume. The algorithm for filtering is framed in the next section.

4.4.2 Algorithmic Steps for BBA Ellipsoidal Filtering

The algorithm we used consisted of the following steps and is in the spirit of Frangi et al.'s approach [73]. The diagram showing the algorithm pipeline is seen in Figure 4.31, left, and discussed below as:

1. *Preprocessing of the MRA data sets.* This consists of changing the anisotropic voxels to isotropic voxels. We used trilinear interpolation

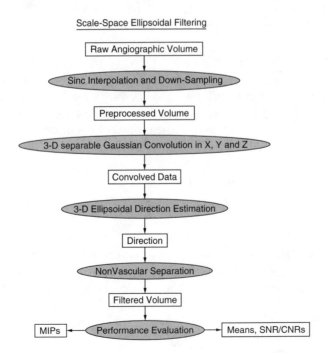

FIGURE 4.31
Algorithm pipeline for the ellipsoidal filter.

for this conversion. The second step in this preprocessing is image resizing. We used the standard wavelet transform method to down-sample the volume to half, primarily for speed concerns.

2. *Convolution of the image volume with the higher-order Gaussian deriva-tive operators:* The computation of the second Derivatives of Gaussian in the Hessian matrix is implemented using three separate convo-lutions with one-dimensional kernels given as:

$$I_{x^i y^j z^k}(\mathbf{x}, \sigma_f) = \frac{d^i}{d\mathbf{x}^i} G(\mathbf{x}, \sigma_f) \otimes \left\{ \frac{d^j}{d\mathbf{y}^j} G(\mathbf{y}, \sigma_f) \otimes \left\{ \underbrace{\underbrace{\underbrace{\frac{d^k}{d\mathbf{z}^k} G(\mathbf{z}, \sigma_f) \otimes I(\mathbf{x})}_{convolution\text{-}1}}_{convolution\text{-}2}}_{convolution\text{-}3} \right\} \right\}$$

(4.26)

where $I(\mathbf{x})$ is the interpolated gray-scale volume; i, j, and k are the nonnegative integers satisfying $i + j + k = 2$; and 3σ was used as the radius of the kernel. G is the Gaussian kernel in the x, y, and z direc-tions. $\frac{d^k}{d\mathbf{z}^k} G(\mathbf{z}, \sigma_f) \otimes I(\mathbf{x})$ is the convolution of the Gaussian kernel with a standard deviation of σ_f. Note that three sets of convolutions are done to obtain the scale-space representation of the gray-scale volume, rather than one convolution in three dimensions.

3. *Running the directional processor for computing the eigenvalues.* This is computed using Jacobi's method.

4. *Computation of the vessel score to distinguish the vessels from non-vessels using the eigenvalues based on connectivity, scale and contrast.* This can be computed using the combination of components that are com-puted using the geometry of the shape, which in turn is a function of the eigenvalues λ_1, λ_2, and λ_3,

$$V(\sigma, \gamma) = \begin{cases} 0 & \text{if } |\lambda_2| > 0 \text{ or } \lambda_3 > 0 \\ \left(1 - exp\left(-\frac{\mathcal{R}_A^2}{2\alpha^2}\right)\right) exp\left(-\frac{\mathcal{R}_B^2}{2\beta^2}\right)\left(1 - exp\left(-\frac{\mathcal{S}^2}{2\epsilon^2}\right)\right) \end{cases}$$

(4.27)

where γ is the Lindeberg constant and α, β, and ϵ are the thresh-olds that control the sensitivity of the filter for the measurements of features of the image such as area, blobness, and distinguishing property given by notations $\mathcal{R}_A^2$, $\mathcal{R}_B^2$, and $\mathcal{S}^2$. The first two geomet-ric ratios are gray-level invariants. This means they remain con-stant under intensity rescaling. The geometrical meaning of $\mathcal{R}_B^2$ is the derivation from a blob-like structure, but cannot distinguish be-tween a line and a plate-like pattern. The $\mathcal{R}_B^2$ is computed as the ratio of the volume of the ellipsoid to the largest cross section-area, which came out to be a fraction $\frac{|\lambda_1|}{\sqrt{|\lambda_2 \lambda_3|}}$. The "blob-term" is at a maximum for a blob-like structure and is close to zero if λ_1, or λ_1 and λ_2, tend to vanish. $\mathcal{R}_A^2$ referred to the largest area of the cross section of the ellipsoid in the plane that was perpendicular to the vessel direction (the least eigenvalue direction). This is computed as the ratio of the two largest second-order derivatives. This ratio basically distinguishes between the plate and line-like structures. Mathematically, it was given as $\frac{|\lambda_2|}{|\lambda_3|}$. The third term helps in distinguishing the vessel and non vessel structures. This term is computed as the magnitude of the derivatives, which is the magnitude of the eigenvalues. This is computed using the norm of the Hessian. The Frobenius matrix norm was used because it was straightforward in terms of the three eigenvalues and was given as $\mathcal{S} = \sqrt{\lambda_1^2 + \lambda_2^2, \lambda_3^2}$.

5. *Repeating the above steps from starting scale, s_{min}, to ending scale, s_{max}.*
6. *Scale optimization to remove the nonvascular and background structures.* The filter optimization was done by finding the best scale σ. This is computed as:

$$\mathcal{V}(\gamma) = \max_{s_{min} \leq s \leq s_{max}} \mathcal{V}(s, \gamma)$$

The volume corresponding to the best scale s_{opt} is the filtered volume.

4.5 Comparisons: Three-Dimensional Median vs. Three-Dimensional Black-Blood Ellipsoidal Filtering

This section presents briefly the previous methods that have been used for filtering the angiographic volumes. They are primarily the Alexander et al. [27] and Sun et al. [26] directional filtering approaches. Alexander et al.'s algorithm is discussed using the object process diagram (OPD), as shown in Figure 4.32. This method exploits the fact that most intracranial vessels are narrower than other structures that appear dark in the image (called black-blood angiography). The main reasons that complicate the vessel segmentation in BBA include:

1. Bone, air, and vessels are all seen as black in intensity.
2. Two neighboring bones can touch each other, thereby making the black region thicker. If they do not touch each other, then they can have gray-level tissues in between.
3. Air pockets are irregular shapes. These can be very large or very small. The very large ones can be longitudinal or circular in nature.

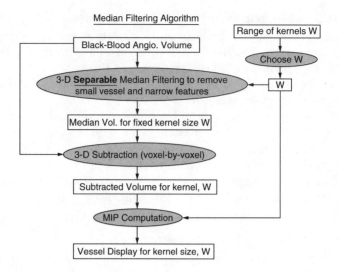

FIGURE 4.32

Protocol for black-blood angiography (BBA) for a three-dimensional FSE MR knee data set. Implementation of Alexander and Parker et al.'s algorithm.

4. The blood vessels are black and sometimes of the same size as that of air pockets or small bony structures. Thus, it is not possible to distinguish between the blood vessels and small air pockets or small bone circular structures.

5. The bone lining (cartilage) is thin in diameter, while the vessels are also thin in diameter. Using median filtering with subtraction will remove both the thin vessels and the thin lining. Similarly, using Gaussian blurring along with subtraction will remove both the thin lining and the thin vessels.

Having discussed the characteristics of BBA, we now present Alexander et al.'s algorithm along with their results. The algorithm consisted of finding the median value of the voxels that constitutes the cube region. Alexander et al. implemented this by applying one-dimensional median filters in three orthogonal directions to the original three-dimensional MRA data set. A median filter kernel (whose width was W) operated by sorting the W values and selecting the value that is in the middle of the sorted list. In this approach, the method first ran the one-dimensional filter in the z-direction, followed by the x- and y-directions. This was done to remove vessels and narrow structures. This process generated the *masked volume*. Because air and bone in the brain were also dark (in BBA), the above mask would preserve the signal contrast of the brain parenchyma and the boundaries between regions of tissues, bone, and air. Thus, the original volume was subtracted from the masked volume to generate the subtracted volume, which had the vessels in it. This algorithm is

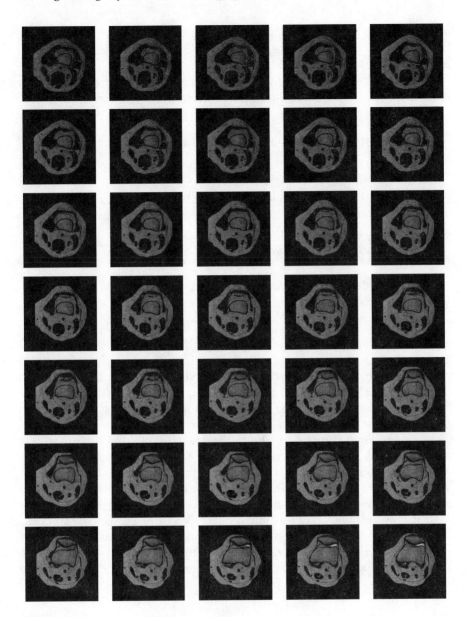

FIGURE 4.33
Axial slices acquired for the black-blood angiography (BBA) data set of the knee.

shown in Figure 4.32. Note that the method needs a kernel whose width is $3W$. Alexander et al. used a kernel size of $9 \times 9 \times 7$ in three different directions. Our protocol consisted of using a BBA of the knee data set of $256 \times 256 \times 147$. Sample slices of the knee data set are shown in Figure 4.33. After median filtering and subtraction, the resultant slices can be seen in Figure 4.34. Finally, MIPs of the subtracted results can be seen in Figure 4.35. We have shown this protocol using different kernel sizes W.

The major *advantage* of the system is that the three-dimensional median filter was separable. The major *disadvantages* of the system are that the method:

1. Was too sensitive to the kernel size W
2. Used a slow sorting method such as heap sort
3. Was only demonstrated for brain BBA and there were no experiments on vasculature in other areas of the body
4. The method did not show any timing issues for a comparison between the separable vs. nonseparable three-dimensional median filter
5. The article did not show any performance evaluation of the technique
6. The method did not remove the background and nonvasculature structures.

Figure 4.37 shows the comparison between the three-dimensional median filter and the three-dimensional ellipsoidal filter presented here for BBA of the knee images. Two orientations were acquired for this experiment: transverse and sagittal. Figure 4.33 shows the transverse slices acquired of the BBA knee data set. The median filter vs. ellipsoidal results of sagittal views from transverse acquired data set are shown in Figure 4.37 (top row). In the second experiment, we acquired the sagittal data set of the same knee. The acquired slices are shown in Figure 4.36. The median vs. ellipsoidal results are shown in Figure 4.37 (bottom row). As seen in Figure 4.37 (top and bottom rows), the background noise was greatly suppressed in the ellipsoidal scale-space filter (ESSF) for both views (right column). Also, the black vessels were more accurately detected with the ellipsoidal filtering method. The greatest advantage of ESSF was the removal of the nonvascular structures, such as the air pockets and bone, which was not done in previous research. Having discussed ellipsoidal filtering in Section 4.4, and the comparison of ellipsoidal filtering with median filtering in Section 4.5, we will next discuss the implementation issues of black-blood angiographic filtering.

4.6   Implementation Issues in Black-Blood Angiography Filtering

The issues related to ellipsoidal filtering include:

1. *Vessel thickness sizes.* It is important to know to what level the largest scale needs to be chosen. If the vessels are very thick, then to filter the

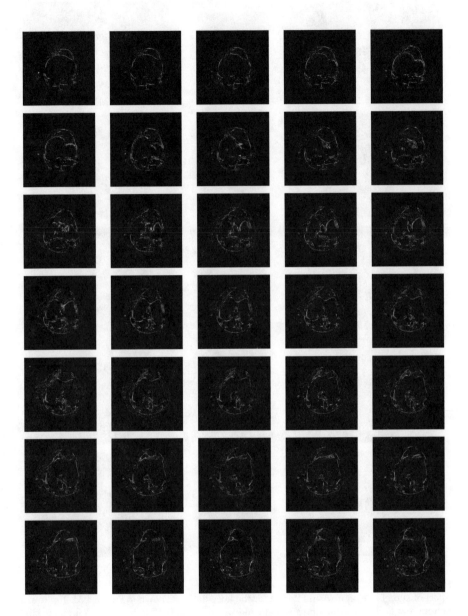

FIGURE 4.34
Protocol for black-blood angiography (BBA) for three-dimensional FSE MR knee data set. Implementation of Alexander and Parker et al.'s algorithm. Subtracted results of the three-dimensional data set, kernel size of $9 \times 9 \times 9$ separable median filter from the raw data set. Only non overlapping vessels are unidentified.

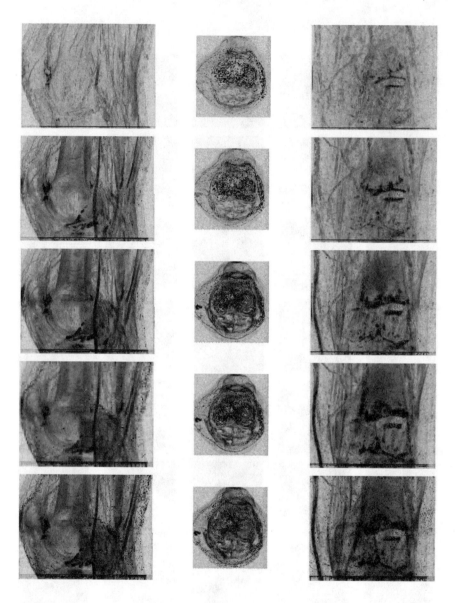

FIGURE 4.35
Effect of kernel size on median filtering for the knee data set shown in Figure 4.33. Top row to bottom row, kernel size one-dimensional window, $W = 5, 7, 9, 11$ and 13. Left Column: Sagittal MIP views. Middle Column: Axial MIP views. Right Column: Coronal MIP views.

largest thickness of vessels, one needs scales on the order of 10. In such cases, it may be better to skip some scales and one can compute the intermediate or alternate volumes that can then be used for scale optimization.

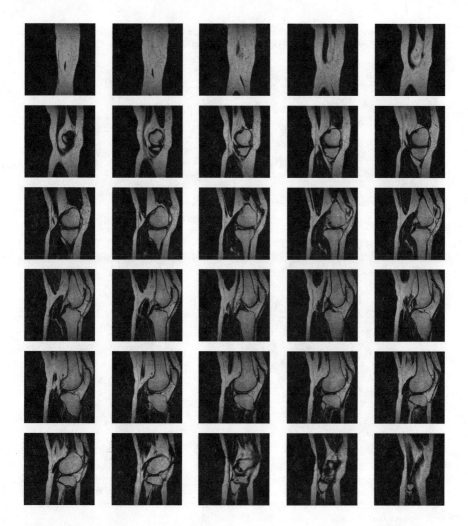

FIGURE 4.36
Sagittal slices acquired for the black-blood angiography (BBA) data set of the knee. Slice positions shown are in increments of five, starting from slice number 25.

2. *Gaussian kernel size.* The width of the Gaussian kernel is given as $W = 1 + 2.0 \times ceil(F \times \sigma)$, where F is the Gaussian fall constant. In our experiments of real and synthetic tests, we took the set of values of 1.5 and 2.5. If the vessels were very thick, using a small value was better justified. For thicker vessels, we took $F = 2.5$.

3. *Separable vs. nonseparable.* Three-dimensional Gaussian convolution was done using separable Gaussian kernels. This means the convolution was implemented in three different directions independently.

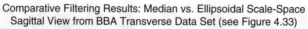

Comparative Filtering Results: Median vs. Ellipsoidal Scale-Space
Sagittal View from BBA Transverse Data Set (see Figure 4.33)

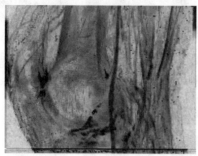
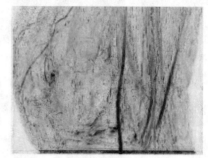

Sagittal View from BBA Sagittal Data Set (see Figure 4.36)

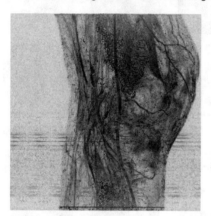
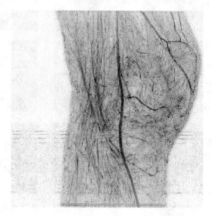

FIGURE 4.37
Comparison between three-dimensional median filtering vs. ellipsoidal scale-space filtering algorithm. Left Column: Three-dimensional median filtering. Right Column: Three-dimensional ellipsoidal filtering. Top Row: Sagittal views from the transverse acquired data set. Bottom Row: Sagittal views from the sagittal acquired data set.

This brought significant speed improvement and reduced the order of complexity from k^3 to $3k$.

4. *ROI computation.* Most of the time, the processing was done with ROI chosen in the volume. This was done by specifying the starting and ending coordinate positions in all three different directions. This saves much computation time, as the eigenvalues and eigen directions were computed for each voxel position.

5. *Effect of large scales.* When the scales were large, there was little blurring of the thin vessels due to the large Gaussian window convolution. As a result, the intensities around the vessels increased and the

vessel tended to be broader. On optimization, these blurred intensities show up and remove the crispness of the thin vessels. Thus, the thin vessels seem to be a little (say, one pixel) broader than expected.

6. *Quality–speed trade-off.* Ellipsoidal filtering is a very powerful technique for the segmentation of tubular structures. The results are very refined and the CNR ratio is very high when run on original MR data sets. But because ellipsoidal filtering requires volume generation at multiple scales, this may take huge computer runtime memory and space. It can be more troublesome if the volumetric data sets are very large. On average, a data set can take up to 7.5 Gigabytes. Five to six volumes can take around 40 Gigabytes and almost freeze the running machine. To avoid this problem, one has to down-sample the data size to have half the image size. This might also bring in some artifacts, which can be removed using Gaussian smoothing. This could also bring blurring to these vessels and the second-order operation can make this more noisy and complicated.

7. *Eigenvalue/direction computations.* The eigenvalues and directions need to be very carefully computed and all need to be estimated to three or four decimal places. We used the computer vision library of Intel (freeware), but we also verified our computer program using Numerical Recipes in C (see [100]).

8. *Three-dimensional interpolation.* We followed a simple three-dimensional trilinear interpolation for interpolating the three-dimensional angiographic volume. This was straightforward. Interested readers can look at the following research articles on voxel shift and sinc interpolation techniques; see [90–99]. In this chapter, we have not discussed the interpolation merits and demerits, as these are discussed elsewhere.

4.7 Conclusions, Challenges, and the Future

4.7.1 Conclusions

The first part of this chapter introduced the importance of vascular image processing and prefiltering. The major part of this chapter focused on scale-space ellipsoidal filtering. We presented several experiments and showed that the SNR and CNR for the filtered MIP were far superior to the raw MIPs. Our results were compared with median filtering. We also presented experiments on BBA and compared our algorithm with Alexander et al.'s (recently published). A full discussion was presented on the implementation issues of scale-space ellipsoidal filtering.

4.7.2   Challenges in BBA

Some of the challenges in vasculature filtering techniques include, the ability (1) to distinguish between the air pockets and bone in comparison to blood vessels in black-blood angiography; (2) to integrate the regularizers in the geometric framework for robust vasculature filtration; (3) to distinguish arteries and veins during the filtration process; (4) to develop methods that can incorporate the local object size in defining the connectedness, object material inhomogeneity, noise, blurring, and background variations.

4.7.3   The Future

We demonstrated using the ellipsoidal scale-space filtering algorithm for black-blood MR angiography. Although the method was successfully demonstrated on more than 20 patient studies and was also compared with existing state-of-the-art filtering algorithms, the method needs further improvements in the computation of the vessel score for each voxel position in the three-dimensional volume. Such methods are called regularizers and, when incorporated into the system, make the system more robust, accurate, and insensitive to variation in the parameters used in MR data acquisition methods. Terms like Fuzzy connectivity, classification, geometric frameworks, and skeletonization of the tubular structures must be brought into the scale-space framework for better filtration. Researchers are working aggressively toward new methods.

Acknowledgments

Thanks are due to Dr. Elaine Keeler from Philips Medical Systems, Inc., Cleveland, OH, and Professor Linda Shapiro, University of Washington, Seattle, for their motivation. Thanks also go to Dr. Larry Kasuboski, Philips Medical Systems, Inc., for his encouragment during the course of this project. Special thanks go also to Marconi/Philips Medical Systems, Inc., for the MR data sets.

References

1. http://www.med.jhu.edu/vascsurg/AAA1A1.html-Anchor-11481/.
2. North American Symptomatic Carotid Endarterectomy Trial (NASCET), *Stroke*, Vol. 22, No. 6, pp. 711–720, 1991.
3. European Carotid Surgery Trialists Collaborative Group, Randomised trial of endarterectomy for recently symptomatic carotid stenosis: final results of the

MRC European Carotid Surgery (ECST), *Lancet,* Vol. 351, No. 9113, pp. 1379–1387, 1998.

4. Wiebers, D. O., Torner, J. C., and Meissner, I., Impact of unruptured intracranial aneurysms on public health in the United States, *Stroke,* Vol. 23, No. 10, pp. 1416–1919, Oct. 1992.

5. Rhim, E. Y., Yuan, C., Mitsumori, L. M., Kaneko, E., Reichenbach, D. D., and Nelson, J. A., MRI of normal and atherosclerotic arteries: analysis of contrast features, *J. Vascular Invest.,* Vol. 3, No. 1, pp. 42–51, 1997.

6. Jara, H. and Barish, M. A., Black-blood MR angiography, *MRI Clinics in N. Am.,* Vol. 7, No. 2, pp. 303–317, May 1999.

7. Zahi, A. F., Fuster, V., Fallon, J. T., Jayasundera, T., Worthley, S. G., Helft, G., Aguinaldo, G. J., Badimon, J. J., and Sharma, S. K., Non-invasive *in-vivo* human coronary artery lumen and wall imaging using black blood MRI, *Circulation,* Vol. 102, pp. 506–510, 2000.

8. Ladak, H. M., Thomas, J. B., Mitchell, J. R., Rutt, B. K., and Steinman, D. A., A semi-automatic technique for measurement of arterial wall from black-blood MRI, *Medical Phys.,* Vol. 28, No. 6, pp. 1098–1107, June 2001.

9. Ingersleben, G. V., Schmiedl, U. P., Hatsukamni, T. S., Neslon, J. A., Subramaniam, D. S., Ferguson, M. S., and Yuan, C., Characterization of atherosclerotic plaques at the carotid bifurcation: correlation of high resolution MR with histology, *Radio Graphics,* Vol. 17, pp. 1417–1423, 1997.

10. Martin, A. J., Gotlieb, A. I., and Henkelman, R. M., High resolution MR imaging of human arteries, *J. Magn. Reson. Imag.,* Vol. 5, pp. 93–100, 1995.

11. Merickel, M. B., Carman, C. S., Brookeman, J. R., and Ayers, C. R., Image analysis and quantification of atherosclerosis using MRI, *Comput. Med. Imag. Graph.,* Vol. 15, No. 4, pp. 207–216, Jul.–Aug. 1991.

12. Merickel, M. B., Berr, S., Spetz, K., Jackson, T. R., Snell, J., Gillies, P., Shimshick, E., Hainer J, Brookeman, J. R., and Ayers, C. R., Noninvasive quantitative evaluation of atherosclerosis using MRI and image analysis, *Arterioscler. Thromb.,* Vol. 13, No. 8, pp. 1180–1186, Aug. 1993.

13. Yuan, C., Beach, K. W., Smith, H. L., and Hatsukami, T. S., *In vivo* measurement of maximum plaque area based on high resolution MRI, *Circulation,* 1998.

14. Yuan, C., Lin, E., Millard, J., and Hwang, J.-N., Closed contour edge detection of blood vessel lumen and outer wall boundaries in black-blood MR images, *J. Magn. Reson. Imag.,* Vol. 17, No. 2, pp. 257–266, 1999.

15. Berr, T. S., Hurt, N. S., Ayers, C. R., Snell, J. W., and Merickel, M. B., Assessment of the reliability of the determination of carotid artery lumen sizes by quantitative image processing of MR angiograms and imaging, *J. Magn. Reson. Imag.,* Vol. 13, pp. 827–835, 1995.

16. Han, C., Hatsukami, T. S., Hwang, J.-N., and Yuan, C., A fast minimal path active contour model, *IEEE Trans. Image Processing,* Vol. 10, No. 6, pp. 865–873, June 2001.

17. Thomas, J. B., Rutt, B. K., Ladak, H. M., and Steinman, D. A., Effect of black blood MR image quality on vessel wall segmentation, *Mag. Reson. Med.,* Vol. 46, pp. 299–304, 2001.

18. Patel, M. R., Klufas, R. A., Kim, D., Edelman, R. R., and Kent, K. C., MR angiography of the carotid bifurcation: artifacts and limitations, *Am. J. Roentgenol.,* Vol. 162, No. 6, pp. 1431–1437, 1994.

19. Yucel, E. K., *Magnetic Resonance Angiography: A Practical Approach*, McGraw-Hill, New York, 1995.

20. Suri, J. S., Liu, K., Reden, L., and Laxminarayan, S., A state-of-the-art review of vascular segmentation algorithms from magnetic resonance angiography data, submitted 2001.

21. Suri, J. S., Singh, S., and Reden, L., Computer vision and pattern recognition techniques for 2-D and 3-D MR cerebral cortical segmentation. I. A state-of-the-art review, to appear in *Int. J. Pattern Anal. Appl.*, Vol. 4, No. 3, Sept. 2001.

22. Suri, J. S., Singh, S., and Reden, L., Fusion of region and boundary/surface-based computer vision & pattern recognition techniques for 2-D and 3-D MR cerebral cortical segmentation. II. A state-of-the-art review, to appear in *Int. J. Pattern Anal. Appl.*, Vol. 4, No. 4, Dec. 2001.

23. Suri, J. S., Setarehdan, S. K., and Singh, S., *Advanced Algorithmic Approaches to Medical Image Segmentation: State-of-the-Art Applications in Cardiology, Neurology, Mammography and Pathology*, first edition, in press, 2001.

24. Wink, O., Niessen, W. J., and Viergever, M. A., Fast delineation and visualization of vessels in 3-D angiographic images, *IEEE Trans. Med. Imag.*, Vol. 19, No. 4, pp. 337–346, 2000.

25. Du, Y. P. and Parker, D. L., Vessel enhancement filtering in three dimensional angiograms using long range signal correlation, *J. Magn. Reson. Imag.*, Vol. 7, No. 2, pp. 447–450, 1997.

26. Sun, Y. and Parker, D. L., Performance analysis of maximum intensity projection algorithm for display of MRA images, *IEEE Trans. Med. Imag.*, Vol. 18, No. 12, pp. 1154–1169, Dec. 1999.

27. Alexander, A. L., Champman, B. E., Tsuruda, J. S., and Parker, D. L., A median filter for 3-D fast spin echo black blood images of cerebral vessel, *Magn. Reson. Med.*, Vol. 43, No. 2, pp. 310–313, 2000.

28. Yu, B. C., Jara, H., Melhem, E. R., Caruthers, S. D., Yucel, E. K., Black-blood MR angiography with GRASE: measurement of flow-induced signal attenuation, *J. Magn. Reson. Imag.*, Vol. 8, pp. 1334–1337, 1998.

29. Alexander, A. L., Busswell, H. R., Sun, Y., et al., Intracranial black-blood MR angiography with high-resolution 3D fast spin echo, *Magn. Reson. Med.*, Vol. 40, pp. 298–310, 1998.

30. Rutt, B. K. and Napel, S., Magnetic Resonance Techniques for Blood-Flow Measurement and Vascular Imaging. *Can. Assoc. Radiologists J.*, Vol. 42; No. 2, pp. 21–30, 1991.

31. Vandermeulen, D., Delaere, D., Suetens, P., Bosmans, H., and Marchal, G., Local filtering and global optimization methods for 3-D MRA image enhancement, in *Proc. Visualization in Biomedical Computing*, pp. 274–288, 1992.

32. Liu, K. and Margosian, P., Utilizing supplementary flow information in dual contrast SIMVA for black-blood MRA, in *Proc. ISMRM 8th Annu. Meeting*, Denver, 2000, p. 1541

33. Liu, K. and Rutt, B. K., Sliding Interleaved kY (SLINKY) Acquisition: a novel 3D TOF MRA technique with suppressed slab boundary artifact, *J. Magn. Reson. Imag.*, Vol. 8, pp. 905–911, 1998.

34. Lin, W., Haacke, E. M., Masaryk, T. J., and Smith, A. S., Automated local maximum-intensity projection with three dimensional vessel tracking, *J. Magn. Reson. Imag.*, Vol. 2, No. 5, pp. 519–526, 1992.

35. Chen, H. and Hale, J., An algorithm for MR angiography image enhancement, *J. Magn. Reson. Imag.*, Vol. 33, No. 4, pp. 534–540, 1995.

36. Chen, H., Li, A., Kaufman, L., and Hale, J., A fast filtering algorithm for image enhancement, *IEEE Trans. Med. Imag.*, Vol. 13, No. 3, pp. 557–564, Sept. 1994.

37. Gerig, G., Kubler, O., and Jolesz, F. A., Nonlinear anisotropic filtering of MRI data, *IEEE Trans. Med. Imag.*, Vol. 11, No. 2, pp. 221–232, 1992.

38. Orkisz, M. M., Bresson, C., Magnin, I. E., Champin, O., and Douek, P. C., Improved vessel visualization in MR angiography by nonlinear anisotropic filtering, *J. Magn. Reson. Med.*, Vol. 37, No. 6, pp. 914–919, 1997.

39. Chen, H. and Hale, J., An algorithm for MR angiography image enhancement, *Magn. Reson. in Med.*, Vol. 33, No. 4, pp. 534–540, 1995.

40. Bezdek, J. C. and Hall, L. O., Review of MR image segmentation techniques using pattern recognition, *Med. Phys.*, Vol. 20, No. 4, pp. 1033–1048, March 1993.

41. Hall, L. O. and Bensaid, A. M., A comparison of neural networks and Fuzzy clustering techniques in segmenting MRI of the brain, *IEEE Trans. Neural Networks*, Vol. 3, No. 5, pp. 672–682, Sept. 1992.

42. Suri, J. S., Liu, K., Reden, L., and Laxminarayan, S., White and black blood volumetric angiographic filtering: ellipsoidal scale-space approach, submitted 2001.

43. Suri, J. S., Liu, K., Reden, L., and Laxminarayan, S., A Revisit of Skeleton vs. Non-Skeleton Approaches for MR and CT Vasculature Segmentation, Internal Report, Philips Medical Systems, Inc., Cleveland, OH, 2001.

44. Suri, J. S., Two dimensional fast MR brain segmentation using a region-based level set approach, *Int. J. Eng. Med. Biol.*, Vol. 20, No. 4, pp. 84–95, July/Aug. 2001.

45. Suri, J. S., Fast WM/GM boundary segmentation from MR images using the relationship between parametric and geometric deformable models, in Suri, Setarehdan, and Singh, Eds., *Advanced Algorithmic Approaches to Medical Image Segmentation: State-of-the-Art Applications in Cardiology, Neurology, Mammography and Pathology*, Dec. 2001, chapter 8.

46. Suri, J. S., Leaking prevention in fast level sets using Fuzzy models: an application in MR brain, *Int. Conf. Information Technology in Biomedicine (ITAB-ITIS)*, pp. 220–226, Nov. 2000.

47. Suri, J. S., White matter/gray matter boundary segmentation using geometric snakes: a Fuzzy deformable model, *Int. Conf. Application in Pattern Recognition (ICAPR)*, Rio de Janeiro, Brazil, March 11–14, 2001.

48. Suri, J. S., Liu, K., Singh, S., Reden, L., and Laximinarayan, S., Shape recovery algorithms using level sets in 2-D/3-D medical imagery: a state-of-the-art review, to appear in *IEEE Trans. Information Technology in Biomedicine (ITB)*, Dec. 2001.

49. Suri, J. S., Wu, D., Reden, L., and Laximinarayan, S., Modeling segmentation issues via partial differential equations, level sets, and geometric deformable models: a revisit, *Int. J. Image and Graphics (IJIG)*, Vol. 1, No. 4, pp. 1–54, Dec. 2001.

50. Suri, J. S., Liu, K., Reden, L., Singh, S., and Laxminarayan, S., Automatic local effect of window/level on 3-D scale-space ellipsoidal filtering on run-off arteries from white blood contrast-enhanced magnetic resonance angiography, *Int. Conf. Pattern Recognition*, 2002.

51. Liu, K., Suri, J. S., and Zhen, X., Recent development of magnet resonance angiography: image segmentation, *Int. Workshop in Angiography Imaging, Signal and Image Processing*, Hawaii, 2002.

52. Edelman, R. R., Mattle, H. P., Wallner, B., Bajkian, R., Kleefied, J., Kent, C., Skillman, J. J., Mendel, J. B., and Atkinson, D. J., Extracranial carotid arteries: evaluation with "black blood" MR angiography, *Radiology*, Vol. 177, No. 1, pp. 45–50, 1990.

53. Edelman, R. R., Chien, D., and Kim, D., Fast selective black blood MR imaging, *Radiology*, Vol. 181, No. 3, pp. 655–660, 1991.

54. Chien, D., Goldmann, A., and Edelman, R. R., High speed black blood imaging of vessel stenosis in the presence of pulsatile flow, *J. Magn. Reson. Imag.*, Vol. 2, No. 4, pp. 437–441, 1992.

55. Toussaint, J. F., Southern, J. F., Foster, V., and Kantor, H. L., T2 contrast for NMR characterization of human atherosclerosis, *Aterioscler Thromb. Vasc. Biol.*, Vol. 15, pp. 1533–1542, 1995.

56. Martin, A. J., Gotlieb, A. I., and Henkelman, R. M., High resolution MR imaging of human arteries, *J. Magn. Reson. Imag.*, Vol. 5, pp. 93–100, 1995.

57. Steinman, D. A. and Rutt, B. K., On the nature and reduction of plaque-mimicking flow artifacts in black blood MRI of the carotid bifurcation, *Magn. Reson. Med.*, Vol. 39, No. 4, pp. 635–641, 1998.

58. De Becker, Jan F. L., Hoogenboom, T. L. M., and Fuderer, M., Method of and device for measuring the velocity of moving matter by means of magnetic resonance, U.S. Patent No. 5,773,975.

59. Mistretta, C. A., Polzin, J. A., and Alley, M. T., Measurement of flow using a complex difference method of magnetic resonance imaging, U.S. Patent No. 5,408,180 (phase-contrast, flow velocity).

60. Doumoulin, C. L., Phase conttrast MR angiography techniques, *Magnetic Resonance Imaging, Clinics of North America*, Vol. 3, pp. 399–411, 1995.

61. Doumoulin, C. L., Souza, S. P., and Walker, M. F., Three-dimensional phase contrast angiography, *Magn. Reson. Med.*, Vol. 9, pp. 139–149, 1989.

62. Bryant, D. J., Payne, J. A., Firmin, D. N., and Longmore, D. B., Measurement of flow with NMR imaging using a gradient pulse and phase difference technique, *J. Comput. Assist. Tomogr.*, Vol. 2, pp. 588–593, 1984.

63. Moran, P. R., A flow velocity zeugmatorgraphic interlace for NMR imaging in humans, *Magn. Reson. Imag.*, Vol. 1, pp. 197–203, 1982.

64. Chien, R. T. and Jacobus, C., Directional derivatives in computer image processing, in *Proc. 3rd Int. Joint Conf. Pattern Recognition*, Coronado, CA, pp. 684–688 1976.

65. Liu, K. and Margosian, P., Multiple contrast fast spin-echo approach to black-blood intracranial MRA: use of complementary and supplementary information, *Mag. Reson. Imag.*, in press.

66. Ogawa, S., Lee, T. M., and Barrere, B., The sensitivity of magnetic resonance image signals of a rat brain to changes in the cerebral venous blood oxygenation. *Magn. Reson. Med.*, Vol. 29, 205–210, 1993.

67. Weisskoff, R. M. and Kiihne, S., MRI susceptometry: image-based measurment of absolute susceptibility of MR contrast agents and human blood, *Magn. Reson. Med.*, Vol. 24, 375–383, 1995.

68. Haack, E. M., Lai, S., Yablonskiy, D. A., and Lin, W., *In vivo* validation of the BOLD mechanism: a review of signal change in gradient echo functional

MRI in the presence of flow, *J. Imaging Systems and Technol.*, Vol 6, 153–163, 1995.

69. Wang, Y., Yu, Y., Li, D., Bae, K. T., Brown, J. J., Lin, W., and Haacke, E. M., Artery and vein separation using susceptibility-dependent phase in contrast enhanced MRA, *J. Magn. Reson. Imag.*, Vol. 12, 661–670, 2000.

70. Frangi, A. F., Niessen, W. J., Hoogeveen, R. M., van Walsum, Th., and Viergever, M. A., Model-based quantification of 3-D magnetic resonance angiographic images, *IEEE Trans. Med. Imag.*, Vol. 18, No. 10, pp. 946–956, Oct. 1999.

71. Frangi, A. F., Niessen, W. J., Nederkoorn, P. J., Elgersma, O. E. H., and Viergever, M. A., Three-dimensional model-based stenosis quantification of the carotid arteries from contrast-enhance MR angiography, *IEEE Workshop of Mathematical Methods in Biomedical Image Analysis (MMBIA)*, pp. 110–118, 2000.

72. Frangi, A. F., Niessen, W. J., Hoogeveen, R. M., van Walsum, Th., and Viergever, M. A., Quantitation of vessel morphology from 3D MRA, in *Medical Image Computing and Computer-Assisted Intervention—MICCAI'99*, Taylor, C. & Colchester, A., Eds., *Lecture Notes in Computer Science*, Springer-Verlag, Berlin, Vol. 1679, pp. 358–367, 1999.

73. Frangi, A. F., Niessen, W. J., Vincken, K. L., and Viergever, M. A., Multiscale vessel enhancement filtering, in *Medical Image Computing and Computer-Assisted Intervention—MICCAI'98*, Wells, W. M., Colchester, A., and Delp, S., Eds., *Lecture Notes in Computer Science*, Springer-Verlag, Berlin, Vol. 1496, pp. 130–137, 1998.

74. Lee, C. K., Automated Boundary Tracing Using Temporal Information, Ph.D. thesis, Department of Electrical Engineering, University of Washington, Seattle, 1994.

75. Sheehan, F. H., Haralick, R. M., Suri, J. S., and Shao, Y., U.S. Patent No. 5,734,739, Method for Determining the Contour of an *In Vivo* Organ Using Multiple Image Frames of the Organ, March 1998.

76. Zavaljevski, A., Dhawan, A. P., Gaskil, M., Ball, W., and Johnson, J. D., Multi-level adaptive segmentation of multi-parameter MR brain images, *Comput. Med. Imag. Graph.*, Vol. 24, No. 2, pp. 87–98, Mar.–April 2000.

77. Johnson, R. A. and Wichern, D. W., *Applied Multivariate Statistical Analysis*, Prentice Hall, 1982.

78. Wells III, W. M., Grimson, W. E. L., Kikinis, R., and Jolesz, F. A., Adaptive segmentation of MRI data, *IEEE Trans. Med. Imag.*, Vol. 15, No. 4, pp. 429–442, Aug. 1992.

79. Gerig, G., Kubler, O., and Jolesz, F. A., Nonlinear anisotropic filtering of MRI data, *IEEE Trans. Med. Imag.*, Vol. 11, No. 2, pp. 221–232, 1992.

80. Joshi, M., Cui, J., Doolittle, K., Joshi, S., Van Essen, D., Wang, L., and Miller, M. I., Brain segmentation and the generation of cortical surfaces, *Neuroimage*, Vol. 9, No. 5, pp. 461–476, 1999.

81. Dempster, A. D., Laird, N. M., and Rubin, D. B., Maximum likelihood from incomplete data via the EM algorithm, *J. R. Stat. Soc.*, Vol. 39, pp. 1–37, 1977.

82. Kao, Y.-H., Sorenson, J. A., Bahn, M. M., and Winkler, S. S., Dual-echo MRI segmentation using vector decomposition and probability technique: a two tissue model, *Magn. Reson. Med.*, Vol. 32, No. 3, pp. 342–357, 1994.

83. Lindeberg, T., Scale-space for discrete signals, *IEEE Pattern Analysis and Machine Intelligence*, Vol. 12, No. 3, pp. 234–254, 1990.

84. Lindeberg, T., On scale selection for differential operators, *Proc. 8th Scandinavian Conf. Image Analysis (SCIA)*, pp. 857–866, 1993.

85. Lindeberg, T., Detecting salient blob-like image structures and their scales with a scale-space primal sketch: a method for focus of attention, *Int. J. Computer Vision*, Vol. 11, No. 3, pp. 283–318, 1993.

86. Lindeberg, T., Edge detection and ridge detection with automatic scale selection, in *Proc. of Computer Vision and Pattern Recognition*, pp. 465–470, 1996.

87. Lindeberg, T., Feature detection with automatic scale-space selection, *Int. J. Computer Vision*, Vol. 30, No. 2, pp. 79–116, 1998.

88. Lindeberg, T., *Scale-Space Theory in Computer Vision*, Kluwer Academic, 1994.

89. Lindeberg, T., Discrete derivative approximations with scale-space properties: a basis for low-level feature extraction, *J. Mathematical Imaging and Vision*, Vol. 3, No. 4, pp. 349–376, 1993.

90. Schanze, T., Sinc interpolation of discrete periodic signals, *IEEE Trans. Signal Processing*, Vol. 43, No. 6, pp. 1502–1503, June 1995.

91. Yaroslavsky, L. P., Signal sinc-interpolation: a fast computer algorithm, *Bioimaging*, Vol. 4, pp. 225–231, 1996.

92. Yaroslavsky, L. P., Efficient algorithm for discrete sinc-interpolation, *Appl. Opt.*, Vol. 36, No. 2, pp. 460–463, Jan. 1997.

93. Candocia F. M. and Principe, J. C., Comments on sinc interpolation of discrete periodic signals, *IEEE Trans. Signal Processing*, Vol. 46, No. 7, pp. 2044–2047, July 1998.

94. Sato, Y., Westin C.-F., Bhalerao, A., Nakajima, S., Tamura, S., and Kikinis, R., Tissue classification based on 3-D local intensity structures for volume rendering, *IEEE Trans. Visualization and Computer Graphics*, Vol. 8, No. 2, pp. 160–180, April–June, 2000.

95. Kober, V., Unser, M., and Yaroslavsky, L. P., Spline and sinc signal interpolations in image geometrical transforms, *Proc. SPIE Fifth Int. Workshop on Digital Image Processing and Computer Graphics (DIP'94)*, Samara, Russia, Vol. 2363, pp. 152–156, August 23–26, 1994.

96. Parker, J. A., Kenyon, R. V., and Troxel, D. E., Comparison of interpolating methods for image resampling, *IEEE Trans. Med. Imag.*, Vol. 2, No. 1, pp. 31–39, March 1983.

97. Hylton, N. M., Simovsky, I., Li, A. J., and Hale, J. D., Impact of section doubling on MR angiography, *Radiology*, Vol. 185, No. 3, pp. 899–902, Dec. 1992.

98. Du, Y. P., Parker, D. L., Davis, W. L., and Cao, G., Reduction of partial-volume artifacts using zero-filled interpolation in three-dimensional MR angiography, *J. Magn. Reson. Imag.*, Vol. 4, No. 5, pp. 733–741, 1994.

99. Chapman, B. E., Goodrick, K. C., Alexander, A. L., Blatter, D. D., and Parker, D. L., Two alternative forced choice evaluations of vessel visibility increases due to zero-filled interpolation in MR angiography, in *Proc. 15th Int. Conf. Information Processing in Medical Imaging, (LNCS)*, Springer-Verlag, Berlin, Vol. 1230, pp. 543–548, 1997.

100. Press, W. H., Flannery, B. P., Teukolsky, S. A., and Vetterling, W. T., *Numerical Recipes in C*, Cambridge University Press, 1988.

5

Segmentation of Retinal Fundus Vasculature in Nonmydriatic Camera Images Using Wavelets

Roberto M. Cesar, Jr. and Herbert F. Jelinek

CONTENTS

5.1 Introduction

Diabetes and its associated complications, including diabetic retinopathy (DR), have been identified as a significant growing global public health problem [1]. Within this context, an important step toward reducing the number of individuals seriously affected by diabetic retinopathy is to simplify the procedure used to diagnose the condition and ensure that early eye examinations become routine for diabetic patients [1–3]. However, large population screening, especially in rural and remote areas, is difficult because of the geographical and economic isolation associated with the cost of visits to specialists and the lack of ophthalmologists available [4, 5]. Studies that trialed nonspecialist health workers in identifying diabetic eye disease have shown that correct identification is no better than random in all cases tested (50) and for identifying earlier stages of proliferation [6]. Introducing a simple and economical means to quantitatively assess the health status of the optic fundus while visiting rural and remote communities would provide support to health workers not specialized in identification of optic fundus pathology and timely, on-the-spot feedback to the individuals being assessed.

Due to the characteristics associated with wavelets, they provide an ideal means to segment vessels of the optic fundus [7, 8]. Previous work using mathematical morphology and describing optic fundus analysis has concentrated on using fluorescein angiograms and identifying the optic disk and "red-spots" in the fundus [9, 10]. Blood vessels in the optic fundus are a complex network of branches that spread out from the optic disk to provide nutrients and oxygen to the fundus. The macula, which is the area of greatest visual acuity, is devoid of blood vessels. In proliferative retinopathy, new blood vessels are formed that emerge from the area of the optic disk and spread toward the macula or emerge from peripheral vessels [11]. To assess this increase in complexity of the vessel patterns, fractal analysis has been successfully applied on fluorescein angiograms [4, 6]. Nonmydriatic images obtained by either scanning Polaroid or 30-mm SLR camera photographs used most often by community health workers present a special problem for segmentation as the resolution is much less and the quality of the images is not always optimal.

This chapter reports on the development of a software tool for community health workers in rural and remote areas for assessing the ocular fundus of diabetics using nonmydriatic cameras. In particular, the use of automated segmentation of nonmydriatic retinal fundus images and vessel pattern analysis is described.

We start by describing some background material from previous approaches in Section 5.2. Section 5.3 describes the image segmentation method based on the wavelet transform. A previous version of the wavelet-based segmentation technique is described in [8]. Our approach for performance assessment of the segmentation technique is described in Section 5.4, and the experimental results obtained by the introduced framework are presented and discussed in Sections 5.5 and 5.6, respectively. The perspectives for future developments of the topics herein described are discussed in the final chapter of this book.

5.2 Bibliographical Background

5.2.1 Automated Isolation of Morphological and Pathological Features in the Fundus

Diabetic retinopathy screening involves the assessment of the optic fundus, concentrating on a number of features that indicate fundus pathology [11]. Previous investigations into automated segmentation of the optic fundus have concentrated on identifying small vessel leakage (microaneurysms) associated with early stages of diabetic eye disease. Because the number of microaneurysms identified is a good indicator of disease progression, these types of automated screening procedures can be very successful in the community [9, 10, 14, 15]. Neovascularization is a feature that is associated with more advanced diabetic retinopathy, characterized by new vessel growth in the fundus and eventually leading to blindness without treatment (Kanski, 1989). The important aspect of automated vessel identification is that it provides clinically relevant data by being sensitive to the presence of new vessels in the fundus. Automated procedures are not required to segment the smallest vessels that can be visually identified, but new vessel growth that is clinically significant and requires attention. Vessel segmentation of fundus vessels using fluorescein has been reported by various research groups [8, 15, 16]. Such approaches have explored different image processing techniques as steerable filters and Hough transform [17], improved thresholding [18], user interaction [19], matched filters [20], and mathematical morphology [16]. Additional research has also focused on detection of blood leakage within the optic disk [21] and registration of temporal images [22].

5.2.2 Assessment of Vessel Branching Pattern Complexity

Combining automated segmentation procedures to isolate the vessel pattern in the fundus with a pool of morphological descriptors that identify several different attributes of branching patterns can provide a clinically useful index for the classification of neovascularization. A number of mathematical techniques have been reported to measure the vessel branching complexity of fluorescein angiograms [3–6, 24]. However, the outcome of these studies is not useful for the analysis of images obtained using nonmydriatic cameras by nonspecialists, as vessels were provided by ophthalmology clinics as angiograms and hand-drawn prior to analysis [26–28].

The medical community has paid increasing attention to shape analysis, with special attention focused on signal processing techniques to analyze shape (e.g., tumor) and temporal (e.g., heart rate variability) signals [29]. For example, Fourier descriptors and wavelets have been successfully applied to two-dimensional shape analysis. In particular, the wavelet transform is widely explored because of its nice scaling properties, which can be used to focus the analyzing tools on shape structures occurring at different scales. Furthermore, differential mother wavelets (e.g., the derivatives of the Gaussian [30]) are also intensively used because some of the main shape features commonly extracted are based on differential measures (e.g., curvature and torsion).

5.3 Image Segmentation Using Wavelets

The wavelet transform is a mathematical tool that has been developed and applied in very different fields such as signal and image processing, astronomy, medicine, and finances, to name but a few [30–32]. This chapter discusses the technique introduced in [8] for segmentation of blood vessels of fundus images using the two-dimensional wavelet transform, and introduces some of the main concepts related to the two-dimensional wavelet transform following the notation used in [30].

5.3.1   Preprocessing

There are different ways of obtaining the ocular fundus image, such as with nonmydiatric cameras or through angiograms [33]. Nonmydiatric cameras generally provide color images and, because the technique developed by Leandro et al. [8] applies to angiogram gray-level images, they need to be properly converted. Another important difference between these two modalities regards resolution, that is, nonmydiatric images capured with Polaroid or SLR cameras generally present lower resolution than angiograms captured with digital equipment, as illustrated in Figure 5.1, which shows an angiogram, and Figure 5.2(a), which shows a nonmydiatric image.

The nonmydriatic color image was converted to gray scale and inverted (i.e., black is converted to white). This inversion in the gray levels was performed so that the vessels, which are darker than the background in the color image, became lighter than the background in the corresponding gray-scale version.

All images were then scaled to a common size so that the same imaging parameters, such as window sizes, could be equally applied to different images. In our implementation, the resizing procedure was applied so that the larger side of the original image becomes 1024 pixels. The other (smaller)

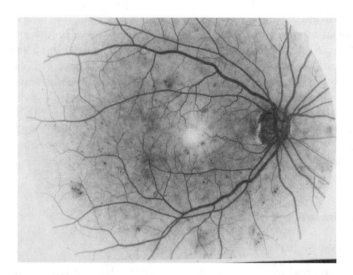

FIGURE 5.1
Example retina angiographic image.

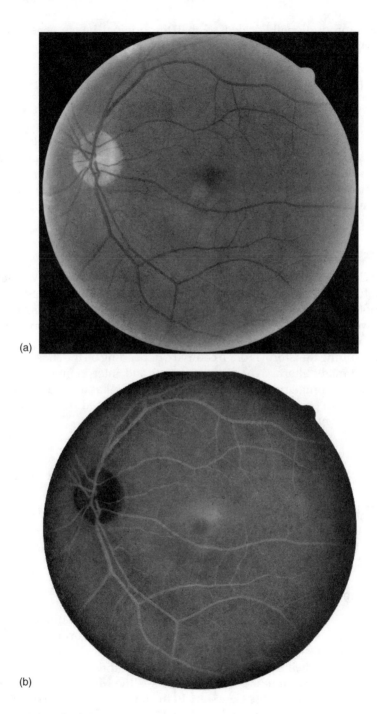

(a)

(b)

FIGURE 5.2 (See color insert.)
(a) Original nonmydiatric image, and (b) gray-scale inverted version.

side was proportionally scaled so that the original image aspect ratio is preserved.

5.3.2 The Wavelet Transform

The gray-level image can be seen as a function $f(x, y)$, $(x, y) \in \mathbf{R}^2$, where $\mathbf{R}^2 = \mathbf{R} \times \mathbf{R}$ denotes the real plane. Formally, the image $f(x, y)$ is represented as a square integrable (i.e., finite energy) function defined over $\mathbf{R}^2$, which is denoted as $f \in L^2$ [31]. We also denote two-dimensional points in the real plane as bold letters (e.g., $\mathbf{x} = (x, y)$). Therefore, we denote $f(\mathbf{x})$ as a gray-level image. The continuous wavelet transform of a two-dimensional signal $f(\mathbf{x})$ can be defined as:

$$W_\psi(\mathbf{b}, \theta, a) = C_\psi^{-1/2} \frac{1}{a} \int \psi^*(a^{-1} r_{-\theta}(\mathbf{x} - \mathbf{b})) f(\mathbf{x}) d^2\mathbf{x}$$

where C, ψ, $\mathbf{b}$, θ, and a are the normalizing constant, the mother wavelet, the translation vector, the rotation angle, and the dilation parameter, respectively. ψ^* denotes the complex conjugate of the mother wavelet ψ, which is a function that is well-localized in the space and frequency domains and always has zero mean (i.e., null DC component) [31].

The resulting transform is often complex, depending on the chosen wavelet. There are many alternatives for visualizing and interpreting the obtained wavelet transform, and the reader is referred to [34] as a good reference on this subject. In particular, the transform can be analyzed from its modulus-phase representation:

$$W_\psi(\mathbf{b}, \theta, a) = M(\mathbf{b}, \theta, a) e^{i\Phi(\mathbf{b}, \theta, a)} \tag{5.1}$$

with

$$M(\mathbf{b}, \theta, a) = |W_\psi(\mathbf{b}, \theta, a)| \quad \text{and} \quad \Phi(\mathbf{b}, \theta, a) = \arg(W_\psi(\mathbf{b}, \theta, a)) \tag{5.2}$$

where $|z|$ and $\arg(z)$ denote the modulus and argument of the complex number $z \in \mathbf{C}$.

5.3.3 Choosing the Right Mother Wavelet

One of the main advantages of the wavelet transform is that different mother wavelets can be adopted, depending on the kind of information to be extracted from the signal. For example, whenever signal singularities have to be detected and their scaling properties analyzed, different wavelets should be employed. An example of such wavelets is the Mexican hat, defined as the second derivative of the Gaussian. In the image processing context, such wavelets are commonly explored for edge detection [35] and multi-scale pyramid formation [36]. In fact, it can be shown that any derivative of the Gaussian can be used as a valid wavelet. For example, the first partial derivatives of the Gaussian, denoted as g_x and g_y, can be used to define mother wavelets, with the respective wavelet transforms denoted as W_{g_x} and W_{g_y}. These transforms allow the creation of a wavelet gradient ∇_W, which has been used for multi-fractal analysis [30]. The wavelet transform for each surface point is actually a vector whose components are the respective wavelet coefficients using g_x and g_y as the mother wavelets.

On the other hand, it is well-known in the literature that local frequency analysis can be better performed by the Morlet wavelet, sometimes also called the Gabor wavelet [37], which can be efficiently tuned to specific frequencies [31, 38]. This property allows the application of this wavelet to detect specific image structures of interest while leaving out undesirable artifacts such as noise. This capability is especially important in filtering out the background noise of the fundus images while detecting the vessels. Furthermore, the Morlet wavelet is known to be directional, in the sense of being effective in selecting orientations. These characteristics of the Morlet wavelet represent its advantages with respect to other standard filters such as the Gaussian and its derivatives. The two-dimensional Morlet wavelet is defined as:

$$\psi_M(\mathbf{x}) = \exp(j\mathbf{k}_0\mathbf{x})\exp\left(-\frac{1}{2}\|A\mathbf{x}\|^2\right)$$

where $j = \sqrt{-1}$ and

$$A = \begin{bmatrix} \epsilon^{-1/2} & 0 \\ 0 & 1 \end{bmatrix}, \quad \epsilon >= 1$$

is an array that defines the anisotropy of the filter, that is, its elongation in a given direction [31]. In other words, the larger ϵ is, the more elongated is the mother wavelet along the x-axis with respect to the y-axis. By varying the rotation parameter θ of the wavelet transform (Equation 5.2), it is possible to orient the elongated wavelet in any desirable direction.

The Morlet wavelet is a complex exponential multiplying a two-dimensional Gaussian, where $\mathbf{k}_0$ is a vector that defines the frequency of the complex exponential in the x- and in the y-directions; that is:

$$\mathbf{k}_0 = \begin{bmatrix} k_x \\ k_y \end{bmatrix}$$

The Morlet wavelet is shown in Figure 5.3a as a surface and in Figure 5.3b as an image. Because this wavelet is represented on a complex number plane, only the real part is shown.

The role played by the wavelet parameters is illustrated in Figure 5.4a–d. When the frequency parameter k_y is increased, the number of wavelet oscillations in the y-direction is also increased, as shown in Figure 5.4a and b, for two larger values of k_y. The effect of changing the elongation parameter is illustrated in Figure 5.4c and d for $\epsilon = 1$ (no elongation) and $\epsilon = 10$ (much more elongated), respectively.

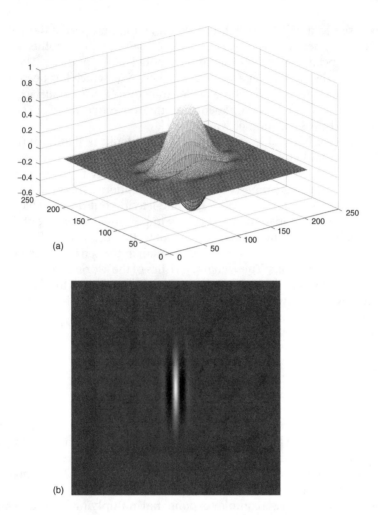

FIGURE 5.3
Morlet wavelet shown as a surface in (a) and as an image in (b).

Figure 5.5a–d illustrates the Morlet wavelets under the effect of varying the wavelet transform scale and rotation parameters a and θ. The size of the mother wavelet is changed by varying the scale parameter a, as shown in Figure 5.5a and b, while its orientation is determined by the rotation parameter, as illustrated in Figure 5.5c and d. It is clear from these considerations that the parameters can be configured in different ways to make the wavelet suitable for analyzing image structures of different shapes, which is explored by the segmentation algorithm explained below.

To apply the Morlet wavelet to detect blood vessels in fundus images, the parameter ϵ was set as a large value (41 in our implementation) to make the

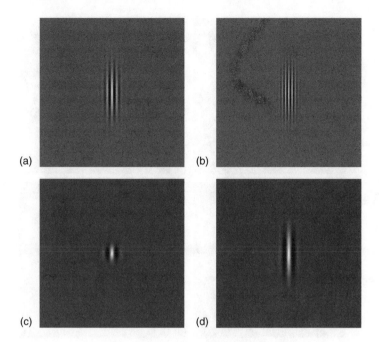

FIGURE 5.4
Morlet wavelet shown for two different frequencies in (a) and (b); and for two different elongations in (c) and (d).

filter elongated. Furthermore, we set

$$\mathbf{k}_0 = \begin{bmatrix} k_x \\ k_y \end{bmatrix} = \begin{bmatrix} 0 \\ 1 \end{bmatrix}$$

That is, a low frequency complex exponential with few significant oscillations. This configuration was chosen so that the transform presents stronger responses for the coefficients associated with the blood vessels.

5.3.4 Detection of Vessels Using Morlet Wavelets

The wavelet transform (Equation 5.2) is defined as a function of the parameters $\mathbf{b}$, θ, and a, and it is important to understand the role played by each parameter in detecting vessels in a fundus image. The translation parameter $\mathbf{b}$ is responsible for shifting the mother wavelet throughout the image and is therefore important in detecting the vessels that may appear anywhere in the image. By varying the orientation parameter θ, an anisotropic mother wavelet selects structures in different orientations. The scale parameter a is important in tuning the wavelet size to the vessel's structure: too large a scale implies that only thick vessels are detected, whereas too small a scale leads to a large amount of false vessels (i.e., noise) detected.

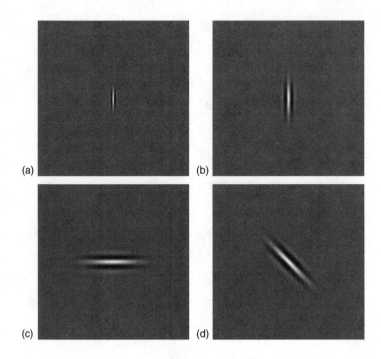

FIGURE 5.5
Morlet wavelet shown for two different scales in (a) and (b); and for two different orientations in (c) and (d).

To detect the blood vessels, the scale and angle parameters (a and θ, respectively) were kept fixed for some *a priori* defined values $a = a_0$ and $\theta = \theta_0$, with the resulting wavelet transform being represented as a two-dimensional function defined in Equation 5.3 (the so-called *position representation* [31]):

$$W_\psi(\mathbf{b}) = C_\psi^{-1/2} \frac{1}{a_0} \int \psi^* \left(a_0^{-1} r_{-\theta_0}(\mathbf{x} - \mathbf{b}) \right) f(\mathbf{x}) d^2\mathbf{x} \qquad (5.3)$$

The transform $W_\psi(\mathbf{b})$ is able to detect vessels oriented at the angle direction θ_0, which can be better understood by observing the resulting $|W_\psi(\mathbf{b})|$ of Figure 5.6, which was obtained from the retina image of Figure 5.2b for $\theta = 0°$. As can be seen, the horizontally oriented vessel segments have been detected by the Morlet wavelet. Figure 5.6b–d shows the analogous results for $\theta = -30°$, $-60°$ and $-90°$, respectively. To segment the blood vessels, the scale parameter was held constant and a series of transforms was calculated for a set of orientations $\theta = 0, 10, 20, 30, \ldots, 180°$. We label these transforms as $W_{\psi,0}(\mathbf{b})$, $W_{\psi,10}(\mathbf{b})$, $\ldots$, $W_{\psi,180}(\mathbf{b})$, respectively.

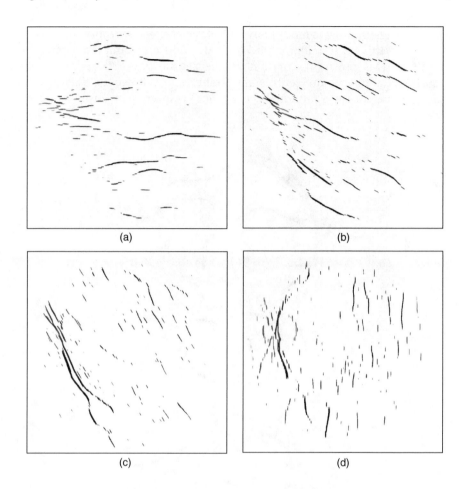

FIGURE 5.6
Wavelet transform of the image in Figure 5.2b calculated using four different wavelets (a–d) with different rotation angles, thus detecting vessels with different orientations.

5.3.5 All Together Now: The Segmentation Algorithm

The last section demonstrated that the transforms $W_{\psi, \theta_0}(\mathbf{b})$, $\theta_0 = 0, 10, ..., 180$ presented stronger responses where the vessels have the same orientation of θ_0. Therefore, if the input image has a vessel at a given position, say $(\mathbf{b}_0)$, locally oriented at a given angle, say $20°$, then $W_{\psi, 20}(\mathbf{b}_0)$ has a strong response, generally larger than the response for all other orientation angles at that position; that is:

$$|W_{\psi, 20}(\mathbf{b}_0)| \geq |W_{\psi, \theta_0}(\mathbf{b}_0)|, \quad \theta_0 = 0, 10, ..., 180, \quad \theta_0 \neq 20$$

This idea was explored by the algorithm to detect all vessels at all orientations. The transforms $W_{\psi, \theta_0}(\mathbf{b})$, $\theta_0 = 0, 10, ..., 180°$ were calculated and the maximum coefficient (in modulus) of the wavelet at each position was taken. We denote this representation as $W_{\psi,\theta_{max}}(\mathbf{b})$, and an example is shown in Figure 5.7. This new representation emphasizes the wavelet response for the vessels in the fundus image. It is important to note, however, that $W_{\psi,\theta_0}(\mathbf{b})$ may present non-zero (although very weak) responses at positions where

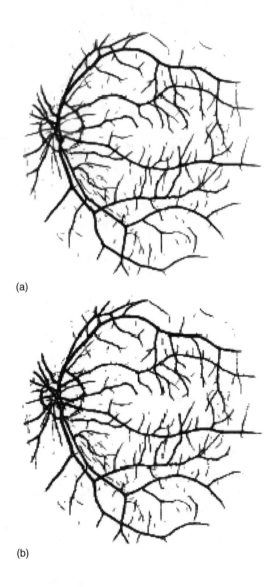

(a)

(b)

FIGURE 5.7
(a) Shows $W_{\psi,\theta_{max}}(\mathbf{b})$ calculated from the image in Figure 5.2b (see also Figure 5.6) while (b) shows the respective adaptive thresholding result.

there are no vessels. To avoid noise due to this, such small coefficients are set to zero. The blood vessels can then be detected by properly segmenting $W_{\psi, \theta_{max}}(\mathbf{b})$, and the framework can be summarized by the Algorithm 1.

ALGORITHM 1 *Algorithm for Blood Vessel Segmentation*

> Set $W_{\psi, \theta_{max}}(\mathbf{b}) = 0$, $\forall \mathbf{b}$
> **for all** $\theta_0 = 0, 10, 20, 30, ..., 180$ **do**
> > Calculate $W_{\psi, \theta_0}(\mathbf{b})$
> > Shrinkage $(W_{\psi, \theta_0}(\mathbf{b}))$
> > Set $W_{\psi, \theta_{max}}(\mathbf{b}) = \max(W_{\psi, \theta_{max}}(\mathbf{b}), W_{\psi, \theta_0}(\mathbf{b}))$
> **end for**
> Find the blood vessels by segmenting $W_{\psi, \theta_{max}}(\mathbf{b})$
> Apply the postprocessing procedures

The *shrinkage* function inside the **for** loop of Algorithm 1 was carried out in order to set the noise coefficients with weak response to 0. This operation is commonly referred to as shrinkage in the wavelet literature [39] (thus the function name) and, in our implementation it was carried out with the help of the adaptive thresholding algorithm explained below.

Different image segmentation algorithms were assessed during the development of the present method, namely, thresholding, adaptive thresholding, edge detection, and semi-interactive region-growing [40, 41]. The adaptive thresholding, adapted from [41], performed best in our experiments and was incorporated into the framework.

Adaptive thresholding is obtained by comparing the value of each position $\mathbf{b}$ with $m - c$, where m is the mean value around b and c is a constant introduced to avoid noisy segmentation along uniform background regions. The size of the neighborhood where the mean value is calculated is an input parameter, together with a small 5×5 window. Wavelet coefficients larger than $m - c$ were associated with blood vessels, while those smaller were considered background.

It is worth emphasizing that the adaptive thresholding technique is applied twice in the above algorithm: (1) in setting the small coefficients of $W_{\psi, \theta_0}(\mathbf{b})$ to zero inside the **for** loop; and (2) in segmenting $W_{\psi, \theta_{max}}(\mathbf{b})$ to detect the fundus vessels.

5.3.6 Postprocessing Phase

Algorithm 1 indicates, as its last step, a postprocessing phase where noise is eliminated from the thresholded transform and the final skeleton of the vessel's branching pattern is obtained. This postprocessing phase, carried out using only binary images, consisted of the following sequence of mathematical morphology operations [40, 41]:

- *Area open*: to remove small objects whose area is less than a given threshold
- *Closing*: to smooth the vessel boundary and minimize the occurrence of small spurious skeleton branches
- *Skeletonization*: to obtain the skeleton (one pixel wide connected structure) of the vessels

These operations have been applied using the Morphology Toolbox [42] and the respective results can be seen in Figure 5.8a and b and Figure 5.9.

5.4   Assessing the Segmentation Results

An important issue regarding the segmentation procedure is how to validate it to assess its feasibility. Clearly, a straightforward way to analyze the segmentation results is by visual inspection. Our segmented images were assessed by clinical specialists who indicated a relatively good fit of the segmented images with the originals.

Despite the importance of such inspection by experts, it is important to devise a methodology to objectively assess the segmentation results based on quantitative measures. Such a methodology is important because it can be applied multiple times and in large scale. Furthermore, it is important to have nonsubjective parameters to draw conclusions about the effectiveness of the segmentation procedure.

Our approach to solve this problem was to compare the wavelets-based segmentation with the corresponding segmentation produced by a human expert. A set of fundus images was segmented by an expert who simply traced the vessels over the images. This set of segmented images can be considered the standard for the assessment framework; that is, the wavelet segmentation should be as similar as possible to the hand-drawn vessels.

To assess how similar each pair of segmented images (i.e., wavelet and hand-drawn segmented) were, a set of shape features was extracted to compose feature vectors used to compare the two groups of segmented vessels. There are several different shape features that can be used [29]; how to choose which are more suitable for each situation is beyond the scope of this chapter. Based on previous experience and on the literature regarding retinal image analysis, the following features have been chosen:

- Area
- Perimeter
- Circularity
- Wavelet entropy
- Correlation dimension

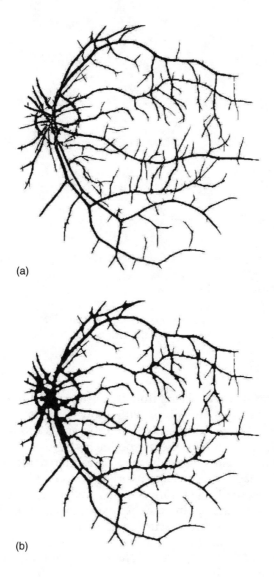

(a)

(b)

FIGURE 5.8
Results of the morphological postprocessing steps from the image in Figure 5.7b: (a) area opening; (b) closing.

The feature values have been normalized to have zero mean and unitary standard deviation. This normalization, commonly referred to as normal transformation [29], allows the comparison between distinct features, such as area, entropy, and fractal dimension. Standard shape features area, perimeter, and circularity have been described in [29]. The wavelet entropy and the correlation dimension are explained in the following subsections.

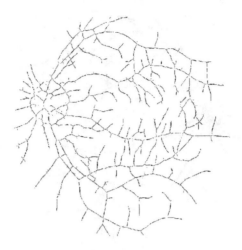

FIGURE 5.9
Continued from Figure 5.8: skeletonization.

Box-counting fractal dimension has also been calculated to compare our results with previously published data, as mentioned in Section 5.5.

5.4.1 Wavelet Entropy

The statistical measures extracted from the histogram of blurred binary images (i.e., binary images convolved with a low-pass filter) have been used for characterizing shape complexity, including applications involving psychophysical experiments [43]. These experiments have used Gaussian convolution as a means of blurring the image to characterize the spatial coverage property of the shape, which is an important concept related to shape complexity (see, for example, [44, 45]). To better understand the role played by such measures, note that an initially binary image (e.g., fundus segmented image where black pixels represent the vessels and white pixels the background) presents a histogram with two peaks corresponding to these extreme gray levels (black and white). The process of blurring the image by Gaussian convolution introduces new gray levels in the original binary image implied by weighted sums among black and white pixels. Now, spatial coverage properties of the vessels network lead to large background regions partially traversed by vessels being blurred by the Gaussian filter (note that the background regions not reached by the vessels are homogeneously white and therefore unchanged by blurring). Therefore, the greater the capacity of the vessel network to fill the surrounding background area, the more the initial binary histogram would spread, the limit being a uniform histogram. The aforementioned statistical measures (especially the entropy and second statistical moment) reflect the spread of the histograms. This same principle is applied to the wavelet measure introduced in this section.

Recently, the use of statistical measures has been extended to include shape measures extracted from the wavelet transform [46]. We extended these features in the experiments reported in this chapter using the entropy of the wavelet coefficients as a new shape measure to characterize the vessels branching pattern. Let p_i be the histogram of the coefficients of the wavelet transform modulus $|W_\psi(\mathbf{b}, \theta_0, a)|$, for fixed orientation and scale a_0 and θ_0, that is, p_i is the relative frequency of the modulus values around i, which represent the bin centers for calculating the histogram. The wavelet entropy is defined as:

$$E = -\sum_i p_i \ln(p_i)$$

The two-dimensional wavelets present a stronger response at the image edges, which, in the present case, correspond to the vessels. Furthermore, because of the local support of the wavelets, there is a direct influence of the interaction between edges on the wavelet responses. Therefore, the wavelet coefficients are related to a measure of spatial coverage of the cell: the more the vessels fill their surrounding area, the more the corresponding wavelet coefficients histogram will spread, as explained above for the blurred image histogram.

5.4.2 Correlation Dimension

We have also explored the correlation dimension as a complexity measure as explained in [7]. This procedure leads to a graph $C(\epsilon)$ from which a log-log plot-based line fitting is able to estimate the correlation dimension [7].

A key issue for most fractal analysis problems is how to calculate the log-log slope, mainly because of the limited fractality of objects found in nature and represented by digital images [29, 48].

Different approaches have been implemented, such as an *a priori* definition of range to fit the line or multi-scale differentiation of the log-log plot [49]. We have developed a new approach for estimating the correlation dimension slope by taking the wavelet transform of the log-log plot using the third derivative of the Gaussian as mother wavelet.

The basic idea underlying this method is that the log-log plot experimentally obtained often presents three main segments [29]. The first segment is associated with a too small analyzing scale, where the shape does not present fractal behavior such as self-similar construction rules; that is, the image resolution is not sufficient to capture the fractal structure. The dimension in this portion tends to 1. The intermediary portion is associated to scales where the shape can be perceived as a fractal structure. The dimension in this intermediary portion is generally larger than 1. Finally, the third segment corresponds to too large scales (indeed, larger than the whole shape itself), and the object is perceived as point, presenting dimension equal to zero.

The log-log plot can be differentiated to detect the different line segments. The first derivative of the log-log plot actually shows the slope of each line segment composing it, while the second derivative presents local maxima at the slope breakpoints; that is, the extremities of the segments. Instead of looking for such maxima points, it is possible to search for the zero-crossings of the third derivative.

It is known that such numerical differentiation of signals can be carried out by the wavelet transform in which each slope breakpoint is taken as a singularity [32, 35]. In this case, the most suitable wavelets are the derivatives of the Gaussian [30] in the sense that the wavelet transform of a signal using the nth derivative of the Gaussian as mother wavelet is related to the nth derivative of a smoothed version of the signal. To apply the wavelet transform, a signal must be formed from the log-log plot, which will be denoted as $\gamma(t)$, where:

$$\gamma = \log(C)$$

and

$$t = \log(\epsilon)$$

The one-dimensional wavelet transform of $\gamma(t)$ is defined as:

$$W_\psi(b, a) = \frac{1}{a} \int \psi^* \left(\frac{t - b}{a} \right) \gamma(t) \, dt$$

$$= \frac{1}{2\pi} \int \widehat{\psi}^*(a\omega) \, \widehat{\gamma}(\omega) \, e^{ib\omega} \, d\omega \tag{5.4}$$

where $b \in \mathbf{R}$ is the translation parameter, $a > 0$ is the dilation parameter, and the hat denotes the Fourier transform (e.g., $\widehat{\psi}(\omega)$ is the Fourier transform of $\psi(t)$). Similar to the two-dimensional case of Equation 5.2, $\psi(t)$ denotes the mother wavelet, which must have a null DC component, as stated by the simplified admissibility condition [38].

In the present case, we want to explore $\psi(t)$ as the third derivative of the Gaussian, which can be more easily expressed in Fourier domain by the application of the wavelet transform of Equation 5.4. Let $g(t)$ denote the Gaussian function:

$$g(t) = e^{-t^2/2}$$

The nth derivative of the Gaussian can be expressed in the Fourier domain as:

$$g^{(n)}(t) = \frac{d^n g(t)}{dt^n} \quad \Leftrightarrow \quad \widehat{g}^{(n)}(\omega) = (i\omega)^n \widehat{g}(\omega) \tag{5.5}$$

where $\widehat{g}(\omega)$ denotes the Fourier transform of the Gaussian. Equation 5.5 is defined by the application of the Fourier derivative property to $\widehat{g}(\omega)$ [29].

Our approach considers two ways of estimating the slope, local (based on a series of line segments) and global (based on fitting the line to the middle portion of the log-log plot), both based on wavelet zero-crossings. A simple example will now be considered to bring some insight to this new approach. Figure 5.10a shows a log-log plot obtained for a triadic Koch curve, with the corresponding wavelet transform for a fixed scale a_0 being shown in Figure 5.10b.

Once a line segment is determined by its extremities, corresponding to a pair of consecutive zero-crossings, the initial and last segments of the log-log plot can be determined from the wavelet transform. Therefore, we fit a line to the middle portion of the log-log plot by excluding the initial and final segments, in order to exclude the aforementioned non-fractal scales (see Figure 5.10c). These segments are defined to be to the left of the first zero-crossing and to the right of the last zero-crossing.

5.5 Experimental Results

As nonmydriatic images capture less of the optic fundus compared to fluorescein angiograms (approximately 30° versus 60°) [4], important information is not included with respect to the vessel branching pattern in the periphery of the posterior pole. However, previous investigations have shown that the retinal vasculature is fractal and that the magnitude of the fractal dimension using the box-counting procedure obtained with varying angle fundus photographs is close to being equal [3]. Therefore, we used the box-counting analysis to establish whether our nonmydriatic images were similar to images previously published using fluorescein angiograms. Previous fractal analysis results were associated with dimension values in the range of 1.63 to 1.75 [4]. Our study obtained a mean dimension value of 1.68 ± 0.04, suggesting that the traces we used were compatible with those previously reported.

Of the 58 images (35 people) analyzed, 15 were diabetic but did not have neovascularization. Images of the optic fundi of diabetics showed either no clinical abnormality or the presence of microaneurysms, hemorrhages, cataract vessel occlusion, and lipid spots. As our aim was to investigate the effectiveness of the segmentation algorithm, our images also included a set of images that was over- or underexposed and other photographic artifacts (i.e., inclusion of eyelid shadow). In addition, six images included morphological features that obstructed the vessel's fundi with strong reflection from the epithelium layer, the presence of hemorrhages and microaneurysms, and photocoagulation laser scars on the retina.

Thus, of 52 images, visual inspection judged 34 images (66%) to represent a good segmentation (e.g., Figure 5.11a and b). Our technique has shown an acceptable level of segmentation even in the presence of vein occlusion and hemorrhage (Figure 5.11c). Seventeen of these included part of the optic disk border (e.g., Figure 5.12a). Errors in segmentation in the remaining 18 images included nonsegmenting of small vessels, especially near the macula (Figure 5.12b); missing segments where vessels run parallel or cross

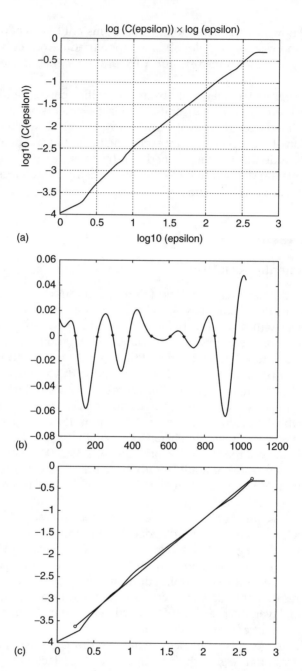

FIGURE 5.10
(a) Log-log plot obtained from the correlation dimension procedure of a triadic Koch curve.
(b) Resulting one-dimensional wavelet transform using the third derivative of the Gaussian as
mother wavelet (the zero-crossings are indicated by "o"). (c) Line fitted to the middle portion,
thus excluding the initial and final nonfractal portions.

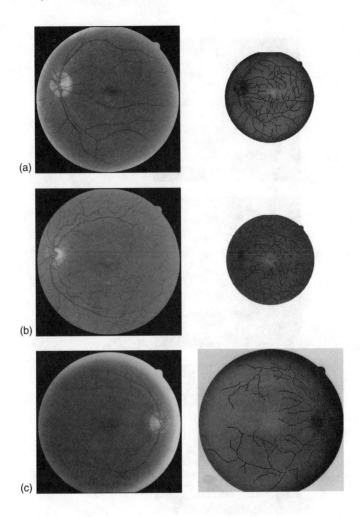

FIGURE 5.11 (See color insert.)
Segmentation results.

(Figure 5.12c); and segments were placed between two original blood vessels that traveled in close proximity to each other (e.g., Figure 5.12d). Of the six images that were suboptimal, four had only minor errors in the segmentation.

In addition to visual inspection of the segmented images, the segmentation algorithm has undergone a performance assessment using the shape features discussed in Section 5.4, that is, area, perimeter, circularity, wavelet entropy, and the correlation dimension. In particular, the latter has been estimated using the wavelet-approach discussed in Section 5.4.2. Each of these shape features has been calculated for each skeleton produced by the wavelet-based segmentation algorithm, as well as for the respective hand-drawn skeleton produced by one of the authors. For each of these features, we will denote

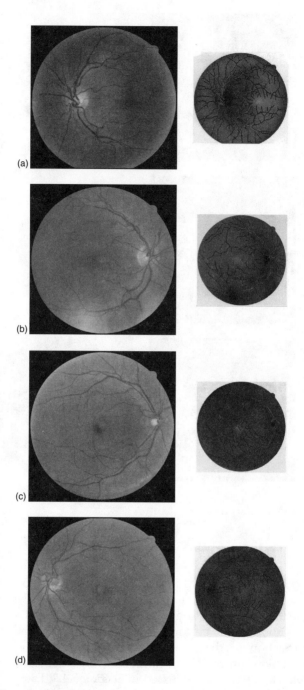

FIGURE 5.12 (See color insert.)
Segmentation results (continued).

$\phi_w(i)$ as the obtained value from the wavelet segmentation of the ith image. Similarly, $\phi_h(i)$ denotes the obtained value from the hand-drawn skeleton of the ith image.

These measures allowed us to assess the segmentation results with respect to the hand-drawn vessel pattern produced by a human operator. The obtained results are summarized in the plots of Figures 5.13 to Figure 5.17. Figure 5.13a shows two superposed plots of $\phi_w(i)$ and $\phi_h(i)$ for the area.

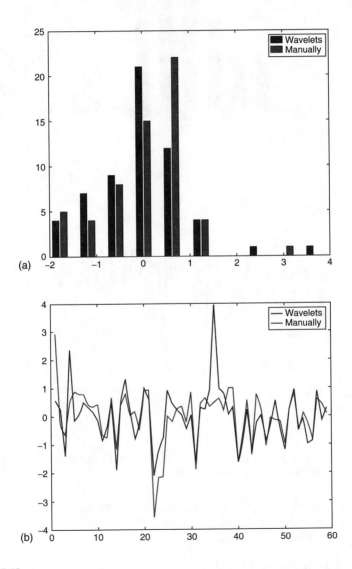

FIGURE 5.13
(a) Superposed plots of $\phi_w(i)$ and $\phi_h(i)$ (refer to the text) for the area feature. (b) Histogram of $\phi_w(i)$ superposed to the histogram of $\phi_h(i)$ for the area feature.

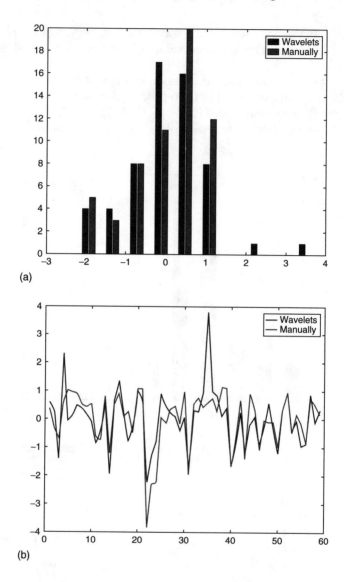

FIGURE 5.14

(a) Superposed plots of $\phi_w(i)$ and $\phi_h(i)$ (refer to the text) for the area feature. (b) Histogram of $\phi_w(i)$ superposed to the histogram of $\phi_h(i)$ for the perimeter feature.

Figure 5.13b is a histogram of $\phi_w(i)$ superposed to the histogram of $\phi_h(i)$, also for the area. The remaining figures present analogous results for the other features; that is:

- Perimeter: Figure 5.14a and b
- Circularity: Figure 5.15a and b

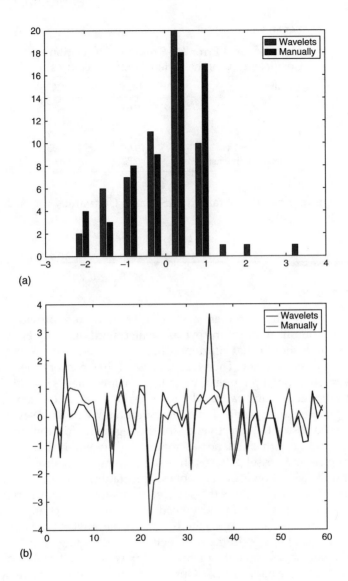

(a)

(b)

FIGURE 5.15
(a) Superposed plots of $\phi_w(i)$ and $\phi_h(i)$ (refer to the text) for the circularity feature. (b) Histogram of $\phi_w(i)$ superposed to the histogram of $\phi_h(i)$ for the circularity feature.

- Wavelet entropy: Figure 5.16a and b
- Correlation dimension: Figure 5.17a and b

To assess these results in a quantitative manner, two different error measures have been calculated to compare each pair (i.e., wavelets and hand-drawn): the mean-squared error *MSE* and the correlation coefficient *CC*.

TABLE 5.1

Mean-Squared Error MSE and the Correlation
Coefficient CC of the Different Shape Features

Feature	MSE	CC
Area	0.65	0.67
Perimeter	0.56	0.72
Circularity	0.58	0.71
Wavelet entropy	0.69	0.65
Correlation dimension	0.72	0.63

Table 5.1 summarizes the obtained MSE and CC values for each feature considered.

5.6 Discussion

The use of a nonmydriatic camera in rural and remote areas provides a means of assessing complications of the eye associated with diabetes. However, research has also shown that untrained health workers are not effective in retinal fundus assessment. Therefore, our work has concentrated on automated segmentation of the retinal vasculature using images obtained from a nonmydriatic camera and captured with a 30-mm SLR Nikon camera. These photographs were then scanned into the computer. We utilized several shape parameters to assess the effectiveness of the segmentation routine with the aim of using some of these shape parameters to differentiate between normal vessel patterns and vessel patterns showing neovascularization.

Despite only 66% showing acceptable segmentation, our segmentation routine can be adjusted to address the detected problems. It is worth mentioning that the obtained results were produced using the same configuration parameters for all images; that is, there was no parameter adjustment from image to image. Our algorithms were better in identifying vessels traveling through hemorrhages and if the picture quality was not optimal compared to the images that were hand-drawn. Optic disk interference can be removed by identifying the disk using appropriate edge detection algorithms and starting the segmentation of the vessels from the border of the optic disk.

In addition to the visual analysis, the results obtained from the shape features of the wavelets and of the hand-drawn skeletons also indicate a successful segmentation. The average correlation coefficient between all measures is 0.61, indicating that the wavelets and the hand-drawn segmentation produced positive correlated features, which is desirable for using such a technique for automatic classification of fundus images. On the other hand, a gap present in the experiments reported in this chapter is the lack of more than one group of subjects (i.e., those with no neovascularization) to verify the effectiveness of

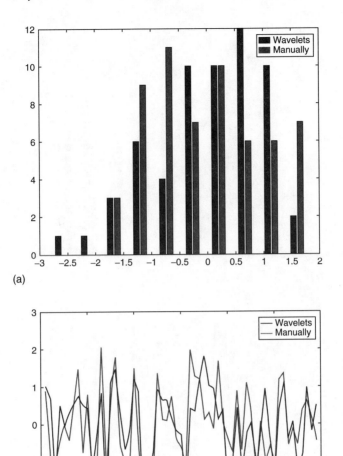

FIGURE 5.16
(a) Superposed plots of $\phi_w(i)$ and $\phi_h(i)$ (refer to the text) for the circularity feature. (b) Histogram of $\phi_w(i)$ superposed to the histogram of $\phi_h(i)$ for the wavelet entropy feature.

the shape features for image classification. The main problem in assessing the segmentation results with one unique group is that there is the possibility of a feature having small *MSE* and *CC* — not because of good agreement between the automatic and human segmentations, but because that feature has a very poor discrimination potential. We feel that this is not the case for the reported experiments because all features presented similar *MSE* and *CC*; but assessing

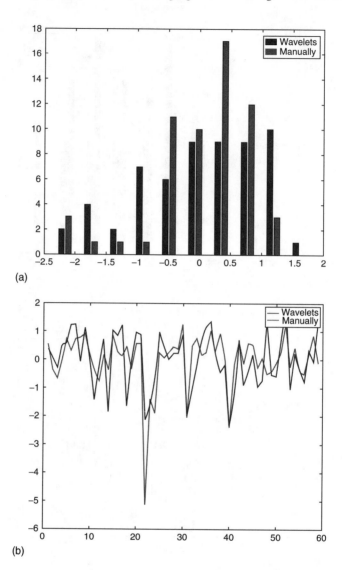

FIGURE 5.17

(a) Superposed plots of $\phi_w(i)$ and $\phi_h(i)$ (refer to the text) for the area feature. (b) Histogram of $\phi_w(i)$ superposed to the histogram of $\phi_h(i)$ for the correlation dimension feature. (c) and (d) represent analogous results for the correlation dimension feature.

the segmentation and the features using more than one group is a problem that remains to be investigated. Currently, we are collecting images with neo-vascularization present in the optic fundus using a nonmydriatic camera.

Our segmentation algorithms differ from previous techniques in that they perform vessel detection and noise filtering in a single pass in an efficient way because of the nice properties of the Morlet wavelet, which is effectively orientation selective and well-localized in the frequency domain. Furthermore, the results reported here have been obtained with nonmydiatric images, which are generally poorer, in terms of resolution, than traditional angiographic images. The method has undergone a thorough assessment by being applied to many images containing different real-life artifacts, such as hemorrhages, as discussed above.

We also extended previous work of analyzing the fundus vessels by including the correlation dimension analysis. The log-log plot slope estimation for this method has been done by line fitting to the middle portion of the plot. This middle portion is determined without user intervention by a wavelets-based technique. The correlation dimension results have been slightly inferior to the others with respect to the MSE and CC error measures. Nevertheless, this fact does not necessarily mean that this is an inferior shape measure for differentiating between normal optic fundi and that with neovascularization present. This is because the better performance of one shape feature with respect to another may also mean that such a feature is less discriminative than the other. This topic remains to be investigated by future research.

A novel parameter introduced here is wavelet entropy. This feature was proposed in the same spirit of the measures extracted from blurred images and the wavelet histogram, which have been previously applied for the characterization of neural morphology (branching patterns too). The entropy is an information theoretic measure able to capture shape complexity and does not present any parameters to be set (which is the case with statistical moments, whose order must be defined empirically). All other traditional feature parameters used (area, perimeter, etc.) provided additional data useful for assessing the segmentation performance.

Our next steps are to deal with optic disk interference and to identify microaneurysms and hemorrhages in order to minimize the interference due to blood vessel leakage. We are also collecting images that display neovascularization, which will allow us to test our segmentation method combined with our pattern analysis tools in order to identify new vessel growth.

Acknowledgments

RMC is grateful to FAPESP (99/12765-2) and to CNPq (300722/98-2, 468413/00-6). HJ was in receipt of a CSU small grant (A5141739605). The authors also wish to acknowledge the contribution of Graeme Frauenfelder, who provided the nonmydriatic images and to the West Australian Lions Clinic for providing the Polaroid and Zeiss images. Dr J. LaNauze from the Albury Eye Clinic provided expert advice. Finally, Jorge J. G. Leandro and Emerson L. N. Tozette helped us with the programs and bibliographic review.

References

1. Taylor, H. R. and Keeffe J. E., World blindness: a 21st century perspective, *Br. J. Ophthalmol.,* Vol. 85, pp. 261–266, 2001.
2. Collective, Research breakthroughs. Diabetic retinopathy group (drg) makes recommendations on diabetic retinopathy, Tech. Rep., Juvenile Diabetes Research Foundation, http://www.jdrf.org/research/feature/res010302.php, 2002.
3. Lee S., Sicari C., Harper C., Taylor H., and Keeffe, J., Program for the early detection of diabetic retinopathy: a two-year follow-up, *Clin. Exp. Ophthalmol.,* Vol. 29, pp. 12–25, 2001.
4. Ariyasu, R., Lee, P., Linton, K., LaBree, L., Azen, S., and Siu, A., Sensitivity, specificity and predictive values of screening tests for eye conditions in a clinic-based population, *Ophthalmology,* Vol. 103, pp. 1751–1760, 1996.
5. Lee, V., Kingsley, R., and Lee, E., The diagnosis of diabetic retinopathy. Ophthalmology versus fundus photography, *Ophthalmology,* Vol. 100, pp. 1504–1512, 1993.
6. Sussman, E., Tsiaras, W., and Soper, K., Diagnosis of diabetic eye disease, *JAMA,* Vol. 247, pp. 3231–3234, 1982.
7. Chen, J. Sato, Y., and Tamura, S., Orientation space filtering for multiple orientation line segmentation, *IEEE Trans. Patt. Anal. and Mach. Intell.,* Vol. 22, No. 5, pp. 417–429, 2000.
8. Leandro, J. J. G., Cesar Jr., R. M., and Jelinek, H., Blood vessels segmentation in retina: preliminary assessment of the mathematical morphology and of the wavelet transform techniques, in *Proc. Brazilian Conf. on Computer Graphics, Image Processing and Vision,* (SIBGRAPI-01, Florianpolis-SC, Out 2001), pp. 84–90, IEEE Computer Society Press, 2001.
9. Cree, M., Olson, J., McHardy, K., Sharp, P., and Forrester, J., A fully automated comparative microaneurysm digital detection system, *Eye,* Vol. 11, pp. 622–628, 1997.
10. Spencer, T., Olson, J., McHardy, K., Sharp, P., and Forrester, J., Image-processing strategy for the segmentation and quantification of microaneurysms in fluorescein angiograms of the ocular fundus, *Computers Biomed. Res.,* Vol. 29, pp. 284–302, 1996.
11. Kanski, J., *Clinical Ophthalmology: A Systematic Approach,* Butterworth-Heinemann, London, pp. 465–479, 1989.
12. Family, F., Masters, B., and Platt, D., Fractal pattern formation in human retinal vessels, *Physica D,* Vol. 38, pp. 98–103, 1989.
13. Landini, G., Murray, P., and Misson, G., Local connected fractal dimensions and lacunarity analysis of 60 degree fluorescein angiograms, *Invest. Ophthalmol. Vis. Sci.,* Vol. 36, pp. 2749–2755, 1995.
14. Hipwell, J., Strachan, F., Olson, J., McHardy, K., Sharp, P., and Forrester, J., Automated detection of microaneurysms in digital red-free photographs: a diabetic retinopathy screening tool, *Diabetic Med.,* Vol. 17, pp. 588–594, 2000.
15. Sinthanayothin, C., Boyce, J., Cook, H., and Williamson, T., Automated localisation of the optic disc, fovea and retinal blood vessels from digital colour fundus images, *Br. J. Ophthalmol.,* Vol. 83, No. 8, pp. 902–912, 1999.

16. Zana, F. and Klein, J., Segmentation of vessel-like patterns using mathematical morphology and curvature evaluation, *IEEE Trans. Image Processing*, Vol. 10, No. 7, pp. 1010–1019, 2001.

17. Englmeier, K.-H. et al., Image processing within ophtel, http://sungria.gsf.de/OPHTEL/ima_proc/ophtel_img_proc.html, 1997.

18. Hoover, A., Kouznetsova, V., and Goldbaum, M., Locating blood vessels in retinal images by piecewise threshold probing of a matched filter response, *MedImg*, Vol. 19, pp. 203–210, March 2000.

19. Gao, X.W., Bharath, A., Stanton, A., Hughes, A., Chapman, N. and Thom, S., Quantification and characterisation of arteries in retinal images, *Comput. Meth. Programs Biomed.*, Vol. 63, No. 2, pp. 133–146, 2000.

20. Chaudhuri, S., Chatterjee, S., Katz, N., Nelson, M., and Goldbaum, M., Detection of blood vessels in retinal images using two dimensional matched filters, *IEEE Trans. Med. Imag.* Vol. 8, No. 3, pp. 263–269, 1989.

21. Li, H., and Chutatape, O., Automatic location of optic disk in retinal images, in *ICIP01*, p. Biomedical Applications ii, 2001.

22. Zana, F. and Klein, J., A multi-modal registration algorithm of eye fundus images using vessels detection and hough transform, *IEEE Trans. Med. Imag.*, Vol. 18, No. 5, pp. 419–428, 1999.

23. Daxer, A., Characterisation of the neovascularisation process in diabetic retinopathy by means of fractal geometry: diagnostic implications, *Graefe's Arch. Clin. Exp. Ophthalmol.*, Vol. 231, pp. 681–686, 1993.

24. Mainster, M., The fractal properties of retinal vessels: embryological and clinical impliations, *Eye*, Vol. 4, pp. 235–241, 1990.

25. McQuellin, C. and Jelinek, H., Characterisation of fluorescein angiograms of retinal fundus using mathematical morphology: a pilot study, in *Proc. 5th Int. Conf. Ophthalmic Photography*, 2002 (accepted).

26. Higgs, E., Harney, B., Kelleher, A., and Reckless, J., Detection of diabetic retinopathy in the community using a non-mydriatic camera, *Diabetic Med.*, Vol. 8, pp. 551–555, 1991.

27. Diamond, J., McKinnon, M., and Barry, C., Non-mydriatic fundus photography: a viable alternative to funduscopy for the identification of diabetic retinopathy in an aboriginal population in rural Western Australia, *Aust. N.Z. J. Ophthalmol.*, Vol. 26, pp. 109–115, 1998.

28. Taylor, R., Lovelock, L., Turnbridge, M., Alberti, K., Brackenridge, R., Stephenson, P., and Young, E., Comparison of non-mydriatic retinal photography with ophthalmology in 2159 patients: mobile retinal camera study, *BMJ*, Vol. 301, pp. 1243–1247, 1990.

29. Costa, L. F. and Cesar, Jr., R. M., *Shape Analysis and Classification: Theory and Practice*, CRC Press, 2001.

30. Arnodo, A., Decoster, N., and Roux, S., A wavelet-based method for multifractal image analysis. I. Methodology and test applications on isotropic and anisotropic random rough surfaces, *Eur. Physical J.* B, Vol. 15, pp. 567–600, 2000.

31. Antoine, J.-P., Carette, P., Murenzi, R., and Piette, B., Image analysis with two-dimensional continuous wavelet transform, *Signal Processing*, Vol. 31, pp. 241–272, 1993.

32. Mallat, S. and Hwang, W., Singularity detection and processing with wavelets, *IEEE Trans. Information Theory*, Vol. 38, pp. 617–643, March 1992.

33. Lee, J.-S., Sun, Y.-N., Chen, C.-H., and Tsai, C.-T., Wavelet based corner detection, *Pattern Recognition*, Vol. 26, No. 6, pp. 853–865, 1993.

34. Grossmann, A., Kronland-Martinet, R., and Morlet, J., Reading and understanding continuous wavelet transform, in [50], 1989.

35. Grossmann, A., Wavelet transforms and edge detection, in *Stochastic Processes in Physics and Engineering*, A. S., B. Ph., H. M., and S. L., Eds., Reidel Publishing, Dordrecht, 1988.

36. Burt, P., and Adelson, E., The laplacian pyramid as a compact image code, *IEEE Trans. Communications*, Vol. COM-31, pp. 532–540, April 1983.

37. Feris, R. S., Krger, V. and Cesar, Jr., R. M., Efficient Real-Time Face Tracking in Wavelet Subspace, in *Proc. Second Int. Workshop on Recognition, Analysis and Tracking of Faces and Gestures in Real-Time Systems, 8th IEEE International Conference on Computer Vision*, (RATFG-RTS — ICCV 2001 — Vancouver, Canada), pp. 113–118, 2001,

38. Antoine, J. P., Barache, D., Cesar, Jr., R. M., and Costa, L. F., Shape characterization with the wavelet transform, *Signal Processing*, Vol. 62, No. 3, pp. 265–290, 1997.

39. Donoho, D. L. and Johnstone, I. M., Ideal spatial adaptation via wavelet shrinkage, *Biometrika*, Vol. 81, pp. 425–455, 1994.

40. Gonzalez, R. C. and Woods, R. E., *Digital Image Processing*, Addison-Wesley, 1992.

41. Fisher, R., Perkins, S., Walker, A., and Wolfart, E., *HIPR — The Hypermedia Image Processing Reference*, John Wiley & Sons, 1996.

42. Systems, S. I., Morphology Toolbox, http://www.mmorph.com/, 2000.

43. Bruno, O., Cesar, Jr., R., Consularo, L., and Costa, L. C., Automatic feature selection for biological shape classification in synergos, in *Proc. Brazilian Conf. on Computer Graphics, Image Processing and Vision*, (SIBGRAPI-98, Rio de Janeiro — RJ, Out 1998), pp. 363–370, IEEE Computer Society Press, 1998.

44. Costa, L. and Consularo, L., The Dynamics of Biological Evolution and the Importance of Spatial Relations and Shapes, in Cantoni, V. and Ges, V. and Setti, A. and Tegolo, D., Eds., *Human and Machine Perception 2*, pp. 1–14. Kluwer Academic/Plenum Publishers, 1999.

45. Panico, J. and Sterling, P., Retinal neurons and vessels are not fractal but space-filling, *J. Comparative Neurol.*, Vol. 361, pp. 479–490, 1995.

46. Jelinek, H., Cesar, Jr, R. M., Leandro, J. J. G., and Spence, I., Automated computational morphometric analysis of the cat retinal α/y, β/x and δ ganglion cells using clustering algorithms, *Visual Neuroscience*, 2002 (in preparation).

47. Grassberger, P. and Procaccia, I., Characterization of strange attractors, *Phys. Rev. Lett.*, Vol. 50, No. 5, pp. 346–349, 1983.

48. Jelinek, H., Bolea, J., and Fernandez, E., Towards a useful fractal analysis methodology in biological research, in *Proceedings of the IV Congreso Iberamericano de Biofísica*, Alicante, Spain, pp. 1–15, 2000.

49. Bianchi, A. G. C., Santos, M. F., Hamassaki-Britto, D. E., and Costa, L. F., How do neurons grow, in *Proc. World Congress on Neuroinformatics*, pp. 386–394, Vienna University of Technology, September 2001.

50. Combes, J.-M., Grossmann, A., and Tchamitchian, P., Eds., *Wavelets, Time-Frequency Methods and Phase-Space* (Proc. Marseille 1987), Springer-Verlag, Berlin, 1989.

6

Automated Model-Based Segmentation, Tracing, and Analysis of Retinal Vasculature from Digital Fundus Images

Kenneth H. Fritzsche, Ali Can, Hong Shen, Chia-Ling Tsai, James N. Turner, Howard L. Tanenbaum, Charles V. Stewart, and Badrinath Roysam

CONTENTS

6.1 Overview

Quantitative morphometry of the retinal vasculature is of widespread interest, directly for ophthalmology and indirectly for diseases involving structural and/or functional changes of the body vasculature. Key points such as bifurcations and crossovers are of special interest to developmental biologists and clinicians examining conditions such as hypertension and diabetes. Segmentation/tracings of the retinal vasculature and the key points, such as bifurcations and crossovers, are also important as spatial landmarks for image registration. Image registration, in turn, has direct applications to change detection, mosaic synthesis, real-time tracking, and real-time spatial referencing. Change detection is important for supporting a variety of clinical trials, high-volume reading centers, and for large-scale screening applications.

The best-available algorithms for segmenting/tracing retinal vasculature are model based, and a variety of models are in use. Depending on the intended application, different algorithmic and implementation choices can be made. This chapter describes some of these models and algorithms and illustrates some of the implementation choices that need to be considered using a real-time algorithm as an example. Also described are methods for extracting key points and a discussion of how vessel morphometric data can be applied. Some methods are presented for generating ground truth or "gold standard" images as well as comparing these against computer-generated results. Finally, some experimental analysis is presented for RPI-Trace and the ERPR landmark determination algorithms developed by our group.

6.2   Introduction

The vasculature in the back of the eye, on the ocular fundus, is a multi-layered structure that supplies the light-sensitive retinal tissue with essential nutrients and assists in the disposal of metabolic waste products [40]. The upper-most layer, referred to hereafter as the "retinal vasculature" is the subject of this chapter.

The retinal vasculature is visible noninvasively using a common clinical instrument known as the fundus camera, or fundus microscope [116]. There are two common types of fundus microscopes: mydriatic and nonmydriatic [61]. Mydriatic instruments are designed assuming that the eyes have been dilated using drops. The nonmydriatic instruments do not require dilation. The mydriatic instruments produce higher-quality images due to the wider field of view enabled by dilation. The nonmydriatic instruments are better suited to initial screening type applications, or in cases when dilation is problematic or impossible. In addition to the above imaging techniques, fluorescence-based angiography methods are in common use as well; fluorescein and indocyanine green (ICG) are the most commonly used dyes. Increasingly, confocal instruments, also known as scanning laser ophthalmoscopes (SLO), are entering clinical use, but are still not as common as the fundus camera [116].

Figure 6.1(a) shows a fundus camera in use. Figure 6.1(b) shows a typical fundus image captured using red-free illumination. The bright round

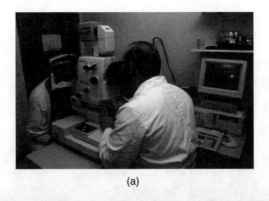

(a)

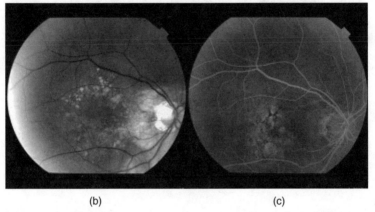

(b) (c)

FIGURE 6.1
Illustrating common retinal imaging methods. Panel (a) shows a fundus camera in use. The lower panels show two images of the same eye containing pathologies. Panel (b) is a retinal image acquired using red-free illumination. The vessels appear darker than the background in this case. Panel (c) was obtained by injecting a patient with fluorescein, and imaging the resulting fluorescence. In this latter image, the vessels appear light against the background. Note in the two panels how the retinal features and pathologies are revealed differently.

structure in this image is known as the optic disk. Retinal arteries and veins are visible as dark linear branched structures. They enter or exit the eye via this location. The darker region in the middle of the image with no vasculature is known as the macula. The center of the macula is largely responsible for acute vision, and is known as the fovea. Many conditions leading to blindness are associated with pathologies of the macular region of the retina. Figure 6.1(c) shows a sample fluorescein angiogram (FA) obtained by injecting a patient with a dye called fluorescein, which fluoresces when excited with light of the appropriate wavelength. The fluorescein travels through the circulatory system and makes the vessels in the retina appear brighter than the surrounding area. Generally, different imaging modalities reveal different layers of the

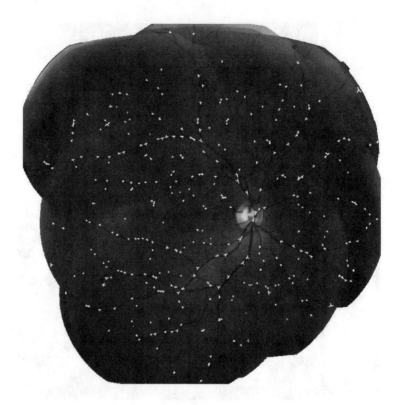

FIGURE 6.2
An automatically generated tracing of the retinal vasculature for a healthy eye, using RPI-Trace, a multi-platform software package developed by the authors. The fundus camera was used to image various portions of the retina, which were montaged (mosaiced) together to form a high-resolution, wide-angle image. The vessel traces are shown in green. The points of bifurcation and crossovers are indicated in white.

overall retinal vasculature at different times. The reader is referred to [40] for a more in-depth description of instrumentation, intra-ocular anatomy, function, and pathologies.

Segmentation and tracing of the retinal vasculature has widespread applicability. Considerable research has been devoted to developing automated algorithms to identify the vasculature structure and differentiate it from other features that may be present in retinal images. Figure 6.2 shows an automatically generated tracing of the retinal vasculature. In this case, the fundus camera only yielded small 30° views of the retina. Multiple such images were combined to form a seamless mosaic (montage) of the retina, which was traced using a software package named RPI-Trace developed by the authors of this chapter.

The quantitative morphology of the retinal vasculature is of direct interest to a number of studies in ophthalmic science. For example, observation and quantification of the development of retinal vasculature in premature infants is important for early detection of serious conditions such as retinopathy of prematurity [40, 108]. Many diseases related to vision loss are associated with abnormalities in the retinal vasculature. Common examples of such abnormalities are hemorrhages, angiogenesis, increases in vessel tortuosity, and blockages. For this reason, the topological and/or morphological changes in the retinal vasculature are of great interest to clinicians. More generally, the retinal vasculature has the unique distinction of being the only part of the body vasculature that is observable noninvasively. Indeed, the retinal vasculature, which is affected by all factors that affect the body vasculature in general, is a unique "window" into the circulatory system. For this reason, it is studied for nonocular conditions as well, such as hypertension [15, 36, 105, 106]. Finally, the structure of the retinal vasculature is distinctive enough to be used as a biometric for identifying persons. However, this type of application is not widespread due to the high performance of iris scanning technology, which has simpler imaging requirements.

Characteristic points of the retinal vasculature, such as bifurcations and crossover points (see Figure 6.3) are of special interest from the standpoint of developmental studies as well as clinical diagnosis. They form an important component of retinal image understanding systems [1]. For example, arteriolar narrowing, "nicking" or blockages of vessels at crossover points, and retinopathy are associated with hypertension (high blood pressure) [55]. Figure 6.3 (right panel) shows an example of artery/vein nicking.

Changes in the retinal vasculature are important indicators of disease states and/or effects of clinical treatments [48, 74]. Change detection is important for supporting a variety of clinical trials, high-volume reading centers, and for

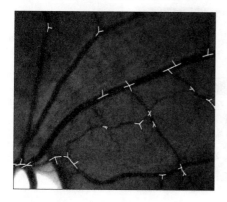 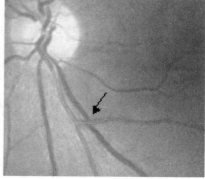

FIGURE 6.3 (See color insert.)
Crossing and branching points of the retinal vasculature. The left panel shows these points as detected by RPI-Trace. The right panel shows an example of vein nicking observed in hypertensive patients caused by an artery exerting pressure on a vein. Automatic location of these interest points may be valuable for clinical diagnosis.

large-scale screening applications. Critical to change detection is the problem of accurate alignment, that is, registration of retinal images that have been captured at different times [11]. Such image capture is performed, for example, during annual checkups. Images are also captured before and after various treatments to observe and document the changes of clinical interest [10, 41]. Finally, image sequences are routinely captured during fluorescein and ICG angiography. The inter-image changes reveal patterns of blood flow in this case. Accurate registration of images ensures that the detected changes (i.e., the difference image) reflects only the real changes, and avoids any artifacts associated with the registration procedure itself. Figure 6.4, panels A and B, shows a pair of images of the same retina taken 30 days apart while the patient was undergoing a clinical treatment. These images have been registered accurately using a sophisticated algorithm developed in this group [22]. The result of detecting the changes are also shown in Figure 6.4C.

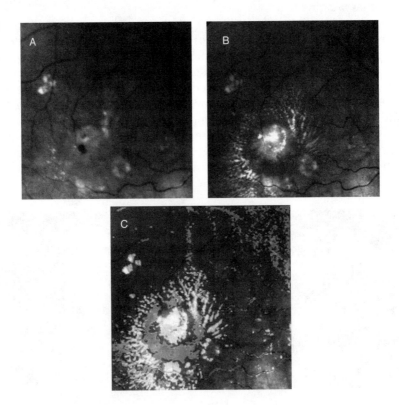

FIGURE 6.4 (See color insert.)
Application of vessel tracing and registration to retinal image change detection. Panels A and B show images captured 30 days apart. Panel C shows the result of registration of the above two images, followed by an automatic segmentation (delineation) of the "difference" image, revealing the regions of change in blue.

An essential first step for retinal image registration is precise detection and localization of landmarks, or feature points [17]. These points must have the following properties to be useful. They (1) must be at fixed locations on the patient's retina; (2) must be present in sufficient numbers in all areas of the retina for effective location determination; (3) must be detectable in different images of the same area of the retina even when the images differ in magnification, focus, and lighting; and (4) must be quickly detectable. Points identifying bifurcations and crossing points of the retinal vasculature, and traces of the vasculature between these characteristic points, generally meet these requirements (with exceptions such as those arising in retinal detachment). That is, the retina appears as a rigid structure unless detached. Physicians have long used vasculature features as spatial references for finding specific locations on the retina during manual examination and surgery. Figure 6.1 shows an automatic tracing of the retinal vasculature with the crossing and branch points highlighted. Section 6.8 describes methods for locating these points with sub-pixel precision and high repeatability.

Image registration has direct applications in addition to change detection [27, 28, 84]. One such application is mosaic synthesis, which requires multiple partial views of the retina to be combined into a single high-resolution synthetic wide-angle view [69, 70]. Retinal mosaics are useful for accurate vessel morphometry taking overlapping views into account, detection of changes at the retinal periphery for conditions such as AIDS CMV [128]. Mosaics are also useful as key elements in building a spatial map [9, 14, 95] of the retina for the purpose of tracking and real-time spatial referencing. Figure 6.5 illustrates retinal image mosaicing and spatial referencing as registration problems. Diagnostic images (panels A through E) are mosaiced together to form a wide-angle spatial map of the entire retina [18–20, 23].

The retinal vasculature has been used for real-time tracking [5, 6] and spatial referencing [95] in the context of laser retinal surgery. Tracking algorithms use the retinal vasculature to register each frame of an image sequence to the next. However, given the tendency of the retina to exhibit large motions [88], tracking is often lost or inaccurate. Whenever this happens, tracking must be reestablished [8, 9]. One method to reestablish tracking is to use the mosaic as a spatial system of reference, as described by Becker et al. [10]. Another approach is to register each image frame to a preestablished mosaic-based map of the retina. This is known as spatial referencing. Shen et al. [95] have described a fast method for spatial referencing using quasi-invariant indexing. In this method, geometric invariants are computed from local constellations of landmarks (crossing and branching points of the retinal vasculature), and looked up in a precomputed indexing database to estimate an initial registration and iterative alignment of the vasculature. This initial registration is subsequently refined using robust estimators. The spatial map consists of mosaics, together with the surgical plans (outlined in panel F) drawn by the physician, and various data structures (quasi-invariant indexing databases) to support fast spatial referencing during surgery.

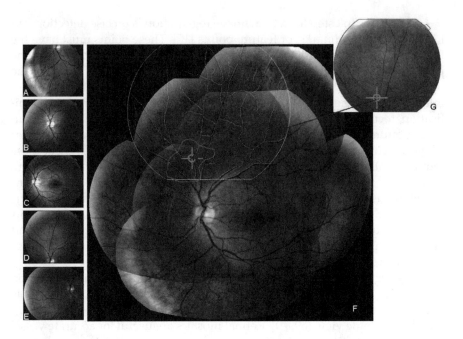

FIGURE 6.5
Two applications of vessel segmentation: mosaicing and spatial referencing. Panels A through E show some of the images taken from the same eye on a single visit. Panel F shows the mosaic (or spatial map) built from these and other images [23] using traces of the vasculature as spatial landmarks, and with a desired treatment area outlined. Panel G simulates an image acquired during a surgical procedure in which the aiming point in G is referenced against the spatial map in real-time to determine the precise location of the laser and check if it is within the desired treatment area before allowing the laser to be turned on [95].

Figure 6.5 illustrates spatial mapping. Panel G simulates an image frame captured by a camera during a surgical procedure. This image is registered onto the spatial map, effectively estimating the location of a laser beam (illustrated by the cross-hairs on panel G) relative to the spatial map. The arrow illustrates this mapping. The vascular traces from the image frame (panel G) are superimposed on the mosaic to show correct registration. Spatial referencing can, for example, determine whether or not the surgical laser is aimed within a desired treatment region. While performing laser retinal surgery, the images that the surgeon is viewing can be processed for vascular landmarks in much the same fashion as they were extracted for registration. These landmarks can then be compared against the landmarks in the mosaic image so as to identify whether the surgical tool is in the correct region. If so, the surgeon can then apply the laser to the desired treatment area, while the spatial referencing algorithms enable a recording of the optical dosage administered to each point. If not, the spatial referencing processor can perform a protective cut-off of the laser.

Thus, the extraction of vessels is vital in providing the landmarks necessary to perform such spatial tasks in computer-assisted surgical instrumentation.

6.3   Retinal Imaging Background

Still digital images and live digital image sequences of the human retina are captured using a digital video camera attached to a fundus camera [42, 85]. Still photography is generally performed with a flash and live imaging is done with continuous illumination. In the former case, imaging noise is lower than in the latter case where less light is available. The confocal imaging case is not considered here [116]. Readers who do not have access to a source of retinal images, such as an ophthalmology clinic, can access large collections of retinal images on CD-ROM [123].

Several aspects of retinal images make automated processing challenging. First, the images are highly variable. Large variability is observed between images from different patients, even if healthy, with the situation worsening when pathologies exist. For the same patient, variability is observed under differing imaging conditions and during the course of treatment. Unlike industrial vision problems where the conditions can be carefully controlled, retinal images are frequently subject to improper illumination, glare, fadeout, and loss of focus. Artifacts can arise from reflection, refraction, and dispersion.

The movement of the eye can result in significant variation, even for a stable, well-seated patient. The eye movements are rapid and significant [88]. The saccadic movements involve sudden jumps up to 15°. These movements occur at speeds ranging from 90 to 180°/sec. The mean peak acceleration can range from 15,000 to 22,000°/sec^2. These movements cannot be fully suppressed, even with medication. Often, medications are considered harmful, and so are not used. These numbers imply that interlaced image sensors are often a poor choice for imaging the vasculature [4]. Most commercial imaging systems, such as the TOPCON ImageNet system, employ non-interlaced digital megapixel cameras. Additionally, movements resulting from a distracted patient, or in response to the irritation induced by the laser, or the involuntary attempt to fixate the fovea on the laser light, all affect the quality of the image. Finally, each image or frame in a video sequence represents a partial view of the retina, and the zoom factor (magnification, scale) can vary from frame to frame, due to either selection of a different magnification setting on the fundus camera or movement of the camera nearer to or farther from the patient's eye (which may be necessary for focusing).

The inherent difficulty of illuminating the retina in a uniform and steady manner for reflectance imaging [100] causes several difficulties. For effective imaging, the retina cannot simply be illuminated by directing a strong light into the patient's eye. In addition to causing patient discomfort, this would generate reflections off the patient's cornea (glare) that can dominate the light reflected from the retina back out the pupil. As a result, another method of retinal illumination is used. Before imaging a patient's retina, the patient is administered eye dilating drops (e.g., Tropicamide ophthalmic solution) to dilate the pupil to allow a large area for light to enter and exit the eye. The fundus camera's illumination is focused to form a ring of light at the anterior (front) of the eye with an unilluminated circle in the center of the pupil. As a result, reflection off the surface of the eye only occurs in the illuminated ring. At the retina, the light ring is out of focus, and the result is diffuse illumination. The aperture of the fundus camera is designed to block the reflected light from the circle of illumination while allowing light from within the unilluminated circle, resulting in a fundus image uncontaminated by reflection or glare from the cornea. Unfortunately, this method does not always work flawlessly. For the retina to be illuminated while preventing glare, the camera must be focused properly on the patient's eye. Movements of the patient's eye, even slight ones, can degrade the focusing. In particular, if the eye moves so that the iris blocks some of the ring of illumination, the total illumination of the retina can drop dramatically. In addition, eye movements can allow some stray reflected or refracted light to be directed into the aperture of the fundus camera. This is seen as a bright glare at the edges of the retinal image. Figure 6.6 shows examples of these possibilities.

When live video imaging is desired, one has to contend with eye movements and the difficulty of providing steady illumination. The factors noted above result in image frames that are often dim, out of focus, motion blurred, or corrupted with optical effects such as glare or nonuniform illumination. In retinal still photography, skilled technicians quickly refocus the camera for optimum illumination for each picture. Images are only taken/saved when the illumination is optimal. Any images with insufficient illumination or excessive glare are simply discarded. Tracing algorithms designed for real-time

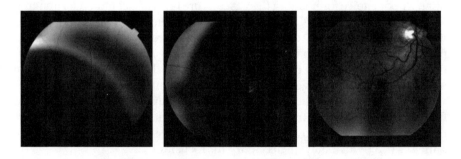

FIGURE 6.6
Some examples of fundus images with nonuniform illumination. Note in the rightmost image how the lower portion of the image is blurred.

online operation do not have this luxury. They must be able to work with image frames with suboptimal illumination, and be able to detect when image quality is too poor for processing, and then reject these frames. They must not only be adaptive enough to be useful and reliable, but also efficient enough to handle high data rates. While much work remains to be done in this area, much progress has been made. Some of the algorithms described in Section 6.5 were designed in the context of such conflicting, practical, and extreme needs.

6.4 Models for Detecting Retinal Vasculature in Digital Imagery

This section describes methods for modeling the appearance of retinal vessels in fundus images in a manner that is sufficient for the purpose of image segmentation. Specifically, we are interested in features of vessels that allow an algorithm to determine if specific pixels in an image are part of the vessel tree or the background. A full physics-based modeling of the image formation process, including the geometry of the vasculature and the imaging systems, could yield more accurate and realistic models, but is beyond the scope of this chapter (see [16, 35, 89, 100]).

Generally, models are applicable only in the context of the image type for which they are developed. For example, in a red-free retinal image (that is, an image taken with a specialized red filter to block out most of the red light), the blood vessels appear to be darker than the local background. In a fluorescein image, dye is injected into the bloodstream, which causes the vessels to appear brighter than the background. Application of the same intensity-based model in both cases will not yield the same results. Fortunately, it is often possible to modify a model that works well at detecting light vessels against a dark background to be able to detect dark vessels against a light background.

Most of the methods described in the literature model the cross-sectional profile of vessels. Figure 6.7 illustrates the idea of a cross section. The conceptual basis for such modeling is the differential behavior of light propagation through vessels, and the reflectance off of the vessel surface, compared to the local background. The following sections review some of the different models used to detect retinal vessels and assume an image in which blood vessels are darker than the surrounding background.

6.4.1 Thresholding

One approach to segmentation of blood vessels is based on the observation that blood vessel pixels are darker than the background pixels. Thus, by identifying all pixels that are darker than some threshold T, you can easily identify

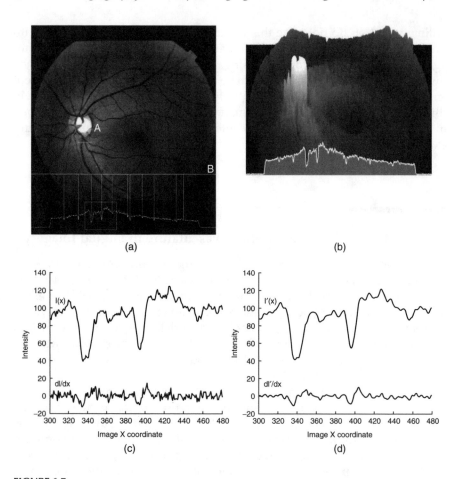

(a)   (b)

(c)   (d)

FIGURE 6.7

Cross-sectional gray-scale profiles of retinal vasculature. Panel (a) shows an image with two marked cross sections, A and B, with the intensity profile of B below the image. Lines are extended from the points where vessels intersect the cross section to the profile below showing how vessels correspond to relative minima on the profile. Panel (b) shows a three-dimensional image where the pixel intensity is used as the value for height and illustrates the resulting intensity profile from a cut along the cross-section B. Panels (c) and (d) show the intensity and derivatives for the actual and smoothed profiles, respectively, for the boxed region shown in panel (a).

all vessel pixels. While attractive in its simplicity, this idea does not generate satisfactory results. First, a method for selecting an appropriate value for the threshold needs to be addressed. Second, retinal images can contain pathologies, are inherently noisy, and the intensity structure is not uniform throughout the entire image. Figure 6.8 exemplifies how the intensity structure varies through an image. So, a threshold that works in one area of an image does not work in another or incorrectly identifies noisy pixels from pathologies or the

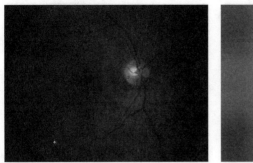

FIGURE 6.8 (See color insert.)
Illustrating the changes in local thresholds indicative of the varying intensity structure across the entire image. For each region center denoted by the x in the right image, a local minimum threshold is calculated. These thresholds are then interpolated for any pixel that is not a region center. The thresholds shown in the image on the right were determined from the image on the left with the thresholds multiplied by 4 for display purposes.

background. Thus, thresholding by itself is not an adequate model of vessel segmentation.

6.4.2   Local Gray-Scale Minima-Based Models

A different way to model the vasculature is from a slight modification to the above dark-pixel observation in that the central portions of vessels correspond to maximum absorption of light and are the *darkest* pixels [29]. Thus, a method of finding the darkest pixels relative to their neighbors should indicate that the pixel is a vessel. The easiest way to find these minima is to consider cross sections, commonly in both the x- and y-directions. By scanning a row or column of pixels and flagging each pixel that is a relative minimum (i.e., its intensity is smaller than its two neighbors), a vessel pixel can be found.

While the simplicity of this model is attractive, it has limitations. First, it is possible to have flat portions of the cross-sectional profile, including in the vessel. Second, the local minima are not unique to vessels — the image background often contains relative minima caused by pathologies, the presence or absence of pigmentation in the retinal tissue, noise from image signal path (through the lens, through the vitreous fluid, etc,), or noise from the camera. Thus, while this model is simple and relatively fast, it often flags as many non-vessel pixels (false positives) as it does vessel pixels. Nevertheless, this model is proven to be useful as a way of obtaining "seed" or "candidate" vessel points from which to initiate a vessel tracing algorithm if coupled with a method to cull out bad points [21]. Figure 6.9 shows a sample result of the local minima model.

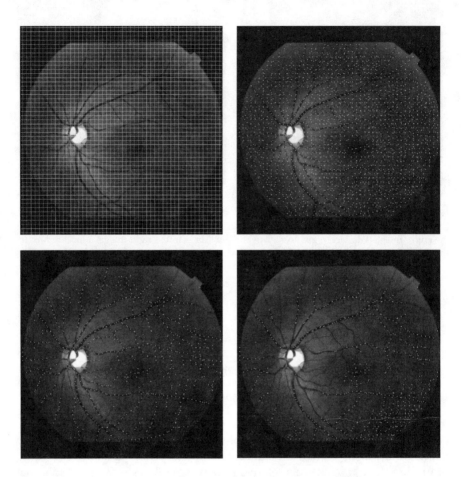

FIGURE 6.9
The performance of three different models detecting retinal vasculature. Panel (a) shows the 50 horizontal and 50 vertical lines used as cross sections to extract profiles to identify vessels. Panel (b) shows local minima only. Panels (c) and (d) show local minima with local and global thresholds, respectively, for $\alpha = 1$ in Equation 6.1.

6.4.3   Combining Local Gray-Scale Minima with Thresholding

The above model can be enhanced by combination with thresholding. From the observation that the intensities (pixel values) of the relative minima in the background region of the image are substantially higher than the local minima found in vessels, a threshold can be selected such that if the relative minimum is higher than the threshold, then that pixel will not be considered as part of a vessel. Only gray-scale local minima with intensities below the threshold should be considered vessel pixels. The trick is in determining an appropriate threshold.

One method is to use a single global threshold value for the entire image. A straightforward method for estimating such a threshold is to examine the intensities of a set of evenly spaced sample points S throughout the image and to use order statistics to arrive at a threshold. First, the intensities of the sample points denoted S are ordered. Then, the median $m(S)$ of these values is computed. Additionally, the median of the absolute deviations of all the points from the median value is then computed and converted to an estimate of the scale and denoted as $s(S)$. The threshold $T_m(S)$ can then be defined as:

$$T_m = m(S) - \alpha s(S) \qquad (6.1)$$

where α is a non-negative weighting factor. A typical value for α is 1.

A somewhat more adaptive approach is to estimate the above thresholds locally. In this approach, the image is tiled into rectangular regions (which may overlap), and the threshold is calculated as above for each such region. For determining T_m for points in between the centers of these rectangular regions, bilinear interpolation can be used. The advantage of using local thresholds is that they are more appropriate due to the change in contrast and lighting conditions observed in a single image but they are computationally more expensive. Results of filtering image pixels over a 50×50 grid using local minima with global and local thresholds computed according to Equation 6.1 are presented in Figure 6.9. The variation in the local threshold across an image is displayed in Figure 6.8.

6.4.4   Hybrid Gray-Scale and Edge-Based Models

As noted above, a purely gray-scale (intensity) based model is inadequate for separating vessel and non-vessel pixels. Even after combined with thresholding as described above, local gray-scale minima are incorrectly identified as vessel pixels. Additional information is needed to perform a more complete separation. Vessel boundaries provide powerful *structural* information for this purpose. All pixels in a blood vessel are bounded on two sides by a pair of prominent boundaries. Applying this idea, for each gray-scale minima detected, areas on either side of the minima can be searched to find edges by looking for oppositely signed derivatives where the derivative at each pixel is computed using the following equation (for a horizontal profile):

$$I'(x, y) = I(x + 2, y) + 2I(x + 1, y) - 2I(x - 1, y) - I(x - 2, y). \qquad (6.2)$$

When the pixel is part of the background or inside a vessel (depending on the vessel width), the derivative should be very close to zero. When a pixel is on the left or right vessel boundary, the derivative magnitude is at its maximum and is negative for the left boundary and positive for the right boundary. Only derivatives with the greatest local magnitude (i.e., local minima or local maxima) are considered as boundary points.

The above edge constraints serve to filter out local gray-scale minima that are not associated with boundary edges. This constraint by itself is not sufficient to distinguish vessel and non-vessel pixels. This can be seen by noting that a pair of edges on opposite sides of the image are obviously too far apart to form a vessel that satisfies the above requirements. Therefore, it is necessary to filter the points based on the distance between the edges. If the oppositely signed derivatives are too far apart to be representative of expected vessel widths, they should not be considered matching boundary points of a vessel and the local minima should be considered background.

This type of bound on expected vessel widths is a powerful constraint. The results of using this method to filter image pixels using 50 evenly spaced vertical and 50 evenly space horizontal cross sections (50×50 grid) can be seen in Figure 6.10. This method improves upon the results shown in Figure 6.8. This is the method used by Shen et al. in their real-time vessel tracing work [96].

Even with a bound on vessel width, the relative minima with edges model is often inaccurate in identifying vessel pixels. Specifically, it is still common to incorrectly label background pixels as vessel by encountering multiple oppositely signed derivatives around a minima within a given distance in the background regions. One method to be more selective is to check if the magnitudes of the oppositely signed derivatives are roughly equal. While this is effective in eliminating some of the false positives, there is still one more step that can be applied to eliminate even more false positives. This involves using a thresholding technique similar to that described in Equation 6.1 above, but applied to the edges and based on the edge strength.

6.4.5 Combining Hybrid Gray-Scale and Edge-Based Models with Thresholds

As can be seen in the results in Figure 6.10, the hybrid gray-scale and edge-based model still incorrectly identifies non-vessel pixels as vessel. One approach to minimizing such false detection of vessel pixels is to establish thresholds based on edge strengths. This threshold would represent the cutoff between what should be considered a vessel boundary and what should just be considered background noise. This threshold can be calculated globally or for local regions using the procedures described earlier. For each sample in a given region R (either a global or local region), the derivatives in four directions, $0°$, $45°$, $90°$, $135°$, are calculated. The mean and standard deviation of these derivatives are descriptive of the contrast for neighboring pixels or potential edge sites within the region and can be used to develop a minimum edge strength threshold, T_e, for an edge within a region R as follows:

$$T_e(R) = \mu_d(R) + \alpha\sigma_d(R), \tag{6.3}$$

where $\mu_d(R)$ is the mean of the all the derivatives in the region, $\sigma_d(R)$ is the standard deviation of the derivatives in the region, and α is some weighting factor applied to the standard deviation. A typical value for α is 1.5.

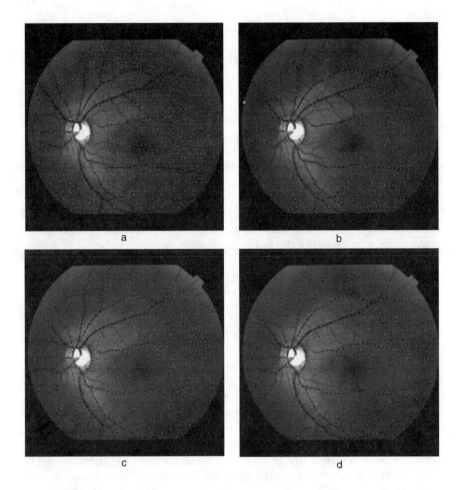

FIGURE 6.10 (See color insert.)
The performance of edge-based vessel models. Panel (a) shows the identified vessels from the vertical and horizontal profiles shown in Figure 6.9(a) using one-dimensional parallel edges within a radius of 11 pixels and edge magnitude within 20%. Panel (b) shows use one-dimensional parallel edges with the same settings as used in panel (a) with the addition of global thresholds for grayscale minima and edge strength. Panel (c) is the same, but with local thresholds. Both (b) and (c) used $\alpha = 1.5$ in Equation 6.3 and $\alpha = 1$ in Equation 6.1. Panel (d) shows vessel points found using two-dimensional parallel edges (with the same local thresholds as panel (c)).

Anything above this threshold would be considered sufficiently strong to be considered an edge.

This threshold, coupled with the gray-scale minima threshold discussed previously, now provides a method for identifying a vessel point in a more selective manner. Thus, for every minima below some threshold, if it has two, roughly equal, oppositely signed derivatives within a defined distance, where the left derivative is negative and the right is positive, if the sum of the magnitudes are greater than $2T_e(R)$, one could consider those points as vessel boundaries. Results from using this model are shown in Figure 6.10.

6.4.6   Models Based on Parallel and Opposite Two-Dimensional Edges

Up until now, our discussions of vessel models have been based entirely on a one-pixel-wide cross-sectional profile. However, there are other, non-one-dimensional properties of vessels that can be used to improve the accuracy of our models. One such property is the observation that while vessels do curve, they are locally straight over short distances. This property allows us to expand the one-dimensional models described above into two-dimensional models.

Consider a vessel that is locally oriented along the vertical (i.e., y) axis over a distance of L pixels. For such a vessel, the right boundary (edge) can be detected using a kernel of the following form:

$$
Length = L = \left\{
\begin{array}{|c|c|c|c|c|}
\hline
-1 & -2 & 0 & 2 & 1 \\
\hline
-1 & -2 & 0 & 2 & 1 \\
\hline
\multicolumn{5}{|c|}{\vdots} \\
\hline
-1 & -2 & 0 & 2 & 1 \\
\hline
\end{array}
\right.
$$

This is the operator used by Can et al. [21], and called "low-pass differentiators" by Sun et al. [110]. The kernel response will be a maximum positive number when the left half of the above kernel is overlaid on a dark vessel and the right half is overlaid on the brighter background. Thus, it yields a maximum response when the column of zeros is on the right boundary of a vertical vessel. A mirror image about the vertical axis of the above kernel has similar response properties, but for the left boundary of the vessel.

The kernel length L is set based on two considerations. First, a higher value of L results in a more sensitive detection of the two-dimensional vessel boundary. Specifically, if the gray-scale contrast between the foreground and background pixels is δ, then the kernel response is simply $3 \times L \times \delta$. This suggests maximizing the length of the kernel L. However, this cannot be done indefinitely, given the curvature of vessels. Another consideration that is important for high-speed tracing applications is the computation cost. Increasing L results in a proportional increase in the computation time. A reasonable trade-off is to fix L for a given application, or a class of images. For example, Can et al. [21] used a value of 6. As an aside, the computations for this kernel are quite efficient. The constants are powers of 2, so it only involves fixed-point shift and add operations.

Vessel boundaries at arbitrary angles can be detected by kernels that are obtained by rotating the kernel in Equation 6.2. Fortunately, a quite coarse descretization of angles is known to be adequate for retinal vasculature based on its known curvature properties. For example, Can et al. [21] used a set of 16 kernels separated by 22.5° for orientations from 0 to 360°, while Chaudhuri et al. [25] used just 12 kernels separated by 15° for orientations from 0 to 180°.

Once the templates for finding vessel boundaries have been created, the task of locating vessel pixels is similar to that described in Section 6.4.4 above. For a pixel to belong to a vessel, there must be edges around a local minima (as indicated by two template responses within a given distance in opposite directions) that are nearly equal. The thresholding criteria described above (T_m and T_e) are also applicable, except that prior to applying the T_e threshold, the response must first be normalized to account for the length. Vessel points identified by these criteria can be seen in Figure 6.10.

6.4.7 Models Based on Gaussian Cross-Sectional Profiles

Another methodology used to model a cross section of a blood vessel is fitting the observed cross-section profile of the vessel with the profile of a predefined curve. Gaussian profiles have been shown to be effective in this regard [25, 26, 127]. For a vessel that is locally oriented along the y-axis (i.e., vertically), and assuming a Gaussian gray-scale profile yields the following model:

$$G(x) = b - c \times e^{-(x-a)^2/2\sigma^2} \qquad (6.4)$$

where a is the center point of the vessel, σ is a parameter representing the width of the vessel, b is the approximate value of the background around the vessel, and c represents the degree of contrast between the vessel and the background (i.e., how dark the vessel is as compared to the background). It can be observed from the images in Figure 6.11 that while not entirely accurate

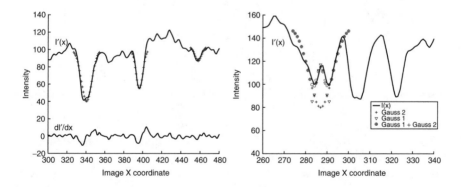

FIGURE 6.11

Illustrating the use of a Gaussian curve to model the gray-scale vessel cross section. The left panel shows how three different Gaussian curves formed using Equation 6.4 with differing values for σ closely approximate the smoothed profile "B" from Figure 6.7. The right panel shows how for a vessel with central reflex obtained from the profile marked "A" in Figure 6.7, two Gaussian curves can be combined to better approximate the vessel profile.

for the entire profile, the Gaussian curve does provide a close fit to portions of a cross section corresponding to the vessel.

The Gaussian model described above can be used to construct matched filters [25]. Constructing a kernel based on the Gaussian profile is challenging. First, because the function in Equation 6.4 is defined for all points (i.e., it is continuous), the spatial extent of the filter must be made finite to enable efficient computation. Commonly, a filter formed from Equation 6.4 is truncated beyond two or three standard deviations; that is, $a - 3\sigma \leq x \leq a + 3\sigma$.

Also, it is convenient to design the kernel such that the template response is zero in a uniform region like background and non-zero over vessels. One such kernel, used by Chaudhuri et al. [25], used a kernel of the following form based on a value for σ of 2:

4	3	2	1	−2	−5	−6	−5	−2	1	2	3	4

The maximum response results when the central entry (i.e., −6) coincides with the center of the vessel. Thus, this template can be applied at all pixels across a cross section, and the point at which the response is maximum can be considered a center point of a vessel.

This filter described above can now be expanded into a two-dimensional model to once again take advantage of the locally straight feature of vessels. This is accomplished in the same manner as described in Section 6.4.6. Once again it becomes necessary to generate a set of templates to account for different orientations of vessels. A sample two-dimensional kernel for a Gaussian profile and a kernel length L is shown below.

$$
Length = L = \begin{cases}
\begin{array}{|c|c|c|c|c|c|c|c|c|c|c|c|c|}
\hline
4 & 3 & 2 & 1 & -2 & -5 & -6 & -5 & -2 & 1 & 2 & 3 & 4 \\ \hline
4 & 3 & 2 & 1 & -2 & -5 & -6 & -5 & -2 & 1 & 2 & 3 & 4 \\ \hline
\end{array} \\
\qquad\qquad\qquad \vdots \\
\begin{array}{|c|c|c|c|c|c|c|c|c|c|c|c|c|}
\hline
4 & 3 & 2 & 1 & -2 & -5 & -6 & -5 & -2 & 1 & 2 & 3 & 4 \\ \hline
\end{array}
\end{cases}
$$

The above model requires an estimate of the scale σ. In the implementation described by Chaudhuri et al. [25], a fixed value of σ was used and determined to be effective even for detecting vessels of varying scales. Figure 6.13 illustrates the effectiveness of an algorithm using this model σ.

Sato et al. [91] propose using multiple Gaussian filters using a small number of σ values (typically three or four different values are used) to account for vessels of different widths. Gang et al. [44] have proposed a method that relies on adaptively estimating the σ value. They point out that the Gaussian filters, while appropriate as vessel models, do not directly permit measurement of the vessel width. They propose an amplitude modified second-order differential Gaussian model of the form:

$$f(x) = \frac{1}{\sqrt{2\pi\sigma^3}}(x^2 - \sigma^2)e^{-x^2/2\sigma^2} \tag{6.5}$$

With this model, there is a linear relationship between the parameter σ and the diameter of the vessel. The notion of vessel diameter used in this model is distinct from one that can be measured by locating the vessel boundaries.

6.4.8 Models for Vessels with a "Hollow" Appearance

Frequently in fundus images, vessels sometimes appear to be "hollow," that is, the walls of the vessels appear as dark pixels and the center of the vessels appear lighter, sometimes as light as the background itself. This is caused by a reflection from or below the surface of the vessel and is known as vessel reflex. Figure 6.12 illustrates this phenomenon and more information can be found in [89, 45]. While some of the previously mentioned models are still successful in identifying these vessels [21], none of the models were developed with this phenomenon specifically in mind. To accurately model these "hollow" vessels, a twin-Gaussian model has been proposed by Gao et al. [45].

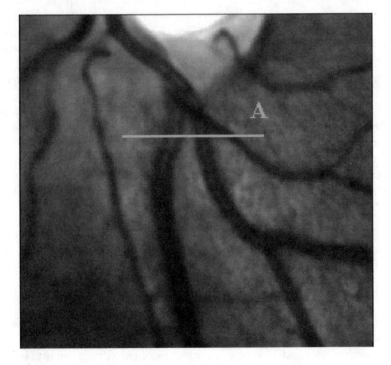

FIGURE 6.12
Magnified portion of the image in Figure 6.7 depicting the central reflex phenomenon, that is, vessels that appear lighter in color in the center, as if they were hollow. This is caused by the reflectance of light on or below the surface of the vessel See [16, 45, 89] for a more detailed explanation.

The first Gaussian in this model is representative of the entire vessel, whereas the second Gaussian represents the reflex and they are combined as follows:

$$C_{model}(x) = C_{vessel}(x) + C_{reflex}(x)$$
$$C_{vessel}(x) = b - c \times e^{-(x-a)^2/2\sigma_1^2} \qquad (6.6)$$
$$C_{reflex}(x) = d \times e^{-(x-\epsilon)^2/2\sigma_2^2}$$

The parameters a, b, and c are as described above in Equation 6.6; d is representative of the relative contrast between the vessel pixels and the reflex pixels, ϵ is the center point of the reflex, and σ_1 and σ_2 are representative of the widths of the vessel and the reflex, respectively. This can be seen in Figure 6.11b. Given this equation for a cross section of a vessel with a central reflex, a filter can be generated for the one-dimensional case and for the two-dimensional case in exactly the same manner as described in the previous section and used to detect the center points of these types of vessels.

This section has summarized some of the models used for retinal vasculature that have been used for vessel segmentation. None of the models is individually fully adequate for all applications and the models presented are not all-inclusive. For example, Pedersen et al. [83] have described a vessel model based on using a six degrees-of-freedom cubic spline and its derivatives to locate the boundaries of vessels. This work is not described here. Overall, a combination of these modeling ideas is considered the best approach to vessel segmentation. Of course, the more sophisticated models are associated with higher computational costs, making them less attractive for real-time applications. With rapid improvements in computing speeds, applications can be expected to incorporate increasingly more sophisticated models. In our experience, the kernels based on low-pass differentiators [21, 96] have proved an excellent trade-off when computation speed is important and provide excellent results. When computation times are not critical, a combination of preprocessing algorithms using the Gaussian model and algorithms based on the low-pass differentiators could also be considered.

6.5 Vessel Extraction Approaches

The models described in the previous section lead to a variety of approaches for conducting segmentation and tracing. In this chapter, the term "vessel segmentation" is used to imply the process of classifying each pixel in the image as either belonging to a vessel or not. The term "vessel tracing" is the closely related but refers to the distinct process of extracting the centerlines of the vessels.

There are two prevalent approaches for extracting vascular structure from retinal images. The first approach requires certain processing to be done for each pixel in the image and will be referred to as pixel processing algorithms. The second approach is known as vectorization or exploratory tracing. These exploratory methods start at an initial point that is determined to be part of a vessel and then "track" that vessel through the image as far as possible. In general, these methods are computationally much faster than pixel processing approaches as only the pixels in the immediate vicinity of the vessel structure are actually "explored" while extracting the vasculature structure. This is the reason they are referred to as "exploratory" algorithms. Both pixel processing and exploratory algorithms are discussed in the following sections.

6.5.1 Pixel Processing-Based Algorithms

The pixel processing-based approaches [49, 53, 86] work by adaptive filtering, morphological preprocessing segmentation, followed by thinning and branch point analysis. These methods require the processing of every image pixel and multiple operations per pixel. When these operations are highly regular, they can be implemented on fast workstations [86] and pipelined accelerators [25]. Other pixel processing approaches involve the use of neural networks [58, 99] and frequency analysis [111] to determine if individual pixels are vessels. Generally, the computational needs of pixel processing methods scale sharply with image size, and are usually unsuitable for fast, real-time processing without special hardware.

The method of Chaudhuri et al. [25] is based on two-dimensional matched filters. These filters are designed to maximize response over vessels and minimize the response in background regions. Prior to matched filtering, the images are smoothed using a 5×5 median filter to reduce the effect of spurious noise. This algorithm uses a Gaussian vessel model similar to that described earlier in Section 6.4. In this case, a vessel profile is described by the Gaussian function

$$f(x, y) = A\left(1 - ke^{-d^2/2\sigma^2}\right)$$

where d is the distance between the point and the center of the vessel, σ is representative of the width of the profile, A is the intensity of the local background, and k is a measure of the contrast between the vessel and the local background. From this profile, a kernel K is developed that is defined by:

$$K(x, y) = -e^{-x^2/2\sigma^2} \quad \text{for } |y| \leq L/2 \tag{6.7}$$

where L is the length of the kernel, which is the parameter associated with the length of a vessel. This algorithm bounds x at $\pm 3\sigma$. The kernel given in the above equation matches (i.e., yields a maximum response for) a vertical vessel that is locally straight. For different orientations, a kernel with $15°$ of angular resolution is constructed by simply rotating it accordingly. The value of L is set to 9, which is experimentally determined to work well with both "normal" and highly tortuous (curvy) vessels. The value of σ is fixed and set to 2.

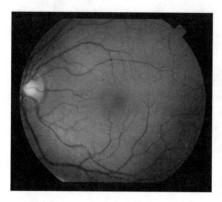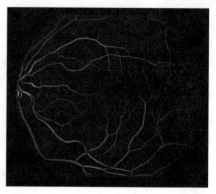

FIGURE 6.13

The use of a matched filter for enhancing vessel-like structures. The left panel shows a retinal image. The panel on the right is the result of matched filtering using the algorithm of Chaudhuri et al. [25].

All the directional kernels are applied at every pixel in an image, with the maximum magnitude response being retained as the value for that pixel in the results image. The results image obtained from this operation can be seen in Figure 6.13. If this maximum is above a certain threshold, the pixel is labeled as vessel. This threshold is determined by selecting the value that maximized the inter-class intensity variance as described in [81].

6.5.1.1 Morphological Filtering-Based Algorithms

The next class of pixel processing algorithms of interest is based on using operators from mathematical morphology [37] as a means of segmenting vessels. A good example is the work of Zana and Klein [125, 126]. This algorithm is based on the idea that the vessels in a fundus image exhibit three identifying traits. First, the shape of the cross section is approximately Gaussian. Second, vessels are piece-wise linear and connected in a tree-like pattern. Third, they have a certain width and cannot be too close together. From these traits, morphological operators and algorithms are designed for classifying the vessel pixels. The first such possible operation would be to use the linearity trait. From this trait, a set of linear structuring elements can be used with opening and top-hat operations, which are discussed below.

Two morphological operations, termed "opening" and "closing," respectively, are based on combinations of erosion and dilation operations. The opening operation is defined as an erosion operation followed by a dilation operation. The closing operation is defined as a dilation operation followed by an erosion operation. If the vessels are known to be darker than the background, a simple gray-scale dilation operation can be realized by a min-filter. Otherwise, a max-filter is used to dilate the bright vessels. For each pixel, the max/min-filter output is the maximum/minimum value of all pixels within the neighborhood of that pixel. For dark vessels, erosion can be implemented by max-filtering.

Another morphological operation used is the "top-hat" operation. This operation is defined as the difference between the original image and the image resulting from an opening operation. This is useful in identifying the parts of the image that disappear as a result of the opening operation.

Recall the three vessel traits from above: the shape of the cross section is approximately Gaussian; they are piece-wise linear and connected in a tree-like way; and they have a certain width and cannot be too close together. Using the linear and width traits, it is possible to brighten/identify the blood vessels by summing the results of a series of top-hat operations that used a linear structuring element. Each top-hat operation would brighten a portion of the vessel structure that corresponded to the orientation of the structuring element. This structuring element would need to be long enough and oriented over a range of different directions to ensure that all vessels in all orientations would be eliminated by the opening operation in the top-hat operation and ultimately brightened (i.e., enhance the contrast between the vessels and the background) by the top hats. However, this process results in noise also being brightened. Another trait, the connectivity of the vessels, needs to be utilized before performing the top-hat operations.

To remove the noise in the image, a geodesic reconstruction [37] is first performed on the image. Performing this operation using twelve 15 pixel $\times$ 1 pixel structuring elements, oriented at every $15°$, results in an image $I'(x, y)$ where all elements in the original image $I(x, y)$ smaller than 15 pixels, such as noise and abnormalities, are eliminated. This operation is also known as a linear opening by reconstruction of size 15. Thus, the sum of the top hats can now be applied to brighten the vessels. At this point, a simple threshold can be applied to separate the vessels from the background but there still exist some background linear features or some bright or dark thin irregular zones that may falsely be identified as vessels. To eliminate these, the Gaussian-like curvature trait of the vessels can be exploited. This is done by computing the Laplacian of the Gaussian (LoG) at all points in $I'(x, y)$ and using its sign as an approximation of the sign of the curvature [101]. By using a Gaussian with a width of 7 pixels and $\sigma = 7/4$, the edges in $I'(x, y)$ can be detected based upon the curvature. If the sign of the curvature is positive, the pixels will be white and negative values will be portrayed in black. Once the LoG image $I''(x, y)$ is calculated, it once again becomes necessary to remove the noise in the background caused by "curves" detected in the previous process. This is done by applying three additional morphological operations in sequence to I''. First, a linear morphological opening by reconstruction of size 15 is performed, followed by a linear closing by reconstruction of size 15 and a linear opening of size 29. The last step is to threshold the resulting image to determine the vessels.

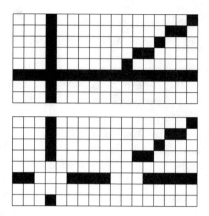

FIGURE 6.14
The breaking of the skeletonized vessels into segments.

Another pixel processing-based method, which can be thought of as a generalization of another morphological algorithm known as the watershed algorithm, is described by Hoover et al. [12]. The first step in this algorithm is to generate a set of seed points (or "queue points") using the matched filter response (MFR) of Chaudhuri et al. [25] to enhance vessels over the background. They used the same matched filter given in Equation 6.7. This MFR is then thresholded where all pixels above the threshold are retained as candidate pixels. These pixels are then thinned to a 1 pixel wide linear structure that represents the vessels. The reader is referred to [3] for a more thorough discussion of thinning. From these thinned pixels, line segments are formed by erasing any point that has more than two adjacent candidate pixels. This, in essence, is deleting any point where a vessel splits into two, or the point where two vessels intersect while keeping any point that is an interior part of a segment as exemplified in Figure 6.14. When this is complete, all segments with fewer than 10 pixels are discarded and the remaining segment endpoints are placed into a queue as "seed" points. These seed points are then used as a starting point in a procedure called "threshold probing." This is an iterative process where the threshold for an area is initially set to the intensity value in the MFR image of the seed pixel for the area. At each iteration, a region is grown from the seed using a conditional paint-fill technique. This paint-fill spreads to all connecting pixels whose values are above the current threshold and should be considered as "candidate" vessel pixels. Once all pixels for a particular threshold are identified, the region is then tested to see if any of the stopping criteria is met. If a criterion is not met, the threshold is decreased by one and the paint-fill technique is once again applied. The stopping criteria and its effect/rationale are as follows.

- *The number of pixels in the region exceeds a maximum number T_{max}. This ensures that the region stops and that other regions are grown (and allows multiple threshold to be used for different regions of the image).*
- *If the threshold reaches zero.*
- *If a region touches two or more previously detected regions.* This helps connect discontinuities on a vessel into a single "identified" region.
- *If a region is at least 30 pixels in size and is "fringing," as defined by the ratio of the number of pixels bordering another region to the total number of points in region.* This ratio must exceed T_{fringe}. This prevents the current region from searching along borders of previously detected regions.
- *If a region is at least 30 pixels in size and seems to be branching too much.* This is determined using the ratio of the total number of pixels in region to the number of branches in the region. This ratio must be less than a threshold T_{tree} where the number of branches in a region is found by calculating the skeleton of the region. This prevents over-branching down false paths, particularly in poor contrast or noisy areas of an image.

Once the iterative probing is complete, the candidate region is labeled as a vessel if it connects two previous regions or has more than T_{min} pixels and less than T_{max} pixels. If the region is labeled a vessel, its endpoints are, in turn, added to the queue of seed points. When one of these "new" seeds is probed, an artificial boundary is placed perpendicularly at the end of the previous vessel region. Its purpose is to prevent the new probing from "fringing" on the previously detected region which forces the new region to grow away from the previous region.

6.5.1.2   *Methods Based on Edge Detection*

An algorithm described by Wang and Lee in [119] uses two basic appro-aches prevalent in edge detection. First, it performs an edge enhancement/thresholding technique to find vessel edges and then applies an edge fitting technique. For the first part of the algorithm, Sobel operators are used to enhance the edges of vessels. These edges are then thinned [3] so that the edge pixel with the lowest intensity value along each cross section of the vessel segments remains. These remaining edge pixels are used as "seeds" in the second part of the algorithm. As discussed in Section 6.4.7, it has been shown that one model of a vessel has a Gaussian-shaped cross section. Such edge models of the vessels can be obtained by local windowing and local thresholding, from which the skeletons of the vessels within the local gray-scale images are extracted [30].

The second part of the algorithm takes the local thresholded image and runs it through a set of twelve 15×15 matched binary filters (i.e., a filter consisting of only zeros and ones) with a single row of ones for each of the 12 cardinal directions (each $15°$ apart). These filters will yield a maximum response when aligned over the vessel boundaries found with the Sobel operators. After convolving these templates with every pixel, the mean and standard deviation can be calculated. Then for each seed pixel, the response of the 12 convolution values can be measured and compared against an experimentally determined threshold. Those responses that are higher than the threshold are considered to be vessel pixels. Those that are lower are considered background. The final step is to use a single linkage region growing technique with locally adaptive thresholds. Overall, this technique emphasizes speed by use of binary valued filters.

Li and Chutatape [67] implement a vessel detector using Kirsch operators in much the same fashion as [119] used Sobel operators and [25] used matched filters [67]. A Kirsch operator is a kernel that represents an "ideal" edge in each of the eight cardinal directions (0 to $360°$, in $45°$ intervals) [101]. It works by applying each of the eight Kirsch templates at each pixel $I(x, y)$ in image I and building I', where each pixel $I'(x, y)$ is the maximum response of the eight Kirsch templates at $I(x, y)$. A threshold is then experimentally derived and each pixel in I' greater than the threshold is considered a vessel.

Feature-based registration is one of the applications where segmentation is commonly used as a primitive. Pinz et al. have described a method for extracting vessels using matching edgels [85]. The purpose of their vessel segmentation algorithm is to extract "enough vessels" to be able to perform registration [9, 22, 23]. It works by first locating edgels (edge pixels) based on the gradient magnitude of a pixel and a locally computed threshold. The next step of the process is to find corresponding "partner" edgels. This is done for each edgel by first identifying a best matching "partner edgel." Potential partners are selected based on two constraints. First, the distance between the two must between 3 and 17 pixels (inclusive) and, second, the angle deviation between the gradient direction of the edgels must be $180 \pm 30°$. For each edgel in the set of potential partners, a cross-section line is used to connect them to the original edgel. The angular differences from the cross-section line to the gradients of the original edgel and the potential partner are computed and summed, and the cross section with the minimum sum determines the appropriate pairing. A common phenomenon known as vessel reflex (discussed in Section 6.4.8) necessitates another step in the process. This vessel reflex sometimes results in a single vessel cross section actually consisting of three pairs of connected edgels (cross sections). These edgels are combined into a single cross section if the orientations of the three are similar and the resulting cross section is below the maximum vessel diameter and the lengths of the two outer crossings are similar.

Once the vessel cross sections have been identified, the next step is to connect them and form vessel centerlines. This is done by connecting the midpoints of adjacent vessel cross sections as long as the following conditions are met:

- The cross-sectional lengths are similar.
- The distance between the cross section is below a certain value.
- The lines connecting consecutive cross sections should be relatively straight.
- The combined cross sections should be almost parallel.
- A cross section can only belong to one midpoint connecting line.

Once connected, short "vessels" are eliminated if the length of the vessel is smaller than the length of the cross section (i.e., the vessel width is larger than the length). The final step is to connect vessels located at crossings or intersections. These are the sites where only vessels are allowed to cross after checking both directions. This is done using the following constraints:

- The vessels to be connected must be longer than the distance to be spanned.
- The vessels to be connected must have similar cross-sectional lengths (vessel widths).
- The resulting connection must be as linear as possible.

Overall, pixel processing approaches are a useful tool, especially if computational speed is not an overriding concern. They can also be useful as preprocessors for the exploratory approaches discussed next.

6.5.2 Exploratory Algorithms

Approaches described in this section are referred to variously as vessel tracking, vectorial tracking, or tracing [21, 26, 109]. These methods work by exploiting local image properties to trace the vasculature starting from an initial point either specified manually or detected automatically. They only process pixels close to the vasculature, avoiding the processing of every image pixel, and so are appropriately called "exploratory algorithms." They have several properties that make them attractive for real-time, live, and high-resolution processing because they can provide useful partial results [96] and are computationally efficient. (As an aside, numerous papers have been published on vectorization of binarized images within the document image processing literature; for example, [57]). These algorithms can be grouped in two categories referred to as semi-automated tracing where user input is needed and fully automated tracing where no user interaction is necessary.

6.5.2.1   Semi-automated Tracing Algorithms

One common type of semi-automated tracing algorithm is where the initial and end points of the vessel (sometimes also the direction and width) are entered manually. These are extensively used in quantitative coronary angiography analysis (QCA) [60, 102, 103, 109, 117, 127]. These algorithms are accurate but are unsuitable for real-time retinal image processing because they require manual input and suffer from high computational time, which is not a compelling constraint in QCA. Another QCA approach requiring initialization of points is the use of "snakes" [60, 104].

The first semi-automatic retinal algorithm is one used for identification and diameter measurement described by Gao et al. [45]. In it, two points c_0 and c_e on a vessel are manually supplied by the user. A line is drawn connecting these points with a direction d_0. The region or neighborhood used for estimating the parameters of their model is limited to three times the estimated vessel profile width. The vessel is modeled as a sum of two Gaussian equations as shown in Equation 6.6, where its parameters are estimated by the nonlinear Levenberg-Marquardt method [87]. The seven unknowns $(a, b, c, d, \epsilon, \sigma_1, \sigma_2)$ are varied from a predetermined set of values and the method works iteratively to minimize a χ^2 cost function to determine the parameters that best fit the profile. Once these best-fit parameters are found, the center point of the vessel can be determined from the value of a. Using this new center point, a second point is found in the same fashion using the perpendicular profile obtained at a point that is 2 pixels away in the previous direction (in this case d_0). This continues until six points are found. The centroid of these six points, c_1, is the center of the first vessel segment whose direction is defined by the vector from the previous center (c_0) to the new center (c_1). This procedure of finding six points to determine the next segment continues until c_e is reached. Another algorithm where start and endpoints are entered manually for tracing retinal vessels in ocular fundus images is given by Pedersen et al. [83].

Another class of semi-automated tracing algorithms is where a manually entered initial point and direction is specified by the user. This tracing algorithm recursively tracks the entire arterial tree [68] using a breadth-first search. This would not be guaranteed to generate complete results for retinal images because the vessels are not necessarily connected, especially in partial views of the retina.

6.5.2.2   Fully Automated Tracing Algorithms

This set of algorithms automatically extracts the vascular tree without user initialization or intervention. They work well for coronary angiograms and have been applied to three-dimensional reconstruction [46, 79, 110]. Most of them [79] utilize the centerline gray-level intensities.

In retinal angiograms, although the blood vessels are darker than the local background, areas like the fovea are also dark relative to the average background. This consideration has motivated the development of algorithms that rely on more localized cues, such as contrast and edge gradients, similar to some of the methods used in QCA [21, 102, 103]. This also enables the algorithms to be more robust to lighting-related artifacts such as glare, dropouts, and overexposed frames that can easily occur in retinal images, especially in images containing pathologies that are generally of most interest.

A Kalman filter-based method that uses Gaussian matched filters is described in [26]. This method utilizes an amplitude-modified, second-order Gaussian model for the blood vessels. The first step of this algorithm is to extract an intensity profile from the circumference of the circular region placed around the optic disk (found using a separate algorithm). This profile is then convolved with the amplitude-modified, second-order Gaussian filter described by Equation 6.5. The points at which the response is a relative maximum are candidate points at which vessels are entering/leaving the optic disk. From this set, the six highest maxima are selected as vessel starting points. These points are placed into a queue and are selected in turn for vessel tracking.

Each vessel segment is defined by three parameters: the width w, the centerline point c, and the direction d. For each step in the tracking process, a Kalman filter [51] is used to give the optimal estimation of the next centerline point (based on the previous location, direction, and supplied tolerances/ covariance). At this estimated location, the Gaussian filter, as described in Equation 6.5, is applied to find the true center. In this process, a value of $w/2$ is used for σ, where the w is the value of the width of the last vessel segment. Once the correct location is found, the new segment's location, direction, and width are updated. The zero crossings of the response are then used to determine width (i.e., width = distance between zero crossings/1.2). At each step, if a branch is detected, its location is added to the start point queue. "This iterative process ends when an endpoint is detected by Gaussian filter and the tracking result is recorded" [51].

While this algorithm is successful at tracing the vessels, its success strongly depends on the initial estimation of the optic disk, which in itself is a hard problem [66]. Additionally, by using the optic disk as the starting location, this algorithm is restricted to the set of retinal images in which the optic disk is present. Another issue not addressed by this algorithm is the fact that all the vessels in the image are not necessarily connected to the optic disk. Another automated tracing algorithm that uses steerable filters is given in [62]. This algorithm also uses the optic disk to initiate the traces and suffers from the same limitations.

Another exploratory algorithm based on vessel models that are based on local gray-scale intensity differences is described by Collorec and Coatrieux [31]. As can be expected, this issue leads to some "hard problems" as noted by Coatrieux et al. [29]. Specifically, they note the difficulty in handling branching and crossover points because they do not conform well to the vessel models, the difficulty of making the algorithms locally adaptive, and the problem of wandering and looping of traces.

6.6   RPI-Trace

Can et al. [21, 96] have addressed the issues noted by Coatrieux et al. using a stricter model for the vessels in an algorithm. Their algorithm and implementation gave birth to what is referred to as RPI-Trace in this chapter. Can et al. overcome two "hard problems" described by Coatrieux et al., namely, (1) robust and accurate handling of branching and crossover points; and (2) improved handling of discontinuous regions by relying on local contrast and edge information (as opposed to gray values), instead of a global intensity threshold. It also overcomes the "wandering and looping" artifact using an improved stopping criterion. Some tracing accuracy improvement is also gained by more accurate angular discretization, more filtering across and along the vessels, and more careful handling of the discrete image space. Computationally, this algorithm is comparably attractive. The very strict rules used by this algorithm for validation and verification of initial seed points allow it to reject many incorrect seed points, thus making up for the higher complexity in the core tracing computations. More recent work has resulted in sub-pixel localization of vessel boundaries, and much improved handling of branching and crossover points.

Can's method relies on a recursive tracing of the vasculature based on a localized model. This approach has been shown to be much faster (e.g., video frame rates are readily achieved), more adaptive, and more practical for implementation on conventional and parallel MIMD computers [4]. It also requires the fewest parameter settings, and provides useful partial results [96], which is discussed in Section 6.7. This fully automated exploratory tracing algorithm proceeds in three stages.

Step 1 (seed point initialization):   The algorithm analyzes the image along a coarse grid (see Figure 6.9a) to gather gray-scale statistics (contrast and brightness levels) and to detect seed locations on blood vessels using the gray-scale minima between opposite-signed, one-dimensional edges described in Section 6.4.5. False seed points are filtered out by testing for the existence of a pair of sufficiently strong parallel edges with opposite gradient values. For this, a set of directional kernels is applied to the seed's neighboring points, radially in 16 directions, in which the kernel used is orthogonal to the radial line, and the two strongest responses are found. This search strategy is illustrated in Figure 6.16. The initial point is filtered out if the two strongest responses do not both exceed a sensitivity threshold T_e given in Equation 6.3, or if the directions of the two strongest edges are not sufficiently similar (within ±22.5°). On average, about 40% of the initial points are filtered out by this procedure.

Step 2 (recursive tracing):   The second stage, illustrated in Figure 6.15, is a sequence of recursive tracing steps that are initiated at each of the filtered seed points, and proceed along vessel centerlines using an update equation

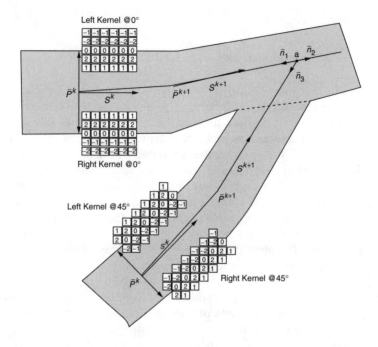

FIGURE 6.15
Illustration of the core tracing step in the exploratory algorithm of Can et al. [21]. The left and right kernels are shown for 45° and 0° on the two left vessel branches. Starting from a point p^k, the direction of maximum response of these kernels defines the direction of the tracing step. Crossing and branching points of the vasculature are detected where traces intersect.

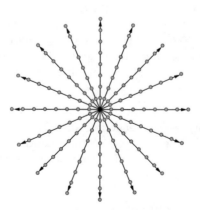

FIGURE 6.16
The radial search strategy used to verify initial points as vessel points at which to initiate tracing in Step 1. Each dot represents a location at which a template perpendicular to the radius is applied to search for an edge.

of the following form:

$$p^{k+1} = p^k + \alpha \left[\cos\left(\frac{2\pi s^k}{N}\right), \sin\left(\frac{2\pi s^k}{N}\right) \right]^T + \beta^k \qquad (6.8)$$

where k is the iteration count, p^k and p^{k+1} denote the current and new locations of the trace, α is a step size, $s^k \in \{0, 1, 2 \ldots N - 1\}$ is an integer index specifying one of N discretized angular directions (usually $N = 16$), and β^k is a lateral displacement vector that centers the new point p^{k+1} on the vessel. In Figure 6.15, this is illustrated for a pair of intersecting vessels. The left and right directional kernels at $0°$ and $45°$ are also illustrated for the lower branch in Figure 6.15. The angle at which the correlation kernels produce the highest response is estimated. These maximum responses are computed by performing a local search along a line perpendicular to the current trace within a neighborhood of size $M/2$, where M is defined as the maximum expected blood vessel width. The next trace point p^{k+1} is determined by taking a step of size α, from the current trace point in the direction s^{k+1}, and applying a correction β that is calculated based on how far p^{k+1} was from the center of the points at which the left and right template responses were found. This new point is kept only if it does not intersect any previously detected vessels, is not outside the image frame, and if the sum of maximum template left and right responses is greater than the sensitivity threshold, which is computed as follows:

$$T = 6L(1 + \lambda|L_{av} - B_{av}|) \qquad (6.9)$$

where L is the length of the template, and L_{av} and B_{av} are the estimates for the average vessel intensity and average background intensity, respectively. Hence, their difference is an estimate of average contrast. λ is a scaling factor between 0 and 1 that can be thought of as a percentage of overall contrast, and the 6 is two times the response of the template for a ridge of one unit high per unit length (i.e., response per contrast increase). Low values for λ make tracing more sensitive to noise whereas high λ values cause tracing to terminate prematurely. Average intensity values for the background and vessel are estimated using the intensity values along the grid lines used for seed point detection.

Step 3 (landmark extraction): The tracing that starts from a seed point continues until the end of the vessel is reached, or until the centerline of the tracing intersects a previously detected vessel centerline. Landmarks are placed at intersections of traces and at locations where three or more centerline traces meet, as shown in Figure 6.30f. In the former case, the location is the actual intersection; in the latter, the location is the centroid of the trace endpoints. These landmarks are characterized by this location and by the orientations of the traces meeting to form the landmark. Example trace results are shown in Figure 6.17, and a composite result containing traces and landmarks is shown in Figure 6.2.

Modifications and improvements to RPI-Trace have been implemented in [93] and by the authors of this chapter. These modifications include:

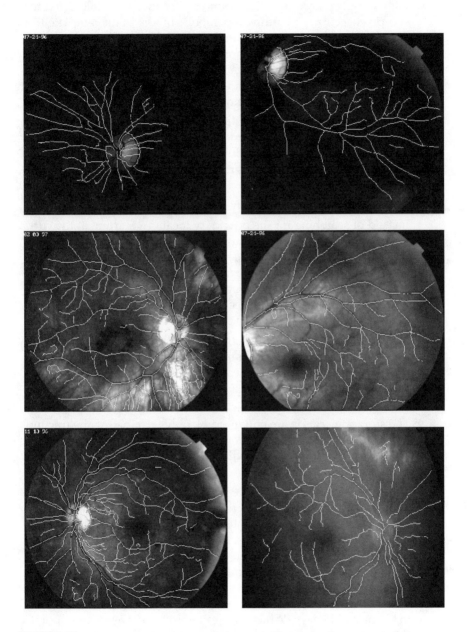

FIGURE 6.17
Results of exploratory tracing [21] on a diverse set of images with varying lighting conditions
and presence of pathologies.

- The centerline, boundary, and seed point locations are computed with sub-pixel accuracy. The boundary locations are calculated to sub-pixel accuracy by fitting a parabolic model to the template response around its maximum, and then finding the location of the peak from the center of this parabola. For certain applications, sub-pixel computation of image centerlines and landmarks gives improved precision for higher-level computer vision tasks such as registration and spatial referencing [94, 95].

- The seed points along the grid lines are determined more accurately. This is achieved using one-dimensional edge detection constraints in addition to intensity constraints and local thresholds, as described in Section 6.4.5. Results of this method are shown in Figure 6.10.

- The local threshold value for T_e, as described in Section 6.4.5, is used in finding each trace point rather than a global threshold.

- Instead of searching for the boundary locations starting at the current trace point and stepping out, the width of the previous locations is used to limit the search space for the boundary location at the current iteration. Based on the current iteration's estimated location of a vessel boundary, the search space is bounded within a fixed distance Δ. Hence, abrupt changes in boundary location between two iterations is prevented and the computational time is reduced.

- Instead of applying a set of templates with fixed length, multiple templates of different lengths are applied, with the resulting responses being normalized based on template length. Detection and localization can be improved simultaneously by longer directional templates [24].

- The stopping criteria are enhanced by only terminating the tracing when several consecutive weak responses are detected, rather than a single weak response. This modification gives additional robustness to the tracing.

- The use of a bin data structure to calculate intersections is added. Two spatial data structures, each representing the area of the original image are created. One is used to track center points and the other is used to track boundary points. In each of these structures, the area of the original image is broken into smaller pieces or "bins." Each bin represents an equivalent area on the original image, typically a 4×4 or 8×8 pixel area. When a center point or a boundary point is found, it is "placed" into the bin that corresponds with its location in the original image. When it is desired to see if a new center point intersects with an existing trace, the appropriate bins are queried. These bins help to reduce the time needed to determine if there is an intersection and can also be used in other algorithms such as registration and spatial referencing.

6.7 Algorithm Design Considerations for Real-Time Tracing

The design of algorithms for real-time vessel tracing are driven by the end objective. Spatial referencing [95] is an excellent application example. Here, the end goal is not the vessel traces by themselves, but rather the results of image registration. The role of the vessel traces is to provide the spatial landmarks needed for the registration. This is an instance of a "hard" real-time system [65] in which the computations must be completed prior to a deadline, or else the system is considered to have failed. A failure represents a loss of tracking, requiring the surgical laser to be switched off [122]. System performance degrades with an excessive number of failures. The computational deadlines are dictated by the frame rate of the imaging camera (usually about 30/sec). Within this deadline, two computations must be completed: landmark extraction and landmark-based image matching. For a given computer system, the computational budget is fixed within this deadline. It is desired to maximize the probability of a successful image match within this budget.

The computational budgeting issues are illustrated in Figure 6.18. The left and right columns show the partial results of two different tracing procedures, captured at 8%, 28%, and 53% of the total computational effort. The only difference between the two procedures is the order in which the vessel segments are traced; they use the same tracing algorithm, the same total amount of computation, and produce the same final result. The partial results in the right column are far more valuable because they have more numerous and more prominent landmarks. Given a high-quality partial result, image matching can be attempted from partial traces. If this is successful (i.e., sufficient confidence exists in the result), then the overall system can be much faster. Even if this is unsuccessful, it can form the basis for a better subsequent matching attempt. The frame cycle time can be subdivided into a series of milestones and the performance of the matching algorithms monitored at each milestone. Failure to reach set milestones can provide an early indication of conditions such as poor image quality (images that are dim, saturated, out of focus, affected by glare, etc.). The idea of utilizing partial results relates to the concept of imprecise computations as proposed by Lin et al. [75] within the real-time scheduling literature. The methods for scheduling the tracing computations in a manner that produces such an early yield of high-quality partial results are described next.

The spatial prioritization scheduling algorithm of Shen et al. [96] aims to maximize the number and quality of the bifurcation and crossover points in the image within a given number of computations. The quality of an individual landmark can be quantified based on the prominence of the intersecting vessels and their contrast, as follows. Suppose a single landmark is formed by the intersection of m vessel segments. Let t_p be the estimated thickness

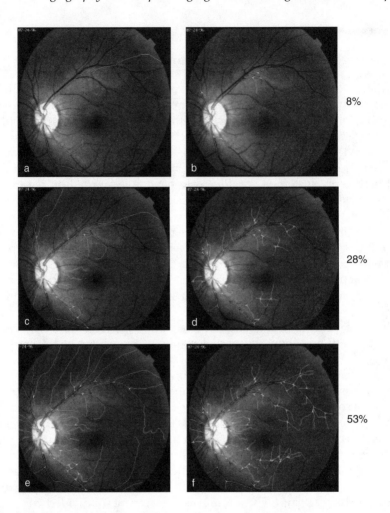

8%

28%

53%

FIGURE 6.18
The impact of scheduling on landmark detection performance for the same level of computational effort (W/W_{total}): (a) a partial result from tracing an image using a poorly scheduled algorithm shows the work wasted on long and unproductive tracing; (b) a partial result from a better scheduled algorithm for the same computational work. The latter is much more productive, having prioritized its efforts in a manner that yields numerous prominent landmarks early. (c–f) Partial results for the two algorithms at 28% and 53% effort.

of segment p, and s_p a measure of its edge strength. Then, the quality of the landmark can be measured as:

$$q = \sum_{p=1}^{m} s_p \cdot t_p \qquad (6.10)$$

The edge strength s_p is estimated using the directional correlation kernels [21] and summarized in the previous section. The quality of a partial result is measured simply by summing the qualities of the individual landmarks constituting it.

The computational effort can be quantified as well. One straightforward method to quantify computational work is to count the processor cycles. However, such a measure is necessarily dependent upon a specific combination of processor, compiler, and other implementation details. An extensive profiling analysis revealed that the vast majority of the processor cycles were expended on computing the response of local correlation kernels. This suggests a simple system-independent measure of computational work: simply count the number of correlation kernel computations. We use the variable w to denote this count. The tracing of the vasculature is carried out through a sequence of computations, with the work (as measured by counting correlation kernels) denoted $w_1, w_2, \ldots, w_N$, that produce a sequence of non-negative incremental results $q_1, q_2, \ldots, q_N$. The quality of the partial result at the completion of w_k is given by:

$$Q_k = \sum_{n=1}^{k} q_n \tag{6.11}$$

where q_n is the quality measure defined in Equation 6.10 for the nth landmark. The cumulative computational effort used to produce the above partial result is given by:

$$W_k = \sum_{n=1}^{k} w_n \tag{6.12}$$

At this point some observations can be made. The sequence of partial results is always of monotonically improving quality; that is, $Q_{k+1} \geq Q_k$. In the terminology of imprecise computation, the tracing algorithm is an "anytime algorithm" [75]. The amount of vasculature in the (finite-size) image is finite. Thus, a definite endpoint exists for the tracing, and the last partial result also represents the complete result. For a given image, and algorithm settings such as the grid size and sensitivity, the quality of the complete result, denoted Q_{total}, and the total computational work W_{total} are both finite and fixed. Finally, the order of tracing of vascular segments has minimal effect on the final result. The above observations suggest that, in principle, one could divide the vasculature arbitrarily into vessel segments and decide the order in which the vessel segments are traced. A scheduling algorithm can decide the starting, stopping, and restarting of the tracing, and choice of seed points. An optimal scheduling algorithm will make decisions that maximize the rate at which the quality of partial results improves.

The monotonically improving quality of a partial result can be described by a growth function $Q(W)$. This function does not have a closed-form expression, and is represented by an empirically derived Q vs. W curve. The quality and total work (Q_{total} and W_{total}) are different for different images, so for comparison and averaging across images, it is advantageous to normalize

Q and W by Q_{total} and W_{total}, respectively. With this in mind, the question of interest is: given a partial computation $W_k / W_{total} \leq 1$, how can the tracing computations be scheduled so that the normalized quality of the corresponding partial result, Q_k / Q_{total}, is maximized for every k? This can also be viewed as maximizing the area under the normalized Q vs. W curve. The fully optimal scheduling algorithm must perform this maximization globally for every partial result — a daunting task. To maximize the optimality criterion just described, the scheduling algorithm must somehow perform just enough tracing to detect each of the landmarks, thereby minimizing the amount of work done. Simultaneously, it should trace around the highest-quality landmarks first, thereby maximizing the quality measure. Unfortunately, achieving this objective requires prior knowledge of the very traces that are sought — an inherently impossible task. This leads to the inevitable conclusion that an optimal schedule can only be computed in hindsight or, equivalently, with perfect foresight. In other words, the optimal schedule is hypothetical. Even with perfect foresight, computation of the optimal schedule is a difficult global combinatorial optimization; for each value of $W_k \leq W_{total}$, one must select a set of landmarks so that the sum of their computational work does not exceed W_k, and the sum of their qualities is the maximum.

Shen et al. [96] described an approximation to the optimal solution known as the preemptive spatial prioritization algorithm. A detailed step-by-step dissection of the optimal schedule for several images reveals that it primarily derives its high performance from advance knowledge of the spatial locations and quality values of the landmarks. It concentrates just-sufficient levels of tracing effort around the most promising landmarks. This observation suggests predicting landmark locations and qualities, and using these to schedule the tracing.

Landmark locations and qualities can be predicted from the initial grid analysis step of exploratory tracing. The parallel edge-based model discussed in Section 6.4.6 can be used to weed out all seed points that do not correspond to a pair of nearly parallel edges, and produce local orientation, strength, and width estimates (Figure 6.19a). Shown in Figure 6.19b through g are cropped and enlarged views of selected boxes formed by the grid lines. In these images, the short lines crossing the grid lines mark the estimated orientations of the initial points. The black dots on these lines indicate the location of the initial points after the filtering. From these images, the presence/absence of landmarks inside the grid box can be guessed even before tracing by analyzing the distributions and orientations of the initial points around the grid box. For example, in Figure 6.19b through d, the orientations of the initial points clearly suggest the existence of at least one landmark inside the grid box. Conversely, in Figure 6.19e and Figure 6.19f, although there are initial points associated with that grid box, their parallel orientations suggest that there is probably no landmark in the grid box. However, not all grid boxes exhibit the simplicity of Figure 6.19b through Figure 6.19f. For instance, the

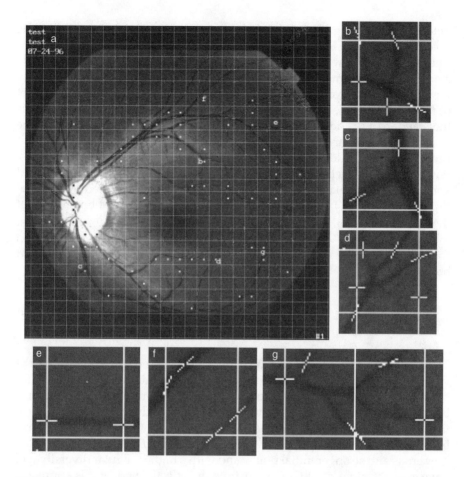

FIGURE 6.19
The basis for spatial prioritization. (a) The small line segments crossing the grid lines indicate the filtered seed points. Their orientations indicate the estimated local vascular orientations. Panels b through g highlight selected regions from panel a. Boxes with the highest 10% of $D(G)$ values are shown marked with a dot in the middle. Panels b through d illustrate cases when the filtered initial points provide strong clues about the presence of landmarks within the grid box. Panels e and f illustrate cases when the initial points suggest the absence of landmarks. Panel g illustrates a more complex case. Although there is no landmark inside this box, a landmark is right beside its left border. This example suggests that one should not only consider the possibility of a landmark inside a box, but also in the box's neighborhood. Notwithstanding such cases, this approach is very successful.

right-hand box in Figure 6.19g shows a more complex case. Although there is no landmark inside this box, a landmark is next to its left border. This suggests that one should not only consider the possibility of a landmark inside a box, but also its neighborhood. On the other hand, errors in seed point detection or filtering can produce misleading conclusions about grid boxes. A computationally simple yet effective measure is needed to capture these intuitions. Primarily, it must rate the likelihood of a landmark occurring inside a grid box and estimate its quality. We choose a weighted angular diversity measure adapted from angular statistics [120]. The angular variance of a set of unit vectors $\{\vec{u}^{(1)}, \vec{u}^{(2)} \cdots \vec{u}^{(K)}\}$ is defined as $1 - \frac{1}{K}\left\|\Sigma_{k=1}^{K}\vec{u}^{(k)}\right\|$, where $\|.\|$ is the standard Euclidean norm. Intuitively, the length of the resultant of the unit vectors is as large as possible K when all the vectors are aligned with each other, and the least possible 0 when they are pointing in opposite directions, cancelling each other out. For the present work, a strength-weighted version of the angular variance is used, and is further weighted by the total number of vectors. Let the number of initial points on a grid box be K. Let the two-dimensional estimates of edge strength be $\hat{s}_{2D}^{(k)}$, $k = 1, 2, \ldots K$, and let the unit vectors $\vec{u}^{(k)} = [\cos\theta^{(k)}, \sin\theta^{(k)}]^{T}$ indicate the local vessel orientation estimates. Then, the strength-weighted angular diversity measure for a grid box G is:

$$D(G) = \sum_{k=1}^{K}\hat{s}_{2D}^{(k)} - \left\|\sum_{k=1}^{K}\hat{s}_{2D}^{(k)}\left[\cos 2\theta^{(k)}, \sin 2\theta^{(k)}\right]\right\| \tag{6.13}$$

The angles must be doubled because the angular diversity between a pair of vectors is maximum when they differ by $\pi/2$, and minimum when they differ by π. In computing the above measure, an initial point is assigned to a grid box if it is located on or sufficiently close to any of the grid lines that form the grid box. Therefore, an initial point may belong to more than one grid box. The grid boxes are prioritized by their values of $D(G)$. Boxes with more numerous and stronger initial points and with a higher angular diversity will have greater values of $D(G)$. To illustrate the effectiveness of this approach, the top 10% of the grid boxes in the priority queue for the image shown in Figure 6.19a are indicated with dots in the center. Note that most of these marked boxes have at least one landmark within or nearby.

Within a grid box, the initial points are prioritized equally. The tracing is preempted after a number of steps that is proportional to the size of a grid box. Upon preemption, the stopping point is inserted back into the priority queue at the same level of priority as the grid box in which the tracing was stopped. An exception occurs when the tracing is preempted in a grid box whose priority is higher than the grid box from which the tracing was initiated. In this case, the tracing is continued until the next preemption. Therefore, this is a preemptive scheduling algorithm with both spatial- and edge strength-based prioritization. Figure 6.20 shows the quality of the partial result Q as a function of computing effort W for a typical image. Overall, this algorithm produced $\approx 400\%$ improvement in the quality of the partial results at a defined milestone (33% of the total tracing), compared to random scheduling.

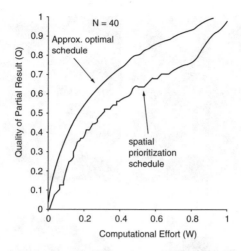

FIGURE 6.20
The growth of the quality of the partial tracing results as a function of the computational effort as measured by the number of kernel operations. The higher curve is an estimate of the optimal schedule, which is hypothetical and unachievable. By mimicking the observed behavior of the hypothetical scheduler, it is possible to approximate its behavior using the preemptive spatial prioritization scheduling algorithm.

6.8 Accurate Extraction of Vessel Bifurcations and Crossovers

Branching and crossover points in neuronal/vascular structures are of special interest from the standpoint of biology and medicine [9, 63]. One such application is the early diagnosis of hypertension by measuring changes in select vascular branching and crossover regions [82, 114]. Another example is the study of early development of the retinal vasculature, and its evolution under various pathologies and applied conditions [39, 77, 80, 97, 112].

Branching and crossover points are also important from a purely image analysis standpoint. The locations of these points, if known to be stable, are valuable as features (i.e., landmarks) for image registration and mosaicing [32, 33, 43, 124]. The pattern of angles of intersection can be used as landmark signatures [9, 10, 22, 23].

Crucial to the performance of image registration algorithms is the accuracy and repeatability with which vascular crossing and branching locations (landmarks) can be extracted, more so than their absolute location [9]. The landmarks, when placed in correspondence, constrain the image-to-image transformation that must be estimated to register the images. Of particular interest, landmark repeatability plays two crucial roles: to reduce the number of possible correspondences between two images and accurately initialize a

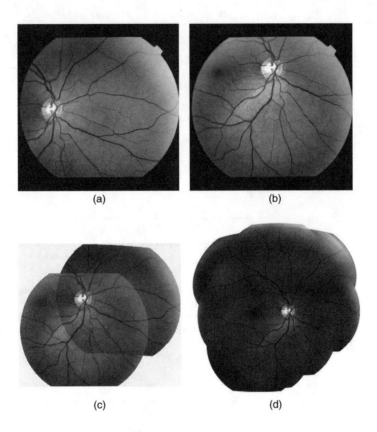

(a)   (b)

(c)   (d)

FIGURE 6.21
Retinal image registration and mosaicing. Panels a and b are fundus images taken at the same time with approximately 50% overlap (c) the results of registering panels a and b, displayed as a mosaic. Panel d is a complete mosaic of the same retina. Accurate registration to sub-pixel accuracy requires precise and repeatable estimation of image features (landmarks), and their signatures (intersection angles and thickness values).

local transformation for registration. The more repeatable the landmarks, the more likely the registration process is to succeed with the least computation.

The design of the landmark extraction technique in the exploratory tracing algorithm in [21] is conceptually simple and effective in terms of detection. However, it suffers from limitations relating to the accuracy and repeatability of estimating the intersection coordinates and angles.

These limitations arise primarily from the fact that the anti-parallel edge model on which the tracing algorithm is based, is no longer valid very close to branching and crossover points due to the rounded nature of the junctions (see Figure 6.22). Consequently, when the recursive tracing steps approach a junction, the estimation of the centerline of the vessels is less accurate. That is, trace points become inaccurate very close to intersections. The peak responses of the left and right templates often occur for many different orientations as they

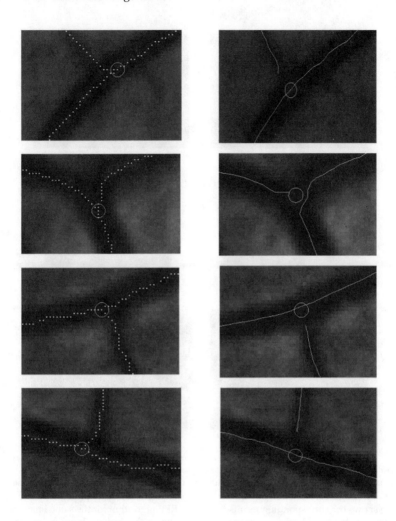

FIGURE 6.22
The issue of landmark location accuracy. The left column shows enlarged close-up views of three landmarks, overlaid with the results of tracing from our earlier algorithm. As the tracing steps approach the intersection, the anti-parallel edges model that holds well for the straight portions of the vasculature fails, leading to errors in estimating the intersection position and angle. The column on the right shows results produced by the enhanced algorithm (ERPR) presented in this section. This algorithm estimates the locations of the intersections, and the angular signatures more accurately using a model. The detected intersection is the center of the overlaid circle.

begin to overlap intensity values from two or more different blood vessels. This may result in uncertain and unreliable placement of centerline points. Finally, errors in estimating the point of intersection have a pronounced effect on the accuracy with which the intersection angles are estimated. The issues related to landmark accuracy are illustrated in Figure 6.22. The issues related to repeatability are illustrated in Figure 6.23.

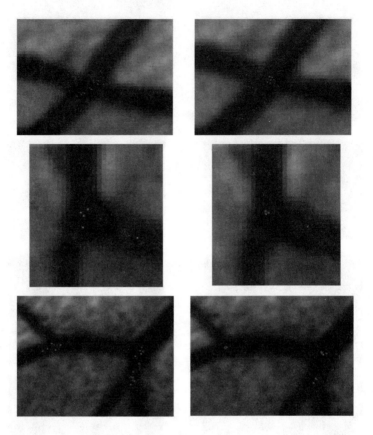

FIGURE 6.23
The issue of landmark repeatability. The dots on the vessels are the landmarks mapped from the fundus images. The left column shows three examples from the original method. The right column shows the corresponding results from the ERPR algorithm for the same image regions. Observe the substantial improvement in the repeatability with which the locations are estimated. This is important for image registration applications, especially with real-time implementations.

Our discussion here leaves out nonexploratory approaches for locating the branching and crossing points using interest operators [9, 59, 72, 76].

6.8.1   A Model for Vessel Bifurcations and Intersections

The failure of the anti-parallel edges model near bifurcations and intersections is the primary source of error. The solution described here is to build an explicit model of the structure of a landmark and an estimation technique that estimates the parameters of this model. The proposed landmark model, illustrated in Figure 6.25, consists of three parts:

1. *A circular exclusion region.* This region models the region of intersection of the blood vessels. In this region, the anti-parallel model of the blood vessels is violated. Therefore, traces computed in this region are not used.

2. *The landmark location.* This is defined as the (x, y) point nearest the extrapolation of the centerlines of the vessels that meet to form the landmark.

3. *Orientation vectors.* The set of blood vessel orientations that meet to form the intersection. These orientations are defined relative to the landmark location.

The exclusion region radius is estimated once, but the other parameters — the landmark location and the blood vessel orientations — are estimated iteratively. The following subsections provide a more detailed description of these items, the estimation algorithms, and the relevant notation.

6.8.1.1 Overview of the Landmark Refinement Algorithm

The starting point for the estimation process is the endpoint of a trace when either it intersects the boundary of another blood vessel or it meets at least two other trace endpoints. From this endpoint, the algorithm gathers information about neighboring traces, estimates the initial landmark point, determines the exclusion radius, and estimates the initial blood vessel orientations. This initializes an iterative process that alternates steps of re-estimating traces and orientations of blood vessels outside the exclusion region, and then re-estimating the landmark point from the blood vessels. Together, these steps ensure that the traces outside the intersection are more accurate, that multiple trace points are used in estimation, and that ultimately the final landmark location is estimated more accurately.

6.8.1.2 Gathering Information About Neighboring Traces

The estimation technique for a single landmark starts from a trace endpoint and a set of neighboring traces. Figure 6.25 illustrates the terminology and notation used here. A *trace* is defined as a sequence of centerline points detected during recursive tracing starting from a single seed point. Let T be the set of all traces (across the entire image), $t \in T$ be a single trace, and $P(t)$ be the sequence of centerline points on trace t. The centerline points on trace t are $p_{t,i}$, and $p_{t,e}$ is the ending centerline point ("endpoint"). The set of neighboring traces, denoted by $N(p_{t,e})$, is the set of other traces having at least one centerline point close to endpoint $p_{t,e}$. Finally, let $w_{t,i} = w(p_{t,i})$ be the width of the blood vessel at each centerline point, computed easily during recursive tracing.

6.8.1.3 Initializing the Landmark Model Parameters

During the initialization process, the landmark location, the exclusion region radius, and the blood vessel orientations are estimated in turn. The exclusion region radius remains fixed throughout the computation.

Initializing the landmark location starts by gathering sets of neighboring traces' trace points. These sets are formed for each trace's end point by searching an area with a radius of 10 pixels for nearby traces. When a nearby trace is found, if its closest trace point is an endpoint, it is included in the set. If the trace's closest point is a mid-point, then the trace is split into two separate traces and the two new endpoints are added to the set. For each set:

- If the set has only two traces, then no landmark is placed here.
- If the set contains only endpoints (at least three), then the initial landmark location, denoted by q^0, is the centroid of the endpoints.
- If the set was made from splitting a trace, the initial landmark location q^0 is set at the split point p. See Figure 6.24a for an example of this.

Next, the exclusion region radius r^* is estimated. Intuitively, the exclusion region should have a diameter at least as wide as the width of the thickest vessel in the intersection. Because the width of a vessel varies, and is less reliable as the vessel approaches the intersection, we define the width of a trace $w(t)$ as the median value of widths of all trace points on t. The exclusion radius r^* is then defined as the maximum of the trace widths for all traces from which a landmark is made. There is no need to refine r^* because it does not depend significantly on the landmark location or other landmark parameters

The final step in initialization is estimating the blood vessel orientations near the intersection. This orientation is denoted $\phi(t)$ for each trace at the landmark. The initial value of this orientation $\phi^0(t)$ is found by fitting a line to points on trace t that are just outside the exclusion region. This is described in more detail below because it is exactly the same computation as used in the iterative procedure.

6.8.1.4 Iterative Estimation of Model Parameters

The trace centerlines, blood vessel orientations, and landmark location are estimated iteratively. The first step in each iteration $j \geq 1$ is to re-estimate the trace centerline points near landmark location q^{j-1}, but outside the exclusion region. This procedure is called *back-trace refinement*, and is illustrated in Figure 6.24. For each trace, a seed point on the boundary of the exclusion region is found, and then the recursive tracing procedure (described by Can's algorithm in Section 6.5.2.2) is run for a small number of steps (e.g., $n = 5$) away from the intersection. The seed point for each trace is simply:

$$q^{j-1} + [r^* \cos \phi^{j-1}(t), r^* \sin \phi^{j-1}(t)] \qquad (6.14)$$

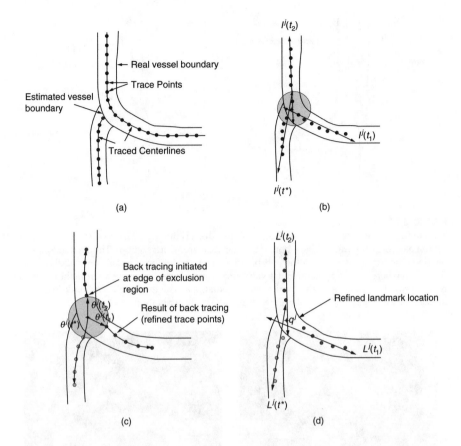

FIGURE 6.24
The steps in estimating model parameters: (a) the result of initial tracing; (b) showing the exclusion region (circle) and method for initializing the back-tracing, lines, denoted $l'(t_1)$, $l'(t_2)$, and $l'(t^*)$ are fit to the previously traced centerline points; (c) showing new traces from back-tracing, initiated from points that are estimated based on the angles of the fitted lines and just outside the exclusion region; (d) the refined landmark location is estimated by fitting lines denoted $L'(t_1)$, $L'(t_2)$, and $L'(t^*)$ and q' finding the point that is closest to these lines.

which is where a ray from the previous landmark location in the previous blood vessel direction intersects the boundary of the exclusion region. For each trace, these new refined trace points and the previous landmark location are used to fit lines and recompute the landmark location. The previous landmark location is added to ensure stability, especially for intersections with acute angles.

6.8.1.5 Simplified Estimation of Landmark Model Parameters

The most expensive (and unstable) part of the estimation process is back-trace refinement. It makes sense to consider the possibility of a simpler algorithm where back-trace refinement is removed from the iterative estimation process

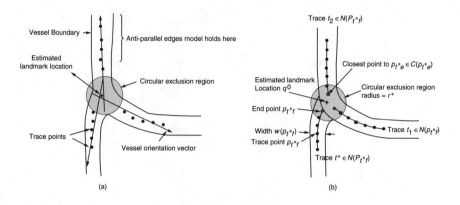

FIGURE 6.25

The landmark (intersection) model. Panel a shows the terminology. The vessels are assumed to exhibit pairs of anti-parallel edges/boundaries far away from intersections. The circular exclusion region is the region over which the anti-parallel edges model for vessels is not valid. It is also the region where the proposed model is valid and useful. Traces farther away from the exclusion region provide estimates of the local vessel orientations. The estimated landmark location is indicated by a star symbol. Panel b shows the mathematical notation.

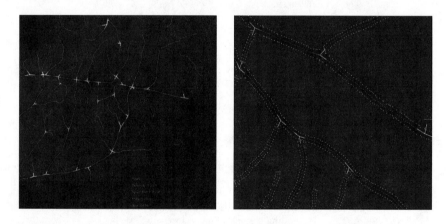

FIGURE 6.26 (See color insert.)

The left panel shows how for a selected vessel, the vessel's morphometric measures (tortuosity, width, area, etc.) can be calculated and displayed. The right panel shows the boundary locations of vessels that are needed to generate these measures.

and only applied at the end. In this simplified process, each iteration contains only two steps: estimation of the lines $L^j(t)$ for each trace in the landmark, followed by estimating q^j from these lines. After the iterative process, a single full iteration is applied, including back-trace refinement, line estimation, and centerline point estimation.

Using the same test criterion as above, if the new location is too far from the previous one, the landmark location is restored to its previous value.

Intuitively, this should work because it should be possible to obtain a reasonably accurate estimate of the landmark location from the traces outside the exclusion region, and allowing final accuracy of the centerline positions, trace orientations, and then landmark position in just a single, full iteration.

6.9   Applications of Vessel Segmentation Data

This section concerns the applications of retinal vessel tracing/segmentation that require specific structural and/or topological measurements to be generated from the images [107]. Typically, these measurements are needed in support of a clinical or biological hypothesis. The focus of these studies is often on quantifying changes effected by agents such as drugs, disease states, aging, development, and clinical treatments.

Commonly sought measurements include vessel widths and lengths [34, 83, 127], tortuosity [50, 52], and angles of intersection at crossing and branch locations. These measurements could be sought separately for arteries and veins, and different parts of the vasculature [56]. The thickness and length measurements are valuable measurements. The boundary length measurements are indicative of the surface area of the retinal vasculature. Means and variances on these quantities are also of common interest. Topological measurements usually involve the study of the above measures as a function of branching order.

Interestingly, most of these measurements are also used in the neurobiology community. Well-implemented software packages are commonly available for generating these measurements. The Neurolucida system (Microbrightfield, Inc., Colchester, VT, www.microbrightfield.com) is a good example of such a package [47, 64]. The file formats used by such packages are widely published. All that remains to leverage these tools is to write out the vessel tracing data into the format accepted by them.

6.10   Implementation Methods

Both hardware and software techniques have been used for retinal vessel tracing. Hardware techniques are useful for pixel processing algorithms when the application of interest requires fast computation, usually for real-time medical vision systems. With the development of fast exploratory algorithms, especially algorithms for intelligent scheduling of the tracing computations, and the rapid improvements in conventional processor technology, the need for specialized hardware is decreasing. A pure software-based approach also offers high levels of flexibility and portability across computing platforms.

Finally, even in pure software implementations, it is now possible to exploit processor features that are specifically aimed at image computing. For example, the Intel Pentium series of computers have a built-in instruction set, known as the MMX Multimedia Extension [13], that enables rapid computation of operations such as correlations. Often, the speedup attained by MMX is a factor of 2 to 3 over a generic implementation.

The modified version of Can's exploratory tracing algorithm described in Section 6.5.2.2 has been implemented for both a command-line and graphical user interfaces (GUIs). Known as RPI-Trace, it is written using a public-domain, open-source image-processing library known as VXL [118] that enables the source code to be compiled under multiple compilers in both Unix-based and Windows-based systems for a variety of commonly used graphical environments (GL, VTK, etc.) with no modifications.

The command-line version of the algorithm is useful for incorporation into an Internet application server or for batch processing of images. Users can upload images to a server, set desired parameters, and immediately download the results of automatic tracing.

Figure 6.27 shows a screen view of the graphical version of this implementation. The graphical user interface (GUI) allows a user to load a gray-scale or color image and, if desired, modify the image by applying local intensity normalization or selecting a specific color channel. The parameters can also be changed using provided menus if parameters other than the default are desired. Once the desired modification is made to the image, the exploratory tracing algorithm can be run in a piecemeal fashion or in its entirety, depending on the menu options selected. Results for each step (seed detection, seed verification, centerline trace identification, landmark determination, landmark refinement) of the algorithm can be toggled on and off and be viewed separately or collectively. The results can be saved in ASCII format for further analysis and can be again loaded directly into the GUI at a future time. Users also have the option of saving selected results as images in multiple formats. The algorithm can be run multiple times for the same or different images, and the results can be viewed by paging up and down through the results. This lends itself to batch processing of a set of images for different parameter settings using the command-line executable. Then, using the GUI, a user can load and view the results for all images in a single batch or for the same image across all the batches and page through the results. Also included in the GUI is the ability to zoom in and out, pan, and display the parameters used to generate the results with the option to make the parameters a permanent part of the results image.

Also included in the GUI is the ability for a user to manually designate vessels as vein, artery, or unknown. As each vessel segment is selected, morphological metrics such as tortuosity, median width, length, and area are computed and displayed. As the segmentation progresses, these metrics are combined to form cumulative statistics for areas and widths for each type of vessel.

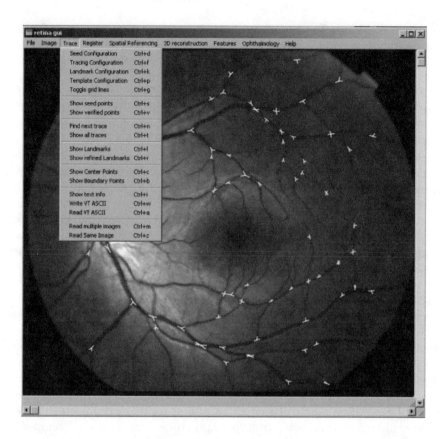

FIGURE 6.27 (See color insert.)
Screen view of the RPI-Trace multi-platform graphical user interface. Shown are the currently options available for tracing vessels.

6.11 Experimental Validation Using Ground Truth Data

Validating the performance of automatic vessel segmentation algorithms is not straightforward, primarily due to the difficulty in identifying the "ground truth," that is, establishing what is the "correct answer" or what *exactly* a computer segmentation is expected to produce. A secondary issue is the fact that, based on the application, the degree or amount of error that is acceptable varies and a way to quantify the error needs to be developed. For example, topological applications for studies of the vasculature may place a high emphasis on detection of all vascular segments or precision in determining the vessel boundaries, possibly to sub-pixel accuracy. On the other hand, applications that require vessel segmentation for registration purposes may have the opposite emphasis. To validate a segmentation algorithm, the ground truth, the definition of what is being compared, and a measure are all required [78].

The arrival at "ground truth" is a known hard problem in image analysis and pattern recognition systems [54]. With retinal images, the ground truth is simply unavailable, and can be approximated by the creation of a "gold standard" to which computer-generated results are measured. In the context of this chapter, we define a gold standard as a binary segmentation, denoted as G, where each pixel, denoted as $G(x, y)$, assumes a value of 0 or 1 for background or vessel, respectively. With such a standard, a computer-generated segmentation, denoted C, can be compared and evaluated against the gold standard G. In evaluating each pixel, there are four possible cases. The case when $C(x, y) = G(x, y) = 0$ is called a "true negative." The case when $C(x, y) = G(x, y) = 1$ is called a "true positive." The case when $C(x, y) = 1$ and $G(x, y) = 0$ is called a "false positive." Finally, the case when $C(x, y) = 0$ and $G(x, y) = 1$ is called a "false negative." The frequency of these cases provides data that can be used as an indication of an algorithm's performance.

Generation of gold standards is often a costly and time-consuming process. In addition, it is known that even expert human observers are subjective and prone to a variety of errors. For example, it is possible for one observer to label a vessel that another missed, and vice versa. This inconsistency is referred to as inter-observer variability. Likewise, the same human observer is very likely to generate different segmentations for the same image, which is known as intra-observer variability. Thus, the use of a single human expert's annotations is unreliable and should be considered inadequate for the purpose of generating a gold standard. Thus, one approach to the creation of a gold standard is to combine multiple human-generated manual segmentations. From a set of multiple observers' manual segmentations H, with each individual segmentation being denoted H_i, we wish to obtain a single binary segmentation G that will be considered the gold standard. We know that these segmentations will differ and thus a strategy for resolution of these differences must be created.

6.11.1 Ground Truth from Conflicting Observers

To determine the best way to combine different observer's segmentation results, one must first consider what constitutes a correct and incorrect vessel segmentation. Essentially, there are three possible ways to define correct vessel segmentation for a particular pixel. A conservative method is to declare pixels to be part of a vessel (or part of the background) when all observers' segmentations agree. If such total agreement exists, then that pixel would be marked as vessel (or background) in the gold standard image. In essence, this amounts to computing a Boolean "AND" of the multiple observer segmentations. A less conservative method would be based on using majority rule. Each segmentation result would contribute a single vote for each pixel when determining if a pixel should be considered a vessel in the gold standard. If 50% or more of the observers have determined a particular pixel to be a vessel, it would be marked a vessel in the gold standard. Note that the "majority" threshold could be set higher or lower as appropriate for the specific application. The least conservative method is to label a pixel in the gold standard as a vessel pixel if it is marked as a vessel in at least one of the observers' results. This last case is equivalent to computing the Boolean "OR" of the multiple observer segmentations.

An alternate approach to the gold standard generation process described above is to generate a modified gold standard in which each pixel is assigned a weight based on the number of observers who segmented that pixel as a vessel. This weight can be considered a probability as described in the next section. Figure 6.28 illustrates the resulting weights or probabilities of a non-binary gold standard formed from five separate hand-traced images.

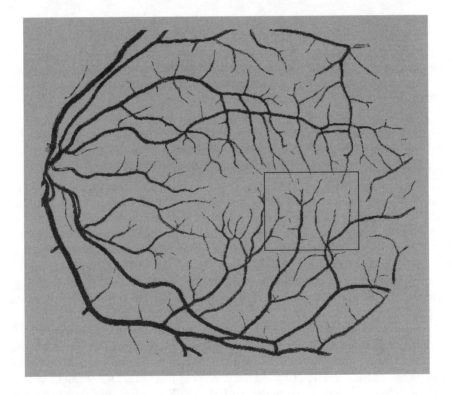

FIGURE 6.28 (See color insert.)
Multi-observer standard image formed from five separate hand tracings (two of the hand tracings courtesy Prof. Adam Hoover). Blue pixels are cases where five observers agree that the pixel is vessel; cyan is four; green is three; red is two; yellow is one; and white is zero.

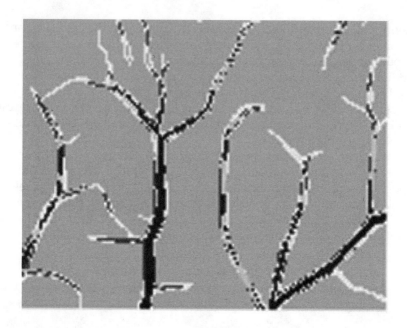

FIGURE 6.29
Enlarged portion of the boxed region in Figure 6.28 with the same color scheme described in Figure 6.28 caption.

6.11.2 Multi-observer (Probabilistic) Gold Standard

Suppose that K is the number of observers ($K = 5$ in Figure 6.28). The segmentation label at each pixel for a computer-generated segmentation $C(x, y)$ can be thought of as a binary random variable V from the set $\{0, 1\}$. A value of $V = 0$ indicates a background pixel, and $V = 1$ indicates a vessel pixel. Let M denote an integer-valued random variable assuming values from the set $\{0, 1, ..., K\}$, indicating the number of observers who have labeled a pixel as a vessel. The joint probability distribution $P_{VM}(v, m)$ can be estimated from the computer-generated segmentation and the manually scored segmentations. This distribution forms the basis for a performance measure S_{vessel} described below.

S_{vessel} was designed so that it assumes values in the interval from 0 to 1, where 1 indicates a perfect score and 0 a complete failure. A perfect score would indicate that all pixels determined by R or more observers to be vessel pixels have also been determined to be vessel pixels in C. A complete failure occurs when all vessel pixels determined by R or more observers are not labeled as vessel pixels in C. It is somewhere between 0 and 1, based on the number of pixels the computer does not label as vessel that are labeled as vessel by R or more observers. Note that in this method, described by Equation 6.15, a missed vessel pixel in C, for which *all* observers agree to be a vessel pixel, carries more weight in determining the final score than a pixel for which only R observers agree. R can be set to any appropriate value and we illustrate a "majority rules" idea in Figure 6.28 by choosing R such that it represents a majority (50% or higher) of the observers ($R = \lceil K/2 \rceil$). Based on these considerations, we define the S_{vessel} as follows:

$$S_{vessel} = \frac{E[M/V = 1; M \geq R]P[V = 1]}{E[M/V = 1, M \geq R]P[V = 1] + E[M/V = 0, M \geq R]P[V = 0]}$$

(6.15)

This simplifies to:

$$S_{vessel} = \frac{\sum_{m \geq R}^{K} m P[V = 1, M = m]}{\sum_{m \geq R}^{K} m P[M = m]}$$

(6.16)

In Equation 6.16, the numerator denotes the expected value of M for all the pixels for which the computer algorithm and R or more observers label as a vessel and can be thought of as the amount of agreement between C and the majority of observers. The denominator represents the average value of M for all the pixels that R or more observers have labeled as a vessel and can be thought of as the "perfect score."

However, S_{vessel} does not take into account another indicator of segmentation performance, namely, the number of false positives, which in our context is the number of pixels falsely identified as vessels. The following second measure accounts for this aspect of segmentation performance:

$$F_{vessel} = \frac{P[V = 1, M = 0]}{P[V = 1, M \geq R]}$$

(6.17)

The numerator is the joint probability that the computer algorithm labeled the pixel to be a vessel and no observers labeled it as a vessel. The denominator is the probability that the computer algorithm labeled it as a vessel, and more than R observers agreed. In this measure, a score of 0 means that there were no false positives. A score of 1 would indicate that an equal number of false positives and true positives was required to achieve the S_{vessel} score.

A special case exists when there is only one observer. In this case, $K = R = 1$, and S_{vessel} and F_{vessel} become:

$$S_{vessel} = \frac{P[V = 1, M = 1]}{P[M = 1]}$$

(6.18)

$$F_{vessel} = \frac{P[V = 1, M = 0]}{P[V = 1, M = 1]}$$

(6.19)

Using the same type of reasoning, it is possible to define similar metrics, denoted $S_{background}$ and $F_{background}$, respectively, for classification of non-vessel pixels, as shown below:

$$S_{background} = \frac{E[M/V = 0, M < R]P(V = 0)}{E[M/V = 0, M < R]\,P(V=0) + E[M/V = 1, M < R]P(V = 1)}$$

(6.20)

and

$$F_{background} = \frac{P(V = 0, M = K)}{P(V = 0, M < R)}.$$

(6.21)

Finally, the above metrics $S_{vessels}$ and $S_{background}$ could be combined simply by averaging to develop an overall score between 0 and 1. The closer a set of the results is to the multi-observer standard, the closer this score will be to 1. Figure 6.30 illustrates these performance measures.

6.11.3 Tracing

While the above measures would work for algorithms for which the goal is the segmentation of the entire vessel from the background, they would not work for algorithms in which the goal is to determine the centerlines of the vessels. For these algorithms, the following approaches can be used. The first approach is to convert a trace result into a segmentation result. This is often possible because most tracing algorithms determine the necessary data, such as vessel width or boundary location for each point found on the trace. Thus, a simple approach would be to segment as vessel points all the corresponding pixels between neighboring trace points based on the widths or vessel boundaries. This segmentation can then be scored as described above.

An alternative approach would be to test each point in the centerline trace against the multi-observer standard. Typically, exploratory algorithms generate results containing a set of center points separated by a fixed or varying step size. Another simple approach to judge the results of a tracing algorithm would be to test for true positives by seeing if a point in the centerline trace matches any non-zero (i.e., vessel) pixel in the multi-observer standard. If it does, it could be scored toward the S_{vessel} measure as described above or simply counted. Likewise, false positives could be scored or counted, and these combined measures could be used to compute measures indicating the algorithm's performance. However, such an approach fails to consider true and false positives because it is debatable as to what exactly constitutes a true negative or false negative. Thus, such an approach should not be considered; an approach that considers true and false negatives is discussed next.

A final approach is to build a trace based upon the multi-observer standard. This trace could be generated by running a tracing algorithm on the

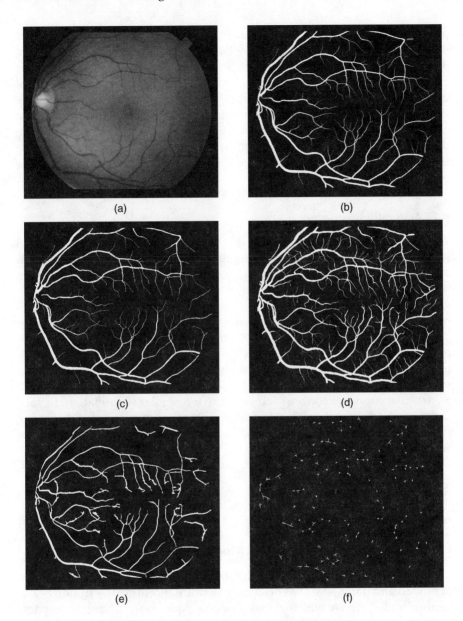

FIGURE 6.30

The measurement of segmentation performance from multiple manual observers. Panel a is the original image. Panel b is the multi-observer gold standard generated from five hand-traced images. Two of these manual traces are shown in panels c and d. Note the significant inter-observer variation. Panel e is a segmentation produced by Hoover's algorithm [53]. For this result, $S_{vessel} = 0.69$, $F_{vessel} = 0.14$, $S_{background} = 0.98$, and $S_{background} = 0.01$. Panel f is a tracing generated by RPI-Trace [21]. This tracing is accompanied by vessel boundary data that is not displayed here. For this result, $S_{vessel} = 0.94$, $F_{vessel} = 0.35$, $S_{background} = 0.94$, and $F_{background} = 0.002$. Based on these scores, the latter algorithm correctly detected more vessel pixels, but with a higher incidence of false positives.

multi-observer standard and then manually editing the results to generate the standard with which to compare tracing results. Once the tracing standard has been determined, false/true positive and false/true negative counts can be determined using a distance tolerance d. A true positive is a trace point in the image to be scored that is within distance d of a trace point in the tracing standard. A false positive is a trace point in the image to be scored that has no corresponding point in the tracing standard within distance d. A false negative would be a trace point in the tracing standard that has no corresponding trace point in the image to be scored within distance d. All others are true negatives.

6.11.4   Synthetic Images

Another avenue to consider when trying to gauge the performance of a vessel segmentation or tracing algorithm is the use of synthetic images. The advantage to such an approach is that ground truth can be absolutely known beforehand. However, in the context of retinal images, no matter how much care and attention is applied in trying to create such a synthetic image, it will never be a true recreation of an actual retinal image and, depending on how constructed, can be argued to favor one model over another. Thus, as a means of comparing algorithms, the use of synthetic images should not be considered. However, they may prove to be useful for a researcher to validate or measure the accuracy of a particular model or empirically test sensitivity of a particular model to factors such as noise or irregular illumination. In such cases, a researcher may wish to test an algorithm's performance with varying degrees of noise, or test the accuracies of morphometric measures such as width or tortuosity.

6.12   Experimental Analysis of Model and Settings for RPI-Trace

This section provides the reader with some insight into the effect the selection of models and parameters has on tracing performance. The description below focuses on RPI-Trace, which is based on the exploratory tracing algorithms described in Section 6.5.2.2. The main adjustable parameters include the density of initial sampling using vertical and horizontal cross sections (grid lines), tracing step size, and the expected maximum width of vessels.

Increasing the number of vertical and horizontal cross sections improves the probability of detecting vessels at the expense of computation. Figure 6.31 shows the linear relationship between the number of detected vessel points and the grid lines. Depicted on this graph are the number of vessel points detected by the one- and two-dimensional parallel edge models, both using the

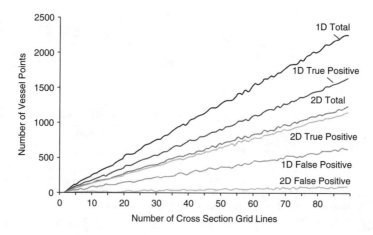

FIGURE 6.31

Graph depicting the results of varying the number of vertical and horizontal cross sections on the one-dimensional parallel edge and two-dimensional parallel edge models described in Section 6.4.6. Both models used local thresholds and the corresponding images with the results are seen in Figure 6.8 and Figure 6.10. This illustrates that there is a trade-off in using the two-dimensional model, in that the the cost of eliminating a large percentage of the one-dimensional false positives results in a loss of true positives.

local minima and edge strength constraints (i.e., local thresholds) described in Section 6.4.6. The number of true positives and false positives, which are found based on comparison against the multi-observer standard (described in Section 6.11) are also depicted. The number of two-dimensional total positives is less than the number of one-dimensional true positives. This implies that the two-dimensional model is more tightly constrained to favor filtering out the false positives at the cost of filtering out some true positives. Notice that the ratio of one-dimensional false positives to true positives is relatively high when compared to the ratio of two-dimensional false positive to true positives.

The graph in Figure 6.32 demonstrates improved detection of vessels, as measured by the number of detected centerline points (trace points), as a function of the grid lines. Also shown are the true positive and false positive counts, again determined by comparison with the multi-observer standard. The rapid increase for a small number of grid lines (less than 5) can be mostly attributed to the thick and long vessels. The subsequent slower increase and leveling off is mostly due to the secondary and tertiary vessels. Figure 6.32, which plots the number of feature points (landmarks) detected as a function of grid size exhibits a similar increase. This can be attributed to the corresponding increase in the number of trace points. As more trace points are found in an image, more trace points are found in the vicinity of landmarks, thus allowing for their detection.

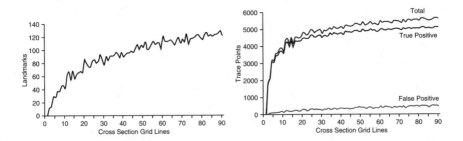

FIGURE 6.32

The graph on the left shows how the number of trace points detected varies as a function of the number of horizontal and vertical cross sections (grid lines). Also shown is the effect the number of grid lines has on the number of true positives and false positives. The graph on the right shows how the number of grid lines affects the number of detected landmarks.

The step size (α in Equation 6.8) is another important settable parameter. Small values of α result in more precise tracing at the expense of more computation. Generally, for a given density of initial sampling grid lines, the computation time decreases linearly [21] with increasing step size α.

6.13   Experimental Assessment of the Impact of Landmark Refinement with the ERPR Algorithm

This section describes experiments measuring the quantitative impact of using the ERPR landmark refinement algorithm described in Section 6.8. The method for measuring the accuracy and repeatability of landmark estimation is based on the image registration algorithm developed in our prior work [22, 23] as a testbed and standard for measuring landmark estimation errors. The average alignment error of this registration algorithm, as measured by the distance between trace centerlines is 0.83 pixels on 1024×1024 images.

The ability to register retinal images with sub-pixel accuracy, *despite errors in estimating the landmark locations (albeit at a high computational price)*, leads to several methods of evaluating the proposed Exclusion Region and Position Refinement (ERPR) algorithm.

- **Repeatability measurement.** For a landmark that appears in two or more images, registering the images places the two different estimated positions in the same coordinate system. This gives us a measure of the repeatability of the landmark position, modulo the transformation error itself.

- **Accuracy measurement.** We can compare the SSD refined positions obtained just prior to convergence to the estimated landmark positions as a further measure of position accuracy.

- We can generate a qualitative, visual indication of the effectiveness of the ERPR technique by transforming many different images of the same landmark into the same coordinate system. Examples of this are shown in Figure 6.23.

The first quantitative measure is the error between the same landmark estimated in registered pairs of images. Let q_1 be the landmark location in image I_1 and q_2 the landmark location in image I_2. Let θ be the estimated registration function mapping I_1 onto I_2, so that $M(q_1;\theta)$ is the mapping of the landmark location into image I_2. The local distance $\|M(q_1;\theta) - q_2\|$ gives one measure of the landmark error. The maximum difference in trace orientations between the mapping of the landmark at q_1 and the landmark at q_2 gives a second measure. By combining these measures over all landmarks in all registered image pairs, we obtain summary statistics on the repeatability of the estimated landmark parameters.

Table 6.1 shows these summary statistics for the original landmark detection technique and for several versions of our new ERPR technique, including the full method, the simplified method using one iteration of backtrace refinement, and a version where back-trace refinement is not used at all. Several conclusions are immediately apparent. First, the ERPR method is twice as repeatable as the original method, both in terms of position and orientation. In fact, it may be higher because of the inherent error in the transformation. Second, there is little difference between the fully iterative ERPR and the simplified version where back-trace refinement is used only once. Third, with no use of back-trace refinement, the results are substantially worse. Based on the latter two conclusions, the remaining experiments will focus exclusively on the ERPR with one step of back-trace refinement.

The second quantitative comparison is between the SSD-refined landmark positions that emerge at the end of registration and the positions estimated by either the original landmark technique or by the ERPR. Using corresponding point locations q_1 and q_2, as above, the SSD step during estimation of θ refines

TABLE 6.1

Landmark Repeatability Experiment

	Location Distance		Max. Orientation Difference	
	Median (pixels)	Mean (pixels)	Median (degrees)	Mean (degrees)
Original	2.0879	2.2117	7.2037	8.6345
ERPR	1.0546	1.3408	3.7587	4.8014
ERPR, simplified	1.0713	1.3317	4.3324	5.4378
ERPR, no back-trace	1.2765	1.5126	5.0371	6.0380

The original Landmark Method is compared to three versions of the new ERPR Method: the full iterative refinement, the simplified version with one step of back-trace refinement, and an even simpler version with no back-trace refinement whatsoever.

TABLE 6.2

Landmark Position vs. SSD Refined Position

	Location Error	
	Median (pixels)	Mean (pixels)
Original	2.04	1.76
ERPR, simplified	1.10	0.72

Comparing the original landmark estimation technique to the new ERPR method with a just one step of back-trace refinement.

the position of q_2 to match the transformation of a small region surrounding q_1. Call the new position q_2'. The error measure is then $\|q_2 - q_2'\|$. Interestingly, this measure is not sensitive to minor errors in the transformation, and therefore an even better measure of the repeatability of the landmark position estimate. The disadvantage is that the SSD refinement gives no orientation accuracy.

The results of this measure taken over all correctly registered pairs from our data set are shown in Table 6.2. Both median and average errors are given. The advantage of the new ERPR method with just a single iteration of back-trace refinement is striking. The average error is 2.5 times lower and the median error is 1.9 times lower.

Overall, the ERPR algorithm reduces the median location error from 2.04 pixels down to 1.1 pixels, while improving the median spread (a measure of repeatability) from 2.09 pixels down to 1.05 pixels. Errors in estimating vessel orientations were similarly reduced from 7.2° down to 3.8°. These improvements are especially significant for real-time image registration applications for which computationally expensive refinement approaches such as sum of squared difference (SSD) registration can be avoided.

6.14   Chapter Summary

This chapter has surveyed some of the published vessel segmentation and tracing algorithms in the specific context of retinal fundus images. While many of the models and algorithms are influenced by related work in other areas of human anatomy, such as cardiac and brain images [110], and dye-injected neuron images [2], the techniques described in this chapter have been developed specifically in the retinal image context. We have attempted to describe some of the considerations of the many models and algorithms in use, in the context of the desired applications.

Among the applications, we broadly recognize two classes: real-time and online vessel tracing applications, and offline applications. In our experience, the online applications are best served by exploratory approaches, while the offline applications are best served by a combination of filtering and exploratory tracing approaches. For the latter, a detailed graph-based output such as the Neurolucida file format [47] provides the most flexibility overall.

We recognize that our classification of algorithms, as reflected in this chapter, is only one of several ways of organizing the body of reported work. Our own work, principally represented by exploratory algorithms, is heavily influenced by the desire to process live image sequences in real-time. It is also influenced heavily by the desire to use conventional off-the-shelf computers rather than specialized hardware whenever possible. Yet another influence on our work is the desire to maintain a common software code base for real-time and offline tracing modules. The former are being incorporated into an ophthalmic instrument under construction. The latter are being adapted for use on an Internet application server. This server enables potential users, especially clinicians, to upload images via the Internet and then download the results of vessel tracing, registration [22], and mosaicing [23].

Much work remains in this field. For example, automatic algorithms for classifying vessels as arteries and veins are still unavailable. Also not available are algorithms that automatically handle normal as well as the "hollow" vessels noted earlier in a reliable manner using multiple models. Finally, there is a continuing need to improve the computational efficiency. For example, the refinement of landmark locations (Section 6.8) is still relatively slow.

More generally, vessel-tracing algorithms have the potential to form the basis for a complete retinal image understanding system. Notwithstanding some prior work in this area [50], much work remains. In the area of real-time tracing, the desire to attain ever higher frame rates (200 frames/sec is considered an appropriate goal given the speed of eye motions [88, 94]). Higher frame rates imply noisier images. Much work remains to be done on handling noisy retinal images in an efficient manner, while using more sophisticated/realistic models of the vasculature that account for the imaging noise, and the varied appearance of the vasculature.

Acknowledgments

Various portions of this research were supported by the National Science Foundation Experimental Partnerships grant EIA-0000417, the Center for Subsurface Sensing and Imaging Systems, under the Engineering Research Centers Program of the National Science Foundation (Award Number

EEC-9986821), the National Institutes for Health grant RR14038, and by Rensselaer Polytechnic Institute.

The authors would like to thank the staff at the Center for Sight, especially photographers Gary Howe and Mark Fish, for assisting with image acquisition. Thanks to Dr. Anna Majerovics for valuable guidance on retinal structure and function, and for numerous images. Thanks also to Matthew Freshman for a part of the retinal photography. Thanks to Dr. Wayne Whitwam and Jay Cohn at the University of Minnesota Medical Center for images and insights related to hypertensive retinopathy. Thanks to Professor Adam Hoover at Clemson University for sharing the manually traced image data, and permission to use this data in this chapter. The authors appreciate the insightful input of Dr. George Nagy at Rensselaer, especially regarding vectorization methods from the document image analysis literature.

Finally, thanks to the other associated members of the RPI Retina Project group, including Chris Carothers, Amitha Perera, Gary Yang, Gang Lin, Mohamad Tehrani, Justin LaPre, and Michal Sofka, for their input, ideas, support, artwork, and friendship.

References

1. Akita, K. and Kuga, H., "A Computer Method of Understanding Ocular Fundus Images," *Pattern Recognition,* Vol. 15, No. 6, pp. 431–443, 1982.
2. Al-Kofahi, K., Lasek, S., Szarowski, D. H., Pace, C., Nagy, G., Turner, J. N., and Roysam B., "Rapid Automated Three-Dimensional Tracing of Neurons from Confocal Image Stacks," *IEEE Trans. Information Technology in Biomedicine,* accepted 2002.
3. Anarim, E., Aydinoglu, H., and Goknar, I. C., "Decision Based Edge Detector," *Signal Processing,* Vol. 35, pp. 149–156, 1994.
4. Balduf, E., "Real-Time Algorithms for a Laser Retinal Surgery System — Implementation on the Silicon Graphics Octane Dual-Processor System," M. S. thesis, Rensselaer Polytechnic Institute, 1998.
5. Barrett, S. F., Jerath, M. R., Rylander, H. G., and Welch, A. J., "Digital Tracking and Control of Retinal Images," *Optical Engineering,* Vol. 33, No. 1, pp. 150–159, 1994.
6. Barrett, S., Wright C., and Jerath, M., "Computer-Aided Retinal Photocoagulation System," *J. Biomed. Opt.,* Vol. 1, pp. 83–91, 1996.
7. Beach, M., Tiedeman, J. S., Hopkins, M., and Sabharwal, Y., "Multi-spectral Fundus Imaging for Early Detection of Diabetic Retinopathy," *Proc. SPIE Conf. Clinical Diagnostic Systems and Technologies,* Vol. 3603, pp. 114–121, 1999.
8. Becker, D., "Algorithms for Automatic Retinal Mapping and Real-Time Location Determination for an Improved Retinal Laser Surgery System," Ph. D. thesis, Rensselaer Polytechnic Institute, August 1995.

9. Becker, D., Can, A., Tanenbaum, H., Turner, J., and Roysam, B., "Image Processing Algorithms for Retinal Montage Synthesis, Mapping, and Real-Time Location Determination," *IEEE Trans. Biomed. Eng.*, Vol. 45, No. 1, 1998.

10. Berger J., Patel T., Shin D., Piltz J., and Stone R., "Computerized Stereo Chronoscopy and Alternation Flicker to Detect Optic Nerve Head Contour Change," *Ophthalmology*, Vol. 107, No. 7, pp. 1316–1320, 2000.

11. Berger, J. and Shin D., "Computer Vision Enabled Augmented Reality Fundus Biomicroscopy," *Ophthalmology*, Vol. 106, No. 10, 1999.

12. Beucher S., "Watershed, Hierarchical Segmentation and Waterfall Algorithm," *Mathematical Morphology and Its Applications to Image Processing*, Serra, J. and Soille, P., Eds., Kluwer Academic, pp. 69–76, 1994.

13. Bistry, D., Ed., *The Complete Guide to MMX Technology*, Intel Corp. and McGraw-Hill Publishing, 1997.

14. Borodkin, M. and Thompson, J., "Retinal Cartography: An Analysis of Two-Dimensional and Three-Dimensional Mapping of the Retina," *Retina — The J. Retinal and Vitreous Diseases*, Vol. 12, No. 3, pp. 273–280, 1992.

15. Boudier, H., Le Noble, J., Messing, M., Huijberts, M., Le Noble, F., and Van Essen, H., "The Microcirculation and Hypertension," *J. Hypertension*, Vol. 10, pp. S147–S156, 1992.

16. Brinchmann-Hansen, O. and Heier, H., "Theoretical Relations between Light Streak Characteristics and Optical Properties of Retinal Vessels," *Acta Opthalmol.*, pp. 33–37, 1986.

17. Brown, L., "A Survey of Image Registration Techniques," *ACM Computing Surveys*, Vol. 24, No. 4, pp. 325–376, 1992.

18. Can, A., "Robust Computer Vision Algorithms for Registering Images from Curved Human Retina," Ph.D. thesis, Rensselaer Polytechnic Institute, 2000.

19. Can, A., Stewart, C., and Roysam, B., "Robust Hierarchical Algorithm for Constructing a Mosaic from Images of the Curved Human Retina," *Proc. IEEE Computer Society Conf. Computer Vision and Pattern Recognition*, Fort Collins, CO, June 1999.

20. Can, A., Stewart, C., Roysam, B., and Tanenbaum, H., "A Feature-Based Technique for Joint, Linear Estimation of High-Order Image-to-Mosaic Transformations: Application to Mosaicing the Curved Human Retina," *Proc. IEEE Computer Society Conf. Computer Vision and Pattern Recognition*, Hilton Head Island, SC, June 2000.

21. Can, A., Shen, H., Turner, J., Tanenbaum, H., and Roysam, B., "Rapid Automated Tracing and Feature Extraction from Live High-Resolution Retinal Fundus Images Using Direct Exploratory Algorithms," *IEEE Trans. Information Technology in Biomedicine*, Vol. 3, No. 2, pp. 125–138, 1999.

22. Can, A., Stewart, C., Roysam, B., and Tanenbaum, H., "A Feature-Based Robust Hierarchical Algorithm for Registration Pairs of Images of the Curved Human Retina," *IEEE Trans. Pattern Analysis and Machine Intelligence*, Vol. 24, No. 3, 2002.

23. Can, A., Stewart, C., Roysam, B., and Tanenbaum, H., "A Feature-Based Algorithm for Joint, Linear Estimation of High-Order Image-to-Mosaic Transformations: Mosaicing the Curved Human Retina," *IEEE Trans. Pattern Analysis and Machine Intelligence*, Vol. 24, No. 3, 2002.

24. Canny, J., "A Computational Approach to Edge Detection," *IEEE Trans. Pattern Analysis and Machine Intelligence*, Vol. 8, No. 6, pp. 679–698, 1986.

25. Chaudhuri, S., Chatterjee, S., Katz, N., Nelson, M., and Goldbaum, M., "Detection of Blood Vessels in Retinal Images Using Two-Dimensional Matched Filters," *IEEE Trans. Medical Imaging*, Vol. 8, No. 3, pp. 263–269, 1989.

26. Chutatape, O., Zheng, L., and Krishman, S., "Retinal Blood Vessel Detection and Tracking by Matched Gaussian and Kalman Filters," *Proc. IEEE Int. Conf. Engineering in Medicine and Biology Society*, Vol. 20, No. 6, pp. 3144–3149, 1998.

27. Cideciyan, A., "Registration of Ocular Fundus Images," *IEEE Engineering in Medicine and Biology*, Vol. 14, No. 1, pp. 52–58, 1995.

28. Clark, T., Freeman, W., and Goldbaum, M., "Digital Overlay of Fluorescein Angiograms and Fundus Images for Treatment of Subretinal Neovascularization," *Retina–J. Retinal and Vitreous Diseases*, Vol. 2, No. 12, pp. 118–126, 1992.

29. Coatrieux, J., Garreau, M., Collorec, R., and Roux, C., "Computer Vision Approaches for the Three-Dimensional Reconstruction: Review and Prospects," *Crit. Rev. Biomed. Eng.*, Vol. 22, No. 1, pp. 1–38, 1994.

30. Cohen, A., Roysam, B., and Turner, J., "Automated Tracing and Volume Measurements of Neurons from 3-D Confocal Fluorescence Microscopy Data," *J. Microsc.*, Vol. 173, Pt. 2, 1994.

31. Collorec, R. and Coatrieux, J. L., "Vectorial Tracking and Directed Contour Finder for Vascular Network in Digital Subtraction Angiography," *Pattern Recog. Lett.*, Vol. 8, No. 5, pp. 353–358, Dec. 1988.

32. Cooper, J., Venkatesh, S., and Kitchen, L., "Early Jump-out Corner Detectors," *IEEE Trans. Pattern Analysis and Machine Intelligence*, Vol. 15, No. 8, pp. 823–829, 1993.

33. Dani, P. and Chaudhuri, S., "Automated Assembling of Images—Image Montage Preparation," *Pattern Recognition*, Vol. 28, No. 1, pp. 431–445, 1995.

34. Delori F., Fitch K., Feke G., Deupree D., and Weiter, J., "Evaluation of Micrometric and Microdensitometric Methods for Measuring the Width of Retinal Vessel Images on Fundus Photographs," *Graefe's Arch. Clin. Exp. Ophthalmol.*, Vol. 226, pp. 393–399, 1988.

35. Denninghoff, K. and Smith, M., "Optical Model of the Blood in Large Retinal Vessels," *J. Biomed. Opt.*, Vol. 5, No. 4, pp. 371–374, 2000.

36. Dimmitt, S., West, J., Eames, S., Gibsin, J., Gosling, P., and Littler, W., "Usefulness of Ophthalmoscopy in Mild to Moderate Hypertension," *Lancet*, pp. 1103–1106, 1989.

37. Dougherty, E. R., *An Introduction to Morphological Image Processing*, Soc. Photo-Optical and Instrumentation. Eng., Bellingham, WA, 1992.

38. Eichel, P., Delp, E., Koral, K., and Buda, A., "A Method for a Fully Automatic Definition of Coronary Arterial Edges from Cineangiograms," *IEEE Trans. Med. Imag.*, Vol. 7, pp. 313–320, 1988.

39. Family, F., Masters, B., and Platt, D., "Fractal Pattern Formation in Human Retinal Vessels," *Physica D*, Vol. 38, pp. 98–103, 1989.

40. Federman, J. L., Ed., *Retina and Vitreous*. The C. V. Mosby Company, St. Louis, 1988.

41. Fine, S., "Observations Following Laser Treatment for Choroidal Neovascularization," *Arch. Ophthalmol.*, Vol. 106, pp. 1524–1525, 1988.

42. Flower, R. and Hochheimer, B., "A Clinical Technique and Apparatus for Simultaneous Angiography of the Separate Retinal and Choroidal Circulation," *Investigative Ophthalmol.*, Vol. 12, No. 4, pp. 248–261, 1973.

43. Francois, D. and Djemel, Z., "Extracting Line Junctions from Curvilinear Structures," *Proc. Geosci. Remote Sensing Symp.*, IGARSS, IEEE 200 International, Vol. 4, pp. 1672–1674, 2000.

44. Gang, L., Chutatape, O., and Krishnan, S., "Detection and Measurement of Retinal Vessels in Fundus Images Using Amplitude Modified Second-Order Gaussian Filter," *IEEE Trans. Biomed. Eng.*, Vol 49, pp. 168–172, 2002.

45. Gao, X., Bharath, A., Stanton, A., Hughes, A., Chapman, N., and Thom, S., "A Method of Vessel Tracking for Vessel Diameter Measurement on Retinal Images," *IEEE Int. Conf. Image Processing*, pp. 881–884, 2001.

46. Garreau, M., Coatrieux, J., Collorec, R., and Chardenon, C., "A Knowledge-Based Approach for 3-D Reconstruction and Labeling of Vascular Networks from Biplane Angiographic Projections," *IEEE Trans. Med. Imag.*, Vol. 10, No. 2, pp. 122–131, 1991.

47. Glaser J. R. and Glaser E., Neuron Imaging with Neurolucida. A PC-Based System for Image Combining Microscopy, *Computerized Medical Imaging and Graphics*, Vol. 14, pp. 307–317, 1990.

48. Goldbaum, M., Kouznetsova, V., Cot, B., Hart, W., and Nelson, M., "Automated Registration of Digital Ocular Fundus Images for Comparison of Lesions," *SPIE: Ophthalmic Technologies III*, Vol. 1877, pp. 94–99, 1993.

49. Goldbaum, M., Katz, N., Chaudhuri, S., Nelson, M., and Kube, P., "Digital Image Processing for Ocular Fundus Images," *Ophthalmol. Clinics N. Am.*, Vol. 3, No. 3, pp. 447–466, 1990.

50. Goldbaum, M., Moezzi, S., Taylor, A., Chatterjee, S., Boyd, J., Huner, E., and Jain, R., "Automated Diagnosis and Image Understanding with Object Extraction, Object Classification, and Inferencing in Retinal Images," *1996 Proc. IEEE Int. Conf. on Image Processing*, Vol. 3, pp. 695–698, 1996.

51. Grewal, M. and Andrews, A., *Kalman Filtering: Theory and Practice*, Prentice Hall, 1993.

52. Hart, W., Goldbaum, M., Cote, B., Kube, P., and Nelson, M., "Automated Measurement of Retinal Vascular Tortuosity," *Proc. AMIA Fall Conf.*, pp. 459–463, 1997.

53. Hoover, A., Kouznetsova, V., and Goldbaum, M., "Locating Blood Vessels in Retinal Images by Piecewise Threshold Probing of a Matched Filter Response," *IEEE Trans. Med. Imag.*, Vol. 19, No. 3, pp. 203–210, 2000.

54. Hu, J., Kahsi, R., Lopresti, D., Nagy, G., and Wilfong, G., "Why Table Ground-Truthing Is Hard," *Proc. Sixth Int. Conf. Document Analysis and Recogniton*, pp. 129–133, 2001.

55. Hubbard, L., Brothers, R., King, W., Clegg, L., Klein, R., Cooper, L., Sharrett, A., Davis, M., and Cai, J., "Methods for Evaluation of Retinal Microvascular Abnormalities Associated with Hypertension/Sclerosis in the Atherosclerosis Risk in Communities Study," *Opthamology*, Vol. 106, No. 12, pp. 2269–2280, 1999.

56. Jagoe, R., Arnold, J., Blauth, C., Smith, P., Taylor, P., and Wootton, R., "Measurement of Capillary Dropout in Retinal Angiograms by Computerized Image Analysis," *Patt. Recog. Lett.*, Vol. 13, pp. 143–151, 1992.

57. Janssen, R. and Vossepoel, A., "Adaptive Vectorization of Line Drawing Images," *Computer Vision and Image Understanding*, Vol. 65, No. 1, pp. 38–56, 1997.

58. Jasiobedzki, P., Williams, C., and Lu, F., "Detecting and Reconstructing Vascular Trees in Retinal Images," *Medical Imaging 1994: Image Processing*, Murray H. Loew, Ed., Vol. 2167, pp. 815–825, 1994.

59. Kitchen, L. and Rosenfeld, A., "Gray Level Corner Detection," *Patt. Recog. Lett.*, Vol. 1, pp. 95–102, 1982.

60. Klein, A., Egglin, T., Pollak, J., Lee, F., and Amini, A., "Identifying Vascular Features with Orientation Specific Filters and B-spline Snakes," *Computers in Cardiol.*, pp. 113–116, 1994.

61. Klein, R., Klein, B., Neider, M., Hubbard, L., Meuer, S., and Brothers, B., "Diabetic Retinopathy as Detected Using Ophthalmoscopy, a Non-mydriatic Camera and a Standard Fundus Camera," *Ophthamology*, Vol. 92 No. 4, pp. 485–491, 1985.

62. Kochner, B., Schuhmann, D., Michaelis, M., Mann, G., and Englmeier, K.-H., "Course Tracking and Contour Extraction of Retinal Vessels from Color Fundus Photographs: Most Efficient Use of Steerable Filters for Model-Based Image Analysis," *Proc. SPIE, Vol. 3338, Medical Imaging 1998: Image Processing*, Kenneth M. Hanson, Ed., pp. 755–761, 1998.

63. Kyriacos, S., Nekka, F., and Cartilier, L., "Insights into the Formation Process of the Retinal Vasculature," *Fractals*, Vol. 5, No. 4, pp. 615–624, 1997.

64. Lambe, E., Krimer, L., and Goldman-Rakic, S., "Differential Postnatal Development of Catacholamine and Serotonin Inputs to Identified Neurons in Prefrontal Cortex of Rhesus Monkey," *J. Neurosci.*, Vol. 20, No. 23, pp. 8780–8787, 2000.

65. Laplante, P., *Real-Time Systems Design and Analysis, An Engineer's Handbook, 2nd edition*, IEEE Press, 1997.

66. Li, H. and Chutatape, O., "Automatic Location of the Optic Disk in Retinal Images," *Proc. IEEE Int. Conf. Image Processing*, pp. 837–840, 2001.

67. Li, H. and Chutatape, O., "Fundus Image Features Extraction," *Proc. Annu. Eng. Bio. Soc., (EMBS) Int. Conf.*, pp. 3071–3073, 2000.

68. Lu, S. and Eiho, S., "Automatic Detection of the Coronary Arterial Contours with Sub-branches from an X-ray Angiogram," *Computers in Cardiol.*, pp. 575–578, 1993.

69. Mahurkar, A., Trus, B., Vivino, M., Kuehl, E., Datiles, M., and Kaiser-Kupfer, M., "Retinal Fundus Photo Montages: A New Computer Based Method," *Investigative Ophthalmol. Visual Sci.*, Vol. 36, No. 4, 1995.

70. Mahurkar, A., Vivino, M., Trus, B., Kuehl, E., Datiles, M., and Kaiser-Kupfer, M., "Constructing Retinal Fundus Photomontages," *Investigative Ophthalmol. Visual Sci.*, Vol. 7, No. 8, pp. 1675–1683, 1996.

71. Markow, M., Rylander, H., and Welch, A., "Real-Time Algorithm for Retinal Tracking," *IEEE Trans. Biomed. Eng.*, Vol. 40, No. 12, pp. 1269–1281, 1993.

72. Mokhtarian, F. and Suomela, R., "Robust Image Corner Detection Through Curvature Scale Space," *IEEE Trans. Patt. Anal. Machine Intell.*, Vol. 20, No. 12, pp. 1376–1382, 1998.

73. Monahan, P., Gitter, K., Eichler, J., Cohen, G., and Schomaker, K., "Use of Digitized Fluorescein Angiogram System to Evaluate Laser Treatment for Subretinal Neovascularization: Technique," *Retina — J. Retinal and Vitreous Diseases*, Vol. 13, No. 3, pp. 187–195, 1993.

74. Murphy, R., "Age-Related Macular Degeneration," *Ophthalmology*, Vol. 93, pp. 969–971, 1986.

75. Natarajan, S., *Imprecise and Approximate Computation*, Kluwer Academic, Boston, 1995.

76. Nayar, S., Baker, S., and Murase, H., "Parametric Feature Detection," *Proc. IEEE Conf. Computer Vision and Patt. Recog.*, pp. 471–478, 1996.

77. Neumann, F., Schreiner, W., and Neumann, M., "Computer Simulation of Coronary Arterial Trees," *Adv. Eng. Software*, Vol. 28, pp. 353–357, 1997.

78. Niessen, W., Bouma, C., Vincken, K., and Viergever, M., "Error Metrics for Quantitative Evaluation of Medical Image Segmentation," *Performance Characterization in Computer Vision*, Klette, R., Stiehl, H., Viergever, M., and Vincken, K., Eds., Kluwer Academic, Dordrecht, The Netherlands, pp. 275–284, 2000.

79. Nguyen, T. and Sklansky, J., "Computing the Skeleton of Coronary Arteries in Cineangiograms," *Comput. Biomed. Res.*, Vol. 19, pp. 428–444, 1986.

80. Onuki, T. and Nitta, S., "Computer Simulation of Geometry and Hemodynamics of Canine Pulmonary Arteries," *Ann. Biomed. Eng.*, Vol. 21, pp. 107–115, 1993.

81. Otsu, N., "A Threshold Selection Method from Grey-Level Histograms," *IEEE Trans. Syst., Man, and Cybernet.*, Vol. 9, pp. 62–66, 1979.

82. Parida, L., Geiger, D., and Hummel. R., "Junctions: Detection, Classification, and Reconstruction," *IEEE Trans. Patt. Anal. Machine Intell.*, Vol. 20, No. 7, pp. 687–698, 1998.

83. Pedersen, L., Grunkin, M., Ersboll, B., Madsen, K., Larsen, M., Christoffersen, N., and Skands U., "Quantitative Measurement of Changes in Retinal Vessel Diameter in Ocular Fundus Images," *Patt. Recog. Lett.*, Vol. 21, pp. 1215–1223, 2000.

84. Peli, E., Augliere, R., and Timberlake, G., "Feature-Based Registration of Retinal Images," *IEEE Trans. Med. Imag.*, Vol. 6, No. 3, 1987.

85. Pinz, A., Bernogger, S., Datlinger, P., and Kruger, A., "Mapping of the Human Retina," *IEEE Trans. Med. Imag.*, Vol. 17, No. 4, pp. 606–619, 1998.

86. Polli, R. and Valli, G., "An Algorithm for Real-Time Vessel Enhancement and Detection," *Comput. Meth. Programs in Biomed.*, Vol. 52, pp. 1–22, 1997.

87. Press, W., Flannery, B., Tenkolsky, S., and Vetterling, W., *Numerical Recipes in C — The Art of Scientific Computing*, Cambridge University Press, Cambridge, England, 1990.

88. Rayner, K., Ed., *Eye Movements and Visual Cognition: Scene Perception and Reading*, Springer Series in Neuropsychology, Springer-Verlag, New York, 1992.

89. Roberts, D., "Analysis of Vessel Absorption Profiles in Retinal Oximetry," *Medical Phys.*, Vol. 14, pp. 124–130, 1987.

90. Rohr, K., "Recognizing Corners by Fitting Parametric Models," *Int. J. Comput. Vision*, Vol. 9, No. 3, pp. 213–230, 1992.

91. Sato, Y., Nakajima, S., Nobuyuki, S., Atsumi, H., Yoshida, S., Koller, T., Gerig, G., and Kikinis, R., "Three-Dimensional Multi-Scale Line Filter for Segmentation and Visualization of Curvilinear Structures in Medical Images," *Med. Image Anal.*, Vol. 2, No. 2, pp. 143–168, 1998.

92. Sebok, T., Roemer, L., and Malindzak, G., Jr., "An Algorithm for Line Intersection Identification," *Patt. Recog.*, Vol. 13, No. 2, pp. 159–166, 1981.

93. Shen, H., "Optical Instrumentation and Real-Time Image Processing Algorithms for Simultaneous ICG and Red-Free Video Angiography of the Retina," M.S. thesis, Rensselaer Polytechnic Institute, 1996.

94. Shen, H., "Indexing Based Frame-Rate Spatial Referencing Algorithms: Application to Laser Retinal Surgery," Ph.D. thesis, Rensselaer Polytechnic Institute, Troy, NY, 2000.

95. Shen, H., Lin, G., Stewart, C. V., Tanenbaum, H. L., and Roysam, B., "Frame-Rate Spatial Referencing Based on Invariant Indexing and Alignment with

Application to Laser Retinal Surgery," *Proc. IEEE Computer Society Conf. Computer Vision and Patt. Recog.,* Kauai, Hawaii, 2001.

96. Shen, H., Roysam, B., Stewart, C. V., Turner, J. N., and Tanenbaum, H. L., "Optimal Scheduling of Tracing Computations for Real-time Vascular Landmark Extraction from Retinal Fundus Images," *IEEE Trans. Information Technol. Biomed.,* Vol. 5, No. 1, 2001.

97. Sherman, T., "On Connecting Large Vessels to Small," *J. Gen. Physiol.,* Vol. 78, pp. 431, 1981.

98. Simoncelli, E. and Farid, H., "Steerable Wedge Filters for Local Orientation Analysis," *IEEE Trans. Image Processing,* Vol. 5, No. 9, pp. 1377–1383, 1996.

99. Sinthanayothin, C., Boyce, J., Cook, H., and Williamson, T., "Automated Localisation of the Optic Disk, Fovea, and Retinal Blood Vessels from Digital Colour Fundus Images," *Br. J. Ophthalmol.,* Vol. 83, No. 8, 1999.

100. Smith, M., Denninghoff, K., Lompado, A., and Hillman, L., "Effect of Multiple Light Paths on Retinal Vessel Oximetry," *Appl. Opt.,* Vol. 39, No. 7, pp. 1183–1193, 2000.

101. Sonka, M., Hlavac, V., and Boyle, R., *Image Processing, Analysis, and Machine Vision,* Brooks/Cole, Pacific Grove, CA, 1999.

102. Sonka, M., Winniford, M., and Collins, S., "Coronary Borders in Complex Images," *IEEE Trans. Med. Imag.,* Vol. 14, No. 1, pp. 151–161, 1995.

103. Sonka, M., Winniford, M., and Collins, S., "Reduction of Failure Rates in Automated Analysis of Difficult Images: Improved Simultaneous Detection of Left and Right Coronary Borders," *Comput. Cardiol.,* pp. 111–114, 1992.

104. Staib, L. and Duncan, J., "Boundary Finding with Parametrically Deformable Models," *IEEE Trans. Patt. Anal. Machine Intelligence,* Vol. 14, No. 11, 1992.

105. Stanton, A., Mullaney, P., Mee, F., O'Brien, E., and O'Malley, K., "A Method of Quantifying Retinal Microvascular Alterations Associated with Blood Pressure and Age," *J. Hypertension,* Vol. 13, No. 1, pp. 41–48, 1994.

106. Stanton, A., Wasan, B., Cerutti, A., Ford, S., Marsh, R., Sever, P., Thom, S., and Houghes, A., "Vascular Network Changes in the Retina with Age and Hypertension," *J. Hypertension,* Vol. 13, pp. 1724–1728, 1995.

107. Stokoe, N. and Turner R., "Normal Retinal Vascular Pattern Arteriovenous Ratio as a Measure of Arterial Calibre," *Br. J. Ophthalmol.,* Vol. 50, No. 21, pp. 21–40, 1966.

108. Stromland , K., Hellstrom, A., and Gustavsson, T., "Morphometry of the Optic Nerve and Retinal Vessels in Children by Computer-Assisted Image Analysis of Fundus Photographs," *Graefe's Arch. Clin. Exp. Ophthalmol.,* Vol. 233, pp. 150–153, 1995.

109. Sun, Y., "Automated Identification of Vessel Contours in Coronary Arteriograms by an Adaptive Tracking Algorithm," *IEEE Trans. Med. Imag.,* Vol. 8, pp. 78–88, 1989.

110. Sun, Y., Lucariello, R., and Chiaramida, S., "Directional Low-Pass Filtering for Improved Accuracy and Reproducibility of Stenosis Quantification in Coronary Arteriograms," *IEEE Trans. Med. Imag.,* Vol. 14, No. 2, 1995.

111. Tan, W., Wang, Y., and Lee, S., "Retinal Blood Vessel Detection Using Frequency Analysis and Local-Mean-Interpolation Filters," *Medical Imaging 2001: Image Processing,* Milan Sonka and Kenneth M. Hanson, Eds., Vol. 4322, pp. 1373–1384, 2001.

112. Toeledo, R., Radeva, P., Von Land, C., and Villanueva, J., "3D Dynamic Model of the Coronary Tree," *IEEE Computers in Cardiol.*, Vol. 25, p. 777, 1998.
113. Trokel, S. L., "Lasers in Ophthalmology," *Optics and Photonics News*, pp. 11–13, 1992.
114. Tso, M. and Jampol, L. M., "Pathophysiology of Hypertensive Retinopathy," *Ophthalmologica*, Vol. 89, p. 1132, 1982.
115. Turner, J., Shain, W., Szarowski, D., Lasek, S., Sipple, B., Pace, C., Al-Kofahi, K., Can, A., and Roysam, B., "Confocal Light Microscopy of Brain Cells and Tissue: Image Analysis and Quantitation," *Acta Histochem. Cytochem.*, Vol. 32, No. 1, pp. 5–11, 1999.
116. Tyler, M. and Saine, P., *Ophthalmic Photography: Retinal Photography, Angiography, and Electronic Imaging, 2nd edition*, Butterworth-Heinemann Medical, 2002.
117. Van Cuyck, P., Gerbrands, J., and Reiber, J., "Automated Centerline Tracing in Coronary Angiograms," *Pattern Recognition Artificial Intelligence*, pp. 169–183, 1998.
118. VXL, *The VXL Book*, http://vxl.sourceforge.net/, 2002.
119. Wang, Y. and Lee, S., "A Fast Method for Automated Detection of Blood Vessels in Retinal Images," *Conf. Record of the Thirty-First Asilomar Conf. on Signals, Systems and Computers*, Vol. 2, pp. 1700–1704, 1997.
120. Watson, G. S., *Statistics on Spheres*, John Wiley & Sons, New York, 1983.
121. Wink, O., Niessen, W., and Viergever, M., "Fast Delineation of Vessels in 3-D Angiographic Images," *IEEE Trans. Med. Imag.*, Vol. 19, No. 4, pp. 337–346, 2000.
122. Wright, C., Ferguson, R., Rylander H., III, Welch, A., and Barrett, S., "Hybrid Approach to Retinal Tracking and Laser Aiming for Photocoagulation," *J. Biomed. Opt.*, Vol. 2, No. 2, pp. 195–203, 1997.
123. Yannuzzi, L., Guyer, D., and Green, R., *The Retina Atlas* (on CD-ROM), Mosby Year Book, Inc., St. Louis, MO, 1998.
124. Zana, F. and Klein, J.-C., "A Multimodal Registration Algorithm of Eye Fundus Images Using Vessels Detection and Hough Transform," *IEEE Trans. Med. Imag.*, Vol. 18, No. 5, pp. 419–428, 1999.
125. Zana, F. and Klein, J.-C., "Robust Segmentation of Vessels from Retinal Angiography," *Proc. Int. Conf. Digital Signal Processing*, pp. 1087–1091, 1997.
126. Zana, F. and Klein, J.-C., "Segmentation of Vessel-like Patterns Using Mathematical Morphology and Curvature Evaluation," *IEEE Trans. Image Processing*, Vol. 10, No. 7, pp. 1010–1019, 2001.
127. Zhou, L., Rzeszotarski, M., Singerman, L., and Chokreff, J., "The Detection and Quantification of Retinopathy Using Digital Angiograms," *IEEE Trans. Med. Imag.*, Vol. 13, No. 4, pp. 619–626, 1994.
128. Martin, D. F., Sierra-Madero J., Walmsley S., Wolitz R. A., Macey K., Georgiou P., Robinson C. A., and Stempien M. J., "A Controlled Trial of Valganciclovir as Induction Therapy for Cytomegalovirus Retinitis," *New Engl. J. Med.*, Vol. 1346, No. 15, pp. 1119–1126, 2002.

7

Atherosclerotic Plaque Imaging Techniques in Magnetic Resonance Images

Zachary E. Miller and Chun Yuan

CONTENTS

7.1 Introduction

The next three chapters describe the imaging techniques, morphologic index, and tissue characterization approaches for the visualization and characterization of atherosclerosis. Noninvasive magnetic resonance imaging (MRI) is ideally suited for such purposes. Plaque characteristics may be useful in determining high risk, or "vulnerable," plaques, which are more likely to cause thromboembolic events leading to heart attacks or strokes [1]. This chapter focuses on the imaging techniques useful in characterizing plaque tissue composition and in determining plaque morphology, and discusses recent findings from using such techniques in plaque characterization. The main focus of this chapter is on the imaging of human carotid atherosclerosis (Figure 7.1).

7.2 Background

Atherosclerotic cerebrovascular disease is the third leading cause of death and the leading cause of major disability among adults in the U.S. today. Angiographic techniques (including ultrasound, x-ray, CT, and MR) are currently used to determine clinical diagnosis; the only information obtained by these

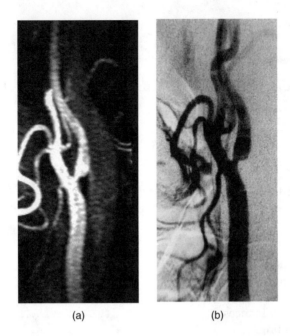

(a)   (b)

FIGURE 7.1
Carotid artery atherosclerosis visualized by MR angiography (a) and x-ray angiography (b). A severe stenosis is seen at the bifurcation (carotid bulb) indicating the location where advance atherosclerosis developed. These images show the overall geometry of the carotid bifurcation and the location where atherosclerosis develops frequently. The MR image is acquired with contrast agent application in a three-dimensional time-of-flight sequence. (Courtesy of J. M. Cai of the PLA General Hospital, Beijing, China.)

methods, however, is the extent of vessel lumen stenosis. Lumen stenosis (the degree to which the vessel is narrowed as a result of plaque growth) is an indirect measure of the severity of atherosclerosis and is not the only indicator of overall plaque burden. As shown in major clinical trials, lumen stenosis predicted one in four strokes in previously symptomatic patients but only one in ten strokes in asymptomatic patients [2–4].

Histological study has shown that a class of plaque (vulnerable plaque) is prone to rupture, causing a thromboembolic event. Such plaque is believed to have a large necrotic lipid-rich core separated by a weakened or ruptured fibrous cap [5–8]. Other plaque features have also been implicated in causing thromboembolic events, such as calcium nodules on the lumen surface and intraplaque hemorrhage [9]. All these are features of the plaques themselves. Additionally, as shown by Glagov, plaque progression may be in the form of outward expansion as compensatory remodeling, creating a significant plaque burden but leaving the lumen relatively unchanged [10, 11].

Measurements of vessel stenosis tell us little about plaque morphology, features, or constituents, all of which may be factors in the "vulnerable" plaque.

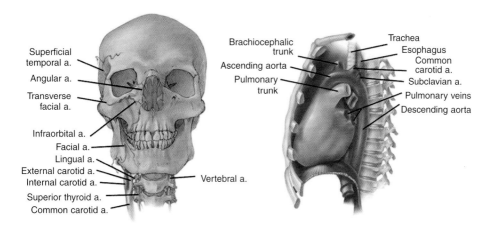

Superficial temporal a.
Angular a.
Transverse facial a.
Infraorbital a.
Facial a.
Lingual a.
External carotid a.
Internal carotid a.
Superior thyroid a.
Common carotid a.
Vertebral a.

Brachiocephalic trunk
Ascending aorta
Pulmonary trunk
Trachea
Esophagus
Common carotid a.
Subclavian a.
Pulmonary veins
Descending aorta

COLOR FIGURE 1.2

Vasculature system for the head and neck and the heart embedded in the skull and chest cavity, respectively. Left: Neck arteries entering the skull area. Right: Aorta seen in the chest cavity. (Courtesy of Professor Fishman, Johns Hopkins University, Baltimore, MD).

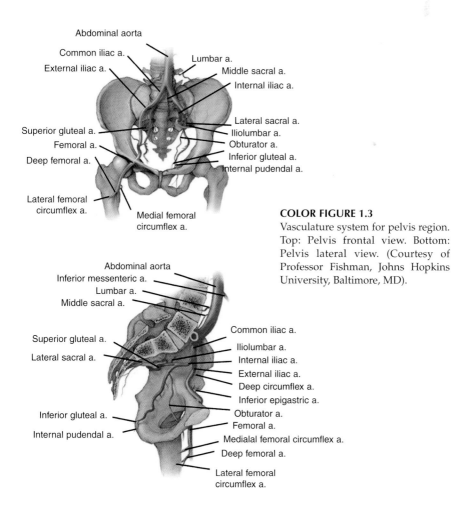

Abdominal aorta
Common iliac a.
External iliac a.
Lumbar a.
Middle sacral a.
Internal iliac a.
Lateral sacral a.
Iliolumbar a.
Obturator a.
Inferior gluteal a.
Internal pudendal a.
Superior gluteal a.
Femoral a.
Deep femoral a.
Lateral femoral circumflex a.
Medial femoral circumflex a.

Abdominal aorta
Inferior messenteric a.
Lumbar a.
Middle sacral a.
Superior gluteal a.
Lateral sacral a.
Common iliac a.
Iliolumbar a.
Internal iliac a.
External iliac a.
Deep circumflex a.
Inferior epigastric a.
Inferior gluteal a.
Obturator a.
Internal pudendal a.
Femoral a.
Medialal femoral circumflex a.
Deep femoral a.
Lateral femoral circumflex a.

COLOR FIGURE 1.3

Vasculature system for pelvis region. Top: Pelvis frontal view. Bottom: Pelvis lateral view. (Courtesy of Professor Fishman, Johns Hopkins University, Baltimore, MD).

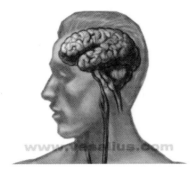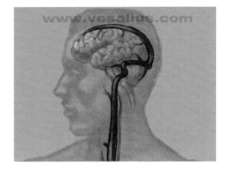

COLOR FIGURE 1.4
Right: The brain and its carotid artery supply. Left: The brain and its major venous drainage. (Courtesy of Vesalius Studios; www.vesalius.com/.)

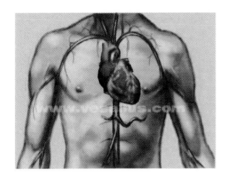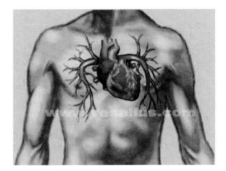

COLOR FIGURE 1.5
Vasculature system in the chest region. Left: Heart and aorta with major upper body branches. Right: The heart and pulmonary arteries. (Courtesy of Vesalius Studios; www.vesalius.com/.)

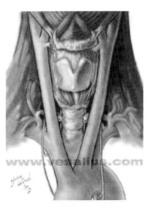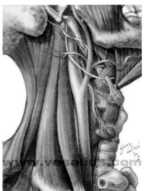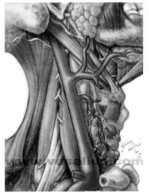

COLOR FIGURE 1.6
Vasculature system in the neck. Left: Anterior view of carotid arteries. Middle: Carotid artery branches. Right: Internal jugular veins and branches. (Courtesy of Vesalius Studios; www.vesalius.com/.)

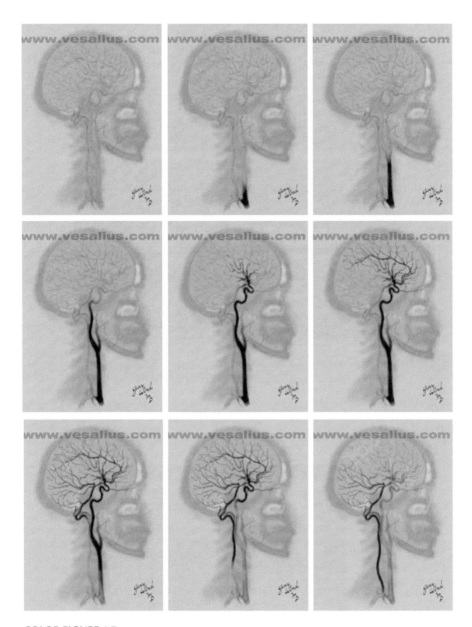

COLOR FIGURE 1.7
Lateral view of a carotid angiogram (arterial to venous). Top to bottom and left to right: shown are only limited angiogram frames: arterial (1–6) and venous (7–9) phases. Also, the density of the vessels and bifurcation can be appreciated. (Courtesy of Vesalius Studios; www.vesalius.com/.)

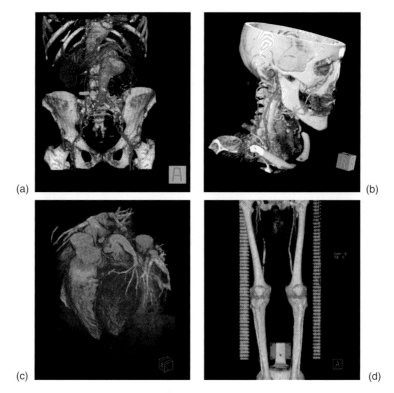

COLOR FIGURE 3.1
Angio studies: (a) abdominal, (b) carotid, (c) cardiac, and (d) peripheral.

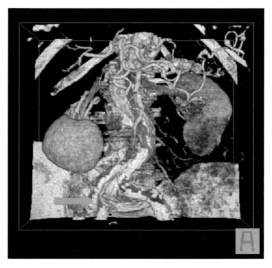

COLOR FIGURE 3.3
Volume-rendered image of contrast-enhanced abdominal CT data.

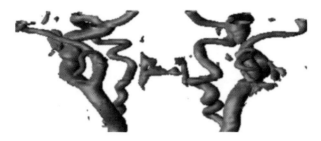

COLOR FIGURE 3.6
This figure illustrates the quality of reconstruction of the vascular structure from MRA images via three-dimensional bubbles [85, 86].

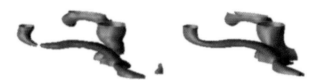

COLOR FIGURE 3.7
This figure illustrates the importance of diffusion process in the three-dimensional bubbles technique. In the reaction process, bubbles cross over the small weak boundary segments, finally causing the vessels to split into pieces. However, in the diffusion process, bubbles do not enter these regions; thus, they reconstruct smooth shapes [86].

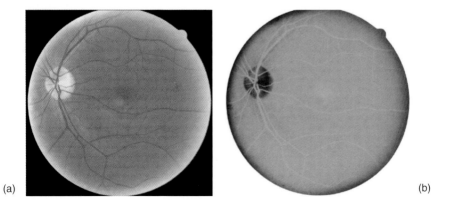

(a)   (b)

COLOR FIGURE 5.2
(a) Original nonmydiatric image, and (b) gray-scale inverted version.

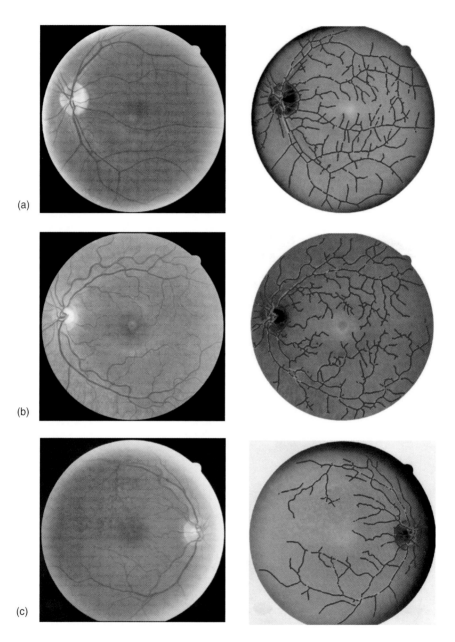

COLOR FIGURE 5.11
Segmentation results.

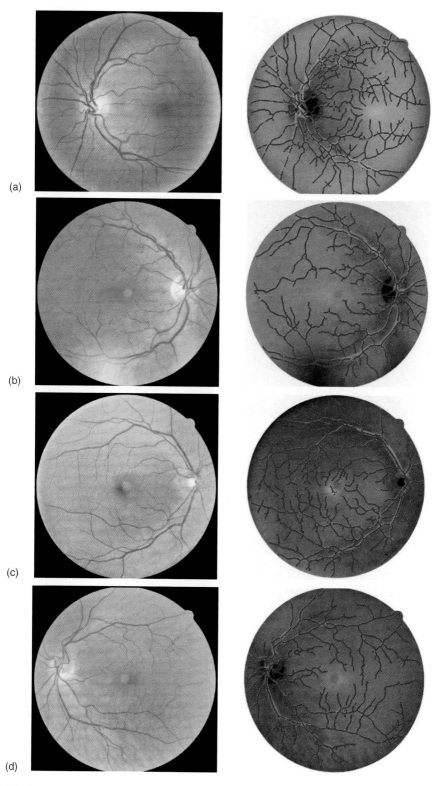

(a)

(b)

(c)

(d)

COLOR FIGURE 5.12
Segmentation results (continued).

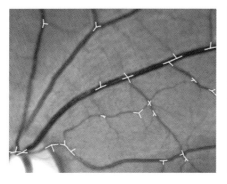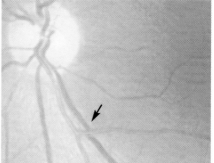

COLOR FIGURE 6.3
Crossing and branching points of the retinal vasculature. The left panel shows these points as
detected by RPI-Trace. The right panel shows an example of vein nicking observed in hypertensive patients caused by an artery exerting pressure on a vein. Automatic location of these
interest points may be valuable for clinical diagnosis.

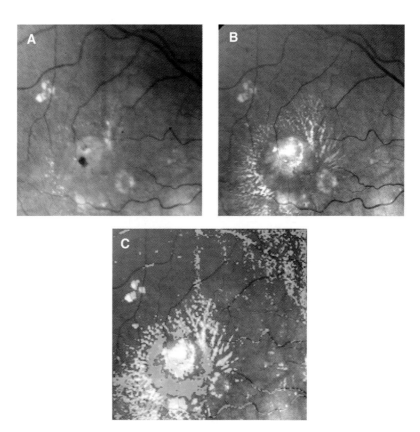

COLOR FIGURE 6.4
Application of vessel tracing and registration to retinal image change detection. Panels A and
B show images captured 30 days apart. Panel C shows the result of registration of the above
two images, followed by an automatic segmentation (delineation) of the "difference" image,
revealing the regions of change in blue.

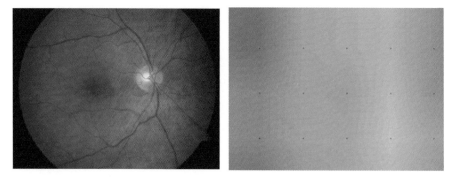

COLOR FIGURE 6.8
Illustrating the changes in local thresholds indicative of the varying intensity structure across the entire image. For each region center denoted by the x in the right image, a local minimum threshold is calculated. These thresholds are then interpolated for any pixel that is not a region center. The thresholds shown in the image on the right were determined from the image on the left with the thresholds multiplied by 4 for display purposes.

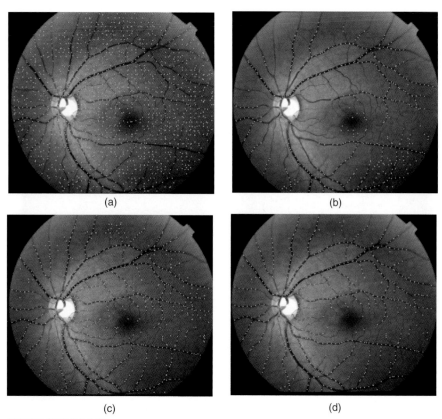

(a)   (b)

(c)   (d)

COLOR FIGURE 6.10
The performance of edge-based vessel models. Panel (a) shows the identified vessels from the vertical and horizontal profiles shown in Figure 6.9(a) using one-dimensional parallel edges within a radius of 11 pixels and edge magnitude within 20%. Panel (b) shows use one-dimensional parallel edges with the same settings as used in panel (a) with the addition of global thresholds for grayscale minima and edge strength. Panel (c) is the same, but with local thresholds. Both (b) and (c) used $\alpha = 1.5$ in Equation 6.3 and $\alpha = 1$ in Equation 6.1. Panel (d) shows vessel points found using two-dimensional parallel edges (with the same local thresholds as panel (c)).

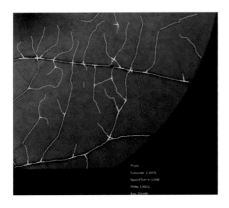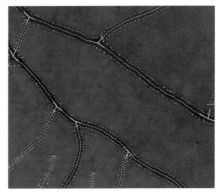

COLOR FIGURE 6.26
The left panel shows how for a selected vessel, the vessel's morphometric measures (tortuosity, width, area, etc.) can be calculated and displayed. The right panel shows the boundary locations of vessels that are needed to generate these measures.

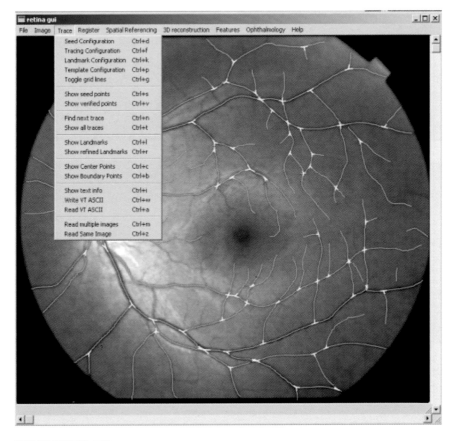

COLOR FIGURE 6.27
Screen view of the RPI-Trace multi-platform graphical user interface. Shown are the options currently available for tracing vessels.

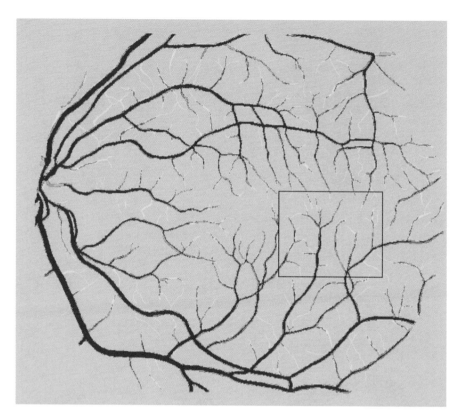

COLOR FIGURE 6.28
Multi-observer standard image formed from five separate hand tracings (two of the hand tracings courtesy Prof. Adam Hoover). Blue pixels are cases where five observers agree that the pixel is vessel; cyan is four; green is three; red is two; yellow is one; and white is zero.

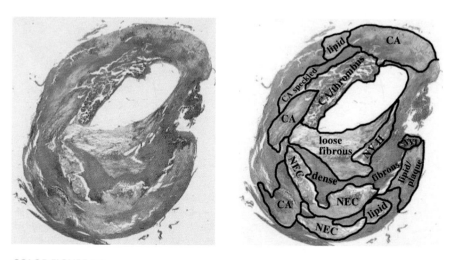

COLOR FIGURE 7.2
A hematoxylin and eosin (H and E) stained slide of an atherosclerotic plaque obtained from the common carotid artery of a patient (a) and outlines of tissue types (b). A typical atherosclerotic plaque usually contains a mixture of different type of tissues as nicely shown in this section and the size of each tissue type can be highly variable (NEC = necrotic core).

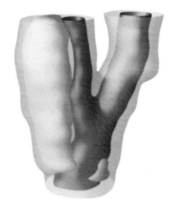 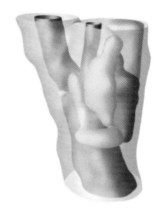

COLOR FIGURE 8.1
Illustration of a vulnerable plaque at the carotid bifurcation showing a large lipid core (yellow) between the outer wall of the artery (opaque) and the lumen (red).

COLOR FIGURE 8.2
A typical carotid artery plaque exhibiting calcification (light blue) and intraplaque hemorrhage (purple) in addition to lipid core (yellow).

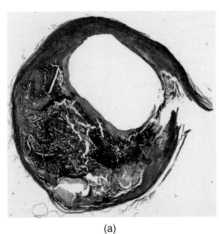

(a)

(b)

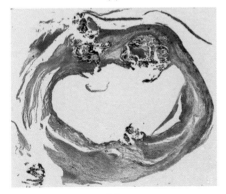

COLOR FIGURE 8.3
Examples of vulnerable plaques: (a) a large plaque with a lipid-rich core (arrow) separated from the lumen by a thin fibrous cap; (b) a plaque with substantial neovasculature in the shoulder region (arrow); and (c) a plaque with calcific nodules (arrow) extruding into the lumen.

(c)

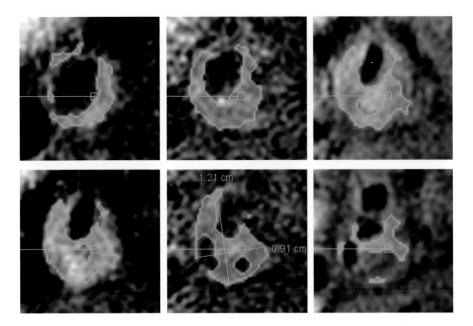

COLOR FIGURE 8.14

Measurement of lipid core volume using ACCENT. The indicated region was selected by a single mouse-click on a region judged to be lipid core. The total region extent was then determined across adjacent images, six of which are shown here.

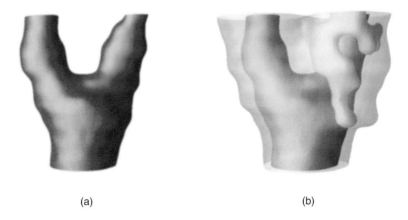

(a)   (b)

COLOR FIGURE 8.17

Resulting model from example in Figure 8.15 and Figure 8.16: (a) artery lumen, and (b) complete model with calcification (light blue) and outer wall (opaque).

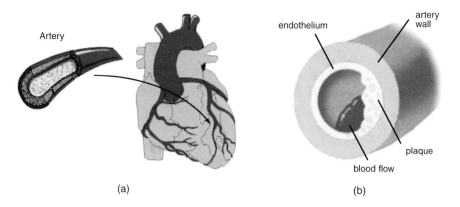

(a)   (b)

COLOR FIGURE 10.1
(a) Coronary arteries as an essential part of the heart, and (b) the morphological structure of coronary vessel.

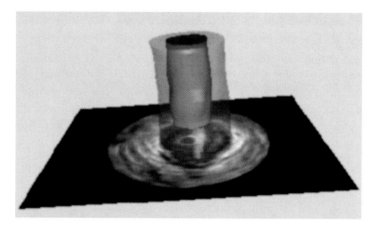

COLOR FIGURE 10.10
Volumetric model of the coronary vessel obtained by interpolating the segmentation of IVUS images.

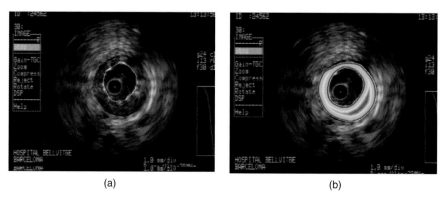

(a)   (b)

COLOR FIGURE 10.17
(a) Segmenting stent and (b) vessel allows measurement of their mutual position.

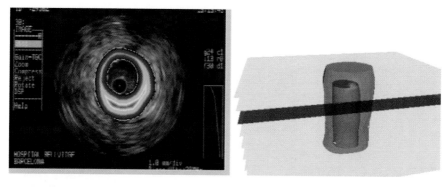

COLOR FIGURE 10.18
(Left) Visualization of the mutual position between stent and (right) vessel in the IVUS plane and space.

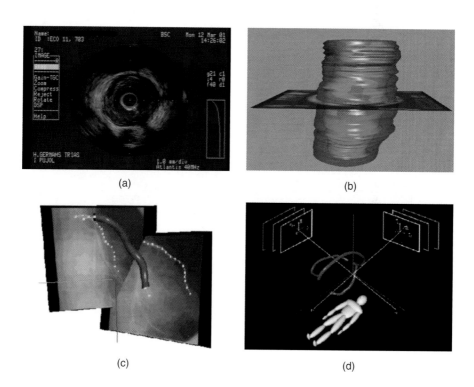

COLOR FIGURE 10.20
(a) Original IVUS image and (b) spatial model of the vessel extracted from IVUS; (c and d) spatial curvature of vessels recovered from biplane angiograms.

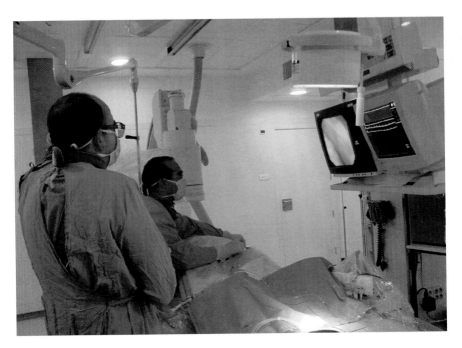

COLOR FIGURE 10.21
Cardiac catheterization laboratory.

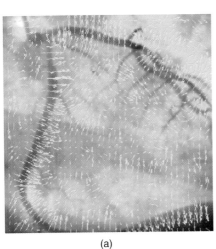
(a)

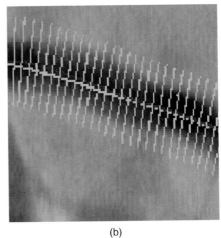
(b)

COLOR FIGURE 10.23
(a) Direction of the first eigenvector of the image structure tensor and (b) training vessel profiles oriented in this direction.

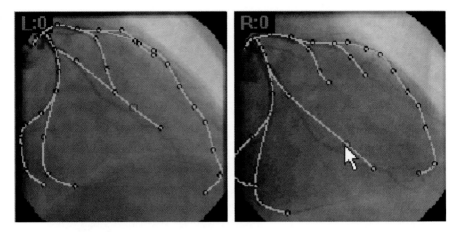

COLOR FIGURE 10.27

A bottom-up strategy to reconstruct vessel centerline is based on user-defined corresponding points in x-ray images.

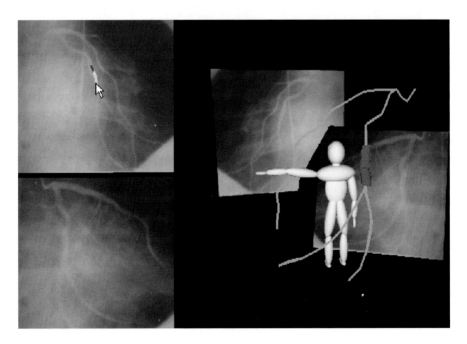

COLOR FIGURE 10.34

Three-dimensional reconstruction of the vessel by biplane snakes allows real three-dimensional measurements.

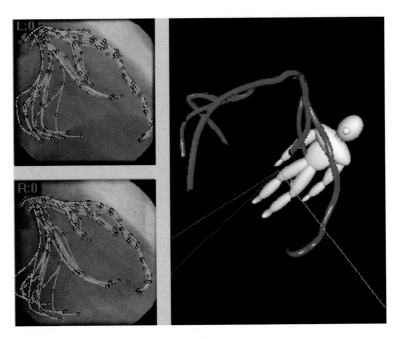

COLOR FIGURE 10.36
Vessel segmentation of angiogram sequences (on the left) and three-dimensional reconstruction of the coronary tree (on the right).

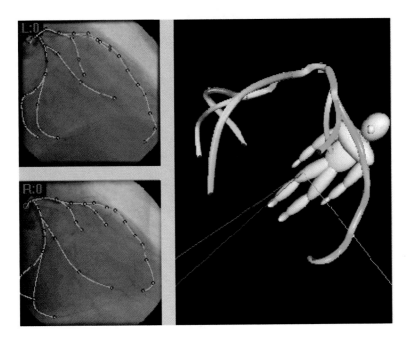

COLOR FIGURE 10.37
Spatial and dynamic model of the coronary tree: red color means high dynamic properties while blue color means static vessel segments.

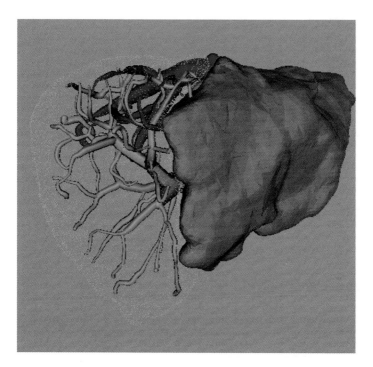

COLOR FIGURE 11.1

Portal and hepatic vein segmentations taken from two contrast CT scans are shown simultaneously for living donor liver transplant planning. *The medical data used to generate this and all of the other images in Chapter 11 were acquired in and provided by the Department of Radiology at The University of North Carolina at Chapel Hill.*

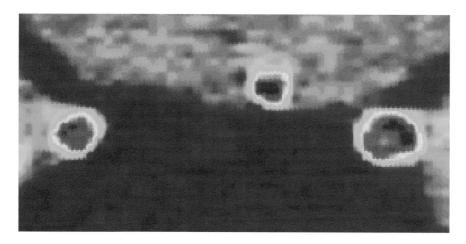

COLOR FIGURE 11.10

An enlargement of a region of an axial time-of-flight MRA slice. Artificial coloring is used to emphasize the different intensities within the carotids, which indicate different flow rates within them. These cross-sectional intensity variations complicate vessel segmentation and may confound vessel registration methods.

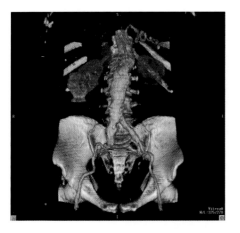

COLOR FIGURE 11.14

This vivid depiction of an abdominal aortic aneurysm was generated on a commercial medical image volume rendering system (Vitrea by Vital Images, Inc.). The user can interactively change the point of view. The points shown and the colors in the image were assigned to the CT data using preset thresholds based on Hounsfield units. These thresholds can be interactively modified. The volume can be trimmed or a region of interest hand-segmented.

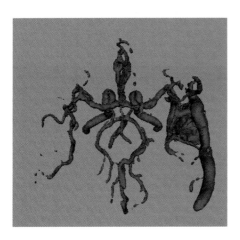

COLOR FIGURE 11.16

In this image, connected components has been applied to segment the vasculature in a ToF MRA volume image. This segmentation can be interactively viewed on standard PC hardware. Embolization planning is facilitated; however, connected components was not able to segment the small vessels in the image.

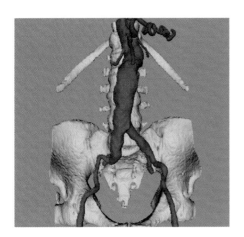

COLOR FIGURE 11.17

By integrating smoothness and connectedness constraints into segmentation via adaptive surface or boundary evolution (shown here) methods, an AAA that abuts the spine can still be segmented from the spine. The spine was still included in this visualization to provide anatomic reference. By isolating the AAA, stent planning is fast and accurate.

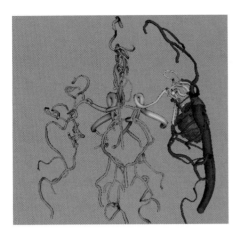

COLOR FIGURE 11.24

The MRA AVM previously depicted in Figure 11.12 and Figure 11.16 is shown here using centerline and radii vessel models, connected component AVM models, and colorings that portray the connectedness of vessels with respect to the AVM. The information content of this image (compared to the information in the other figures) is arguably much more directed to the clinical task at hand: embolization planning.

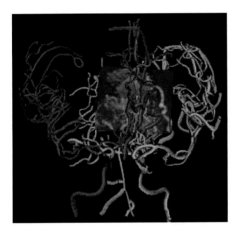

COLOR FIGURE 11.25

This figure is a clear illustration of the power of segmentation when the form of the segmentation (here centerlines and radii) enable functional information to also be captured and displayed. Specifically, coloring is used to illustrate what distal trees are being fed by the right and left carotids and the basilar. Additionally, the AVM is segmented but then volume rendered to allow the fuzzy borders of the nidus to be fully appreciated.

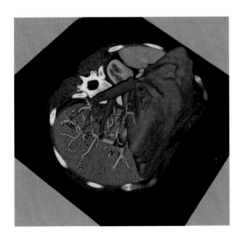

COLOR FIGURE 11.26

From CT images taken with contrast, the liver parenchyma is segmented via connected components and the vessels are segmented using dynamic-scale centerline and radius modeling. Segmented vessels are then reconstructed into vascular trees corresponding to the portal and hepative venous systems. Transplant surgeons interact with these visualizations to specify a cutting path for lobe resection. Here, a portion of the liver to be donated is shown. Vascular patency can be verified. Vessel cross-sectional areas can be compared with those of the recipient to estimate risk of thrombosis.

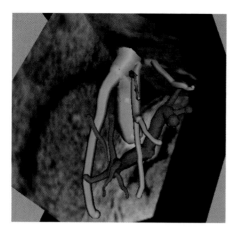

COLOR FIGURE 11.27
The dynamic-scale centerline and radius vessel segmentation system is robust such that without modification it can be used to extract vessel from three-dimensional ultrasound data.

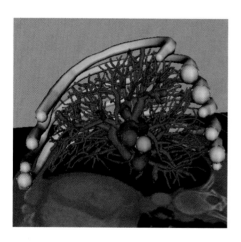

COLOR FIGURE 11.28
The vessels, bronchi, and ribs depicted in this figure were segmented using the dynamic-scale centerline and radius method. Such visualizations can be rapidly interacted with on a standard PC using inexpensive graphics cards (designed for running computer games). Such visualizations are effective for partial lung transplant planning.

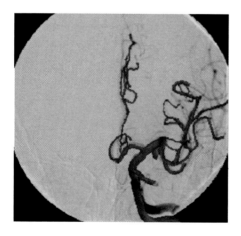

COLOR FIGURE 11.29
Trigeminal neuralgia is characterized by extreme pain on one side of the patient's face. It can be treated by ablating the corresponding nerve but this requires the insertion of a needle through the same opening in the skull that the carotid artery passes through. By performing a feature-based three-dimensional-to-two-dimensional registration of the preoperative MRA with intra-operative biplane digital subtraction angiograms, the three-dimensional position of the needle can be reconstructed and shown in correspondence with the patient's orientation on the table and with respect to the patient's vasculature and anatomy capture in the preoperative CT. The procedure is made safer for the patient.

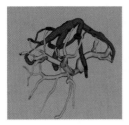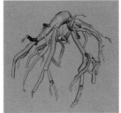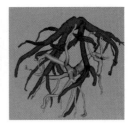

COLOR FIGURE 11.30

Left and middle: The vessels extracted from the arterial and venous phase contrast CT images from a potential liver donor. The first scan captures the portal network and some of the hepatic network. The second captures the hepatic network. Despite few corresponding vessels, the portal models can be registered with the hepatic image (the hepatic models are only shown for illustration; they are not used during registration). Right: After registration, the models from both scans can be fused to get a single complete view of the liver vasculature. These models drive the definition of liver lobes resected during transplantation.

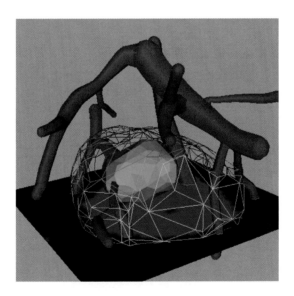

COLOR FIGURE 11.31

A small section from a lung CT image volume containing a tumor. The tumor was modeled using connected components. The vessels were modeled using dynamic-scale centerlines and radii. The tumor was then artificially enlarged (shown in wireframe) and the data was rotated and translated and then given to be registered with the prior vascular models. Despite the enlarged tumor obscuring multiple vessels, the final registration was excellent. Tumor growth can be detected and quantified.

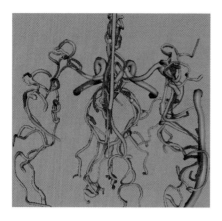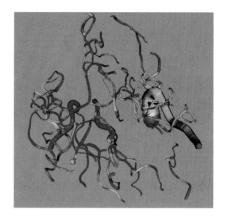

COLOR FIGURE 11.32

Two visualizations of the effect of radiation and surgery on intracranial vessels containing a tumor (an AVM). Left: Pre- and post-treatment vessels are shown registered. On the image right, near the treatment site, there are local vascular displacements. The large wireframe vessel is missing in the posttreatment image. Right: Shading encodes the distance from pre-treatment vessels to nearest postsurgery vessels. The ends of some vessels are colored because of differences in extraction. Long, bright vessels indicate areas of large anatomic change; the tumor bears the majority of the effects of treatment. Visualizations of such vascular changes help physicians determine treatment effectiveness.

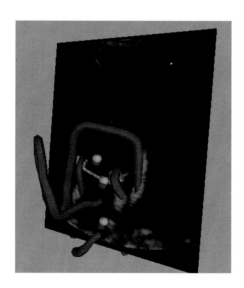

COLOR FIGURE 11.33

Portal and hepatic vein segmentations taken from two contrast CT scans are shown simultaneously for living donor liver transplant planning. A visualization of the effect of radiation and surgery on intracranial vessels containing a tumor (an AVM). Shading encodes the distance from pre-treatment vessels to nearest postsurgery vessels. Ends of some vessels are colored because of differences in extraction. Long, bright vessels indicate areas of large vascular/anatomic change/shift; the tumor bears the majority of the effects of treatment. Visualizations of such vascular changes help physicians determine treatment effectiveness.

MRI provides an excellent, noninvasive way to visualize carotid vessel stenosis, providing detailed information on plaque composition and size. Information that can be determined from visualizing carotid arteries with MRI includes: plaque compositions (such as necrotic lipid core and fibrous cap), total plaque area and volume, lumen area and wall thickness, and plaque distribution. It is hoped that the acquisition of this extra data will enable us to pinpoint plaques that are more susceptible to rupture, that is, the vulnerable plaques.

In the future, this MR plaque imaging technique may be used to select optimal treatment for carotid atherosclerosis. More specifically, the selection of patients for surgical (carotid endarterectomy [CEA]) vs. nonsurgical treatment. CEA has been shown to be effective in preventing strokes in symptomatic patients with carotid stenosis [2]. In patients who are asymptomatic however, the efficacy of CEA is not as clear [4]. Since 60% of CEAs are performed on asymptomatic patients (roughly 84,000 per year in the U.S.), a great deal of unnecessary surgery may be taking place. Improved imaging methods may help in determining the ideal treatment and clinical outcomes for asymptomatic patients by providing more information about carotid atherosclerotic plaque. MRI is a strong candidate for this purpose, as it is noninvasive and capable of distinguishing plaque morphology and features.

MR plaque imaging, as a noninvasive technique, can also be used serially in monitoring the progression of atherosclerosis or changes of such lesion under medical treatment. Results from such serial studies may provide valuable information about plaque progression and/or regression *in vivo* in humans, which have been difficult to obtain from animal model studies or pathological evaluation.

7.2.1 Atherosclerosis

Atherosclerosis is a disease of the large and medium-sized arteries that is characterized by progressive intimal accumulation of lipid, protein, and cholesterol esters [12]. Although considered a systemic disease, it has a propensity for a segmental distribution, being found most commonly at major arterial bifurcations and at points of marked arterial angulation. Predominant sites of involvement include the coronary arteries, the superficial femoral artery, the infrarenal aorta, and the carotid arteries at the area of the common carotid bifurcation.

Traditionally, the degree of artery stenosis, or narrowing, has been targeted as the marker of a vulnerable plaque, and considered to cause either a complete arterial occlusion or ischemic event in the brain. However, in 1988, Ambrose and Little demonstrated in angiographic studies that mild-to-moderate coronary artery stenosis may lead to acute myocardial infarction and suggested that lumen narrowing was not the sole predictor for thrombotic events [13, 14]. Based on histopathologic studies, Davies, Falk, Fuster, and others have suggested that plaque erosion and disruption was the critical feature in these moderately stenotic, vulnerable lesions [5, 7, 15]. Falk noted that greater than 75% of major coronary thrombotic events were precipitated by atherosclerotic plaque rupture [5]. This plaque rupture resulted in exposure of thrombogenic subendothelial plaque constituents. Bassiouny, Davies, Falk, and others showed that the morphology of the unstable plaques that were at risk for disruption typically contained a large acellular core that was separated from the lumen by a thin fibrous cap. In addition, the size of the lipid core and the degree of neovascularization within the plaque may be important determinants of plaque instability [5, 7, 13–16]. Because plaques in the cervical carotid arteries are histologically similar to those in the coronary circulation, it is believed that similar events underlie the development of neurologic symptoms in patients with asymptomatic carotid disease [17]. Carotid angiography, however, does not characterize plaque morphology, with the exception of luminal ulceration [18], and degree of stenosis is not associated with the presence of intraplaque hemorrhage or a necrotic core [19]. Tissue compositions such as recent hemorrhage, lipid-rich necrotic cores, fibrous caps and intimal tissue, calcification, and neovasculature may all play a role in plaque rupture. To date, however, relatively little is known about plaque progression. Noninvasive, reproducible techniques that perform accurate visualization of the carotid vessel wall will enable us to further study plaque evaluation over time.

7.2.2   Current Imaging Modalities

Although several imaging modalities are currently attempting to visualize atherosclerotic plaque, no imaging modality is used clinically to monitor carotid plaque changes and progression *in vivo*.

7.2.2.1   X-Ray

X-ray angiography, especially digital subtraction angiography, is currently the standard for assessing lesions in the coronary, carotid, and peripheral arteries. X-ray angiography is capable of visualizing stenosis and irregular luminal surface; however, it provides no information on vessel wall or plaque compositions, such as fibrous cap or lipid core, thus making it useless in studying plaque morphology and characterization [20]. X-ray angiography is a highly invasive and expensive procedure, making it unsuitable for serial studies over time. As discussed previously, ipsilateral stroke rate, even in patients with severely stenotic vessels, is relatively low, suggesting that the amount of luminal narrowing may not represent the optimal means of assessing clinical risk.

7.2.2.2   Ultrasound

Doppler ultrasound is also widely used clinically to measure lumen stenosis in carotid arteries. First introduced by Saturma and Koenko in 1957 for detecting elevated blood velocities in carotid stenoses, it did not come into widespread use until after 1975, when a quantitative examination protocol was developed by Strandness and others [21–23]. Many investigations have also been made using B-mode ultrasound, developed about the same time, to measure or identify atherosclerotic plaque size, size of the fibrous cap, wall thickness, and plaque compositions or ulceration. Success with plaque characterization has been mixed.

One of the measurements to gain widespread acceptance is the intima-media thickness (IMT) in the common carotid artery (CCA) [24], which has been used in several clinical trials [25–28]. Thickness from 200 to 2000 microns can be measured using ultrasound probes with wavelengths of 200 microns (7.5 MHz). The IMT measurement is accepted as a validated measurement of atherosclerosis. In a landmark study, increased IMT was correlated to coronary artery disease (CAD) and stroke in older adults without a history of cardiovascular disease [29].

IMT measurement, although conducted at the CCA, is not a direct measure of carotid atherosclerosis. An exciting opportunity exists that direct measurement of carotid atherosclerosis can be combined with the ultrasonic IMT measurement, which may provide a clearer picture of atherosclerotic progression, not only in carotid but also in coronary and other vascular beds.

Ultrasound has been used to differentiate "stable" from "unstable" plaque. Here, "unstable" plaque refers to plaque that is associated with past neurological symptoms, in order to predict future neurological events. The stability of the plaque is thought to be related either to mechanical or flow-dynamic motion during the cardiac cycle or plaque composition. Plaque compositions have been identified based on the echogenicity of the plaque, displayed as mean pixel brightness in B-mode carotid artery images [30], median pixel brightness [31], integrated backscatter of the radio frequency (RF) echo, and echo attenuation rate at different frequencies in endarterectomy samples [32–35], pathology samples [36], and carotid artery images [37–40]. Plaque materials that have been identified include calcium, hemorrhage, necrosis, and lipid and fibrous tissue. Intravascular ultrasound images (IVUS) of pathological samples have also been analyzed [41].

It is generally agreed that unstable plaques are likely to have hypoechoic regions [42, 43], or low ultrasound echogenicity [31, 40, 44]. Calcium can significantly limit detection of plaque components by causing bright echoes, thus shadowing other echoes deep into the plaque [45]. Hemorrhage has been associated with strong echoes, while fibrous plaques have been associated with weak echoes [46]. Fibrous plaques exhibit larger echo brightness dependent on the incident angle of the ultrasound beam [47], implying an ordered structure in such tissues. Tissues with high elastin content produce strong echoes [48].

Although visual analysis of plaque in B-mode ultrasound has been the basis for most plaque characterization efforts, quantitative analysis has been hampered by a high degree of inter-operator and exam variability [49–51].

Inter-exam variability can be reduced by quantitatively comparing plaque with neighboring tissues with known echogenecities, such as blood or adventitia [52], but overall the results for identifying unstable plaques "has been largely unsuccessful" [53].

7.2.2.3 CT

Computed tomography angiography (CTA) has been used clinically to evaluate carotid stenosis. An iodine-based contrast agent is, in general, needed in such studies. With the introduction of multi-slice and ultrafast CT, the imaging time of a CTA scan is significantly reduced while retaining excellent spatial resolution. In addition to luminal stenosis, CT has been shown to be able to detect the presence of calcification and ulceration, and measure plaque density. Additionally, electron beam CT and ultrafast CT have been able to characterize calcium in coronary arteries [54–57]. CT and CTA, however, emit significant amounts of radiation, making them unsuitable for serial *in vivo* studies. Some patients may also experience adverse reactions to contrast agents commonly injected with CTA imaging. A review of current literature conducted on Medline found few attempts to characterize tissue compositions beyond calcium, density, and stenosis [58–62].

7.3   Challenges For MRI

Many challenges exist in carotid MR imaging. Perhaps the two most significant challenges are obtaining the right temporal and spatial resolutions necessary to properly visualize plaque compositions, and postprocessing techniques required to analyze plaque progression. In this chapter, we discuss the technical challenges, imaging approaches (both hardware and software) taken to face such challenges, and results from using such imaging techniques for plaque morphology evaluation and tissue characterization. Postprocessing techniques for plaque quantification are discussed in Chapters 8 and 9.

7.3.1   Characterization Goal

Plaque characterization MRI is a relatively new field. Thus, the goals have been to (1) to develop a validation technique such that MR images taken from atherosclerotic plaques *in vivo* can be correlated to histological examination of plaque specimens, (2) explore hardware and software approaches such that both vessel luminal and outer wall boundaries can be accurately identified on the images and detailed information of plaque compositions visualized, and (3) determine the accuracy and reproducibility of plaque features identified by MRI.

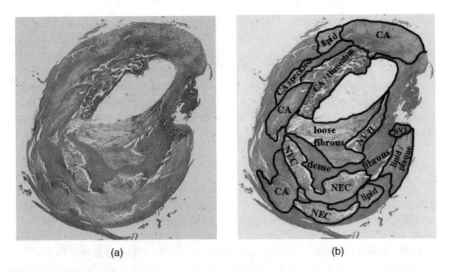

(a) (b)

FIGURE 7.2 (See color insert.)
A hemosidron and eosion (H and E) stained slide of an atherosclerotic plaque obtained from the common carotid artery of a patient (a) and outlines of tissue types (b). A typical atherosclerotic plaque usually contains a mixture of different type of tissues as nicely shown in this section and the size of each tissue type can be highly variable (NEC = necrotic core).

7.3.2 Size

Atherosclerotic plaques in the carotid are usually centered at the bifurcation with a coverage of 2 to 5 cm. Plaques are heterogeneous mixtures of fibrous connective tissue, lipid, blood, and blood products, thrombus, necrosis, and calcification. Histological examination of plaques reveals components such as surface erosions, ruptures, and calcific nodules, which although only 100 μm in size can produce clinically relevant events. It is apparent that a higher resolution than the current 1×1 mm^2 pixel size is needed. In general, the carotid artery is a superficial structure that surface coils can be fully utilized to improve the signal-to-noise (SNR) performance of the scanner (Figure 7.2).

7.3.3 Flow, Motion

It has been documented extensively that MR signal is sensitive to both flowing blood and motion. Flow-enhanced techniques (such as those used in MR angiography) have been very effective in depicting the luminal boundary of the vessel, and hence vessel narrowing. In the meantime, flow suppression techniques have been used extensively in many clinical applications where tissues neighboring flowing blood need to be examined, such as in the evaluation of myocardium. The carotid bulb, where most carotid atherosclerosis develops, presents unique challenges for both flow enhancement and suppression because of the complicated flow patterns that can occur at this site [63]. Thus, an effective plaque imaging technique must provide effective flow suppression or enhancement at the carotid bulb in order to provide distinct signal between flowing blood and the surrounding wall. Motion during an MR scan, especially swallowing, can cause significant artifacts in images. This provides a technical challenge for plaque imaging: how to acquire high-resolution images with good SNR in a short time so that a patient can sustain a comfortable and still position.

7.3.4 Tissue Contrast

As described briefly above, plaques can be a highly complicated heterogeneous mixture of fibrous tissues of varying densities and organization containing lipid, calcium, and intraplaque hemorrhage of different ages. Microvessels associated with plaque activity penetrate the plaque at various locations, bringing inflammatory cells and macrophages to sites of luminal rupture and erosion. The fibrous cap separates the main contents of the necrotic core from the lumen and is composed of collagen bundles or other fibrous tissues. Juxtaluminal calcification can obscure the true lumen boundary and requires time-of-flight sequences to unmask it. It quickly becomes clear that all the MR contrast weightings must be evaluated to accurately characterize the atherosclerotic plaque.

7.4 Technical Advances

7.4.1 Hardware: Phased-Array Carotid Coil and Headholder

The typical in-plane spatial resolution of 1×1 mm^2 obtained with a 1.5T clinical scanner for head or body imaging is too large to satisfactorily detect the small volumes of the major plaque components present in carotid lesions. For example, evaluation of histologically processed endarterectomy specimens revealed mean values for the volume of individual plaque components (lipid core, fibrous intimal tissue, and calcification) ranging from 0.3 mm^3 and up [64]. Although submillimeter voxel sizes can be achieved with whole-body 1.5T scanners, the use of a phased-array surface coil appears to be necessary to generate an acceptable SNR for the high-resolution images required for carotid plaque characterization.

The carotid arteries are superficial structures whose length is greater than their distance from the surface. This configuration is well suited for the use of phased-array (PA) surface coils, which are composed of several adjacent small surface coils that collect data simultaneously. For the purposes of carotid plaque imaging, a dedicated PA coil assembly, with overall dimensions of 6.4×10.8 cm, was constructed [65]. The assembly consists of two separate sets of coils to allow imaging of both carotid arteries during an exam. Each coil

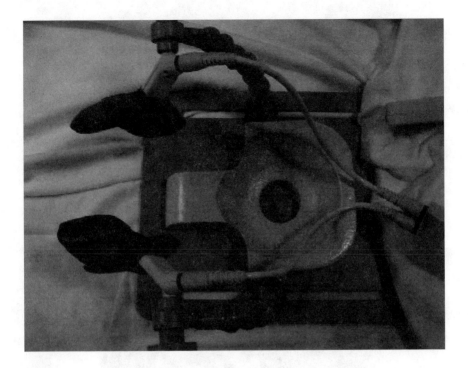

FIGURE 7.3
A top-view picture of the phased-array carotid coil and the accompanying headholder currently in use at the University of Washington Diagnostic Imaging Sciences Center. The phased-array coil is designed to be able to acquire images of both the left and right carotid arteries simultaneously. Two support arms are designed to hold the coils in a fixed position. The headholder is designed to be firm enough to support a subject's head and keep it in a stable position, and soft enough to limit "hot spot" formation within the MR scan.

is made of a soft flexible material that can be comfortably fitted and secured about the neck of the patient. With this coil assembly, an effective longitudinal coverage of up to 5 cm can be obtained. Studies of the performance of these PA coils in normal volunteers demonstrated a 37% improvement in the SNR when compared to commercially available 3-inch surface coils. (Figure 7.3 and Figure 7.4). This greater SNR enables acquisition of diagnostic images of the common internal and external carotid arteries with a best voxel size of $0.25 \times 0.25 \times 2.0$ mm^3 (0.125 mm^3). In addition to the carotid phased-array assembly, a custom-designed headholder was constructed using vacuum-formed PVC plastic. The headholder provides support for the occiput and neck, which not only improves patient comfort but also facilitates repeatable scan positioning and reduces patient movement (Figure 7.3).

Since the introduction of these types of PA coils, similar PA coils have been developed and used for the same purposes of carotid plaque characterization [66, 67]. Additionally, these types of coils have been used in

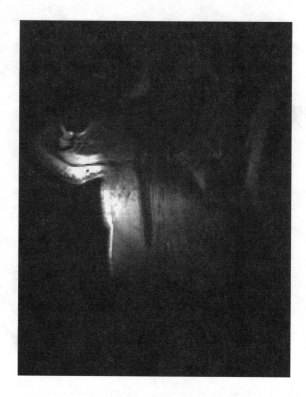

FIGURE 7.4
A sagittal SE MR image of a normal volunteer's head and neck that shows the sensitivity map of the phased-array coil, which covers up to 8 cm longitudinal region.

(1) clinical trials to evaluate the effects of lipid-lowering on human atherosclerotic lesions [68], and (2) assessment of vessel wall thickness measurement [69]. Currently, there are two commercial companies marketing such coil designs (Pathway Medical, Redmond, WA, and Machnet, Utrecht, the Netherlands).

7.4.2   Imaging Sequences

High spatial resolution imaging results in relatively long scan times (several seconds to a few minutes); therefore, the design of MR imaging sequences must consider the contrast weightings that are important for plaque tissue characterization, effective ways for flow enhancement or suppression, so that vessel walls can be highlighted, and techniques to reduce the effects of motion and flow artifacts. Fortunately, for most 1.5T whole-body scanners with which the carotid imaging is likely to be conducted, echo-planar capabilities are available. The gradient amplifiers and higher slew rates supported by these systems allow for shorter echo times and echo spacing (in fast-spin-echo sequences). These features reduce the overall scan times of the pulse sequences used and, as a result, minimize the effects of motion and flow artifacts. Pulse sequences designed for vascular imaging can generally be described as either black or bright blood techniques, depending upon the signal of the flowing blood relative to the surrounding soft tissues. In this section we review the techniques available for plaque imaging and discuss the benefits and weaknesses of each.

7.4.2.1 Flow-Enhanced Gradient Echo Sequence

Flow-enhanced techniques refer to the gradient echo-based imaging sequences that are typically used to acquire MR angiograms. The enhancement (bright blood) is due to the time-of-flight (TOF) effects of blood flow. Techniques such as gradient recalled echo (GRE), spoiled gradient recalled echo (SPGR), TOF, and true FISP are all variations of such techniques. With flow enhancement, the lumen appears hyperintense relative to the adjacent vessel wall. Compared to spin echo (SE) sequences, bright blood techniques can produce images with shorter TE and TR times. The lack of a spin echo in these sequences creates a T_2^*-sensitive tissue signal that appears to improve the visualization of the intimal calcifications and fibrous cap, which in general is a dense structured layer of collagen [70, 71]. Faster scanning also allows the acquisition of high-resolution, three-dimensional data sets that should improve plaque characterization [72].

As shown in Figure 7.5, by properly selecting the imaging parameters (TR, TE and flip angle), a three-dimensional TOF technique can provide a significant amount of information on atherosclerotic plaque at the carotid bifurcation. In particular, bright blood techniques can detect the presence of collagen

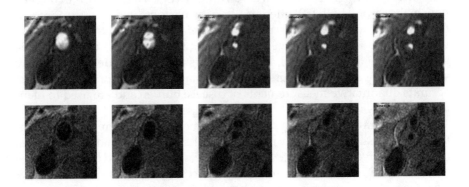

FIGURE 7.5
A set of three-dimensional TOF images (top row) and corresponding two-dimensional FSE T1W images (bottom row) of a diseased right carotid artery centered at the bifurcation (the imaging parameters are listed in Table 7.2). The luminal narrowing and the presence of atherosclerotic plaque can be identified in both the top and bottom raw images. This set of images demonstrates the important role that a modified three-dimensional TOF technique can play in the characterization of atherosclerotic plaque.

fibrous cap [70], calcium, and intraplaque hemorrhage [73], and lumen and outer wall boundaries [74]. A great advantage of bright blood techniques is their extensive clinical use in MRA applications. That is, by properly selecting imaging parameters, MRA applications can be adopted for plaque imaging and provide critical information on tissue compositions and plaque morphological distribution, as well as lumen narrowing.

7.4.2.2 Flow-Suppressed Spin Echo (or Fast Spin Echo [FSE]) Techniques

T2 or T1 weighted SE images were the first to be used to identify individual plaque components [75, 76]. SE or FSE techniques are very effective in generating images with excellent soft tissue contrast. These techniques are the backbones for both plaque tissue characterization and morphological evaluation. The use of these techniques, however, requires effective flow suppression, thus the term "black-blood" (BB) techniques [77]. These BB techniques are ideal for plaque imaging because the conspicuity of the vessel wall is increased when adjacent to a hypointense lumen, and the echo (TE) and repetition (TR) times can be varied to optimize visualization of specific plaque constituents. The major disadvantages of black-blood SE techniques are the relatively long scan times, and that these sequences are based on two-dimensional data acquisition with slice thicknesses that vary between 2 and 5 mm.

Common flow-suppression techniques employed with black-blood imaging involve (1) the use of presaturation radio frequency bands applied along the direction of arterial blood flow with a SE sequence or (2) a double-inversion recovery (DIR) sequence [78]. When presaturation techniques are used, which are less effective than DIR with slowly flowing blood, the complex flow in the carotid bulb [79] often results in artifacts created by unsuppressed flow. Artifacts may be misinterpreted as representing signal from a diseased vessel wall and lead to an overestimation of the size of the atherosclerotic lesion [63]. On the other hand, DIR sequences tend to provide excellent flow suppression, as shown in Figure 7.6. These images typically provide the most accurate quantitative measurements of disease burden and are used to identify soft cores *in vivo* [73].

The main drawback of DIR is a long scan time because DIR requires sequential slice acquisition. A recently proposed dual-slice DIR technique [80] utilizes one nonselective and two slice-selective inversions, followed by consecutive excitation and readout for corresponding slices. Within this approach, however, the further increase in the number of slices acquired per one TR-interval may be difficult due to the long delay between the readout of signal from last slices and the moment of nulling the signal from blood. Yarnykh et al. introduced an alternative multi-slice DIR technique based on the short inversion time (TI) and the simultaneous inversion of an entire imaged volume [81]. In this technique, within the double-inversion pulse pair, the slice-selective

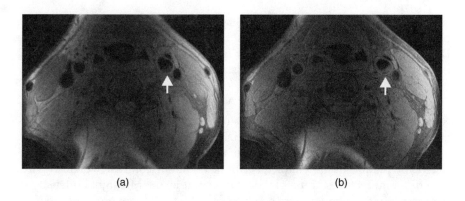

(a)   (b)

FIGURE 7.6
Comparison of the effectiveness of two flow-suppression techniques at the carotid bulb of a normal volunteer: (a) a cross-sectional image taken with DIR SE technique [800/14/16; TR (ms)/TE (ms)/field-of-view (cm)] with TI = 650 ms; (b) taken from the same location with flow saturation band applied superior and inferior to the region of imaging with same imaging parameters. Notice the significant residual flow signals in (b) that could easily be interpreted as part of the vessel wall, which means this normal subject had significant atherosclerosis (arrows). Such mistakes can be easily corrected using the DIR technique in image (a).

pulse is applied to the entire slice pack. TI can be chosen short enough to provide imaging of several slices within TR. A postacquisition delay is used after an echo train to adjust the equal intervals between nonselective inversion pulses, while the number N of slices per TR may vary. For any N, the magnetization of inflowing blood approaches zero at:

$$TI(N) = -T_1 \ln\left[0.5\left(1 + e^{-\frac{TR}{T_1 N}}\right)\right]$$

where $T_1 = 1200$ ms in blood. By design, at all N, DIR provided significantly better blood suppression than presaturation techniques. For N up to 4, the overall image quality remained sufficient for clear delineation of vessel wall. That is, this technique affords a factor of 4 on time saving with good blood flow suppression.

Blood suppression by DIR presumes complete outflow from an imaging volume during TI. Clearly, this requirement constrains an available number of slices per TR because an increase of N leads to an increase of slab thickness and a decrease of TI. However, a drop in the signal from tissues provides a more strict limitation of the proposed technique in the application to thin-slice carotid artery imaging than the incomplete outflow. Even with six slices we obtained satisfactory flow suppression in CA, whereas the visualization of vessel wall worsened due to the reduced signal. The last effect is caused by a combined action of multiple inversions, off-resonance saturation produced by a train of refocusing pulses, and slice cross-talks. The inversion pulses are responsible for about half of the total signal loss, as seen from a comparison between DIR and presaturation scans. Based on these results, the multi-slice DIR method can be safely applied for high-resolution PD- and T2-weighted imaging of carotid arteries with acquisition of three to four slices per TR.

7.4.2.3　Tissue Characterization: The Need for Multiple Contrast Weighting

Recent studies have shown that a combination of different contrast weightings is necessary for noninvasive characterization of plaque morphology [82, 102]. T1-, T2-, PD-, gradient echo, and other contrast schemes have all been evaluated for plaque tissue characterization. Different contrast weightings reveal different features of the plaque. For example, the MR signal intensity of hemorrhage is dependent on the structure of hemoglobin and its oxidation state [83]. Recent hemorrhage with short T1 and long T2 shows a hyperintensive signal intensity on all contrast weighted images, and is readily identified. Calcified tissues, which have very little water and appear dark on all contrast weightings, are easily detected. Calcification on the plaque surface or calcific nodules extending into the lumen is difficult to detect due to low signal intensity, which is easily masked on black-blood sequence (SE or FSE T1, PD- and T2-weighted) [73] but they are easily detected on bright-blood sequence (TOF). In an *ex vivo* study [82], fibrocellular tissue and thrombus appeared relatively dark on PD-weighted images. Calculating relaxation parameters (such as the actual T2 of the components) is useful for the differentiation. In addition, diffusion-weighted MRI is a good technique for identifying thrombus and hemorrhage in plaque [84]. There are, however, still significant problems in obtaining high-resolution diffusion images *in vivo* because of the problems of motion and low SNR of these images. For different types of lipids [85], MR signal patterns (from T1-, T2-, and proton density-weighted images) could be used to readily distinguish each lipid type from surrounding porcine aortic media. Table 7.1 summarizes plaque tissue contrast based on carotid lesions.

7.4.2.4　Contrast Enhancement and Quadruple IR Technique

A combination of black-blood (BB) T1-weighted imaging with contrast enhancement (CE) offers a high potential for various cardiovascular applications, in particular, for high-resolution MRI of atherosclerotic plaque [86]

TABLE 7.1

Contrast of the Main Components of Atherosclerotic Plaque

Plaque Component	MR Contrast Weighting			
	TOF	T1W	IW	T2W
Recent hemorrhage	++	+ to +/−	Variable	Variable
Lipid-rich necrotic core	+/−	++	+	Variable
Intimal calcification	−−	−−	−−	−−
Fibrous tissue	+/− to −−	+/−	+	Variable

(see section below). However, due to significant shortening of the T1 relaxation time in blood, traditional BB methods such as double-inversion recovery (DIR) [78] or side-band saturation cannot guarantee an absence of flow artifacts on postcontrast images, which is especially important for quantitative analysis.

As shown in simulation and phantom studies, DIR provides efficient suppression of blood signal within a narrow range of T1 values at any chosen inversion time TI. Thus, DIR is prone to flow artifacts caused by variations of T1 in blood after a contrast administration. Additionally, DIR is characterized by strong (up to 20% of relative change) dependence of a steady tissue signal on TI. It has been demonstrated that this dependence is determined mainly by the magnetization transfer effect induced by the pair of inversion pulses. While the DIR technique should be applied with different TI for pre- and postcontrast scans to obtain satisfactory blood suppression, it may cause misinterpretation of the contrast enhancement in weakly enhancing tissues [87].

Yarnykh et al. [87] introduced a novel quadruple-inversion recovery (QIR) technique consisting of two DIR blocks followed by inversion delays TI_1 and TI_2. Within each DIR block, a slice-selective adiabatic inversion pulse is applied immediately after a nonselective rectangular pulse. Longitudinal magnetization of blood outside an imaging slice in the presence of the QIR preparation is described by:

$$M_z = \frac{1 - e^{-TR/T_1} - 2e^{-TI_2/T_1} + 2e^{-(TI_1+TI_2)/T_1}}{1 - e^{-TR/T_1}}$$

which has two zero solutions at predefined TR, TI_1 and TI_2. By properly choosing these parameters, signals from tissues with a wide range of T1 relaxation times can be suppressed. That is, the QIR technique provides efficient blood suppression over a wide range of T1 values. This technique is now being used for pre- and postcontrast enhancement MR studies of atherosclerotic plaque.

7.5 Main Findings

7.5.1 Reproducibility

For statistical significance, investigations performed to improve the delineation of clinical risk or assess the efficacy of new interventions typically require large multi-center population-based studies or clinical trials [88, 89]. Thus, along with the growing evidence that MRI can characterize plaque morphology, studies are also needed to assess the quantitative capabilities and the reproducibility of MR techniques before they can be utilized for these investigations.

The ability to serially image the same segments of carotid plaque and the reproducibility of quantitative measures of plaque burden obtained at

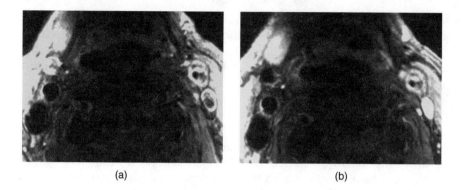

(a)   (b)

FIGURE 7.7

Assessment of reproducibility: (a) and (b) were proton density weighted images taken of a diseased left common carotid artery at two independent MR scans one hour apart. The imaging parameters were 3RR/20/13 (TR/TE/FOV). These images showed that the contrast features of plaque tissues were highly reproducible.

different times were evaluated in a recent experiment [90]. Using the carotid bifurcation as an internal landmark, image slices of the same vessel segment can be reproducibly obtained at different exam times. A comparison of two images of a left CCA obtained from different exams performed on the same day demonstrates the reproducibility of this method of slice prescription (Figure 7.7).

7.5.2   Lipid Core/Hemorrhage

According to AHA classification methods for atherosclerotic plaques, a large lipid core is a feature that is commonly associated with advanced plaque [9]. MR is capable of detecting soft lipid cores in carotid atherosclerotic plaque. A study was conducted to evaluate differential contrast-weighted images, specifically a multi-spectral MR technique, to improve the accuracy of identifying the lipid-rich necrotic core and acute intraplaque hemorrhage *in vivo* [73]. In this study, 18 patients scheduled for carotid endarterectomy underwent a preoperative carotid MRI examination in a 1.5T GE Signa scanner using a protocol that generated four contrast weightings (T1, T2, proton density, and three-dimensional time of flight). MR images of the vessel wall were examined for the presence of a lipid-rich necrotic core and/or intraplaque hemorrhage. Ninety cross sections were compared with matched histological sections of the excised specimen in a double-blind fashion. The overall accuracy (95% CI) of multi-spectral MRI was 87% (80% to 94%), sensitivity was 85% (78% to 92%), and specificity was 92% (86% to 98%). There was good agreement between MRI and histological findings, with a value of $\kappa = 0.69$ (0.53 to 0.85).

Multi-spectral MRI can identify the lipid-rich necrotic core in human carotid atherosclerosis *in vivo* with high sensitivity and specificity. This MRI technique provides a noninvasive tool to study the pathogenesis and natural history of carotid atherosclerosis. Furthermore, it will permit a direct assessment of the effect of pharmacological therapy, such as aggressive lipid lowering, on plaque lipid composition. An recent exciting study demonstrates the capability of MRI in monitoring the effects of lipid-lowering as well as monitoring changes in lipid composition [68]. Based on following eighteen asymptomatic hypercholesterolemic patients with three serial multi-contrast BB MRI in one year, Corti et al. [68] showed significant reductions in vessel wall thickness and vessel wall area without changes in lumen area of the diseased carotid and aortic arteries. This study shows that critical information on vascular remodeling, as manifested by reduced plaque burden, is provided by high-resolution MRI *in vivo*.

In a case-control study examining the effects of prolonged intensive lipid-lowering therapy on the characteristics of carotid atherosclerosis, multiple-contrast MRI again proved very useful [91]. This study, based on studying the plaque compositions and burden obtained from MRI from a group of 16 coronary artery disease patients, showed that prolonged intensive lipid-lowering therapy is associated with a markedly decreased lipid content and increased calcium. This study is the first *in vivo* documentation of such long-term effects of lipid-lowering medicine.

7.5.3 Fibrous Cap

In a 1998 study, Winn et al. [92] reported the performance of T2-weighted MR imaging in detecting atherosclerotic fibrous caps and in depicting their integrity. Twenty atherosclerotic lesions removed by carotid endarterectomy were imaged on a 1.5-T system using T2-weighted spin-echo sequences. The MR images were reviewed independently by four blinded interpreters for fibrous caps and ruptures. The results obtained from the observers were then graded against histologic findings using receiver-operating characteristic (ROC) curve analysis. The area under the ROC curve for fibrous cap detection was 0.80, indicating that T2-weighted MR imaging was a good but not definitively diagnostic test for detecting *ex vivo* fibrous caps. The ROC curve for fibrous cap characterization yielded an area of 0.75, indicating that T2-weighted MR imaging was a fair but not highly diagnostic test for depicting fibrous cap integrity. A definite reading for detection of fibrous caps or rupture was fairly specific (90% and 98%, respectively) but not very sensitive (37% and 12%, respectively). This study concludes that T2W MR imaging is more useful for ruling out disease than for confirming its presence.

Hatsukami et al. [70] were the first to report the use of a three-dimensional-TOF bright-blood imaging technique to identify unstable fibrous caps in atherosclerotic human carotid arteries *in vivo*. The images were acquired with spoiled gradient echo (SPGR) mode with a low flip angle to better visualize both flowing blood and soft tissue. The contrast of these images were more T_2^* and proton density weighted. In a study of 22 preoperatively imaged

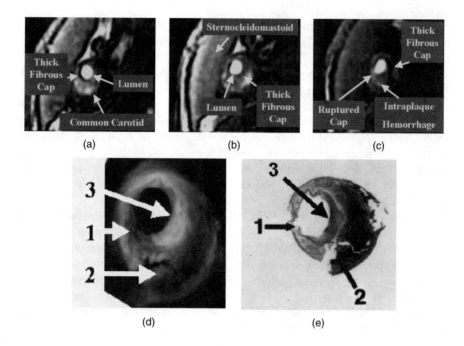

FIGURE 7.8

Plaque with fibrous cap rupture on gross section, histologic section, and MR images (see Table 7.2 for imaging parameters): (a) through (c) three contiguous, transverse, three-dimensional TOF images of a diseased right common carotid artery; (d) gross section location corresponding to (a) through (c); (e) low-power photomicrograph of histologic section (Masson trichrome stain, ×10). In (d) and (e), there is an area of cap rupture (arrow 1) across from a region where the fibrous cap is thick (arrow 3). The site of cap rupture corresponds to a region where the hypointense band is absent, and a hyperintense region is seen adjacent to the lumen on MR images. The hyperintense region is a region in the plaque core on MR images that corresponds to regions of recent intraplaque hemorrhage on gross and histologic cross sections (arrow 2). The fibrous cap is composed of a dense layer of collagen that appears hypointense in (a) through (c). (Reprinted with permission from [93].)

endarterectomy patients, these authors found that the histological state of the fibrous cap correlated well ($\kappa = 0.83$) with the appearance of a hypointense juxtaluminal band seen in the TOF images. Hypothesizing that the layered organization of the fibrous cap was responsible for the relative signal loss in the MR images, they were able to prospectively characterize the *in vivo* state of the fibrous cap as being intact and thick, intact and thin, or ruptured (Figure 7.8).

These findings, together with the reported advantages of plaque characterization based on multiple different contrast-weighted images, led to a subsequent, larger study that was designed to evaluate the ability of multi-contrast MR to characterize the *in vivo* state of the fibrous cap [94]. In this work, an imaging protocol was employed that produced four different contrast weightings — three-dimensional-TOF; T1-weighted double-inversion recovery (DIR) SE sequence; and PD and T2-weighted images from a shared-echo SE technique — at each imaged location of the carotid arteries of 18 endarterectomy patients. In agreement with the work of Hatsukami et al., the results also demonstrated a strong correlation between the MR image findings and the histological state of the fibrous cap ($\kappa = 0.71$). The authors, however, were able to show that the availability of the three SE contrast weightings facilitated image interpretation in 17 of the 91 image locations, and with the larger sample size were able to report test performance statistics (sensitivity of 81%, specificity of 90%) for noninvasively identifying unstable fibrous caps *in vivo*.

The clinical relevance of examining fibrous cap is clearly demonstrated in a study that evaluated whether MRI identification of fibrous cap thinning or rupture is associated with a history of recent transient ischemic attack (TIA) or stroke [95]. Fifty-three consecutive patients (mean age, 71 years; 49 male) scheduled for carotid endarterectomy were recruited after obtaining informed consent. Twenty-eight subjects had a recent history of TIA or stroke on the side appropriate to the index carotid lesion, and twenty-five were asymptomatic. Preoperative carotid MRI was performed in a 1.5T GE Signa scanner that generated T(1)-, PD-, and T(2)-weighted and three-dimensional time-of-flight images. Using previously reported MRI criteria, the fibrous cap was categorized as intact-thick, intact-thin, or ruptured for each carotid plaque by blinded review. There was a strong and statistically significant trend showing a higher percentage of symptomatic patients for ruptured caps (70%) compared with thick caps (9%) ($P = 0.001$ Mann-Whitney test for cap status versus symptoms). Compared with patients with thick fibrous caps, patients with ruptured caps were 23 times more likely to have had a recent TIA or stroke (95% CI = 3, 210). Thus, MRI identification of a ruptured fibrous cap is highly associated with a recent history of TIA or stroke.

7.5.4 Contrast Enhancement

Recent studies have shown that gadolinium-based contrast agents can penetrate into the arterial wall, including the adventitia layer of the artery which marks the outer wall boundary (Figure 7.9) [96–98]. This is useful because although noncontrast MR imaging has been able to identify many plaque constituents in advanced atherosclerosis, some tissues, such as neovasculature, defy detection. A study was performed to determine if a gadolinium-based contrast agent provides additional information for characterization of human plaque tissues, particularly neovasculature [97].

Noncontrast-enhanced carotid artery images from 18 patients scheduled for carotid endarterectomy and two normal volunteers were used to identify regions of fibrous tissue, necrotic core, or calcification, using established criteria. Then, the percent change in T1-weighted images after contrast enhancement was calculated for each region. The results showed statistically significant

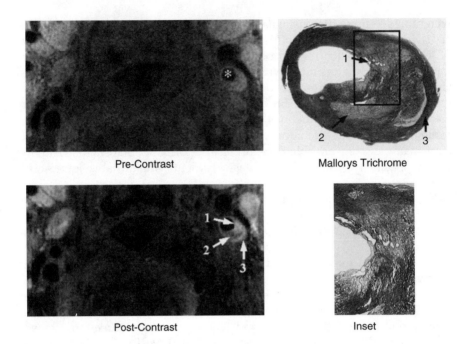

Pre-Contrast   Mallorys Trichrome

Post-Contrast   Inset

FIGURE 7.9

Pre- and post-CE images show regional variation in contrast enhancement. A region of strong enhancement adjacent to the lumen (arrow 1) indicates neovasculature associated with a ruptured fibrous cap, identifying this as a highly vulnerable plaque. Also indicated are a necrotic core with minor enhancement (arrow 2) and an enhancing region of neovasculature near the outer wall (arrow 3). The presence of neovasculature was confirmed in the corresponding histology slice, which is also shown. (permission pending [86]).

differences in mean intensity change between tissues, with the largest increase found in fibrous tissue (79.5%) and the smallest in necrotic core (28.6%). Additionally, histological analysis showed that a subset of fibrous regions rich in plaque neovascularization could be identified using a threshold of 80% enhancement (sensitivity = 76%, specificity = 79%). The ability of contrast-enhanced MRI to identify neovascularization and potentially improve differentiation of necrotic core from fibrous tissue further establishes MRI as a viable tool for *in vivo* study of atherosclerotic plaque. Additionally, it seems to have the ability to improve quantitative measurements of the lumen and outer wall areas. Further studies are ongoing to reveal and quantify the strengths of contrast enhancement.

7.5.5   Atherosclerotic Vessel Wall Area Measurement

Unlike lumen stenosis, plaque volume is considered a direct measure of the size and severity of the atherosclerotic disease. Because MR is able to identify the adventitia boundary in transverse images of the vessel wall, MR imaging could provide a means of measuring the total volume of the diseased vessel wall and accurately determining plaque burden [64].

With the excellent contrast produced between diseased portions of the vessel, the lumen, and the adventitia, initial experiments designed to evaluate the quantitative capabilities of MR have been based on *in vivo* measures of plaque burden. One such study compared the cross-sectional areas of imaged carotid plaques measured preoperatively with similar area measurements made of the excised endarterectomy specimens imaged *ex vivo*. A Bland-Altman analysis performed on the paired *in vivo* and *ex vivo* measurements of the same vessel segments demonstrated a strong correlation between the two values [64]. These results provide evidence of the quantitative capabilities of MR for measuring total plaque volume and disease burden.

Recently, another study was performed [74] that attempted to determine whether gadolinium contrast enhancement was useful in improving quantitative measurement of the carotid outer wall boundary area with bright-blood three-dimensional TOF MRI. Eleven patients scheduled for carotid endarterectomy underwent pre- and post-contrast MRI of their carotid arteries no more than 3 days prior to surgery. Pre- and post-contrast images were measured with an in-house developed quantitative vascular analysis tool (QVAT) [99, 100]. QVAT uses a semi-automated snake algorithm to detect contour boundaries and calculate area. After surgery, another three-dimensional TOF scan was conducted *ex vivo* on the excised plaque as a reference for carotid wall volume measurement. The MR scan of this surgical specimen was performed at body temperature (37°C) within 4 hours of the surgery while the specimen was submerged in saline. One reviewer used QVAT to evaluate *in vivo* images, while another reviewer used QVAT to evaluate *ex vivo* images. The images were evaluated independently to avoid potential bias.

The pre- and post-contrast images were then compared to *ex vivo* images of CEA specimens to determine accuracy. Results were good, with nine cases showing improved outer wall delineation with the addition of the contrast agent, and seven cases showing improved lumen definition. Measurement results showed a significant difference between pre- and post-contrast MWA measurement, with the mean absolute difference in MWA of pre- and *ex vivo* measurements significantly larger than that of post- and *ex vivo* (p = 0.02). The wall volume mean absolute difference between pre- and *ex vivo* measurements is also significantly larger than that between post and *ex vivo*, which is 41.81 mm^3 and 32.73 mm^3, respectively (p = 0.004). Both results show that post-contrast area and volume measurements have a closer association with the *ex vivo* measurements than the pre-contrast images.

A recent study analyzed the precision of quantitative measurements for both lumen and vessel wall areas of human carotid arteries [101]. Based on data obtained from two independent MR scans conducted on eight patients within 2 weeks, the error of lumen area measurement was 6.2%, 9.2% and 9.7% for T1W, SDW, and T2W images, respectively. This error was estimated based on the mean and standard deviation of area measurement from pooled locations using standard analyses of variance. Wall area measurement error was 10.8%, 10.9%, and 12% for the three contrast weightings. Errors in wall volume measurement ranged from 4 to 6% across different contrast methods. This study shows that the vessel wall volume can be accurately measured. This study also shows that among the many factors that might impact the area measurement, the precision of area measurements correlates strongly with the image quality.

7.6 State-of-the-Art Protocol

Studies by our group and others show that a combination of different contrast weightings are necessary for noninvasive characterization of plaque morphology [67, 82, 93, 102]. Based on extensive testing of normal volunteers and endarterectomy patients, a standardized, multi-contrast imaging protocol was developed [102]. This protocol accomplishes several objectives. First, it acquires high-resolution axial images of both carotid arteries in each subject with a range of techniques, including black blood and bright blood. Second, it provides an oblique view of the carotid artery to better visualize the location of carotid bifurcation and demonstrate plaque distribution. Third, it uses the common carotid bifurcation as an internal landmark to reproducibly prescribe slice locations for serial studies. Finally, it restricts the total exam time to an average of 45 minutes (including contrast agent application). A zero-filled Fourier transform is employed to minimize partial volume artifacts [103]. The resulting protocol uses three imaging sequences (three-dimensional TOF, multiple-slice DIR, and QIR) to generate four different contrast weightings at each slice location. The best voxel size achieved was $0.25 \times 0.25 \times 2.0$ mm^3 for the black and bright blood sequences, and $0.78 \times 0.78 \times 2.0$ mm^3 in the oblique views (Table 7.2; Figure 7.10).

TABLE 7.2

MRI Parameters for State-of-the-Art Protocol

	Weighting				
Parameter	**Oblique PDW**	**3-D TOF**	**PDW**	**T2W**	**T1W**
Sequence	DIR-FSE	GRE	DIR-FSE	DIR-FSE	QIR-FSE
Plane	Oblique	Axial	Axial	Axial	Axial
TR (msec)	1800	23	2400	3000	800
TE (msec)	Minimum	3.8	Minimum	50	Minimum
TI (msec)	270	N/A	260	230	500
FOV (cm)	16	16	16	16	16
Thickness (mm)	2	1–2	2	2	2
Matrix	256 × 256	256 × 256	256 × 256	256 × 256	256 × 256

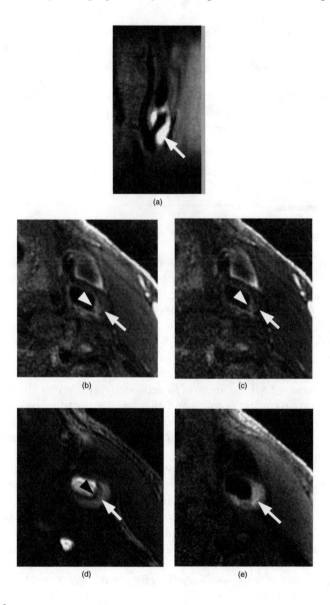

FIGURE 7.10

A set of images taken from a patient with moderate carotid stenosis: (a) an oblique FSE view of the left carotid artery; (b) and (c) are cross sectional images near the carotid bifurcation taken with FSE (PDW, T2W); (d) is a 3D TOF image of the same location which shows both bright lumen and the plaque (arrow); (e) is a DIR FSE image of the same location (T1W). The imaging parameters for the oblique image were: 600/10/20/2/256x256 with flow suppression and for (b)-(e) are summarized in Table 7.2. The lesion is eccentric and caused a minor lumen stenosis. By comparing black and bright blood images, one can find at least two distinct tissue regions in the plaque: the arrows point to a hyperintense (d, e) and hypointense (b, c) region of recent intraplaque hemorrhage and the arrowheads point to a hypointense (d) and hyperintense (b, c) area of fibrous tissue. The tissue contrast in (b) and (c) are similar.

Fat suppression is applied in all imaging sequences to remove strong signals from subcutaneous fat. An interesting fact is that perivascular fat, mainly composed of triglycerides, has a different appearance in MR than lipids found in atherosclerotic plaque, which consist primarily of cholesterol esters and free cholesterol [75, 85]. Thus, fat suppression has little impact on tissue contrast within atherosclerotic plaque [85, 104]. Cardiac gating was found to reduce flow and motion artifacts and may be helpful to improve image quality in long TE and TR sequences.

7.7   Discussion

Over the past decade, significant advances have been made in our understanding of vascular biology and the pathology of atherosclerosis. We now accept the importance of plaque burden, morphology, and composition as appropriate objectives for noninvasive examination and no longer rely solely on the degree of luminal narrowing to assess the severity of atherosclerotic disease. As discussed in this chapter, MR imaging holds much potential for developing into a modality that can be used to quantitatively characterize plaque morphology *in vivo*. Preliminary studies have demonstrated the ability of multi-contrast MR techniques to prospectively identify the major components of human carotid plaques and characterize the morphologic features associated with the vulnerable lesion (unstable fibrous caps, necrotic cores, intimal calcifications, and intraplaque hematomas). Although the sample sizes of these studies were limited, continued patient recruitment and a growing number of studies performed at different institutions will hopefully establish the accuracy of these techniques. Nonetheless, the results and the associated technical developments described open an exciting new era in vascular imaging and raise hopes that we may soon be able to (1) noninvasively and prospectively identify a vulnerable plaque, thereby allowing more timely intervention, and (2) quantitatively monitor changes in disease burden and biologic markers of instability to enhance our understanding of the pathogenesis of the disease and to better evaluate the efficacy of new therapies.

The high spatial resolution images presented in this chapter can be generated with 1.5T clinical scanners and phased-array surface coils. Currently, pulse sequences consisting of both black- and bright-blood techniques are recommended to characterize carotid plaque morphology *in vivo*; however, ongoing *ex vivo* experiments may demonstrate the utility of additional sequences like the three-dimensional-true FISP or magnetization transfer. As the work from multiple institutions shows, the techniques described can readily be transferred to whole-body scanners from the major manufacturers with minimal changes.

The state of carotid imaging and noninvasive plaque characterization is rapidly advancing as an increasing number of institutions begin experimental studies and develop imaging protocols. This growing interest will hopefully produce the resources and patient sample sizes needed to realize the potential of MR for developing into a means of prospectively identifying the vulnerable plaque.

In this chapter, we have described imaging techniques and major findings for the characterization of atherosclerosis in human carotid arteries. In principle, these imaging techniques can be applied to other human vascular beds prone to atherosclerosis. Indeed, a number of recent publications have documented such studies of imaging aortas, femoral and iliac, and even coronary arteries [35, 67, 68, 105–107].

Coronary artery plaque characterization is considered the "holy grail" of MR imaging due to the size of the vessel, complicated orientation, and most of all the complicated motion of blood, heart, and breathing. Keeping these difficulties in mind, there are a number of studies using novel cardiac phased-array coil design and black-blood imaging to visualize coronary plaques [107]. More interestingly, a recent study by Botnar et al., using double inversion in conjunction with a hemidiaphragmatic navigator technique, showed that coronary wall thickness and wall area measured from MR images were significantly greater in patients with angiographic identified coronary atherosclerotic disease. The in-plane resolution achieved was 0.5×1 mm. The authors suggest that this DIR-navigator technique may have potential applications in patients with known or suspected atherosclerotic CAD or for serial evaluation after pharmacological intervention. These technical advances clearly demonstrate the future potential of MRI in coronary imaging.

References

1. Association for Eradication of Heart Attack — AEHA, www.vulnerableplaque. org, 2001.
2. NASCET, Beneficial effect of carotid endarterectomy in symptomatic patients with high-grade stenosis, North American Symptomatic Carotid Endarterectomy Trial Collaborators, *N. Engl. J. Med.*, 1325, 445–453, 1991.
3. Randomised trial of endarterectomy for recently symptomatic carotid stenosis: final results of the MRC European Carotid Surgery Trial (ECST) [see comments], *Lancet*, 351, (9113), 1379–1387, 1998.
4. ACAS Clinical Advisory: carotid endarterectomy for patients with asymptomatic internal carotid artery stenosis, *Stroke*, 25, (12), 2523–2524, 1994.
5. Falk, E., Why do plaques rupture?, *Circulation*, 86, (6 Suppl.), III30–42, 1992.
6. Leen, E. J., Feeley, T. M., et al., "Haemorrhagic" carotid plaque does not contain haemorrhage, *Eur. J. Vasc. Surg.*, 4, (2), 123–128, 1990.

7. Fuster, V., Stein, B., Ambrose, J. A., Badimon, L., Badimon, J. J., and Chesebro, J. H., Atherosclerotic plaque rupture and thrombosis. Evolving concepts, *Circulation*, 82(3 Suppl.), II47–59, 1990.

8. Davies, M. J. and Woolf N., Atherosclerosis: what is it and why does it occur?, *Br. Heart J.*, 69(1 Suppl.), S3–S11, 1993.

9. Virmani, R., Kolodgie, F. D., et al., Lessons from sudden coronary death: a comprehensive morphological classification scheme for atherosclerotic lesions, *Arterioscler. Thromb. Vasc. Biol.*, 20, (5), 1262–1275, 2000.

10. Glagov, S., Weisenberg, E., Zarins, C. K., Stankunavicius, R., and Kolettis, G. J., Compensatory enlargement of human atherosclerotic coronary arteries, *N. Engl. J. Med.*, 316, (22), 1371–1375, 1987.

11. Glagov, S., Bassiouny, H. S., Giddens, D. P., Zarins, C. K., Pathobiology of plaque modeling and complication, *Surg. Clin. North Am.*, 75, (4), 545–556, 1995.

12. Ross, R., The pathogenesis of atherosclerosis: a perspective for the 1990s, *Nature*, 362, (6423), 801–809, 1993.

13. Little, W. C., Canstantinescu, M., Applegate, R. J., et al., Can coronary angiography predict the site of a subsequent myocardial infarction in patients with mild-to-moderate coronary artery disease?, *Circulation*, 78, (5 Pt. 1), 1157–1166, 1988.

14. Ambrose, J. A., Tannenbaum, M. A., Alexopoulos, D., et al., Angiographic progression of coronary artery disease and the development of myocardial infarction, *J. Am. Coll. Cardiol.*, 12, 56–62, 1988.

15. Davies, M. J. and Thomas A. C., Plaque fissuring — the cause of acute myocardial infarction, sudden ischaemic death, and crescendo angina, *Br. Heart. J.*, 53, 363–373, 1985.

16. Bassiouny, H. S., Sakaguchi, Y., Mikucki, S. A., et al., Juxtalumenal location of plaque necrosis and neoformation in symptomatic carotid stenosis, *J. Vasc. Surg.*, 26, (4), 585–594, 1997.

17. Plutzky, J., Atherosclerotic plaque rupture: emerging insights and opportunities, *Am. J. Cardiol.*, 84, (1A), 15J–20J, 1999.

18. Edwards, J. H., Kricheff, I. I., Riles, T., and Imparato A., Angiographically undetected ulceration of the carotid bifurcation as a cause of embolic stroke, *Radiology*, 132, 369–373, 1979.

19. Mann, J. M. and Davies M. J., Vulnerable plaque: relation of characteristics to degree of stenosis in human coronary arteries, *Circulation*, 94, 928–931, 1996.

20. Topol, E. J. and Nissen S. E., Our preoccupation with coronary luminology: the dissociation between clinical and angiographic findings in ischemic heart disease, *Circulation*, 92, 2333–2342, 1995.

21. Roederer, G. O., Langlois, Y. E., Jaeger, K. A., et al., A simple spectral parameter for accurate classification of severe carotid disease, *Bruit*, 8, 174–178, 1984.

22. Kohler, T., Langlois, Y., Roederer, G. O., et al., Sources of variability in carotid duplex examination: a prospective study, *Ultrasound Med. Biol.*, 11, (4), 571–576, 1985.

23. Langlois, Y. E., Roederer, G. O., and Strandness D. E., Jr., Vascular ultrasound: ultrasonic evaluation of the carotid bifurcation, *Echocardiography*, 4, (2), 141–159, 1987.

24. Pignoli, P., Ultrasound B-mode imaging for arterial wall thickness measurement, *Atherosclerosis Rev.*, 12, 177–184, 1984.

25. Riley, W. A., Barnes, R. W., Evans, G. W., and Burke G. L., Ultrasonic measurement of the elastic modulus of the common carotid artery. The Atherosclerosis Risk in Communities (ARIC) Study, *Stroke,* 23, (7), 952–956, 1992.

26. Howard, G., Sharrett, A. R., Heiss, G., et al., Carotid artery intimal-medial thickness distribution in general populations as evaluated by B-mode ultrasound. ARIC Investigators, *Stroke,* 24, (9), 1297–1304, 1993.

27. Burke, G. L., Evans, G. W., Riley, W. A., et al., Arterial wall thickness is associated with prevalent cardiovascular disease in middle-aged adults. The Atherosclerosis Risk in Communities (ARIC) Study, *Stroke,* 26, (3), 386–391, 1995.

28. Chambless, L. E., Folsom, A. R., Clegg, L. X., et al., Carotid wall thickness is predictive of incident clinical stroke: The Atherosclerosis Risk in Communities (ARIC) Study, *Am. J. Epidemiol.,* 151, (5), 478–487, 2000.

29. O'Leary, D. H., Polak, J. F., et al., Carotid-artery intima and media thickness as a risk factor for myocardial infarction and stroke in older adults. Cardiovascular Health Study Collaborative Research Group, *N. Engl. J. Med.,* 340, (1), 14–22, 1999.

30. Aly, S. and Bishop C. C., An objective characterization of atherosclerotic lesion: an alternative method to identify unstable plaque, *Stroke,* 31, (8), 1921–1924, 2000.

31. Biasi, G. M., Mingazzini, P. M., Baronio, L., et al., Carotid plaque characterization using digital image processing and its potential in future studies of carotid endarterectomy and angioplasty, *J. Endovasc. Surg.,* 5, (3), 240–246, 1998.

32. Noritomi, T., Sigel, B., Swami, V., et al., Carotid plaque typing by multiple-parameter ultrasonic tissue characterization, *Ultrasound. Med. Biol.,* 23, (5), 643–650, 1997.

33. Bridal, S. L., Beyssen, B., Fornes, P., Julia, P., and Berger G., Multiparametric attenuation and backscatter images for characterization of carotid plaque, *Ultrasonic Imaging,* 22, (1), 20–34, 2000.

34. Lee, D. J., Sigel, B., Swami, V. K., et al., Determination of carotid plaque risk by ultrasonic tissue characterization, *Ultrasound. Med. Biol.,* 24, (9), 1291–1299, 1998.

35. Raynaud, J. S., Bridal, S. L., Toussaint, J. F., et al., Characterization of atherosclerotic plaque components by high resolution quantitative MR and US imaging, *J. Magn. Reson. Imaging,* 8, (3), 622–629, 1998.

36. Bridal, S. L., Fornes, P., Bruneval, P., and Berger G., Correlation of ultrasonic attenuation (30 to 50 MHz and constituents of atherosclerotic plaque), *Ultrasound Med. Biol.,* 23, (5), 691–703, 1997.

37. Takiuchi, S., Rakugi, H., Masuyama, T., et al., Clinical implications of ultrasonic tissue characterization for atherosclerotic carotid intima-media, *Nippon Ronen Igakkai Zasshi,* 37, (2), 137–142, 2000.

38. Noritomi, T., Sigel, B., Gahtan, V., et al., *In vivo* detection of carotid plaque thrombus by ultrasonic tissue characterization, *J. Ultrasound Med.,* 16, (2), 107–111, 1997.

39. Chan, K. L., Quantitative characterization of carotid atheromatous plaques using ultrasonic rf A-scan data, *Ultrasonics,* 33, (2), 163–164, 1995.

40. Urbani, M. P., Picano, E., Parenti, G., et al., *In vivo* radio frequency-based ultrasonic tissue characterization of the atherosclerotic plaque, *Stroke,* 24, (10), 1507–1512, 1993.

41. Prati, F., Arbustini, E., Labellarte, A., Dal Bello, B., Mallus, M. T., Sommariva, L., Pagano, A., and Boccanelli A., Intravascular ultrasound insights into plaque composition, *Z. Kardiol.,* 89, Suppl. 2, 117–123, 2000.

42. Pourcelot, L., Tranquart, F., De Bray, J. M., Philippot, M., Bonithon, M. C., and Salez F., Ultrasound characterization and quantification of carotid atherosclerosis lesions, *Minerva Cardioangiol.*, 47, (1–2),15–24, 1999.
43. Iannuzzi, A., Wilcosky, T., Mercuri, M., Rubba, P., Bryan, F. A., and Bond M. G., Ultrasonographic correlates of carotid atherosclerosis in transient ischemic attack and stroke, *Stroke*, 26, (4), 614–619, 1995.
44. Geroulakos, G., Domjan, J., Nicolaides, A., et al., Ultrasonic carotid artery plaque structure and the risk of cerebral infarction on computed tomography, *J. Vasc. Surg.*, 20, (2), 263–266, 1994.
45. Wolverson, M. K., Bashiti, H. M., and Peterson G. J., Ultrasonic tissue characterization of atheromatous plaques using a high resolution real time scanner, *Ultrasound Med. Biol.*, 9, (6), 599–609, 1983.
46. Widder, B., Paulat, K., Hackspacher, J., et al., Morphological characterization of carotid artery stenoses by ultrasound duplex scanning, *Ultrasound Med. Biol.*, 16, (4), 349–354, 1990.
47. Hiro, T., Leung, C. Y., Karimi, H., Farvid, A. R., and Tobis J. M., Angle dependence of intravascular ultrasound imaging and its feasibility in tissue characterization of human atherosclerotic tissue, *Am. Heart J.*, 137, (3), 476–481, 1999.
48. Gussenhoven, E. J., Essed, C. E., Lancee, C. T., et al., Arterial wall characteristics determined by intravascular ultrasound imaging: an *in vitro* study, *J. Am. Coll. Cardiol.*, 14, (4), 947–952, 1989.
49. Arnold, J. A., Modaresi, K. B., Thomas, N., Taylor, P. R., and Padayachee T. S., Carotid plaque characterization by duplex scanning: observer error may undermine current clinical trials, *Stroke*, 30, (1), 61–65, 1999.
50. de Bray, J. M., Baud, J. M., Delanoy, P., et al., Reproducibility in ultrasonic characterization of carotid plaques, *Cerebrovasc. Dis.*, 8, (5), 273–277, 1998.
51. Montauban van Swijndregt, A. D., Elbers, H. R., Moll, F. L., de Letter, J., and Ackerstaff, R. G., Ultrasonographic characterization of carotid plaques, *Ultrasound Med. Biol.*, 24, (4), 489–493, 1998.
52. Sabetai, M. M., Tegos, T. J., Nicolaides, A. N., Dhanjil, S., Pare, G. J., and Stevens J. M., Reproducibility of computer-quantified carotid plaque echogenicity: can we overcome the subjectivity?, *Stroke*, 31, (9), 2189–2196, 2000.
53. Estes, J. M., Quist, W. C., Lo Gerfo, F. W., and Costello P., Noninvasive characterization of plaque morphology using helical computed tomography, *J. Cardiovasc. Surg. (Torino)*, 39, (5), 527–534, 1998.
54. Fayad, Z. A. and Fuster V., Clinical imaging of the high-risk or vulnerable atherosclerotic plaque, *Circ. Res.*, 89, (4), 305–316, 2001.
55. Callister, T. Q., Raggi, P., et al., Effect of HMG-CoA reductase inhibitors on coronary artery disease as assessed by electron-beam computed tomography, *N. Engl. J. Med.*, 339, (27), 1972–1978, 1998.
56. Becker, C. R., Kleffel, T., et al., Coronary artery calcium measurement: agreement of multirow detector and electron beam CT, *Am. J. Roentgenol.*, 176, (5), 1295–1298, 2001.
57. Ohnesorge, B., Flohr, T., et al., Cardiac imaging by means of electrocardiographically gated multisection spiral CT: initial experience, *Radiology*, 217, (2), 564–571, 2000.
58. Anderson, G. B., Ashforth R., et al., CT angiography for the detection and characterization of carotid artery bifurcation disease, *Stroke*, 31, (9), 2168–2174, 2000.

59. Binaghi, S., Maeder, P., et al., Three-dimensional computed tomography angiography and magnetic resonance angiography of carotid bifurcation stenosis, *Eur. Neurol.*, 46, (1), 25–34, 2001.

60. Moll, R. and Dinkel H. P., Value of the CT angiography in the diagnosis of common carotid artery bifurcation disease: CT angiography versus digital subtraction angiography and color flow Doppler, *Eur. J. Radiol.*, 39, (3), 155–162, 2001.

61. Klingebiel, R., Busch, M., et al., Multi-slice CT angiography in the evaluation of patients with acute cerebrovascular disease — a promising new diagnostic tool, *J. Neurol.*, 249, (1), 43–49, 2002.

62. Walker, L. J., Ismail, A., et al., Computed tomography angiography for the evaluation of carotid atherosclerotic plaque: correlation with histopathology of endarterectomy specimens, *Stroke*, 33, (4), 977–981, 2002.

63. Steinman, D. A. and Rutt, B. K., On the nature and reduction of plaque-mimicking flow artifacts in black blood MRI of the carotid bifurcation, *Magn. Reson. Med.*, 139,(4), 635–641, 1998.

64. Yuan, C., Beach, K. W., Smith, L. H., Jr; and Hatsukami T. S., Measurement of atherosclerotic carotid plaque size *in vivo* using high resolution magnetic resonance imaging, *Circulation*, 98, (24), 2666–2671, 1998.

65. Hayes, C. E., Mathis, C. M., and Yuan C., Surface coil phased arrays for high-resolution imaging of the carotid arteries, *J. Magn. Reson. Imag.*, 6, (1), 109–112, 1996.

66. Ouhlous, M., Lethimonnier, F., Dippel, D. W., van Sambeek, M. R., van Heerebeek, L. C., Pattynama, P. M., and van der Lugt, A., Evaluation of a dedicated dual phased-array surface coil using a black-blood FSE sequence for high resolution MRI of the carotid vessel wall, *J. Magn. Reson. Imag.*, 15, (3), 344–351, 2002.

67. Quick, H. H., Debatin J. F., and Ladd M. E., MR imaging of the vessel wall, *Eur. Radiol.*, 12, (4), 889–900, 2002.

68. Corti, R., Fayad, Z. A., Fuster, V., Worthley, S. G., Helft, G., Chesebro, J., Mercuri, M., and Badimon, J. J., Effects of lipid-lowering by simvastatin on human atherosclerotic lesions: a longitudinal study by high-resolution, noninvasive magnetic resonance imaging, *Circulation*, 104, (3), 249–252, 2001.

69. Thomas, J. B., Rutt, B. K., Ladak, H. M., and Steinman D. A., Effect of black blood MR image quality on vessel wall segmentation, *Magn. Reson. Med.*, 46, (2), 299–304, 2001.

70. Hatsukami, T. S., Ross R., et al., Visualization of fibrous cap thickness and rupture in human atherosclerotic carotid plaque *in vivo* with high-resolution magnetic resonance imaging, *Circulation*, 102, (9), 959–964, 2000.

71. Aoki, S., Aoki, K., Ohsawa, S., Nakajima, H., Kumagai, H., and Araki T., Dynamic MR imaging of the carotid wall, *J. Magn. Reson. Imag.*, 9, (3), 1999.

72. Coombs, B. D., Rapp, J. H., Ursell, P. C., Reilly, L. M., and Saloner, D., Structure of plaque at carotid bifurcation: high-resolution MRI with histological correlation, *Stroke*, 32, (11), 2516–2521, 2001.

73. Yuan, C., Mitsumori, L. M., Ferguson, M. S., Polissar, N. L., Echelard, D., Ortiz, G., Small, R., Davies, J. W., Kerwin, W. S., and Hatsukami T. S., *In vivo* accuracy of multispectral magnetic resonance imaging for identifying lipid-rich necrotic cores and intraplaque hemorrhage in advanced human carotid plaques, *Circulation*, 104, (17), 2051–2056, 2001.

74. Zhang, S. X., Luo, Y., and Yuan C., Measurement of carotid wall volume and maximum area using contrast enhanced 3D MRI, *RSNA*, 441, 2001.

75. Toussaint, J. F., Southern, J. F., Fuster, V., and Kantor H. L., T2-weighted contrast for NMR characterization of human atherosclerosis, *Arterioscler. Thromb. Vasc. Biol.*, 15, (10), 1533–1542, 1995.

76. Yuan, C., Murakami, J. W., Hayes, C. E., et al., Phased-array magnetic resonance imaging of the carotid artery bifurcation: preliminary results in healthy volunteers and a patient with atherosclerotic disease, *J. Magn. Reson. Imag.*, 5, (5), 561–565, 1995.

77. Finn, J. P. and Edelman R. R., Black-blood and segmented k-space magnetic resonance angiography, *Magn. Reson. Imag. Clin. North. Am.*, 1, (2), 349–357, 1993.

78. Edelman, R. R., Chien, D., Kim, D., et al., Fast selective black blood MR imaging, *Radiology*, 181, (3), 655–660, 1991.

79. Milner, J. S., Moore, J. A., Rutt, B. K., and Steinman D. A., Hemodynamics of human carotid artery bifurcations: computational studies with models reconstructed from magnetic resonance imaging of normal subjects, *J. Vasc. Surg.*, 28, (1), 143–156, 1998.

80. Song, H. K., Wright, A. C., Wolf, R. L., and Wehrli F. L., Multislice double inversion pulse sequence for efficient black-blood MRI, *Magn. Reson. Med.*, 47, (3), 616–620, 2002.

81. Yarnykh, V. and Yuan, C., Feasibility of multi-slice black-blood double inversion-recovery images, *ISMRM*, Hawaii, 2002.

82. Shinnar, M., Fallon, J. T., Wehrli, S., et al., The diagnostic accuracy of *ex vivo* MRI for human atherosclerotic plaque characterization, *Arterioscler. Thromb. Vasc. Biol.*, 19, (11), 2756–2761, 1999.

83. Bradley W. G., Jr., MR appearance of hemorrhage in the brain, *Radiology*, 189, (1), 15–26, 1993.

84. Toussaint, J. F., Southern, J. F., Fuster, V., and Kantor H. L., Water diffusion properties of human atherosclerosis and thrombosis measured by pulse field gradient nuclear magnetic resonance, *Arterioscler. Thromb. Vasc. Biol.*, 17, (3), 542–546, 1997.

85. Yuan, C., Petty, C., O'Brien, K. D., Hatsukami, T. S., Eary J. F., and Brown B. G., *In vitro* and *in situ* magnetic resonance imaging signal features of atherosclerotic plaque-associated lipids, *Arterioscler. Thromb. Vasc. Biol.*, 17, (8), 1496–1503, 1997.

86. Yuan, C., Kerwin, W. S., Ferguson, M. S., Polissar, N., Zhang, S., Cai, J., and Hatsukami, T. S., Contrast-enhanced high resolution MRI for atherosclerotic carotid artery tissue characterization, *J. Magn. Reson. Imag.*, 15, (1), 62–67, 2002.

87. Yarnykh, V. and Yuan C., Quadruple inversion-recovery: a method for quantitative contrast-enhanced black-blood imaging, *ISMRM*, Hawaii, 2002.

88. Kuller L. H., AHA Symposium/Epidemiology Meeting: discussion — why measure atherosclerosis?, *Circulation*, 87SII, II34–II37, 1993.

89. Probstfield, J. L., Byington, R. P., Egan, D. A., Espeland, M. A., Margitic, S. E., Riley, W. A., and Furberg C. D., Methodological issues facing studies of atherosclerotic change, *Circulation*, 87SII, II74–II81, 1993.

90. Yuan, C., Schmiedl, U. P., Maravilla K. R., et al., MR imaging of human carotid plaques: assessment of reproducibility and reader variability, *Abs. Radiol.*, 201, 134, 1996.

91. Zhao, X. Q., Yuan, C., et al., Effects of prolonged intensive lipid-lowering therapy on the characteristics of carotid atherosclerotic plaques *in vivo* by MRI: a case-control study, *Arterioscler. Thromb. Vasc. Biol.*, 21, (10), 1623–1629, 2001.

92. Winn, W. B., Schmiedl, U. P., et al., Detection and characterization of atherosclerotic fibrous caps with T2-weighted MR, *Am. J. Neuroradiol.,* 19, (1), 129–134, 1998.

93. Yuan, C., Mitsumori, L. M., Beach, K. W., and Maravilla, K. R., Carotid atherosclerotic plaque: noninvasive MR characterization and identification of vulnerable lesions, *Radiology,* 221, (2), 285–299, 2001.

94. Yuan, C., Mitsumori, L. M., et al., *In vivo* accuracy of multispectral magnetic resonance imaging for identifying lipid-rich necrotic cores and intraplaque hemorrhage in advanced human carotid plaques, *Circulation,* 104, (17), 2051–2056, 2001.

95. Yuan, C., Zhang, S. X., et al., Identification of fibrous cap rupture with magnetic resonance imaging is highly associated with recent transient ischemic attack or stroke, *Circulation,* 105, (2), 181–185, 2002.

96. Aoki, S., Nakajima, H., Kumagai, H., and Araki T., Dynamic contrast-enhanced MR angiography and MR imaging of the carotid artery: high resolution sequences in different acquisition planes, *Am. J. Neuroradiol.,* 21, 381–385, 2000.

97. Yuan, C., Kerwin, W. S., Ferguson, M. S., Polissar, N., Zhang, S., Cai., J., and Hatsukami, T. S., Contrast-enhanced high resolution MRI for atherosclerotic carotid artery tissue characterization, *J. Magn. Reson. Imag.,* 15, 62–67, 2002.

98. Lin, W., Abendschein, D. R., et al., Contrast-enhanced magnetic resonance angiography of carotid arterial wall in pigs, *J. Magn. Reson. Imag.,* 7, (1), 183–190, 1997.

99. Yuan, C., Lin, E., et al., Closed contour edge detection of blood vessel lumen and outer wall boundaries in black-blood MR images, *J. Magn. Reson. Imag.,* 17, (2), 257–266, 1999.

100. Zhang, S. X., Hatsukami, T. S., et al., Comparison of carotid vessel wall area measurements using three different contrast-weighted black blood MR imaging techniques, *J. Magn. Reson. Imag.,* 19, (6), 795–802, 2001.

101. Kang, X. J., Polissar, N. L., Han, C., Lin, E., and Yuan C., Analysis of the measurement precision of arterial lumen and wall areas using high resolution magnetic resonance imaging, *Mag. Res. Med.,* 44, 968–972, 2000.

102. von Ingersleben, G., Schmiedl, U. P., et al., Characterization of atherosclerotic plaques at the carotid bifurcation: correlation of high-resolution MR imaging with histologic analysis–preliminary study, *Radiographics,* 17, (6), 1417–1423, 1997.

103. Du, Y. P., Parker, D. L., Davis, W. L., and Cao, G., Reduction of partial-volume artifacts with zero-filled interpolation in three-dimensional MR angiography, *J. Magn. Reson. Imag.,* 4, (5), 733–741, 1994.

104. Mohiaddin, R. H. and Longmore D. B., MRI studies of atherosclerotic vascular disease: structural evaluation and physiological measurements, *Br. Med. Bull.,* 45, (4), 968–990, 1989.

105. Fayad Z. A. and Fuster V., Characterization of atherosclerotic plaques by magnetic resonance imaging, *Ann. N.Y. Acad. Sci.,* 902, 173–186, 2000.

106. Botnar, R. M., Stuber, M., Kissinger, K. V., Kim, W. Y., Spuentrup, E., and Manning W. J., Noninvasive coronary vessel wall and plaque imaging with magnetic resonance imaging, *Circulation,* 102, (21), 2582–2587, 2000.

107. Fayad, Z. A., Fuster, V., Fallon, J. T., Jayasundera, T., Worthley, S. G., Helft, G., Aguinaldo, J. G., Badimon, J. J., and Sharma, S. K., Noninvasive *in vivo* human coronary artery lumen and wall imaging using black-blood magnetic resonance imaging, *Circulation,* 102, (5), 506–510, 2000.

8

Analysis and Visualization of Atherosclerotic Plaque Composition by MRI

William S. Kerwin and Chun Yuan

CONTENTS

8.1 Introduction

Medical imaging techniques have advanced to the point that structures within artery walls can now be resolved *in vivo*. These imaging techniques can thus be used to directly view atherosclerotic lesions and potentially to derive quantitative measurements of lesion composition. The purpose of this chapter is to investigate image processing tools for analyzing lesion composition. Because the tools are most advanced for MRI of carotid artery atherosclerosis, the focus of the chapter is on that application [1].

The motivation for this work is derived from histological investigations that have established the concept of a "vulnerable plaque," characterized by a thin fibrous cap separating a soft lipid core from the vessel lumen [2, 3]. A plaque of this type is illustrated in Figure 8.1. Such vulnerable plaques are thought to be prone to rupture, leading to thromboembolic complications such as heart attacks and strokes. If the features associated with plaque vulnerability could be measured by noninvasive imaging, the risk of rupture for a particular lesion could be quantified and used in the assessment of treatment options.

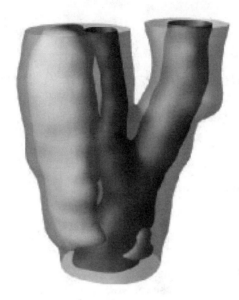

FIGURE 8.1 (See color insert.)
Illustration of a vulnerable plaque at the carotid bifurcation showing a large lipid core (yellow) between the outer wall of the artery (opaque) and the lumen (red).

Additionally, compositional measurements could be used in serial studies to assess the effect of therapy on plaque composition and stability.

In general, plaque structure is more complex than the preceding picture suggests, especially for the large lesions of the carotid arteries. Other compositional features implicated in plaque rupture include the high densities and sizes of neovasculature [4], calcific nodules extruding into the lumen [5], and foci of inflammatory infiltrate such as macrophages [6]. The plaque illustrated in Figure 8.2 is thus more typical, and tools for measuring all of these features are desirable. Such measurements are "compositional indexes" of the disease.

A number of analytical tools have been suggested for measuring plaque composition indexes. These tools can be placed into the following four categories:

1. Global tools for characterizing plaque composition as a whole (Section 8.4)

2. Interactive plaque characterization tools (Section 8.5)

3. Automated plaque characterization tools (Section 8.6)

4. Tools for three-dimensional plaque analysis (Section 8.7)

Each of these approaches is discussed in the indicated section. Before presenting the tools, the goals of plaque characterization are discussed in Section 8.2. Specifically, a set of compositional indexes is presented that would be of

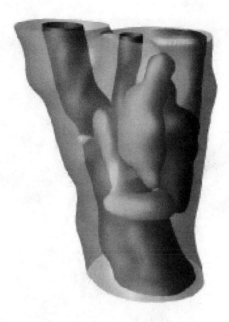

FIGURE 8.2 (See color insert.)
A typical carotid artery plaque exhibiting calcification (light blue) and intraplaque hemorrhage (purple) in addition to lipid core (yellow).

value if extracted from medical images. Next, in Section 8.3, imaging strategies are briefly discussed and the evidence is presented for using MRI over other modalities to measure these indexes. Finally, after discussing the four categories of measurement tools, the chapter closes with some concluding remarks in Section 8.8 on the future of compositional indexes of atherosclerosis.

8.2 Quantifying the Vulnerable Plaque

Figure 8.3 depicts histological specimens from three different carotid plaques. The first example has a thin fibrous cap separating a lipid-rich core from the lumen. The second exhibits calcified nodules extruding into the lumen. The third has large, densely packed neovasculature in the shoulder region of the plaque. Although these plaques show considerable compositional variability, all have been characterized as vulnerable because of these features.

Assuming that the features of vulnerable plaque can be resolved *in vivo* by medical imaging, the features could conceivably be used to identify patients in need of aggressive treatment, monitor progression, or evaluate drug response. For such purposes, the features should be characterized by continuous or quasi-continuous measurements. This has led to the concept of

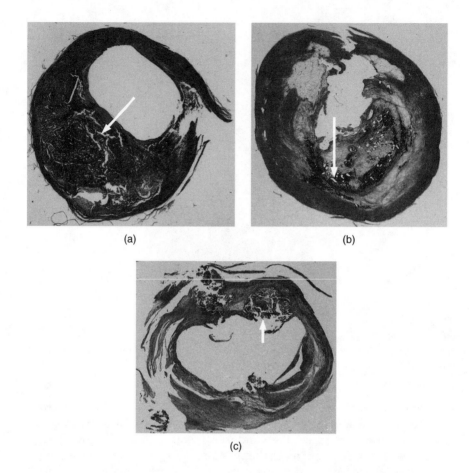

(a)   (b)

(c)

FIGURE 8.3 (See color insert.)
Examples of vulnerable plaques: (a) a large plaque with a lipid-rich core (arrow) separated from the lumen by a thin fibrous cap; (b) a plaque with substantial neovasculature in the shoulder region (arrow); and (c) a plaque with calcific nodules (arrow) extruding into the lumen.

lesion indexes, defined as continuous, mutually independent quantities that characterize plaque vulnerability [7].

8.2.1 Morphological versus Compositional Indexes

The standard for quantitative characterization of atherosclerotic arteries is percent stenosis. Most often, this index of luminal narrowing is measured via digital subtraction angiography (DSA) or duplex ultrasound. In the carotid arteries, for example, percent stenosis is the recommended criterion used to select surgical candidates [8]. Stenosis quantifies the effect of atherosclerosis on the lumen, but not the plaque itself. Thus, the correlation between stenosis and negative outcomes is somewhat weak [8].

Direct measurements of the plaque size and shape are promising alternatives to lumen stenosis, which are being developed as methods for imaging the vessel walls improve. For example, carotid intimal media thickness (IMT) measured by ultrasound has been established as a risk factor for heart attack and stroke [9]. Carotid IMT has also been used as an indicator of progression for clinical trials [10]. Additional morphological indicators under investigation are discussed in Chapter 9. Again, however, plaque morphology does not necessarily equate to plaque vulnerability.

Lumen stenosis and IMT are both examples of *morphological* indexes of atherosclerotic disease. Ideally, the techniques presented in this chapter will establish indexes of plaque *composition*. The combination of morphological and compositional indexes will then provide a detailed description of the plaque that can be used for risk factor analysis, segregation of patients into surgical and nonsurgical groups, or assessment of therapeutic response.

Currently, the calcium score provided by computed tomography (CT) is the most widely accepted compositional index [11]. The extent of high-density regions in CT images of vessel walls associates with the extent of calcification [12], correlates with stenosis [13], and can be used as a risk factor for heart attack and stroke [14]. Further techniques must be developed to assess the integrity of the fibrous cap and the size of the lipid core, both of which are thought to be more telling than the extent of calcification. Whether CT can be used to obtain such compositional indexes is uncertain. Ideally, a single imaging technique will be developed to simultaneously measure all relevant morphological and compositional indexes.

8.2.2 A Set of Compositional Indexes

The following list summarizes compositional indexes that may be important for characterizing plaque vulnerability:

Total lipid content: the total volume of lipid within a lesion

Fractional lipid content: the volume of lipid as a fraction of total plaque volume

Total calcification volume: the total volume of calcifications within a lesion

Juxtaluminal calcification volume: the volume of calcifications that are directly adjacent to the lumen

Vascularity: the percentage of the plaque tissue comprised of neovasculature

Inflammation: the number of inflammatory cells (e.g., macrophages) per unit volume

Average cap thickness: the average thickness of the fibrous cap separating the plaque core from the lumen

Relative surface area of thinned cap: the ratio of the surface area of thinned fibrous cap to the total lumen surface area

Complexity: the number of different tissue regions within the plaque

All these indexes could be measured if the plaque was divided up by tissue type. Measuring plaque composition is, therefore, equivalent to plaque segmentation. Once segmentation is complete, computing the indexes is simply a matter of computing volumes of different regions. The list of tissue types to be segmented includes lipid-rich core, necrotic core, fibrous tissue, loose fibrous matrix, calcification, intraplaque hemorrhage, thrombus, and neovasculature.

8.3 Imaging Methods: The Case for MRI

To segment plaque and measure compositional indexes *in vivo*, an imaging technique is needed that is sensitive to differences in atherosclerotic plaque composition. A number of imaging techniques have been explored. CT, in addition to providing a calcium score, also provides measures of plaque density useful for tissue differentiation. In one study, predominantly fibrous plaques were shown to have densities typical of tissue, whereas plaques with large lipid/necrotic cores tended to have low or patchy densities [15]. In an *ex vivo* experiment, however, the ability of CT to distinguish tissue components proved inferior to MRI even for calcifications [16].

The ability of ultrasound to characterize plaque composition has also been extensively studied. The fact that different components of atherosclerotic plaques have different echogenicities is well-established [17]. This behavior has been used with intravascular ultrasound (IVUS) to segment plaques into soft, hard, and shadow (calcification) regions [18]. Echogenicity has also been used as the comparison variable for a randomized drug trial [19]. The greatest drawbacks for ultrasound techniques are, however, limited view angles for external probes and a high degree of invasiveness for IVUS. Investigations into the ability of B-mode ultrasound to fully characterize plaque composition have had limited success [20].

Nuclear medicine provides some unique alternatives for quantifying atherosclerotic plaque. Radiolabeled species that bind to specific components of atherosclerotic plaque, such as intra-arterial thrombus, have been demonstrated [21]. Such techniques show great promise for quantifying individual components of plaque, but nuclear medicine is unlikely to provide a complete picture of plaque structure.

None of these methods has shown the potential for characterizing plaque composition exhibited by MRI. *Ex vivo* studies have shown sensitivities and specificities verging on 100% for the identification of lipid, fibrous plaque, calcifications, and thrombus [22, 23]. *In vivo* studies have shown that MRI reveals the state of the fibrous cap [24] and the presence of lipid cores or intraplaque hemorrhage [25]. Preliminary investigations with injected contrast agents indicate that MRI may uniquely be able to detect neovasculature [26, 27]. These techniques are also beginning to be used in the evaluation of drug effects [28].

The success of MRI in characterizing plaque composition derives from its excellent contrast between soft tissues, which provides excellent anatomical and compositional detail. Contrast can also be changed by adjusting any of several imaging parameters. Multiple images with different contrast weightings can thus be combined for increased sensitivity to tissue differences. Additionally, MRI is noninvasive and does not use ionizing radiation, making it ideal for serial studies.

Figure 8.4 demonstrates the ability of MRI to characterize atherosclerotic plaque in the carotid artery. The images shown form a "multispectral" data set, including T1-weighted (T1W), T2-weighted (T2W), proton-density-weighted

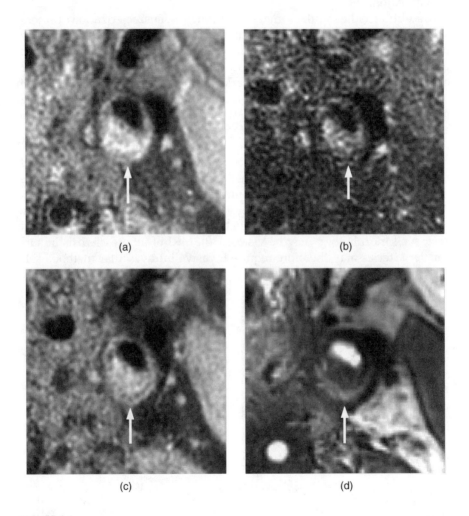

(a)   (b)

(c)   (d)

FIGURE 8.4
MRI appearance of atherosclerotic plaque using four standard contrast weightings: (a) T1W, (b) T2W, (c) PDW, and (d) TOF.

(PDW), and time-of-flight (TOF) images. These images are the standard set used to identify specific atherosclerotic tissue types. The details of the MRI sequences used to generate these images are described in Chapter 7.

Identification of tissue types is performed using established rules that relate intensity characteristics to tissue types, some of which are summarized in Table 7.1. For example, in Figure 8.4, the plaque is very bright on T1W, corresponding to lipid core. Histological examination of the corresponding endarterectomy specimen verifies this demarcation (the matched histology section for these images is shown in Figure 8.3a). The availability of the endarterectomy specimen also permits high-resolution *ex vivo* imaging of plaque for validation.

In addition to the standard image weightings for characterization of atherosclerosis, a number of other MRI techniques are also addressed in Chapter 7. In the current chapter, special attention will be paid to injected contrast agents, used to highlight tissue types. In Figure 8.5, for example, a T1W image after contrast agent application shows marked enhancement of a plaque rich in neovasculature and loose matrix. Dynamic imaging of contrast agent arrival may also allow tissues to be identified by the rate at which they absorb the agent.

The remainder of this chapter addresses techniques for analyzing such MRI data sets. MRI does have some disadvantages for plaque imaging, which makes characterization of vessels other than the carotid arteries difficult. Preliminary results in the aorta are promising [29] and other large arteries are likely targets as well. Imaging of coronary artery wall composition, on the other hand, requires higher-resolution techniques to be developed, although basic wall morphology may be visible [30]. MRI of atherosclerosis in such smaller arteries may therefore require invasive intravascular methods [31].

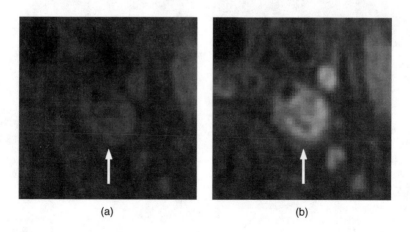

(a)   (b)

FIGURE 8.5
Contrast enhanced T1W MRI of a carotid artery (arrow): (a) before contrast agent injection and (b) after contrast agent injection (same window and level settings).

Which imaging technique will ultimately emerge as the gold standard for identifying plaque composition remains to be seen. Because MRI has emerged as an early leader, at least for large vessels, this chapter focuses on that modality. Many of the techniques outlined here, nevertheless, are equally applicable to other modalities.

8.4   Global Measurements of Composition

Several approaches for quantifying plaque composition can be classified as "global measurements," meaning that they can be computed from the plaque as a whole. If, for example, a certain tissue type has low image intensity, then plaques containing large amounts of that tissue will have lower average intensities than plaques containing little or none. The average plaque intensity could thus be taken as a simple global measurement indicative of composition.

This concept has led to various investigations of plaque composition based on global measurements. Perhaps the most straightforward is T_2 dependence of the plaque. T_2 is the spin-spin relaxation time and image intensity is proportional to:

$$e^{\frac{-TE}{T_2}}$$

where the echo time TE is selected by the user. By obtaining several images with different echo times, parametric maps of T_2 can be extracted. A simpler and more repeatable measurement related to T_2 takes only the ratio of images with long TE ($\approx$50 msec) and short TE ($\approx$10 msec). This technique is facilitated by dual echo sequences, which permit both images to be acquired simultaneously. In one study, this ratio was associated with levels of serum markers for inflammation [32].

Another factor that has been considered is the magnetization transfer ratio (MTR), which measures the amount of signal reduction due to the presence of magnetically presaturated macromolecules. In *ex vivo* experiments, the MTR was shown to vary by tissue type [33]. This has not, however, led to an index of composition.

The attraction of such global measurements is the ease of the analysis. They do not require explicit identification of tissue types, counting instead on the average impact of the different tissues. Also, measurements from multiple contrast weightings (e.g., short and long TE) can be combined without the need to correct for changes in patient position. Global measurements are thus well-suited for clinical applications.

The drawback of most global measurements, however, is that they do not provide specific information regarding which tissues are present or their relative abundance. For example, a plaque with an intermediate ratio between long and short TE images may indicate a uniform, intermediate value of T_2 or a mix of tissues with high and low values of T_2. Ideally, compositional indexes will have an interpretation that directly relates to plaque composition. Fortunately, some global measurements are showing promise as specific indexes of plaque composition, as will now be shown.

8.4.1   Vascularity

One tissue-specific characteristic that can be measured globally by MRI is vascularity. The ingrowth of neovasculature into atherosclerotic plaque is believed to be a pathway for destabilizing inflammation [34] and plaques with substantial neovasculature are therefore thought to be unstable. This belief is further supported by histological studies relating size of neovessels to patient symptoms [4, 35]. In MRI, the density of vasculature is commonly measured with dynamic contrast-enhanced (DCE) techniques that can readily be applied to atherosclerotic lesions [36].

Some of the difficulties with DCE MRI, however, are that the rapid imaging techniques required to capture the dynamic behavior of contrast agents, as well as motion of the patient during acquisition, lead to noise and jitter in the image sequences. For the carotid arteries, substantial reduction of noise and jitter has been demonstrated using the Kalman filtering, registration, and smoothing (KFRS) algorithm [37]. Briefly, the KFRS algorithm recursively registers images in the sequence and temporally smooths the intensity of individual pixels to eliminate noise.

Once the images have been prepared for analysis, the amount of neovasculature can be measured in a variety of ways. The simplest method is to measure the relative area under the time intensity curve (AUC) [38]. The formula for the AUC is:

$$\text{AUC} = \sum_{n=1}^{N} I_n - I_0$$

where I_n is the intensity of a pixel or region at the nth time frame and I_0 is the pre-contrast intensity. Essentially, AUC integrates the effect of the contrast agent over time.

The utility of the AUC comes from the following characteristic of contrast agent concentration versus time $C(t)$. If we integrate:

$$\int_0^\infty C(t)dt$$

the result is proportional to the partial volume p into which the contrast agent penetrates, regardless of the rate of uptake [39]. Therefore, assuming image intensity is linearly related to $C(t)$, the AUC is proportional to p as well.

The partial volume of tissue into which the contrast agent penetrates can thus be measured by taking the ratio of the AUC from tissue and that from blood, measured in the vessel lumen (where $p = 1$). That is:

$$p(\text{tissue}) = \frac{\text{AUC(tissue)}}{\text{AUC(blood)}}$$

This value is then presumed to be indicative of the vascularity of the tissue.

This behavior is demonstrated in the following example [27]. DCE MRI sequences from ten subjects with advanced carotid atherosclerosis were obtained prior to endarterectomy. The images were obtained with a spoiled gradient-recalled echo sequence (TR = 100 msec; TE = 3.4 msec; flip = 60°; thickness = 3 mm; matrix = 256 × 128; field of view = 16 cm) and a time separation of 20 sec between acquisitions. A gadolinium-based contrast agent (Omniscan, Nycomed-Amersham, Oslo) was injected coincident with the second acquisition and sequences containing a total of ten images each were obtained. After endarterectomy, the removed specimens were stained, sectioned, and matched to the location of the dynamic sequence. The total area of neovasculature as a percentage of the total plaque area was then measured from the matched histological section. Figure 8.6 shows a comparison of the neovasculature area and the ratio of the plaque AUC to the blood AUC. A correlation of 0.8 between these measurements indicates that the AUC does indeed indicate the amount of neovasculature ($p < 0.01$).

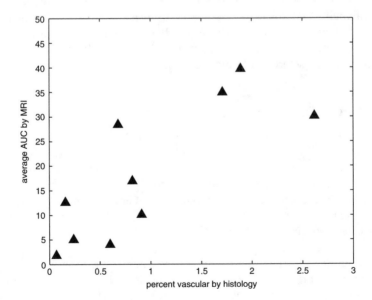

FIGURE 8.6
Association between fractional area of neovasculature measured in histology and the ratio of plaque AUC to blood AUC.

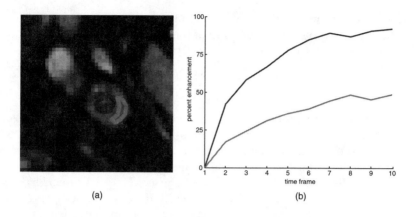

(a)   (b)

FIGURE 8.7

Fast versus slow enhancement: the intensity versus time curves for the regions indicated in (a) are plotted in (b). They show a region of slow enhancement (green) and one of combined fast and slow enhancement (red).

These results may show even stronger correlation if the AUC approach is replaced by one that distinguishes between rapidly enhancing and slowly enhancing tissues commonly encountered in DCE MRI [40]. Such behavior is also encountered in atherosclerotic plaques, as illustrated in Figure 8.7. The difference in behavior may be attributable to the presence of neovasculature (fast enhancing) versus semi-permeable tissues such as loose fibrous matrix (slow enhancing). Separating these two behaviors may permit global measurement of both vascularity and permeability. A useful model specifically applied to atherosclerotic plaque is still under development.

8.4.2   Percent Enhancement

Injected contrast agents can also be used in the steady state to measure plaque composition. T1W DIR Images taken 10 to 20 minutes after contrast agent injection show patchy regions of enhancement compared to pre-contrast images. The percent enhancement has been shown to be highest for regions rich in neovasculature [26]. The average percent enhancement has also shown to be related to levels of serum markers for inflammation [32]. These results suggest that a tissue-specific parameter related to percent enhancement will be forthcoming.

One notable feature evident after contrast agent injection is enhancement of the outermost rim of the vessel wall as shown in Figure 8.8. This enhanced rim has been observed in T1W, TOF, and DCE images [26, 41, 42]. The amount of enhancement and the thickness of the enhanced region varies from patient to patient and from location to location within a patient. Such variation is believed to indicate the extent of the vasa vasorum within the adventitia

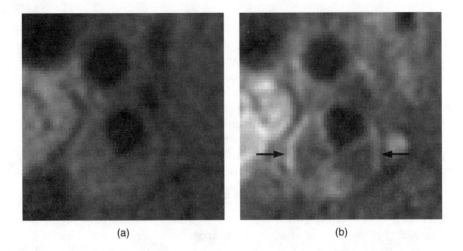

(a) (b)

FIGURE 8.8
Outer rim enhancement: (a) T1W image before injection of contrast agent; (b) 10 minutes after contrast agent injection, an enhanced rim is evident (arrows).

of the vessel. Although the clinical relevance is unknown, extensive vasa vasorum may be related to extensive neovasculature or inflammation within the plaque. Such markers for plaque vulnerability may therefore be measured using outer rim enhancement.

Two basic measurements of outer rim enhancement have been explored: thickness and percent enhancement. In one study, the thickness of the rim showed a distinct correlation with patient age, but was not tied to the state of disease [41]. In another study, the percent enhancement of the outer rim was tied to the number of large vessels in the adventitia, counted after resection of the carotid artery [42]. The two measurements had a correlation coefficient of 0.7 ($p < 0.03$). The significance of this result and outer rim enhancement in general is uncertain because the study was limited to one patient for whom the resected artery was available and because the implications of large vessels in the adventitia are unknown.

Although outer rim enhancement is of uncertain relevance, its measurement has some distinct advantages. First, the measurement can combine data from two separate image acquisitions (before and after contrast agent injection) without a one-to-one correspondence of points in the two images. Thus, patient motion is not an issue. This advantage arises because the outer rim can be identified without ambiguity in the two images. A second advantage is that this measurement comes from a consistent tissue region — the adventitia — not the complicated plaque region. These advantages suggest that outer rim enhancement may be more repeatable and more closely tied to a specific plaque feature than other global measurements. The significance of this measurement therefore warrants further study.

8.4.3 Heterogeneity

Another global measurement that has been proposed seeks to measure plaque heterogeneity [7]. An unstable plaque may undergo a series of subclinical disruptions, such as intraplaque hemorrhages, that lead to a comparatively complicated structure. Plaques with more complicated structures are therefore likely to pose greater risk for future disruptions. Because plaque complexity manifests itself in MRI as greater heterogeneity of signal, plaque complexity can be measured by quantifying the heterogeneity of the image.

One caveat is, however, that the classical "vulnerable plaque" is actually quite uniform, consisting primarily of a large lipid core. Such a uniform plaque would appear homogeneous on MRI, despite the fact that it is highly unstable. Measures of heterogeneity should, therefore, be combined with other measures of composition for assessing risk. An alternative use of heterogeneity arises in serial studies of progression. Changes in heterogeneity may indicate changes in plaque structure in response to therapy, even when the gross morphology appears unchanged.

One means of measuring heterogeneity is to use information theory. For example, the average "information content" over the lesion has been used as a measure of complexity [7]. Information content is defined as:

$$\frac{1}{2} \log_2 \frac{P_s(x, y) + P_n}{P_n}$$

where $P_s(x, y)$ is the power (intensity) of the pixel at (x, y) and P_n is the noise power. Another potential measure of heterogeneity is entropy, defined as:

$$\sum_m p[m] \log p[m]$$

where $p[m]$ is the probability of a pixel having intensity m. This probability is estimated from the histogram of intensity values within the lesion. The drawback of these measurements is that they depend on the system gain and contrast-to-noise level, making them difficult to normalize. Thus, the comparison of values across patients and over time is questionable.

8.5 Interactive Analysis of Plaque Composition

The global measurements discussed in the preceding section avoid the problem of segmenting the plaque by tissue type. They are, however, imprecise and only able to capture certain aspects of plaque composition. For computing all of the compositional indexes, all plaque components must be individually identified.

A suite of programs developed specifically for the analysis of atherosclerotic plaque by MRI is the quantitative vascular analysis system (QVAS) [43].

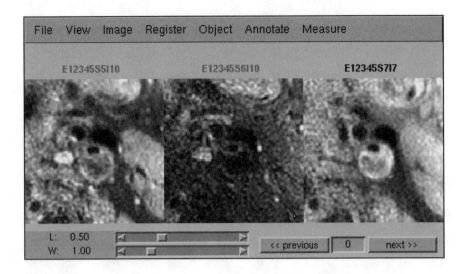

FIGURE 8.9
QVAS interface.

QVAS allows the user to interactively identify the boundaries of tissue regions, assign tissue types, and measure lesion indexes. Figure 8.9 shows the user interface for QVAS.

Using QVAS, any number of images can be displayed, nominally to view different contrast weightings of the same artery. Image processing tools permit the user to zoom in on the region of interest and adjust the brightness and contrast. A two-dimensional coil correction algorithm [44] can also be applied to produce a uniform intensity across the image. Images can then be processed to extract lesion indexes.

8.5.1 Contour Tools

The primary role of QVAS is drawing contours to delineate tissue regions. Several types of contour drawing tools are included:

Shapes: basic objects, such as ellipses

B-spline contours: closed curve selected by a series of mouse-clicks and connected via a B-spline

Active contours: closed curve that automatically conforms to local edge features in the image

Connectors: B-spline curve segment selected by a series of mouse-clicks and constrained to connect at both ends to previously drawn contours

Active connectors: a connector that automatically conforms to local edge features

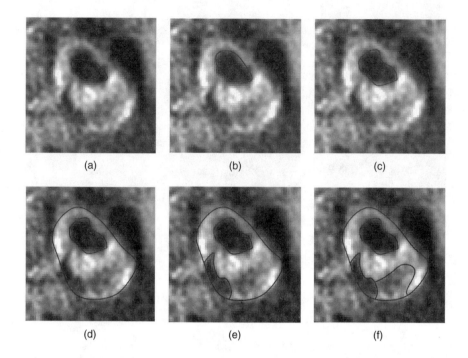

FIGURE 8.10

Example of constructing a coupled-contour mesh: (a) an ellipse is drawn, (b) the ellipse is manually deformed, (c) the resulting contour is activated and conforms to the lumen, (d) an active contour is used to define the outer wall boundary, (e) a connector with both ends on the outer wall contour delineates a calcification, and (f) a connector from the calcification to the outer wall delineates a lipid core.

The result of using these tools is a "coupled-contour mesh," defined as a set of contours and their dependent connectors.

Once a contour is drawn, it can be manually adjusted, activated, or deleted. Thus, for example, an ellipse can be converted into an active contour that deforms to match local edge features. Such manipulations are illustrated in Figure 8.10, which shows the use of these tools to construct a coupled-contour mesh on an image of an atherosclerotic carotid artery. If a contour with dependent connectors is adjusted or deleted, those connectors are also adjusted or deleted as appropriate. When completed, the positions of the contours can be saved, retrieved, and readjusted at any time.

All contours are B-spline based, so that:

$$x(l) = \sum_{k=1}^{K} a_k B_k(l)$$

$$y(l) = \sum_{k=1}^{K} b_k B_k(l)$$

where $B_k(l)$ are the cubic B-spline bases, a_k and b_k are the spline coefficients, and the coordinates $(x(l), y(l))$, $l \in [0, L]$ define the contour. When activated, the spline coefficients are adjusted to maximize the function:

$$\int_0^L \frac{\|\nabla I(x(l), y(l))\|^2}{\sqrt{(dx/dl)^2 + (dy/dl)^2}} dl$$

which is the average squared magnitude of the image gradient along the contour. The value of this function will be maximum when the contour conforms to edges. The smoothness of the contour is controlled by the total number of coefficients K, which can be adjusted by the user.

The contours can also be copied and pasted to other images in the series or images with different contrast weightings. Pasting contours from other images in the series is useful for rapidly identifying similar features in adjacent images. In many cases, a feature can be identified simply by pasting and activating the corresponding contour from the previous image. Pasting contours from different contrast weightings is useful for identifying the location of a tissue that is apparent in one contrast weighting but not visible in another.

To assist in properly locating a feature from a different contrast weighting, QVAS also includes several registration tools, including manual shifting of the images, and two automated techniques. In one, contours identified in two sets of images are aligned [45]. For example, the lumen can be identified in two series, in which case the best alignment of the lumen is found. In the second automated registration technique, the images themselves are registered by aligning edge maps [46]. Whichever registration method is used, the result is a mapping function that determines precisely where a contour from one series should be pasted into another.

8.5.2   Labeling

Once the contouring tools have been used to identify region boundaries, a tissue label can be assigned to any defined region. The assignment can be tied directly to a closed contour, for example, the outer wall boundary. In that case, all enclosed structures are also included within the region. Alternatively, a label can be assigned to any connected region of pixels delineated by closed contours and connectors. In that case, a region is grown from a user selected point to include any pixel that does not lie on the other side of a contour. Examples of labeled regions are shown in Figure 8.11. Contour-specific labels (i.e., outer wall) are shown with a line connecting the label to the contour.

Labeling is assisted by an automated tissue identifier that selects probable labels based on previous assignments. The choice of labels is accomplished by comparing amount of overlap, sizes, and statistics (mean, variance) of regions identified in adjacent images. The label of the region with the best match is copied to the unknown region. This permits the QVAS user to rapidly work through a stack of images spanning the artery and assign labels. The resulting labels can be saved and modified at any time.

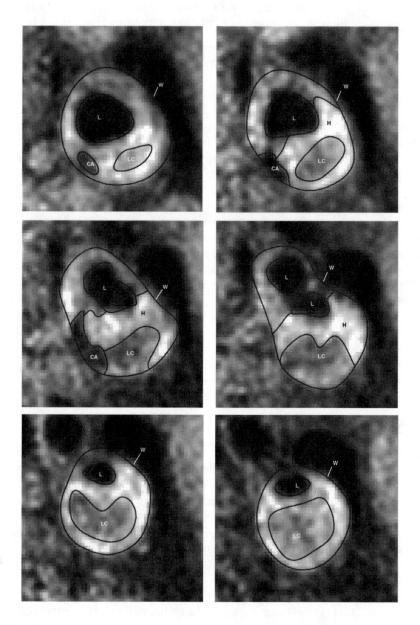

FIGURE 8.11
Labeling of coupled-contour meshes at six locations in a carotid artery. Classification: L = lumen, LC = lipid core, H = hemorrhage, W = outer wall, and CA = calcification.

Along with the tissue labeling, several additional features are also included within QVAS for annotation purposes. First, the user can place lines, arrows, and text within images. These can then be saved in a variety of image formats for incorporation in reports. The labeled regions can also be exported for use with a three-dimensional modeling program (see Section 8.7).

8.5.3   Measurement

The final set of tools available in QVAS allows the user to make the lesion index measurements. For any contour, the length and enclosed area can be computed. For any region, the mean and standard deviation of image intensity can be computed. For any two contours, the average, maximum, and minimum thickness between the contours can be computed. Finally, the volume of any tissue type can be computed.

To illustrate how these measurement tools can be used, suppose the fractional lipid content is desired. The user can then compute the volume of the outer wall (V_w), the lumen (V_l), and the lipid core (V_{lc}). The fractional lipid content is then given by:

$$\frac{V_{lc}}{V_w - V_l}$$

Eventually, the most important indexes will be determined. At that point, QVAS will be able to automatically extract all relevant indexes from the contour and label data. The output will be a report characterizing the atherosclerotic lesion.

8.6   Automated Analysis of Plaque Composition

The interactive QVAS system described in the previous section permits the user to identify tissues within the atherosclerotic plaque. Thus, it provides the necessary tool for computing compositional indexes. The interactive nature of QVAS, however, leads to subjectivity in the tissue classification and rather long analysis times. The foremost goal in compositional analysis of plaque is, therefore, to introduce automated processing steps that extract the same information as QVAS without the need for human interaction.

In short, automated plaque analysis means grouping pixels with similar image characteristics and identifying the corresponding tissue type. Toward this end, a number of investigators have used various unsupervised segmentation techniques to cluster pixels in individual images, including a watershed approach [47]. These single-image techniques have not, however, shown the ability to reliably determine specific tissue types.

The difficulty in assigning tissue types to segmented clusters of pixels arises because only one contrast weighting is being used in the segmentation. Therefore, variability in the imaging configuration, such as positioning of MR coils, leads to variability in the absolute signal received from patient to patient and from scan to scan. Also, the ability to distinguish tissue types varies with the imaging protocol. For example, the fibrous cap may be most visible on TOF images, whereas neovasculature is most visible on contrast-enhanced T1W images.

Both challenges can be overcome using multispectral clustering techniques that combine information from images with different contrast weightings. Multi-spectral techniques, by their nature, utilize the most informative contrast weightings for identification of each tissue. In addition, multi-spectral techniques permit tissues to be identified based on relative intensities rather than absolute levels. These advantages of multi-spectral clustering techniques have been demonstrated in *ex vivo* experiments, which show excellent results in identifying tissues in excised plaques [22].

Use of multi-spectral techniques *in vivo*, however, introduces a new set of problems. Most notably, patient motion between acquisitions misaligns the features between contrast weightings. Because even large plaques have features with dimensions on the order of millimeters or less, patient motion has to be limited or corrected to within fractions of a millimeter. Another problem is that the surface coils used to increase resolution in plaque imaging lead to rapid variations in intensity. To prevent the segmentation algorithm from separating tissues based on the coil inhomogeneity rather than true intensity differences, coil correction must be performed.

Thus, automated analysis of plaque images requires not just segmentation, but also registration and coil correction. In the case of atherosclerotic plaque, these challenges are largely unresolved. Here, the steps needed for automated processing are outlined, including the requirements that must be met for each.

8.6.1   Coil Correction

The problem of coil correction is illustrated in Figure 8.12. Surface coils are placed as close as possible to the carotid arteries to maximize the contrast to noise ratio. The signal, however, rapidly falls off with distance from the coil, leading to a steep brightness gradient across the artery. Mathematically, the signal is given by:

$$I(x, y) = B(x, y)M(x, y)$$

where $M(x, y)$ is the "true" image and $B(x, y)$ is the coil profile. The goal in coil correction is to find an approximation $\hat{B}(x, y)$, and then estimate the true image

$$\hat{M}(x, y) = I(x, y)/\hat{B}(x, y)$$

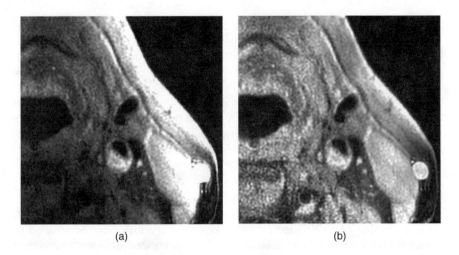

(a)   (b)

FIGURE 8.12
Coil inhomogeneities and correction: (a) original image of the neck exhibits washed-out features toward the right of the image and dim features toward the left; (b) the same image after coil correction, demonstrating improved signal homogeneity across the image.

A number of techniques for coil correction exist, including a wavelet based technique developed specifically for carotid artery imaging [44]. This and similar approaches attempt to determine $B(x, y)$ directly from the image. In practice, they are only able to approximate $B(x, y)$ up to a constant scale factor. This scale factor can vary from image to image or contrast weighting to contrast weighting. As a result, comparative intensity measurements (such as percent enhancement) can be invalidated by coil correction.

For plaque characterization, a coil correction method is needed that corrects inhomogeneities, while preserving relative intensity levels between images. This will be accomplished by deriving a single three-dimensional approximation $\hat{B}(x, y, z)$ of the coil profile based on all image weightings. All images can then be corrected by applying the same profile, thereby preserving relative intensities.

8.6.2   Registration

The need for registration arises as a result of patient motion. Suppose that two volume images $I_1(x, y, z)$ and $I_2(x, y, z)$ have been acquired. If the patient moved between acquisitions, then the tissue located at position (x, y, z) in I_1 has moved to $T(x, y, z)$ in I_2 for some one-to-one transformation T. Our goal in registering the images is to determine the transformation $T(x, y, z)$ that best aligns the anatomy in the source image $I_1(x, y, z)$ with the anatomy in the target image $I_2(x, y, z)$. We can then estimate the image that would have been obtained if no motion had occurred, which is $I_2(T(x, y, z))$.

The implication of this statement is that we must first estimate $T(x, y, z)$, and then interpolate the discrete image I_2, because $T(x, y, z)$ will not, in general, lie exactly at the location of an image pixel.

Although many registration algorithms exist [46, 48], registration of the carotid arteries presents some difficulties. First, the structures of interest are small, making close alignment extremely important. Second, the motion of the neck is quite complex requiring free-form transformations. Third, structures of interest often change dramatically from image to image along the artery, making interpolation difficult if not impossible.

8.6.3 Multi-spectral Segmentation

Once the problems of coil correction and registration have been resolved, any of a number of multi-spectral segmentation algorithms can be applied to identify clusters of similar pixels. The goal is to extract clusters of pixels that have similar intensities and that form a contiguous region. The best approach for clustering pixels will emerge once the preprocessing issues have been resolved.

The identified pixel clusters must also be given a tissue label, such as fibrous cap, lipid core, or calcification. For each cluster, the average intensity values are available from each contrast weighting. Together, these values form a feature vector **f**, and the goal of tissue identification is to determine which tissue is historically most similar to **f**. In making this determination, care must be taken to account for the fact that the magnitude of **f** may depend on the imaging environment (for example, the distance from the artery to the imaging coil). Therefore, the direction of **f** may be more telling than the absolute magnitude.

8.6.4 Example

Although all of these challenges have been addressed to some extent, no one has put them together into a working system for analyzing plaque. To demonstrate how plaque analysis will ultimately work, a program called ACCENT (Confirma, Inc., Kirkland, WA) can be employed. Originally developed for cancer staging, ACCENT incorporates many of the tools required for computing compositional indexes, including multi-spectral segmentation and volume measurement [49].

Figure 8.13 and Figure 8.14 illustrate how automated plaque analysis will ultimately be conducted. In this case, three contrast weightings are available: PDW, T1W, and T2W. Fortunately, patient motion was small in this case, allowing proper registration to be performed using only manual alignment of the images. The multi-spectral segmentation algorithm produced the clusters shown in Figure 8.13d. One cluster was then selected by the user as a probable lipid core and its complete extent across all images was determined, as shown in Figure 8.14. The volume of this region was 0.47 cc.

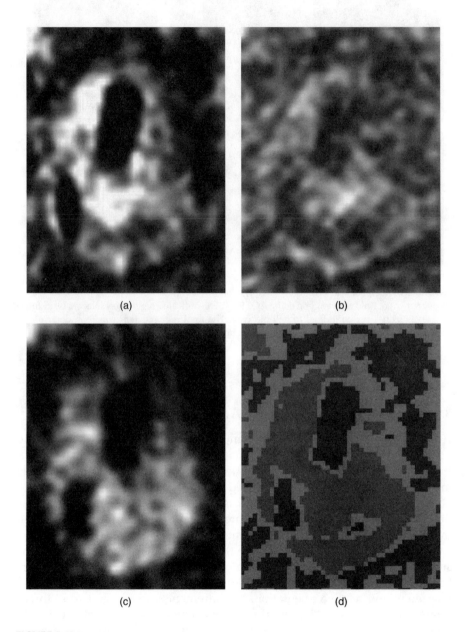

(a)

(b)

(c)

(d)

FIGURE 8.13
Demonstration of multi-spectral segmentation of atherosclerotic plaque using ACCENT: (a) PDW image, (b) T2W image, (c) T1W image, and (d) multi-spectral segmentation result.

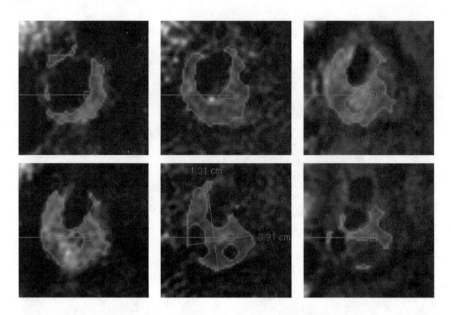

FIGURE 8.14 (See color insert.)
Measurement of lipid core volume using ACCENT. The indicated region was selected by a single mouse-click on a region judged to be lipid core. The total region extent was then determined across adjacent images, six of which are shown here.

8.7   Three-Dimensional Plaque Analysis

A final topic for consideration in compositional analysis of atherosclerotic plaque is converting the tissue information extracted from the images into a three-dimensional model of the plaque. For example, the plaques depicted in Figures 8.1 and 8.2 were constructed from MRIs of actual carotid arteries. To construct such models, a method is required to convert the segmentation data, whether from QVAS or more automated techniques, into surface meshes delineating the structures of interest.

One primary reason for working in three dimensions is that volume measurements are likely to be more accurate and reproducible. This benefit arises because three-dimensional models reduce the variation due to image plane placement and relative orientation. Measurements can also be tied to three-dimensional anatomical landmarks. Increased accuracy is especially valuable for serial studies seeking to identify small changes in plaque burden over time. The models also give the potential for localizing and displaying regions of change.

Another advantage of three-dimensional models is the potential to use them for surgical planning. In endarterectomy, the presence of a calcification in an apparently healthy region of vessel can play an important role in determining where to place clamps or cuts, as well as the extent of the plaque to be removed. Knowing such structural information prior to surgery would likely reduce complications.

To generate a three-dimensional model from the segmentation data, several potential problems must be addressed. First, the sampling of the plaque by MRI is comparatively coarse, with perhaps ten axial images spanning the length of a plaque and tissue regions often consisting of only a handful of pixels in any one image. Second, regions composed of the same tissue are not necessarily connected, and a robust method is needed to determine when regions should be connected. Finally, some regions exist only in one image and must be extrapolated into three dimensions.

Although many methods exist for generating three-dimensional models from segmentation data (e.g., [50, 51]), most fail when one or more of the above problems is encountered. To construct the models in this chapter, a method was developed that handles all of the special cases. The details are presented here.

8.7.1   Surface Model Construction

A tissue region can be defined by a membershiop function $m(x, y, z)$ that equals 1 inside the region and 0 outside the region. The boundary surface exists at the interface between $m(x, y, z) = 1$ and $m(x, y, z) = 0$. Segmentation results from the methods described earlier in this chapter sample the membership function at pixel locations, thereby providing a discrete membership function $m[i]$ defined at each pixel location i. The goal of surface model construction can thus be framed as one of approximating the continuous $m(x, y, z)$ given the discrete $m[i]$.

The approximated membership function $\hat{m}(x, y, z)$ can be found by minimizing the energy function:

$$
\int_{\Re^3} \left[\left(\frac{\partial^2 \hat{m}}{\partial x^2} \right)^2 + \left(\frac{\partial^2 \hat{m}}{\partial y^2} \right)^2 + \left(\frac{\partial^2 \hat{m}}{\partial z^2} \right)^2 \right.
$$

$$
\left. + 2 \left(\frac{\partial^2 \hat{m}}{\partial x \partial y} \right)^2 + 2 \left(\frac{\partial^2 \hat{m}}{\partial x \partial z} \right)^2 + 2 \left(\frac{\partial^2 \hat{m}}{\partial y \partial z} \right)^2 \right] dx\, dy\, dz
$$

$$
+ \frac{1}{\lambda} \sum_i [m[i] - \hat{m}(x_i, y_i, z_i)]^2 \tag{8.1}
$$

where λ is a smoothing parameter. The integral portion of this expression is a rotationally invariant energy, which is analogous in two dimensions to the bending energy of a thin metal plate and penalizes abrupt variations in the approximated membership function. The second term controls the extent to which the approximated membership function matches $m[i]$, with perfect matching as $\lambda \to 0$. Note that the solution to this minimization problem takes on a continuum of values, making it akin to a "Fuzzy" membership function [52].

The function that minimizes Equation 8.1 is given by the three-dimensional smoothing thin-plate spline:

$$\hat{m}(x, y, z) = a_0 + a_1 x + a_2 y + a_3 z + \sum_i r_i w_i$$

where r_i is the distance from (x, y, z) to (x_i, y_i, z_i) [53]. The optimal weights a_0, a_1, a_2, a_3, and w_i are found by solving the set of simultaneous linear equations:

$$\hat{m}(x_i, y_i, z_i) - \lambda w_i = m[i] \tag{8.2}$$

for all i and:

$$\sum_i w_i = \sum_i w_i x_i = \sum_i w_i y_i = \sum_i w_i z_i = 0. \tag{8.3}$$

From the approximated membership function, an isosurface is extracted to produce a three-dimensional surface model of the object given by the set of points:

$$S = \{(x, y, z) | \hat{m}(x, y, z) = v\}$$

for some value v. The approximated membership function, in addition to being continuous in space, also takes on a continuum of values. Thus, an infinite number of isosurfaces exists, depending on the choice of v. The optimal v for isosurface generation can be taken to be that which minimizes the cardinality of the set:

$$\{ i \mid m[i] = 1, \hat{m}(x_i, y_i, z_i) < v\} \bigcup \{ i \mid m[i] = 0, \hat{m}(x_i, y_i, z_i) > v\} \tag{8.4}$$

that is, the number of pixels that belong to the object and fall outside the surface plus the number of pixels that do not belong to the object and fall inside the surface.

The rationale for selecting this overall approach is as follows. The resulting isosurface can only be convoluted or contain sharp bends if $\hat{m}(x, y, z)$ contains sudden variations. The thin-plate spline formulation of $\hat{m}(x, y, z)$, however, precludes such sudden variations. Thus, this method places an implicit smoothness constraint on the surface.

In practice, computational considerations require two simplifications. First, the thin-plate spline is computed only for a finite set of points at a finer grid spacing than the original data. Second, the values used to compute the thin-plate spline at each point are taken only from a local neighborhood of the point, nominally $10 \times 10 \times 4$, where the smaller number of locations in the z-dimension (4 vs. 10) reflects the coarser resolution of images perpendicular to the image slices. This leads to a convolutional implementation for interpolating the membership function [54].

Once the refined membership function is computed, the surface of the object is constructed using the isosurface algorithm from Open Visualization Data

Explorer (IBM Corporation, White Plains, NY). The value used to construct the isosurface is found by minimizing Equation 8.4.

8.7.2 Example

Figure 8.15 through Figure 8.17 illustrate the steps in generating a surface model of a carotid plaque. The input in this example is a data set consisting of ten images with 0.25-mm pixels and 2.0-mm image separations. The outer boundary, lumen, and calcified regions were identified using QVAS. The refined membership functions were then generated using $\lambda = 50$, measuring distances in units of pixels, and up-sampling by a factor of two in-plane and four between-image planes. Note that the model produced a realistic rendering of the calcification despite a relatively complex shape.

8.8 Conclusion

Identifying and quantifying the contents of atherosclerotic plaque will greatly benefit research and clinical investigations of atherosclerosis. First, it will enable the evolution of individual atherosclerotic plaques to be studied over time. In contrast, many conclusions are currently based on population studies of different plaques, rather than serial studies of the same plaques [2, 3, 5]. Second, the effects of drugs on plaque contents can be directly measured. Such studies are already underway [28]. Finally, plaque contents can ultimately be used in addition to stenosis for clinical decisions. For these applications, the analysis of plaque composition must be quantitative to make objective rather than subjective judgments.

At present, global indexes of plaque composition, such as calcium score, are nearing acceptance as markers of atherosclerotic disease beyond stenosis. The advantage of global indexes is their comparative ease of extraction from images because they do not require advanced processing such as registration. Such measurements should appear more and more often in scientific and clinical studies of atherosclerosis.

More specific measurements of plaque composition, on the other hand, are likely to come in the near future from interactive tools such as QVAS. QVAS enables complete plaque characterization to be performed by users familiar with the appearance of atherosclerotic tissues in MRI. Studies currently underway with QVAS are likely to determine the specific characteristics of atherosclerotic plaque associated with progression, regression, and development of symptoms.

Once the key quantitative markers of atherosclerosis are identified, the ultimate challenge will be developing methods to rapidly extract the measurements from MRI. The measurements must be repeatable, user independent,

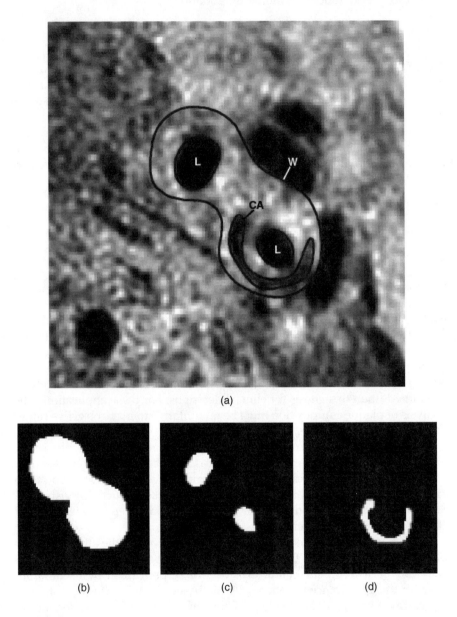

FIGURE 8.15
Membership functions: (a) region boundaries created using QVAS, (b) artery membership function, (c) lumen membership function, (d) calcification membership function.

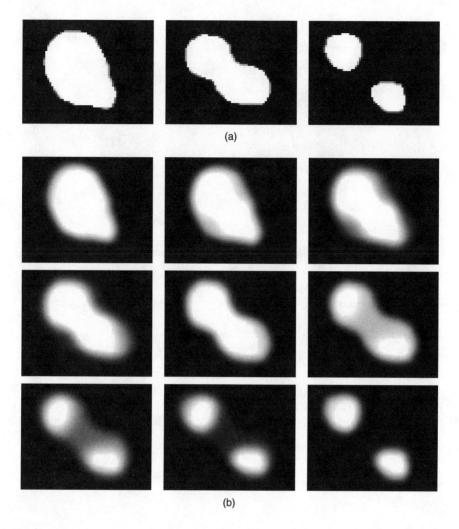

(a)

(b)

FIGURE 8.16
Refining the membership function: (a) lumen membership function for three consecutive images at the carotid bifurcation, and (b) refined membership function with the same coverage showing additional interpolated slices.

and accurate. Accomplishing these goals requires that the obstacles to automated processing of plaque images be overcome.

In summary, this chapter reviewed the basic goals for analyzing plaque composition by MRI. Early developments toward this end were reviewed, including an interactive system called QVAS. The next generation of QVAS will need to be highly automated to be adopted for routine clinical or research use. The remaining obstacles for such automated processing were presented.

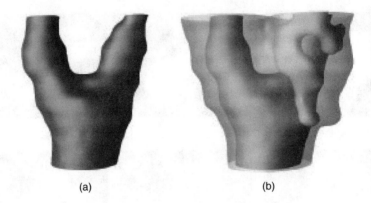

(a)   (b)

FIGURE 8.17 (See color insert.)
Resulting model from example in Figure 8.15 and Figure 8.16: (a) artery lumen, and (b) complete model with calcification (light blue) and outer wall (opaque).

Acknowledgments

The authors thank Marina Ferguson, Thomas Hatsukami, Chao Han, Dongxiang Xu, and Jenq-Neng Hwang for their contributions to this work. Additionally, appreciation is given to Confirma, Inc., for use of ACCENT. Financial Support for the research was provided by grants from the National Institutes of Health (R01-HL56874) and from Astra Zeneca Pharmaceuticals.

References

1. Yuan, C., Mitsumori, L. M., Beach, K. W., and Maravilla, K. R., Carotid atherosclerotic plaque: noninvasive MR characterization and identification of vulnerable lesions, *Radiology*, Vol. 221, No. 2, pp. 285–299, 2001.
2. Davies, M. J. and Thomas, A. C., Plaque fissuring: the cause of acute myocardial infarction, sudden ischaemic death, and crescendo angina, *Br. Heart J.*, Vol. 53, pp. 363–373, 1985.
3. Falk, E., Stable versus unstable atherosclerosis: clinical aspects, *Am. Heart J.*, Vol. 138, No. 5 Pt. 2, pp. S421–S425, 1999.
4. McCarthy, M. J., Loftus, I. M., Thompson, M. M., Jones, L., London, N. J., Bell, P. R., Naylor, A. R., and Brindle, N. P., Angiogenesis and the atherosclerotic carotid plaque: an association between symptomatology and plaque morphology, *J. Vasc. Surg.*, Vol. 30, No. 2, pp. 261–268, 1999.
5. Virmani, R., Kolodgie, F. D., Burke, A. P., Farb, A., and Schwartz, S. M., Lessons from sudden coronary death: a comprehensive morphological classification

scheme for atherosclerotic lesions, *Arterioscler. Thromb. Vasc. Biol.*, Vol. 20, No. 5, pp. 1262–1275, 2000.

6. Glagov, S., Bassiouny, H. S., Giddens, D. P., and Zarins, C. K., Pathobiology of plaque modeling and complication, *Surg. Clin. North Am.*, Vol. 75, No. 4, pp. 545–556, 1995.

7. Yuan, C., Kang, X., Xu, D., and Hatsukami, T., Lesion index: a quantitative measure of atherosclerotic lesion complexity and progression in MR images, *Proc. ISMRM*, p. 85, 1999.

8. ECST Collaborative Group, Randomised trial of endarterectomy for recently symptomatic carotid stenosis: final results of the MRC European Carotid Surgery Trial (ECST), *Lancet*, Vol. 351, No. 9113, pp. 1379–1387, 1998.

9. O'Leary, D. H., Polak, J. F., Kronmal, R. A., Manolio, T. A., Burke, G. L., and Wolfson, S. K., Carotid artery intima and media thickness as a risk factor for myocardial infarction and stroke in older adults, *N. Engl. J. Med.*, Vol. 340, No. 1, pp. 14–22, 1999.

10. Wiklund, O., Hulthe, J., Wikstrand J., Schmidt, C., Olofsson, S. O., and Bondjers, G., Effect of controlled release/extended release metoprolol on carotid intima media thickness in patients with hypercholesterolemia: a 3-year randomized study, *Stroke*, Vol. 33, No. 2, pp. 572–577, 2002.

11. Rumberger, J. A., Brundage, B. H., Rader, D. J., and Kondos, G., Electron beam computed tomographic coronary calcium scanning: a review and guidelines for use in asymptomatic persons, *Mayo Clin. Proc.*, Vol. 74, No. 3, 1999.

12. Sutton-Tyrrell, K., Kuller, L. H., Edmundowicz, D., Feldman, A., Holubkov, R., Givens, L., and Matthews, K. A., Usefulness of electron beam tomography to detect progression of coronary and aortic calcium in middle-aged women, *Am. J. Cardiol.*, Vol. 87, No. 5, pp. 560–564, 2001.

13. Rumberger, J. A., Sheedy, P. F., Breen, J. F., and Schwartz, R. S., Electron beam computed tomographic coronary calcium score cutpoints and severity of associated angiographic lumen stenosis, *J. Am. Coll. Cardiol.*, Vol. 29, No. 7, pp. 1542–1548, 1997.

14. Vliegenthart, R., Hollander, M., Breteler, M. M., van der Kuip, D. A., Hofman, A., Oudkerk, M., and Witteman, J. C., Stroke is associated with coronary calcification as detected by electron-beam CT: The Rotterdam Coronary Calcification Study, *Stroke*, Vol. 33, No. 2, pp. 462–465, 2002.

15. Oliver, T. B., Lammie, G. A., Wright, A. R., Wardlaw, J., Patel, S. G., Peek, R., Ruckley, C. V., and Collie, D. A., Atherosclerotic plaque at the carotid bifurcation: CT angiographic appearance with histopathological correlation, *Am. J. Neuroradiol.*, Vol. 20, No. 5, pp. 897–901, 1999.

16. Halliburton, S. S. and Paschal, C. B., Atherosclerotic plaque components in human aortas contrasted by *ex vivo* imaging using fast spin-echo magnetic resonance imaging and spiral computed tomography, *Invest. Radiol.*, Vol. 31, No. 11, 1996.

17. Barzilai, B., Saffits, J. E., Miller, J. G., and Sobel, B. E., Quantitative ultrasonic characterization of the nature of atherosclerotic plaques in human aorta, *Circ. Res.*, Vol. 60, No. 3, 459–463.

18. Zhang, X., McKay, C. R., and Sonka, M., Tissue characterization in intravascular ultrasound images, *IEEE Trans. Med. Imag.*, Vol. 17, No. 6, pp. 889–899, 1998.

19. Incandela, L., Belcaro, G., Nicolaides, A. N., Cesarone, M. R., DeSanctis, M. T., Corsi, M., Bavera, P., Ippolito, E., Griffin, M., Geroulakos, G., Sabetai, M.,

Ramaswami, G., and Veller, M., Modification of the echogenicity of femoral plaques after treatment with total triterpenic fraction of Centella asiatica: a prospective, randomized, placebo-controlled trial, *Angiology*, Vol. 52 (Suppl. 2), pp. S69–S73, 2001.

20. Estes, J. M., Quist, W. C., Lo Gerfo, F. W., and Costello, P., Noninvasive character-ization of plaque morphology using helical computed tomography, *J. Cardiovasc. Surg. (Torino)*, Vol. 39, No. 5, pp. 527–534, 1998.

21. Vallabhajosula, S. and Fuster, V., Atherosclerosis: imaging techniques and the evolving role of nuclear medicine, *J. Nucl. Med.*, Vol. 38, No. 11, pp. 1788–1796, 1997.

22. Shinnar, M., Fallon, J. T., Wehrli, S., Levin, M., Dalmacy, D., Fayad, Z. A., Badimon, J. J., Harrington, M., Harrington, E., and Fuster, V., The diagnostic accuracy of *ex vivo* MRI for human atherosclerotic plaque characterization, *Arterioscler. Thromb. Vasc. Biol.*, Vol. 19, pp. 2756–2761, 1999.

23. Yuan, C., Hatsukami, T. S., and O'Brien, K. D., High-resolution magnetic reso-nance imaging of normal and atherosclerotic human coronary arteries *ex vivo*: discrimination of plaque tissue components, *J. Invest. Med.*, Vol. 49, No. 6, pp. 491–499, 2001.

24. Hatsukami, T. S., Ross, R., Polissar, N. L., and Yuan, C., Visualization of fibrous cap thickness and rupture in human atherosclerotic plaque *in vivo* with high-resolution magnetic resonance imaging, *Circulation*, Vol. 102, No. 9, pp. 959–964, 2000.

25. Yuan, C., Mitsumori, L. M., Ferguson, M. S., Polissar, N. L., Echelard, D., Ortiz, G., Small, R., Davies, J. W., Kerwin, W. S., and Hatsukami, T. S., *In vivo* accuracy of multispectral magnetic resonance imaging for identifying lipid-rich necrotic cores and intraplaque hemorrhage in advanced human carotid plaques, *Circulation*, Vol. 104, pp. 2051–2056, 2001.

26. Yuan, C., Kerwin, W. S., Ferguson, M. S., Polissar, N., Zhang, S., Cai, J., and Hatsukami, T. S., Contrast-enhanced high resolution MRI for atherosclerotic carotid artery tissue characterization, *J. Magn. Reson. Imag.*, Vol. 15, pp. 62–67, 2002.

27. Kerwin, W. S., Ferguson, M. S., Hatsukami, T. S., and Yuan, C., Analysis of dynamic contrast-enhanced MRI of carotid atherosclerosis quantifies plaque neovasculature, *Proc. ISMRM*, 2002.

28. Zhao, X. Q., Yuan, C., Hatsukami, T. S., Frechette, E. H., Kang, X. J., Maravilla, K. R., and Brown, B. G., Effects of prolonged intensive lipid-lowering therapy on the characteristics of carotid atherosclerotic plaques *in vivo* by MRI: a case-controlled study, *Arterioscler. Thromb. Vasc. Biol.*, Vol. 21, No. 10, pp. 1623–1629, 2001.

29. Fayad, Z. A., Nahar, T., Fallon, J. T., Goldman, M., Aguinaldo, J. G., Badimon, J. J., Shinnar, M., Chesebro, J. H., and Fuster, V., *In vivo* magnetic resonance eval-uation of atherosclerotic plaques in the human thoracic aorta, a comparison with transesophageal echocardiography, *Circulation*, Vol. 101, pp. 2503–2509, 2000.

30. Fayad, Z. A., Fuster, V., Fallon, J. T., Jayasundera, T., Worthley, S. G., Helft, G., Aguinaldo, J. G., Badimon, J. J., and Sharma, S. K., Noninvasive *in vivo* human coronary artery lumen and wall imaging using black-blood magnetic resonance imaging, *Circulation*, Vol. 102, pp. 506–510, 2000.

31. Rogers, W. J., Prichard, J. W., Hu, Y. L., Olson, P. R., Benckart, D. H., Kramer, C. M., Vido, D. A., and Reichek, N., Characterization of signal properties in

atherosclerotic plaque components by intravascular MRI, *Aterioscler. Thromb. Vasc. Biol.*, Vol. 20, pp. 1824–1830, 2000.

32. Weiss, C. R., Arai, A. E., Bui, M. N., Agyeman, K. O., Waclawiw, M. A., Balaban, R. S., and Cannon, R. O., Arterial wall MRI characteristics are associated with elevated serum markers of inflammation in humans, *J. Magn. Reson. Imag.*, Vol. 14, No. 6, 698–704, 2001.

33. Kerwin, W. S., Ferguson, M. S., and Yuan, C., Use of magnetization transfer imaging to identify atherosclerotic plaque components: evaluation on carotid endarterectomy specimens, *J. Cardiovsc. Magn. Reson.*, Vol. 3, No. 2, p. 61, 2001.

34. de Boer, O. J., van der Wal, A. C., Teeling, P., and Becker, A. E., Leucocyte recruitment in rupture prone regions of lipid-rich plaques: a prominent role for neovascularization?, *Cardiovasc. Res.*, Vol. 41, No. 2, pp. 443–449, 1999.

35. Mofidi, R., Crotty, T. B., McCarthy, P., Sheehan, S. J., Mehigan, D., and Keaveny, T. V., Association between plaque instability, angiogenesis and symptomatic carotid occlusive disease, *Br. J. Surg.*, Vol. 88, No. 7, pp. 945–950, 2001.

36. Tofts, P. S. and Kermode, A. G., Measurement of the blood-brain barrier permeability and leakage space using dynamic MR imaging. 1. Fundamental concepts, *Magn. Reson. Med.*, Vol. 17, No. 2, pp. 357–367, 1991.

37. Kerwin, W. S., Cai, J., and Yuan, C., Noise and motion correction in dynamic contrast-enhanced MRI for analysis of atherosclerotic lesions, *Magn. Reson. Med.*, Vol. 47, No. 6, pp. 1211–1217, 2002.

38. Evelhoch, J. L., Key factors in the acquisition of contrast kinetic data for oncology, *J. Magn. Reson. Imag.*, Vol. 10, No. 3, pp. 254–259, 1999.

39. Buxton, R. B., Frank, L. R., and Prasad, P. V., Principles of diffusion and perfusion MRI, in Edelman, Hesselink, and Zlatkin, Eds., *Clinical Magnetic Resonance Imaging*, W. B. Saunders Co., Philadelphia, pp. 233–270, 1996.

40. Ludemann, L., Hamm, B., and Zimmer, C., Pharmacokinetic analysis of glioma compartments with dynamic Gd-DTPA-enhanced magnetic resonance imaging, *Magn. Reson. Imag.*, Vol. 18, No. 10, pp. 1201–1214, 2000.

41. Aoki, S., Aoki, K., Ohsawa, S., Nakajima, H., Kumagai, H., and Araki, T., Dynamic MR imaging of the carotid wall, *J. Magn. Reson. Imag.*, Vol. 9, No. 3, pp. 420–427, 1999.

42. Kampschulte, A., Kerwin, W. S., Ferguson, M. S., Hatsukami, T. S., and Yuan, C., Evidence of adventitial enhancement in carotid atherosclerosis visualized by MRI, 2002 (submitted).

43. Kerwin, W., Han, C., Chu, B., Xu, D., Luo, Y., Hwang, J. N., Hatsukami, T., and Yuan, C., A quantitative vascular analysis system for evaluation of atherosclerotic lesions by MRI, in Niessen and Viergever, Eds., *Medical Image Computing and Computer-Assisted Intervention*, Springer, Berlin, pp. 786–794, 2001.

44. Han, C., Hatsukami, T. S., and Yuan, C., A multi-scale method for automatic correction of intensity non-uniformity in MR images, *J. Magn. Reson. Imag.*, Vol. 13, No. 3, pp. 428–436, 2001.

45. Rosas-Romero, R., Hwang, J. N., and Yuan, C., Tracking of 3D objects with non-rigid deformation estimation in medical images, *Proc. Int. Conf. Imaging Science and Technology*, 1998.

46. Kerwin, W. S. and Yuan, C., Active edge maps for medical image registration, *Proc. SPIE*, Vol. 4322, pp. 516–526, 2001.

47. Han, C., Kerwin, W., Miller, Z., Hwang, J. N., Hatsukami, T., and Yuan, C., Image segmentation based on watershed and evolutionary computation, *Proc. ISMRM*, 2002.
48. Hawkes, D. J., Algorithms for radiologic image registration and their clinical application, *J. Anat.*, Vol. 193, pp. 347–361, 1998.
49. Wyman, B. T., Stork, C. L., Price, R. E., Hazle, J. D., Gavin, P. R., Tucker, R. L., and Smith, J. P., Evaluation of automatic guided specific tissue segmentation using VX-2 tumor in the rabbit, *Proc. ISMRM*, p. 581, 2000.
50. Xu, C., Pham, D. L., Rettmann, M. E., Yu, D. N., and Prince, J. L., Reconstruction of the human cerebral cortex from magnetic resonance images, *IEEE Trans. Med. Imag.*, Vol. 18, No. 6, pp. 467–480, 1999.
51. Haig, T. and Attikiouzel, Y., Segmentation of serial contours for biomedical applications, *J. Elec. Electronic. Eng. - Aus.*, Vol. 10, pp. 36–42, 1990.
52. Pham, D. L. and Prince, J. L., Adaptive fuzzy segmentation of magnetic resonance images, *IEEE Trans. Med. Imag.*, Vol. 18, No. 9, pp. 737–752, 1999.
53. Wahba, G., *Spline Models for Observational Data*, SIAM, Philadelphia, 1990.
54. Kerwin, W. S. and Yuan, C., Three dimensional surface models of carotid atherosclerosis, *Proc. Signal and Image Processing*, 2002.

9

Plaque Morphological Quantitation

Chao Han and Chun Yuan

CONTENTS

9.1 Background

According to the National Center for Health Statistics, cardiovascular disease is the leading cause of death in the United States. Carotid atherosclerosis is one of the main causes of stroke. Improved methods of diagnosis, treatment, and prevention of these diseases would result in significant improvement in quality of life and decrease in healthcare costs [1].

Traditionally, the degree of lumen stenosis is used as a morphological marker for high-risk (vulnerable) plaques. Clinically, x-ray, CT, ultrasound, and MR angiography are used to determine lumen stenosis. The determination of lumen stenosis lacks a unified approach, as evidenced by the two methods of stenosis quantification in the North American Symptomatic Carotid Endarterectomy Trial (NASCET) [2] and the European Carotid Surgery Trial [3]. Regardless of which method is used, two clinical trials (the North American Symptomatic Carotid Endarterectomy Trial and the Asymptomatic Carotid Atherosclerosis Study) demonstrate that lumen narrowing is a poor indicator of vulnerability, predicting only one out of four strokes in symptomatic patients [2] and one out of ten in asymptomatic patients [4].

Some studies indicate the importance of plaque morphological factors (in addition to stenosis) in determining thromboembolic risk. Specifically, ultrasonographic studies show that plaque thickness is a better predictor of transient ischemic attacks than vessel stenosis [5, 6]. Unfortunately, ultrasound measurement of plaque thickness is not highly reproducible, with coefficients of variation between 13.8 and 22.4% [7]. Further evidence of the importance of plaque morphology was documented in a study by NASCET investigators showing increasing risk for stroke with ulcerated plaques compared to nonulcerated plaques with similar degrees of stenosis [8]. These results suggest that a comprehensive, quantitative analysis of plaque morphology, including lumen stenosis, wall thickness, and ulceration, will better identify vulnerable plaques.

Recent studies have shown that magnetic resonance imaging (MRI) is capable of identifying plaque constituents and measuring plaque morphology [1, 9]. MR plaque imaging may therefore be a unique technique that can characterize plaque morphology and tissue constituents in one examination, assessing both aspects of vulnerable plaque.

Some challenges in calculating the indexes still exist in developing plaque morphological quantitation: (1) accurate tracing lumen and wall boundaries, (2) a reasonable definition of carotid wall thickness, (3) accurate computation of lumen surface roughness, and (4) a reasonable definition of plaque burden descriptors.

9.2   Active Contour Model

Boundary extraction is one of the fundamental tasks in computer vision and image processing. Many methods [11] have been proposed for various types of images. Although the edges of objects in images can be easily shown by Canny [12] or Laplacian [13] methods, correct contour detection requires high-level knowledge and this calls for the active contour method [11]. How to convert high-level knowledge into exerting energy (or force) in the contour detection has become one of the most important tasks within the active contour model research in recent years.

The active contour model, also termed "snake" because of the nature of its evolution, is a sophisticated approach to contour extraction and image interpretation. The determination of the presence of an object contour depends not only on the local image force at a specific point, but also on the properties of a contour's shape. An active contour model, introduced by Kass et al. [14], has been used considerably and studied in the last decade. In this approach, an energy-minimizing contour is controlled by a combination of the following two components: one controls the smoothness of the contour and the other attracts the contour toward the object boundary. Although the implementation of this approach is sensitive to its initial position and is vulnerable to image noise, it provides a powerful interactive tool for image segmentation and has been investigated extensively among the model-based techniques [11].

Caselles et al. [21] proposed a geodesic active contour model based on a level set method developed by Osher and Sethian [22]. They have proven that a particular case of the classical energy snake model is equivalent to finding a geodesic or minimal distance path in a Riemannian space with a metric derived from the image content. This means that under a specific framework, boundary detection can be considered equivalent to finding a path of minimal weighted length via an active contour model based on geodesic or local minimal distance computation. Nevertheless, no method has been proposed for finding the minimal paths within their geodesic active contour model.

Cohen et al. [23] proposed a global minimal path approach, based on fast marching method [24], for their active contour models. It detects the global minimum energy path between two endpoints. Although this approach requires user intervention to mark some initial endpoints on the true boundary, it does permit a better handling of the noise than the other active contour models [23, 25]. Nevertheless, little attention is paid to how to design an "ideal potential" to determine the precise contour. In contrast, Gerger et al. [15] further took advantage of *a priori* knowledge of initial endpoints to design a potential window as the search constraints for their dynamic programming active contour model.

Moreover, Mortensen and Barrett [26] proposed an intelligent scissors approach to detect the optimal path within a weighted graph between two endpoints, based on Dijkstra's graph search method [27]. Dijkstra's graph search method is similar to the fast marching method [24] in the sense that both methods search for a running cost to find the shortest path, but their basic philosophies differ. Dijkstra's graph search method uses a grid with prescribed weights to find an optimal path. The fast marching method, on the other hand, is a computational technique that approximates the solution to nonlinear Eikonal equations. Although graph search methods solve minimal path problems much more directly than the fast marching method, they suffer from "metrication errors." That is, a rectangular grid with an equal unit weight entered for each link will produce multiple paths between the two endpoints with the same cost [23, 24]. Therefore, changing the structure of the grid is very important for reducing the "metrication error" frequently encountered in the classical graph search methods.

In this section, a fast minimal path active contour model is presented using a graph search method based on a defining potential window between two endpoints. A potential window defines a narrow band with a list of displacement vectors that are nearly perpendicular to the desired boundary, based on conic curves [30, 31]. The points on the displacement vectors have been resampled, based on the original rectangular grid, to reduce the "metrication errors" between two endpoints. In the potential window, a minimal path approach is conducted based on the classical A* graph search method [32, 33]. The A* method is essentially Dijkstra's method with an additional heuristic that can be used to add intelligent information for the path search. There are four steps for implementing the new approach:

1. Some initial endpoints are placed on or near the desired boundary through an interactive interface.

2. A potential window is defined between two endpoints and a list of displacement vectors is created for the later graph search method.

3. The boundary is searched according to the minimal path principle over the potential windows.

4. The searched boundary is calibrated to reduce the sensitivity of the search results on the selected initial endpoints using a "wriggling" procedure.

All steps are performed automatically, except for Step 1, placing the initial endpoints.

The potential window systematically provides a reasonable framework for the later graph search method. Therefore, the new minimal path active contour model has the following distinct features:

1. The "wriggling" procedure can make the contour evolve in a direction nearly perpendicular to the actual contour. This is similar to the contour evolution process in the geodesic active contour model [21].

2. Search time is decreased.

3. The "metrication error" [23, 24] occurring in the classical graph search method is reduced.

4. It satisfies the consistent property as the grid is refined. These features can significantly reduce "metrication error" and make the artery outer-wall boundary tracing stable and robust even when the MR image boundaries are unclear.

9.2.1 Energy Formulation for Minimal Path Active Contour Model

The classical snake [14], proposed by Kass et al., has the following energy formulation:

$$E(c) = \alpha \int_{\Omega} |C'(v)|^2 dv + \beta \int_{\Omega} |C''(v)|^2 dv - \lambda \int_{\Omega} |\nabla I(C(v))| dv \qquad (9.1)$$

where α, β, and λ are real positive weighting constants; $\Omega \in [0, 1]$ is the parameterization interval for contour C; and ∇I is the gradient of the image. Solving the problem of snakes results in finding the contour C that E minimizes for a given set of the constants α, β, and λ. Let $\beta = 0$ and $-|\nabla I|$ be replaced by $g(|\nabla I|)^2$; the energy function becomes:

$$E(c) = \alpha \int_{\Omega} |C'(v)|^2 dv + \lambda \int_{\Omega} |g(\nabla I(C(v))|)^2 dv \qquad (9.2)$$

where g is a potential that is strictly decreasing, so that $g(r) \longrightarrow 0$ as $r \longrightarrow \infty$. Caselles et al. [21] deduce a new formula for minimizing Equation 9.2 in a Riemannian space as follows:

$$Min \int_\Omega g(|\nabla I(C(v))|) * |C'(v)|dv \qquad (9.3)$$

where the Euclidean length of the contour C is : $L(C) = \int_\Omega |C'(v)|dv = \int_\Omega ds$. From Equation 9.3, the classical energy minimization can be transformed to the search of a global minimal path over the weighting Euclidean of length ds weighted by $g(|\nabla I(C(v))|)$. In this section, we build upon this formulation to design a new minimal path approach for contour extraction.

9.2.2 The New Minimal Path Formulation

From Equation 9.3 we know that the classical snake method can be realized by the minimal path approach, whose main contribution to the classical snake method is the complexity reduction in the high-order gradient computing and the avoidance of the minimization from the corresponding Euler equation [14]. Cohen and Kimmel [23] defined a slightly different active contour model for the minimal path approach:

$$Min \int_\Omega (w + g(|\nabla I(C(v))|)) * |C'(v)|dv \qquad (9.4)$$

where w is a constant parameter, used for measuring the length of the contour. We would like to use Equation 9.3 to introduce our minimal path approach with a potential window, which will be defined in a later section, to control the contour evolution. Here, we define the potential $g(\nabla I)$ as the following explicit form:

$$g_i(\nabla I(C_i)) = \frac{1}{1 + |\nabla I(C_i)|^p} \qquad (9.5)$$

where i is a point on the contour C, and $p = 1$ or 2. The potential $g_i(\nabla I)$ is used for attracting the contour to the high gradient area. The Euclidean distance between neighboring points, (x_i, y_i) and (x_{i-1}, y_{i-1}) on the contour, is defined as:

$$s_i = \sqrt{(x_i - x_{i-1})^2 + (y_i - y_{i-1})^2} \qquad (9.6)$$

Plugging Equations 9.5 and 9.6 into Equation 9.3, the minimal path is thus defined as follows:

$$\arg\min_{c_1,c_2,...,c_n}\left(\sum_{i\in\Omega} g_i * s_i\right) \qquad (9.7)$$

where Ω is the target contour for the minimal path search.

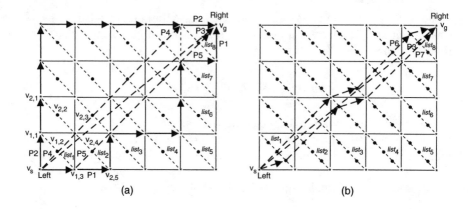

FIGURE 9.1

Node format for the graph-based search methods and path from the lower left to the upper right corner.

9.2.3 Basic Graph Search Procedure

Although the classical graph-based search methods, such as dynamical programming, Dijkstra, and A^* method, are more efficient than level set methods, they suffer from the "metrication errors" [23, 24], which are caused by image pixel format. The classical graph-based search methods consider an image as a graph with a rectangular grid in which each pixel is a node. Under the assumption that a rectangular grid is given with an equal unit weight for each entered link, various Manhattan shortest paths with the same cost between two endpoints are obtained by the graph search methods with an inconsistent property [24]; for example, the cost of the shortest path $P1$ is equal to the cost of $P2$ from the lower left to the upper right corners of the graph in Figure 9.1, but the analytic path is a straight-line diagonal $P3$. This inconsistent property indicates that refinement of this rectangular grid will not produce a solution that converges on the analytic path.

To overcome this problem, a new graph search scheme is introduced. As shown in Figure 9.1a, a list of displacements, produced by connecting the old nodes, are nearly perpendicular to the line between two endpoints, and are used to reformulate the nodes for the later graph search. Some new nodes are inserted between the old nodes on the displacements (e.g., $v_{2,2}$ and $v_{2,4}$ are new nodes in the second displacement in Figure 9.1a). For simplicity, we shall denote the kth displacement as $list_k$.

The basic graph search procedure is from one node on $list_k$ to a set of nodes collectively represented by the next $list_{k+1}$, rather than row-by-row and/or column-by-column in the classical graph search method. Based on the new node connection, the basic graph search procedure will produce a unique solution, for example, the shortest path in Figure 9.1a from the lower left to the upper right corner is path $P4$ using Dijkstra method, although path $P5$ has the same cost as $P4$. This is because the Euclidean distance between nodes

TABLE 9.1

Costs of the Shortest Paths under Conditions of Equal Unit Weight and unit Euclidean Distance between Old Neighboring Nodes in Figure 9.1

Paths	$P1$ or $P2$	$P3$	$P4$ or $P5$	$P6$ or $P7$
Cost	9.0	6.4031	6.6569	6.5308

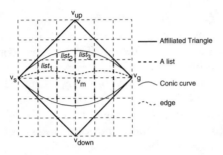

FIGURE 9.2
Construction of potential window from two conic curves.

is not isotropic while using the basic graph search procedure, so that $P4$ can be distinguished from the others. In Figure 9.1b, the shortest path is path $P6$. Comparing Figure 9.1a with the one new interpolated node and Figure 9.1b with the three new interpolated nodes between two old nodes, the shortest paths $P6$ and $P7$ more closely approximate the optimal path $P3$ than paths $P4$ and $P5$ do. Table 9.1 lists the cost of these shortest paths under conditions of equal unit weight and unit Euclidean distance between old neighboring nodes. These comparisons demonstrate that the new node connection has a consistent property; that is, the approximate solution can converge to the analytic solution while the grid is being refined. The new node connection not only reduces the "metrication errors" existing in the classical graph search methods, but also provides a way to design a new contour evolution model, for example, the "wriggling" method (to be discussed later), due to the existence of a unique solution at each search step between the selected endpoints. This unique property promises that the search result is stable and optimal.

Here, the *lists* between the two selected endpoints are constructed using two conic curves [30, 31] (to be described later), as shown in Figure 9.2, which start at one endpoint and indicate toward the other endpoint and form a potential window, that is, define a limited area to speed up the search. The $list_k$ in the window contains displacements that connect the corresponding k^{th} node on two sides of the conic curves. The *lists* produced by this method are nearly perpendicular to the desired boundary.

There are two frequently used graph-based algorithms: one is the graph search, the other is dynamic programming. The latter method often suffers from being stuck in an undesirable local minimal energy point, resulting in an incorrect contour. The A^* method of graph search is thus chosen to design our new minimal path active contour model in this section because heuristic information can help to constrain the search, and thus avoid the local minimum problem.

9.2.4   The "Wriggling" Evolution of a Contour

We know that the basic minimal path active contour model requires the selected endpoints on the desired boundary, because the boundary search takes place between the two selected endpoints. The searched contour is sensitive to the initial nodes. To reduce this problem, a "wriggling" procedure is designed to evolve the contour toward the true boundary along a direction nearly perpendicular to the contour. The "wriggling" procedure is realized by repeating the basic minimal path approach between two newly selected endpoints on the searched contour. Only two new endpoints are selected on the searched contour at each "wriggling" step.

Before describing the "wriggling" procedure, we need to introduce three concepts: wriggle-arc, precedence-contour, and successor-contour. The arc distance between the newly selected endpoints is termed the wriggle-arc. The new wriggled contour is termed the precedence-contour, and the other contour that doesn't wriggle at this step is termed the successor-contour. At each "wriggling" step, only one precedence-contour exists on the contour; the other contour is the successor-contour.

The "wriggling" evolution of a contour can be described as follows. Two endpoints are chosen from the original contour to start the evolution. Then, two new endpoints are chosen with an appropriate wriggle-arc: one on the precedence-contour and the other on the successor-contour. The new precedence-contour is defined based on the two most recently selected endpoints. Keeping a consistent direction along the contour (e.g., the clockwise direction), the algorithm continuously chooses two new endpoints: one on the precedence-contour and the other on the successor-contour for the next "wriggling" step. While this basic procedure repeats, the contour evolves under the control of the active contour model energy and heuristic information.

An example of choosing the endpoints for "wriggling" evolution of a contour is shown in Figure 9.3. After a search for the first minimal path is finished using the user-selected initial endpoints, the original contour is defined. The two endpoints a_1, a_0 are chosen from the contour for initial "wriggling" evolution of contour with appropriate wriggle-arc. The precedence-contour can be defined based on the endpoints a_1, a_0 using the basic minimal path search. For the next wriggle step, one endpoint b_1 is chosen on the precedence-contour and the other b_0 on the successor-contour. The new "wriggling" evolution is conducted between b_1, b_0. If we remain in the same direction of evolution and repeat the selection procedure — one on the precedence-contour and the other on the successor-contour (e.g., c_1, c_0 endpoints) — then the "wriggling" contour will gradually evolve in a direction nearly perpendicular to the contour.

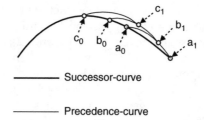

Successor-curve

Precedence-curve

FIGURE 9.3
The wriggling procedure using the minimal path approach. The coarse curve is the old path and
the fine curve is the new minimal path. Only two vertices are chosen while a wriggling procedure
is conducted. When the previous wriggling procedure is finished, we can choose one vertex on
the new wriggled curve and the other vertex on the searched curve.

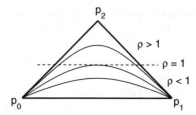

FIGURE 9.4
Different types of conic curves with respect to parameter ρ.

9.2.5 Construction of Potential Window

Given a guiding triangle with vertices p_0, p_1, p_2 and a scalar ρ, a parametric cubic curve can closely approximate a segment of conic polynomial. The
general equation is as follows [30, 31]:

$$p = F_0 \cdot p_0 + F_1 \cdot p_1 + F_2 \cdot \rho \cdot (p_2 - p_0) + F_3 \cdot \rho \cdot (p_1 - p_2) \quad (9.8)$$

where

$$\begin{aligned}
F_0 &= (2u^3 - 3u^2 + 1) \\
F_1 &= (-2u^3 + 3u^2) \\
F_2 &= 4(u^3 - 2u^2 + u) \\
F_3 &= 4(u^3 - u^2)
\end{aligned} \quad (9.9)$$

When $\rho(\rho \in [0, 1])$ is varying and p_0, p_1, p_2 are fixed, the parametric cubic
conic curve represents the following shapes: ellipse, $0 \leq \rho < 0.5$; parabola,
$\rho = 0.5$; and hyperbola, $0.5 < \rho \leq 1$, as shown in Figure 9.4.

To construct the potential window, we need two parametric cubic conic
curves to connect the two end nodes. Thus, two triangles are required to

construct the two curves. The steps to construct the triangles are: (1) connect two endpoints to form a segment (e.g., connect v_s and v_g in Figure 9.2); (2) find the middle point on the segment, (e.g., v_m in Figure 9.2); (3) rotate the segment 90° around the middle point; and (4) connect each endpoint of the segment with the two new endpoints of the rotated segment to construct two triangles (e.g., a triangle with vertices (v_s, v_g, v_{up}) and a triangle with (v_s, v_g, v_{down}) in Figure 9.2). Based on the two generated triangles, the two conic curves are obtained. The dense lists are acquired by connecting the corresponding points on the two curves, as shown in Figure 9.2. The one parameter is used to control the width of the potential window.

9.2.6 Basic Minimal Energy Path Approach

From Equation 9.7 we know that locating an object boundary is accomplished by searching for the path of minimal energy between connected nodes. Here, we use the classical A^* heuristic graph search method [32, 33] to perform the minimal path search. The A^* method iteratively constructs a minimal energy path from a start node v_s to a goal node v_g by extending the best partial path available at each step of the iteration. The node v_p selected for expansion at each step is determined according to an evaluation function $\widehat{g}(v_p)$, which is an estimate of the energy of a path from v_s to v_g, constrained to pass through v_p. The evaluation function $\widehat{g}(v_p)$ can be expressed as:

$$\widehat{g}(v_p) = \widehat{d}(v_p) + \widehat{h}(v_p) \tag{9.10}$$

where $\widehat{d}(v_p)$ is an estimate of the energy of a minimal path from v_s to v_p, and $\widehat{h}(v_p)$ is an estimate of the energy of a minimal path from v_p to v_g. When $\widehat{h}(v_p)$ is set to zero for all nodes, the A^* method becomes the Dijkstra's method [27].

In this new minimal path approach, the potential window is defined as the search area for reducing the computing complexity and the new node connection is also proposed for reducing the "metrication error". Assume that there are M lists $\{list_i, i = 1, \ldots, M\}$ between the nodes v_s and v_g, and there are n_i points, which are expressed as the set $\{V_{n_i}\}$, on the $list_i$. At step 1, we find the point nearest to v_s (i.e., v_s with energy $\widehat{d}_1 = 0$). After $(i - 1)$ steps, where $i < M$, assume that the energy $\widehat{d}_1, \ldots, \widehat{d}_{i-1}$ corresponding to the i nearest points are found. Also assume that those points are numbered $i, \ldots, i - 1$ as they are found, with the starting node as point 1. Then the problem is to find the next nearest point:

$$Minimize(\widehat{d}_{i-1} + \widehat{h}_{i-1,i}) \tag{9.11}$$

where $i - 1$ represents a point v_{i-1} that is already settled, and i is a new point $v_i \in \{V_{n_i}\}$ on the $list_i$. To find the optimal path, it is only the energy $\widehat{h}_{i-1,i}$ that is to be minimized. Here, $\widehat{d}_{i-1}$ is defined as the energy of path from v_s to v_{i-1} given by the accumulation of the arc energy along the path leading v_{i-1} to v_s. $\widehat{h}_{i-1,i}$ is an estimate of the minimal energy from v_{i-1} to v_g through a single

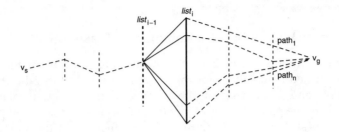

FIGURE 9.5
Basic minimal path approach from $list_{i-1}$ to $list_i$.

point v_i on the $list_i$. Therefore, at step i, there are n_i paths through all points $\{V_{n_i}\}$ on the $list_i$ from v_{i-1} to v_g, (see in Figure 9.5). Because the difference in energy from points $\{V_{n_i}\}$ to v_g is caused by the starting step's energy, we can only choose the limited steps path energy $\widehat{h}_{i-1,i}$ from v_{i-1} to v_g in practice to speed up the search, which is denoted as $\widehat{h}_{i-1,i,t}$.

Suppose that a positive energy $E(v_{k-1}, v_k)$ is attached to the arc, which connects a point v_{k-1} on the $list_{k-1}$ to a point v_k on the $list_k$; then the minimal arc from the old point v_{k-1} to a new point v_k can be expressed as:

$$S(v_{k-1}, v_k) = \min_{v_k} E(v_{k-1}, v_k), \quad v_k \in \{V_{n_k}\} \tag{9.12}$$

where $E(v_{k-1}, v_k) = g_k * s_k, \ k \in n_k$.
Therefore,

$$\widehat{h}_{i-1,i,t} = s(v_{i-1}, v_i) + s(v_i, v_{i+1}) + \cdots + s(v_{t-1}, v_t) \tag{9.13}$$

where t is a limited step for heuristic search. From Equations 9.12 and 9.13, the basic minimal path approach between two endpoints is realized by repeating the basic graph search procedure. Only one point is chosen per list. The minimal energy path is a desired contour, which is composed of the chosen points from the lists.

In summary, the new minimal path search algorithm can be implemented using the following steps:

1. Mark some initial endpoints on or near the boundary of the desired object.
2. Connect iteratively between the pair of endpoints using the basic minimal path approach.
3. Refine the searched boundary with the wriggling procedure using the minimal path principle.
4. Compare the new energy of the minimal path with the old energy of the minimal path of the desired boundary. If the absolute of the energy difference is less than a threshold, then exit; otherwise go to step 3.

9.3   Accurate Lumen Surface Roughness Measurement

Lumen surface quality is one characteristic used to characterize flow distur-
bances generated by small lesions of atherosclerosis. In turn, the characteristics of flow and shear stress on the artery wall are thought to play an important role in the pathogenesis of atherosclerosis and in the development of
complications such as plaque rupture [35, 36]. Mean curvature and Gaussian
curvature are a set of local differential-geometric shape descriptors in classical differential geometry [37]. Gaussian curvature represents intrinsic surface
geometry, whereas mean curvature is extrinsic at individual surface points.
Here, we have chosen the Gaussian curvature to characterize the lumen surface quality of the carotid artery, referred to as roughness.

With the development of medical imaging, high-resolution magnetic resonance imaging (MRI) can produce accurate geometric images of the carotid
artery [38, 39]. The carotid lumen of MR images can be expressed as a stack
of cross-sectional contours, after it is segmented.

Based on these contours, there exist two ways [40] to calculate the roughness
of the lumen surface: one is based on local surface fitting and the other is
based on surface triangulation. In the local surface fit methods, a continuous
differentiable function is used to fit given discrete data, and its derivatives are
computed analytically to evaluate roughness. The drawback of local surface
fit methods is that no compatibility constraints are imposed on these local
surfaces so that the net continuous surfaces interpretation is meaningful; that
is, one needs to make *a priori* assumptions about the digital surface, such as a
surface smoothness assumption, fit window size, and weighting scheme in the
fit window. Making assumptions of these types is contrary to the data-driven
goal of using as few *a priori* assumptions as possible. On the other hand, in
practice, it becomes much more difficult to define constraints for the surface fit,
in part due to the thickness of MR slices; that is, the distance between pixels on
same slice is much smaller than those between slices. In contrast, the discrete
surface triangulation methods can avoid explicit derivative estimates, but the
key problem with these methods becomes finding an appropriate approach
to express the surface with triangles.

To accurately reconstruct the triangulation surface from a set of cross-
sectional contours, two problems need to be addressed. One is the representation of contour; the other is surface optimal tiling. For contour representation, some articles [42, 43] have proposed capturing the contour features.
For surface optimal tiling, Keppel [43] proposed maximizing the volume criterion to tile triangulation surface between two convex contours. This method
requires the decomposition of concave parts of the contours into convex
parts and associating them with the corresponding convex parts on the adjacent contour. Fuchs et al. [44] chose the minimizing surface area criterion to
optimally reconstruct surface triangulation with an approach that is more
intuitive [45]. Nevertheless, there are few articles that consider these two

problems together. Meyers [46] provides a multi-resolution method based on the size of wavelet coefficient constructing a tiling between a pair of planar contours. The amount of detail lost is controlled by appropriate choice of the threshold value. However, this method is not an accurate way to represent the contour because the size of the wavelet coefficient is not enough to characterize the contour properties.

This section presents an accurate roughness measurement method for carotid arteries using the surface triangulation expression. This method is divided into the three sub-problems: (1) representation of contours, (2) optimal surface tiling, and (3) computation of roughness. The B-spline smoothing kernel [47] is used to cope with the noise and to accurately capture the contour features for their representation. The optimal graph-based triangulation tiling technique [43, 45] is used to reconstruct the triangulation surface based on the contour representation. Roughness is computed from triangulating surface without using explicit derivative estimates [40].

9.3.1 Contour Representation

For a given sequence $g(k) \in l_2$, a polynomial B-spline is defined as follows [47]:

$$g(t) = \sum_k c(k)\beta^n(t - k), \quad t \in R, \quad c \in \ell^2 \tag{9.14}$$

where $\beta^n(t)$ is the symmetrical B-spline of order n:

$$\beta^n = \sum_{j=0}^{n+1} \frac{(-1)^j}{n!} \binom{n+1}{j} \left(t + \frac{n+1}{2} - j\right)^n \mu\left(t + \frac{n+1}{2} - j\right), \quad (t \in R) \tag{9.15}$$

where

$$\mu(t) = \begin{cases} 0 & t < 0 \\ 1 & t \geq 0 \end{cases}$$

and $c(k)$ are the spline coefficients used to interpolate the given sequence $g(k)$. The derivative of a given sequence $g(k)$ is formally obtained by differentiating its continuous B-spline representation (Equation 9.14).

$$\frac{\partial g(t)}{\partial t} = \sum_{k=-\infty}^{+\infty} d^{(1)} * c(k)\beta^{n-1}\left(t - k + \frac{1}{2}\right) \tag{9.16}$$

$$\frac{\partial g^2(t)}{\partial t^2} = \sum_{k=-\infty}^{+\infty} d^{(2)} * c(k)\beta^{n-2}(t - k) \tag{9.17}$$

where $d^{(1)}(k) = \delta_0(k) - \delta_0(k - 1)$ and $d^{(2)} = \delta_0(k + 1) - 2\delta_0(k) + \delta_0(k - 1)$ are the first-order and second-order finite difference operators, respectively.

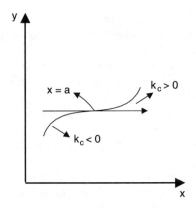

FIGURE 9.6
Information about the sign of cross curvature. If the curvature is positive, then the curve is concave up; if the curvature is negative, then it is concave down; if the curvature changes sign at a point, the curve has a point of inflection there, where the curvature is zero.

For a planar contour $\{r(t) = (x(t), y(t))|t = 1, 2, \ldots, n\}$, the curvature is achieved using the following equations [47]:

$$k(t) = \frac{x'y'' - y'x''}{(\sqrt{x'^2 + y'^2})^3} \qquad (9.18)$$

where the primes denote differentiation computed from Equations 9.16 and 9.17. Therefore, the local concavo-convex direction and the localization of inflection can be confirmed from the property of contour curvature. Figure 9.6 gives information about the sign of cross curvature.

According to the contour curvature, the original contour is represented by a polygonal contour that is used to construct a triangulation surface. The error generated by approximating the original contour is controlled by the predefined threshold. The procedure for representing the original contour is as follows: (1) the original contour is divided into N parts; (2) the maximum curvature point is selected as the vertex within each part; (3) if the area between the line that connects two neighboring vertices and the corresponding contour is bigger than the threshold, a new vertex is inserted with maximum curvature around the middle part of these two vertices. This operation is repeated until the area between neighboring vertices is smaller than the threshold, as shown in Figure 9.7.

9.3.2 Graph-Based Triangulation Tiling

An optimizing algorithm with the maximizing volume criterion [43], proposed by Keppel, can be used to construct the triangulation surface. This method is delimited by the polyhedron surface computed between two

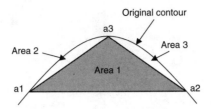

FIGURE 9.7
Approximation of an original contour. The area between vertices a1, a2 and the corresponding contour is a summation of Area 1, Area 2, and Area 3. The area between vertices a1, a3 and the corresponding contour is Area 2. The area between vertices a2, a3 and the corresponding contour is Area 3. Through refining, the approximate error will converge to zero.

convex contours. Thus, all initial vertices should be expressed as convex on the contour. The initial vertices procedure for the triangulation tiling is as follows:

1. Two adjacent contours are extracted from a stack of the polygonal contours.
2. The vertices on the contour are decomposed into vertices subsets of exclusively and alternately convex or concave according to curvature attributes.
3. The concave subsets are transferred to convex subsets by reversing their sequence.

For two adjacent convex polygonal contours, $A_1, A_2, A_3, \ldots, A_m$ and $B_1, B_2, B_3, \ldots, B_n$, their pentahedrons are defined as:

$$P^a = A_i A_{i+1} B_j O_A O_B \quad and \quad P^b = A_i B_j B_{j+1} Q_A Q_B \qquad (9.19)$$

where Q_A and Q_B are the center of polygonal contour, as shown in Figure 9.8. The total volume for the two polygonal contours is written as:

$$V_{TOT} = \sum_a Vol(P^a) + \sum_b Vol(P^b) \qquad (9.20)$$

where

$$P^a (A_i A_{i+1} B_j O_A O_B) = T_1^a (A_i A_{i+1} B_j O_B) + T_2^a (A_i A_{i+1} O_A O_B) \quad (9.21)$$
$$P^b (A_i B_j B_{j+1} O_A O_B) = T_1^b (A_i B_j B_{j+1} O_A) + T_2^b (B_j B_{j+1} O_A O_B) \quad (9.22)$$

Therefore, the total volume is a summation of four kinds of tetrahedrons:

$$V_{TOT} = \sum_a Vol\left(T_1^a\right) + \sum_b Vol\left(T_1^b\right) + c_a + C_b \qquad (9.23)$$

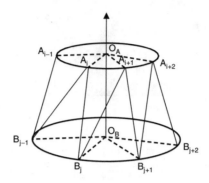

FIGURE 9.8
Volume for the two polygonal contours.

where the two last terms are constant: $c_a = \sum_{i=1}^{m-1} T_2^a (A_i A_{i+1} O_A O_B)$ and $C_b = \sum_{j=1}^{n-1} T_2^b (B_j B_{j+1} O_A O_B)$.

The volumes of the tetrahedrons T_1^a and T_1^b are given by:

$$Vol\left(T_1^a \left(A_i A_{i+1} B_j O_B\right)\right) = \frac{1}{3} (\overrightarrow{O_B A_i} \times \overrightarrow{O_B A_{i+1}}) \overrightarrow{O_B B_j} = v_{i,j}^a \qquad (9.24)$$

$$Vol\left(T_1^b \left(A_i B_j B_{j+1} O_A\right)\right) = \frac{1}{3} (\overrightarrow{O_A B_j} \times \overrightarrow{O_A B_{j+1}}) \overrightarrow{O_A A_i} = v_{i,j}^b \qquad (9.25)$$

where

$$V_{i,j}^a = \frac{1}{3}(Z^B - Z^A)\left(x_i^A y_{i+1}^A - x_{i+1}^A y_i^A + x_j^B y_i^A - x_i^A y_j^B\right) \qquad (9.26)$$

$$V_{i,j}^b = \frac{1}{3}(Z^B - Z^A)\left(x_j^B y_{j+1}^B - x_{j+1}^B y_j^B + x_i^A y_j^B - x_j^B y_i^A\right) \qquad (9.27)$$

and

$$P_i = \left(x_i^P, y_i^P, Z_i^P\right), \quad i = 1, 2, \ldots, m \qquad (9.28)$$

$$Q_i = \left(x_j^Q, y_j^Q, Z_j^Q\right), \quad i = 1, 2, \ldots, n \qquad (9.29)$$

The total volume of the polyhedron, expressed by its Cartesian coordinates, can be rewritten explicitly as:

$$V_{TOT} = \sum_{i,j} V_{i,j}^a + \sum_{i,j} V_{i,j}^b + constant \qquad (9.30)$$

The procedure that finds the triangulation surface between two adjacent convex polygonal contours can be thought of as a "maximum cost graph" search, where each arc represents the volume of the polyhedron [45].

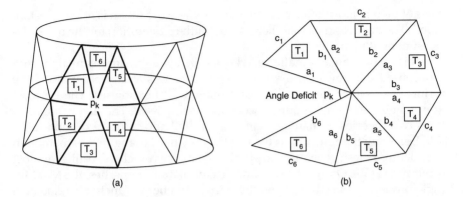

FIGURE 9.9
Discrete Gaussian curvature at a point using angle deficit.

9.3.3 Computation of Gaussian Curvature

Suppose that we look at point P_k on the triangularization of a surface; it is the vertex for T_n different triangles, as shown in Figure 9.9. We assume that the lengths of sides of the ith triangle are a_i, b_i, c_i, where c_i is the length of the side opposite the point of interest and $a_{i+1} = b_i$. The angle deficit at the point c_i is then given by:

$$\Delta_k = 2\pi - \sum_{i=1}^{T_n} \phi_i \tag{9.31}$$

where

$$\phi_i = \cos^{-1}\left(\frac{a_i^2 + b_i^2 - c_i^2}{2a_i b_i}\right) \tag{9.32}$$

The Gaussian curvature at a point is computed based on angle deficit as:

$$K(x) = \frac{2\Delta_k \delta(x - x_k)}{\sum_{i=1}^{N} A_i} \tag{9.33}$$

where

$$A_i = \sqrt{s(s - a_i)(s - b_i)(s - c_i)}, \quad s = \frac{a_i + b_i + c_i}{2} \tag{9.34}$$

and where $\delta(\cdot)$ is the Dirac delta function.

9.4 Thickness Measurement

Wall thickness measurement is a critical factor in determining the atherosclerotic plaque distribution, progression, and regression. Based on the thickness, a set of vascular-shaped descriptors can be developed to distinguish different types of plaque morphology. So far, the thickness definition is not well established. The key reason is that there is no standard definition for the thickness measurement in mathematics.

In this section, an automatic vessel wall thickness measurement algorithm is proposed that can measure vessel wall thickness at any point along the perimeter of either luminal or vessel outer wall boundaries. The only assumption is that a single boundary cannot overlap itself. This algorithm combines two theories: Denaulay triangulation [48] and multi-resolution tiling [49]. Delaunay triangulation is the most widely used triangulation method in unstructured mesh generation in graphics and gives excellent results for most applications [50]. One of the Delaunay triangulation properties, the MaxMin angle property, is used to define the minimum energy function to calculate thickness in this section. The triangulation MaxMin angle lemma provides a way, from theory, to define a minimal energy function based on triangulation angles, which makes geometry computation stable and consistent. The multi-resolution tiling method provides a way to realize the triangulation MaxMin angle lemma to compute vessel wall thickness and make thickness computation stable and unique.

9.4.1 Minimum Energy Function

MaxMin Angle Lemma [48]
Among all triangulations of a finite set $s \subseteq R^2$, the Delaunay triangulation maximizes the minimum angle.

This implies that the smallest angle in any triangulation is no larger than the smallest angle in the Delaunay triangulation. The elementary operation of Delaunay triangulation is edge flipping. Edge flipping does not decrease the smallest angle in a triangulation.

A minimal energy function to compute thickness based on maximizing the minimum angle in a set of triangulations $s \subseteq R^2$ is defined as:

$$\min_{\theta} \left(\frac{1}{\sum_{i=1}^{N} \theta_i} \right) \tag{9.35}$$

where θ_i is a minimum angle in the triangle i, and N is the number of triangulations in $s \subseteq R^2$. The procedure to calculate thickness is to minimize the energy function.

9.4.2 Tiling Optimization

If ab is a "suspect" edge and belongs to two triangles, abc and abd, whose union is a convex quadrangle, then we can flip ab and cd. Formally, this means that ab, abc, and abd are removed from the triangulation and new cd, acd, and bcd are added to the triangulation, as in Figure 9.10. The picture of a flip resembles

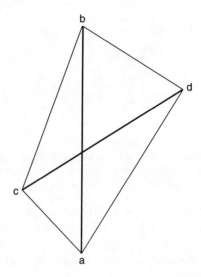

FIGURE 9.10
Edge flipping *ab* to *cd*. Edge flipping does not decrease the smallest angle in Delaunay triangulation.

a tetrahedron with the front and back superimposed. The edge flipping is an elementary operation to convert an arbitrary triangulation to the Delaunay triangulation. The algorithm uses a stack and maintains the invariant that unless an edge is locally Delaunay, it resides on the stack. Initially, all "suspect" edges are pushed on the stack and repeat the following operation.

While stack is non-empty do
    Pop ab from stack and unlabel it;
    If ab not locally Delaunay then
        flip ab to cd;
        for xy ∈ {ac, bd} do
            if xy unlabeled then
                label xy and push it on stack
            endif
        endfor
    endif
endwile

9.4.3   Multi-resolution Tiling

Multi-resolution analysis offers a new approach to optimize the tiling problem. The first step is to reduce the size of the problem using multi-resolution analysis to find low-resolution approximations for the original contours. Detail is then added to the low-resolution tiling by inserting edges at newly

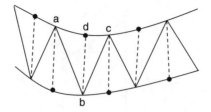

FIGURE 9.11

Insert new vertices and edges from the lower resolution level. For example, vertex *d* is inserted into triangle *abc* in the lower resolution level, which becomes a quadrilateral *abcd*. The inserted edge *bd* split the quadrilateral into two new triangles *abd* and *dbc*.

added vertices and improving the tiling by local edge flipping under control of the minimal energy function. The steps of multi-resolution tiling are as follows:

1. Decompose each contour into a set of low-resolution versions based on wavelet analysis.
2. Compute tiling for the pair of low-resolution contours using the "greedy" method [50].
3. Label all cross edges as "suspect" edges and put them into a stack.
4. Optimize the tiling by flipping the local edge under control of the minimal energy function.
5. Insert a new vertex on both contours at triangle edge of the tiling from the lower resolution level so that the former triangles are now quadrilaterals.
6. Construct an edge from the inserted vertex to the quadrilateral vertex on the other contour, splitting the quadrilateral into two triangles, as shown in Figure 9.11.
7. Label all the old cross edges as "suspect" edges and put them into a stack.
8. Optimize the tiling by flipping the local edge under control of the minimal energy function.
9. Repeat from step 5 to step 9 until the original resolution is reached.

9.5   Carotid Artery Morphological Description

There is clear evidence that carotid artery morphology has strong links to plaque stability [5, 6]. Quantitative morphological descriptors, in conjunction with quantitative measurements of plaque tissue type, will provide a reliable and sensitive means of understanding, monitoring, and predicting the progression of carotid artery atherosclerosis and its effect on the brain.

Morphological description refers to the methods that result in numeric morphological descriptors and is a step subsequent to morphological representation. A morphological description method generates a morphological descriptor vector (also called a feature vector) from a given shape. The goal of description is to uniquely characterize the shape using its morphological descriptor vector. Previous work established the carotid artery MR image reproducibility of *in vivo* measurements of area and volume [51] and their correlation with *ex vivo* measurements. Specifically, volume measurements matched to within 4 to 6% and cross-sectional measurements matched to within 5 to 11%. This provides partial validation of the use of MRI to extract morphological descriptors, but many other descriptors remain to be established and validated.

In this section, a set of carotid artery morphological descriptors is defined based on lumen boundary, wall boundary, and wall thickness. Boundary tracing and thickness computing have been discussed previously. The morphological description includes area descriptors, lumen boundary descriptors, wall boundary descriptors, wall thickness descriptors, complexity thick-lumen descriptors, complexity lumen-wall descriptors, and complexity thick-wall descriptors. The area descriptors show lumen and wall area, as well as their ratio. The lumen boundary descriptors, wall boundary descriptors, and wall thickness descriptors, respectively, demonstrate shape variance themselves. The complexity thick-lumen descriptors, complexity lumen-wall descriptors, and complexity thick-wall descriptors demonstrate their relative variance.

9.5.1 Formulation of Morphological Descriptors

Suppose that a contour has N vertices, the edges connect the vertices in the order $[(x_1, y_1), (x_2, y_2), \ldots, (x_n, y_n)]$, and last vertex is connected to the first vertex. The area of a contour is defined as:

$$Area = \left(\frac{1}{2} \sum_{i=1}^{N} x_i y_{i \oplus 1} - x_{i \oplus 1} y_i \right) \cdot p_x \cdot p_y \qquad (9.36)$$

where $i \oplus 1$ is $(i + 1) \bmod n$, and p_x and p_y are the pixel size. A radius of a contour is defined as a distance from the centroid to a point on the contour. The centroid of a contour is defined as:

$$Centroid(x, y) = \{Centroid(x), Centroid(y)\} = \left\{ \frac{1}{N} \sum_{i=1}^{N} x_i, \frac{1}{N} \sum_{i=1}^{N} y_i \right\} \qquad (9.37)$$

A radius i of a contour is defined as:

$$Radius(i) = \sqrt{(x_i - Centroid(x))^2 \cdot p_x^2 + (y_i - Centroid(y))^2 \cdot p_y^2} \qquad (9.38)$$

A minimum radii of a contour is defined as:

$$MinRadii = \frac{1}{2\sigma} \sum_{i=l_{min}-\sigma}^{l_{min}+\sigma} Radius(i) \tag{9.39}$$

where σ is the neighborhood around the minimum radius location l_{min}:

$$l_{min} = \arg \min_{i=1,2,...,N} (Radius(i)) \tag{9.40}$$

A maximum radii of a contour is defined as:

$$MaxRadii = \frac{1}{2\sigma} \sum_{i=l_{max}-\sigma}^{l_{max}+\sigma} Radius(i) \tag{9.41}$$

where σ is the neighborhood around the maximum radius location l_{max}:

$$l_{max} = \arg \max_{i=1,2,...,N} (Radius(i)) \tag{9.42}$$

A mean of radii of a contour is defined as:

$$MeanRadii = \frac{1}{N} \sum_{i=1}^{N} Radius(i) \tag{9.43}$$

Similarly, suppose that a wall thickness is available with number M. The minimum wall thickness, maximum wall thickness, and mean thickness are defined as:

$$MinThick = \frac{1}{2\sigma} \sum_{i=t_{min}-\sigma}^{t_{min}+\sigma} Thickness(i) \tag{9.44}$$

$$MaxThick = \frac{1}{2\sigma} \sum_{i=t_{max}-\sigma}^{t_{max}+\sigma} Thickness(i) \tag{9.45}$$

$$MeanThick = \frac{1}{M} \sum_{i=1}^{M} Thickness(i) \tag{9.46}$$

where σ is the neighborhood around the minimum thickness location and maximum thickness location:

$$t_{min} = \arg \min_{i=1,2,...,N} (Thickness(i)) \tag{9.47}$$

$$t_{max} = \arg \max_{i=1,2,...,N} (Thickness(i)) \tag{9.48}$$

9.5.2 Morphological Descriptors

9.5.2.1 Area Descriptors

Area descriptors include lumen area (*LumenArea*), outer-wall boundary area (*OuterArea*), wall area (*WallArea*), and the ratio of lumen area to outer-wall boundary area (*LORatio*). The lumen area and outer-wall boundary area are computed from Equation 9.36. The wall area and the ratio are computed from:

$$WallArea = OuterArea - LumenArea \qquad (9.49)$$

$$LORatio = LumenArea/OuterArea \cdot 100\% \qquad (9.50)$$

The *LumenArea*, *OuterArea*, and *WallArea* demonstrate the artery physical area size, and the *LORatio* shows the level of artery stenosis.

9.5.2.2 Lumen Boundary Descriptors

Lumen boundary descriptors include the mean of lumen boundary radii (*MeanLRadii*), minimum lumen boundary radii (*MinLRadii*), maximum lumen boundary radii (*MaxLRadii*), the ratio of minimum lumen boundary radii to maximum lumen boundary radii (*LMMRadii*), the ratio of minimum lumen boundary radii to mean of lumen boundary radii (*LMinDev*), and the ratio of mean of lumen boundary radii to maximum lumen boundary radii (*LMaxDev*). The *MeanLRadii*, *MinLRadii*, and *MaxLRadii* are computed, respectively, from Equations 9.39, 9.41, and 9.43. The *LMM Radii*, *LMinDev*, and *LMaxDev* are calculated from:

$$LMMRadii = (1.0 - MinLRadii/MaxLRadii) \cdot 100\% \qquad (9.51)$$

$$LMinDev = (1.0 - MinLRadii/MeanLRadii) \cdot 100\% \qquad (9.52)$$

$$LMaxDev = (1.0 - MeanLRadii/MaxLRadii) \cdot 100\% \qquad (9.53)$$

The *MeanLRaii*, *MinLRadii*, and *MaxLRadii* demonstrate the physical radius size, and the *LMMRadii*, *LMinDev*, and *LmaxDev* show the level of relative variances between the *MeanLRadii*, *MinLRadii*, and *MaxLRadii*.

9.5.2.3 Outer-Wall Boundary Descriptors

Outer-wall boundary descriptors include the mean of outer-wall boundary radii (*MeanWRadii*), minimum outer-wall boundary radii (*MinWRadii*), maximum outer-wall boundary radii (*MaxWRadii*), the ratio of minimum outer-wall boundary radii to maximum outer-wall boundary radii (*WMMRadii*), the ratio of minimum outer-wall boundary radii to mean of outer-wall boundary radii (*WMinDev*), and the ratio of mean of outer-wall boundary radii to maximum outer-wall boundary radii (*WMaxDev*). The *MeanWRadii*, *MinWRadii*, and *MaxWRadii* are computed, respectively, from Equations 9.39, 9.41, and 9.43. The *WMMRadii*, *WMinDev*, and *WMaxDev* are calculated from:

$$WMMRadii = (1.0 - MinWRadii/MaxWRadii) \cdot 100\% \quad (9.54)$$

$$WMinDev = (1.0 - MinWRadii/MeanWRadii) \cdot 100\% \quad (9.55)$$

$$WMaxDev = (1.0 - MeanWRadii/MaxWRadii) \cdot 100\% \quad (9.56)$$

The *MeanWRaii*, *MinWRadii*, and *MaxWRadii* demonstrate the physical radius size, and the *WMMRadii*, *WMinDev*, and *WMaxDev* show the level of relative variances between the *MeanWRaii*, *MinWRadii*, and *MaxWRadii*.

9.5.2.4 Wall Thickness Descriptors

Wall thickness descriptors include the mean of wall thickness (*MeanThick*), minimum wall thickness (*MinThick*), maximum wall thickness (*MaxThick*), the ratio of minimum wall thickness to maximum wall thickness (*TMMThick*), the ratio of minimum wall thickness to mean of wall thickness (*TMinDev*), and the ratio of mean of wall thickness radii to maximum wall thickness (*TMaxDev*). The *MeanThick*, *MinThick*, and *MaxThick* are computed, respectively, from Equations 9.44, 9.45, and 9.46. The *TMMThick*, *TMinDev*, and *TMaxDev* are calculated from:

$$TMMThick = (1.0 - MinThick/MaxThick) \cdot 100\% \quad (9.57)$$

$$TMinDev = (1.0 - MinThick/MeanThick) \cdot 100\% \quad (9.58)$$

$$TMaxDev = (1.0 - MeanThick/MaxThick) \cdot 100\% \quad (9.59)$$

The *MeanThick*, *MinThick*, and *MaxThick* demonstrate the physical wall thickness size, and the *TMMThick*, *TMinDev*, and *TMaxDev* show the level of relative variances between the *MeanThick*, *MinThick*, and *MaxThick*.

9.5.2.5 Complexity Thick-Lumen Descriptors

Complexity thick-lumen descriptors include the ratio of minimum thickness to mean of lumen radii (*MinTR*), the ratio of maximum thickness to mean of lumen radii (*MaxTR*), and the ratio of mean of thickness to mean of lumen radii (*MeanTR*). The *MinTR*, *MaxTR*, and *MeanRT* demonstrate the level of relative variance between thickness and lumen radii.

$$MinTR = MinThick/MeanLRadii \cdot 100\% \quad (9.60)$$

$$MaxTR = MaxThick/MeanLRadii \cdot 100\% \quad (9.61)$$

$$MeanTR = MeanThick/MeanLRadii \cdot 100\% \quad (9.62)$$

9.5.2.6 Complexity Lumen-Wall Descriptors

Complexity lumen-wall descriptors include the ratio of minimum lumen radii to mean of wall radii (*MinLW*), the ratio of maximum lumen radii to mean of wall radii (*MaxLW*), the ratio of mean of lumen radii to mean of wall radii (*MeanLW*), and ratio of distance between lumen centroid to outer-wall boundary centroid to mean of wall radii (*EccentricityW*). The *MinLW*, *MaxLW*, and *MeanLW* demonstrate the level of relative variance between lumen radii and wall radii. The *EccentricityW* demonstrates the level of relative variance of eccentric distance between lumen boundary and outer-wall boundary to mean of wall radii.

$$MinLW = MinLRadii/MeanWRadii \cdot 100\% \tag{9.63}$$

$$MaxLW = MaxLRadii/MeanWRadii \cdot 100\% \tag{9.64}$$

$$MeanLW = MeanLRadii/MeanWRadii \cdot 100\% \tag{9.65}$$

$$EccentricityW = Dist/MeanWRadii \cdot 100\% \tag{9.66}$$

where

$$Dist = \sqrt{(x_W - x_L)^2 \cdot p_x^2 + (y_W - y_L)^2 \cdot p_y^2} \tag{9.67}$$

and the (x_L, y_L), (x_W, y_W) are the lumen centroid and outer-wall boundary centroid, respectively, and p_x, p_y are the pixel size.

9.5.2.7 Complexity Thick-Wall Descriptors

Complexity thick-wall descriptors include the ratio of minimum wall thickness to mean of wall radii (*MinTW*), the ratio of maximum wall thickness to mean of wall radii (*MaxTW*), and the ratio of mean of wall thickness to mean of wall radii (*MeanTW*). The *MinTW*, *MaxTW*, and *MeanTW* demonstrate the level of relative variance between wall thickness and wall radii.

$$MinTW = MinThick/MeanWRadii \cdot 100\% \tag{9.68}$$

$$MaxTW = MaxThick/MeanWRadii \cdot 100\% \tag{9.69}$$

$$MeanTW = MeanThick/MeanWRadii \cdot 100\% \tag{9.70}$$

9.6 Experimental Results

An example of morphological quantitation is presented in this section. Figure 9.12 shows a series of patient's carotid MR images with extracted contours. Slide 6 is the bifurcation of the common carotid artery. Figure 9.13a is a three-dimensional model with rendered surface shadow. Figure 9.13b is

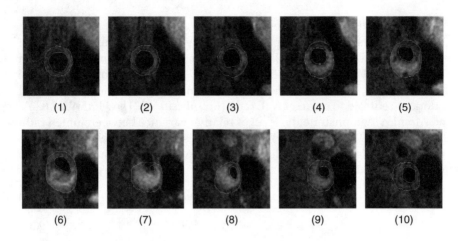

FIGURE 9.12
An example morphological quantitation showing ten consecutive slices with lumen and outer wall contours.

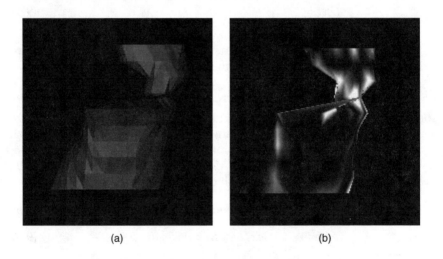

FIGURE 9.13
Three-dimensional model rendered from contours in Figure 9.12.

a three-dimensional model with Guassian curvature mapping. The whiter the surface, the bigger the curvature. Figure 9.14 shows the estimated wall thickness. The bright lines express the maximum and minimum thickness, respectively. Table 9.2 summarizes morphological descriptors calculated from lumen boundary, outer-wall boundary, and wall thickness in this example.

TABLE 9.2

Morphological Descriptors Calculated from Patient Images in Figure 9.12

No.	Lumen Area	Outer Area	LO Ratio	Wall Area	MeanLRadii	MinLRadii	MaxLRadii	LMMRadii
1	26.256	57.872	45.40%	31.616	2.893	2.665	3.069	13.20%
2	25.951	58.34	44.50%	32.389	2.878	2.666	2.945	9.50%
3	22.37	65.918	33.90%	43.548	2.672	2.342	2.932	20.10%
4	17.912	72.538	24.70%	54.626	2.403	2.195	2.661	17.50%
5	15.091	78.223	19.30%	63.132	2.19	1.838	2.518	27.00%
6	14.985	89.102	16.80%	74.117	2.226	1.652	2.816	41.30%
7	1.81	66.142	2.70%	64.331	0.759	0.646	0.81	20.20%
8	6.731	57.278	11.80%	50.546	1.481	1.148	1.941	40.90%
9	8.789	56.118	15.70%	47.33	1.681	1.522	1.89	19.50%
10	14.169	52.516	27.00%	38.347	2.132	1.911	2.348	18.60%

TABLE 9.2

Continued

No.	LMinDev	LMaxDev	MeanWRadii	MinWRadii	MaxWRadii	WMMRadii	WMinDev	WMaxDev
1	7.90%	5.70%	4.318	4.09	4.453	8.20%	5.30%	3.00%
2	7.40%	2.30%	4.332	4.017	4.617	13.00%	7.30%	6.20%
3	12.30%	8.90%	4.598	4.329	4.849	10.70%	5.80%	5.20%
4	8.60%	9.70%	4.815	4.19	5.351	21.70%	13.00%	10.00%
5	16.10%	13.00%	5.001	4.465	5.433	17.80%	10.70%	8.00%
6	25.80%	20.90%	5.35	4.532	6.101	25.70%	15.30%	12.30%
7	14.80%	6.30%	4.605	4.024	5.115	21.30%	12.60%	10.00%
8	22.50%	23.70%	4.289	3.833	4.765	19.60%	10.60%	10.00%
9	9.40%	11.10%	4.247	3.555	4.621	23.10%	16.30%	8.10%
10	10.40%	9.20%	4.097	3.733	4.478	16.60%	8.90%	8.50%

TABLE 9.2
Continued

No.	MeanThick	MinThick	MaxThick	TMMThick	TMinDev	TMaxDev	MinTR	MaxTR
1	1.414	1.061	1.93	45.00%	25.00%	26.70%	36.70%	66.70%
2	1.444	1.092	1.805	39.50%	24.40%	20.00%	37.90%	62.70%
3	1.92	1.221	3.084	60.40%	36.40%	37.70%	45.70%	115.40%
4	2.433	1.203	4.072	70.50%	50.60%	40.20%	50.10%	169.50%
5	2.846	1.188	5.009	76.30%	58.30%	43.20%	54.20%	228.70%
6	3.251	1.35	6.003	77.50%	58.50%	45.80%	60.70%	269.70%
7	4.134	0.815	6.783	88.00%	80.30%	39.10%	107.40%	894.00%
8	2.935	1.077	5.488	80.40%	63.30%	46.50%	72.70%	370.70%
9	2.603	0.938	4.254	78.00%	64.00%	38.80%	55.80%	253.10%
10	1.983	0.726	2.982	75.70%	63.40%	33.50%	34.00%	139.80%

TABLE 9.2
Continued

No.	MeanTR	MinLW	MaxLW	MeanLW	EccentricityW	MinTW	MaxTW	MeanTW
1	48.90%	61.70%	71.10%	67.00%	1.80%	24.60%	44.70%	32.70%
2	50.20%	61.60%	68.00%	66.40%	4.40%	25.20%	41.70%	33.30%
3	71.90%	50.90%	63.80%	58.10%	13.20%	26.60%	67.10%	41.80%
4	101.30%	45.60%	55.30%	49.90%	21.30%	25.00%	84.60%	50.50%
5	130.00%	36.80%	50.30%	43.80%	30.30%	23.80%	100.20%	56.90%
6	146.00%	30.90%	52.60%	41.60%	43.50%	25.20%	112.20%	60.80%
7	544.90%	14.00%	17.60%	16.50%	60.40%	17.70%	147.30%	89.80%
8	198.20%	26.80%	45.30%	34.50%	49.00%	25.10%	128.00%	68.40%
9	154.90%	35.80%	44.50%	39.60%	32.70%	22.10%	100.20%	61.30%
10	93.00%	46.60%	57.30%	52.00%	26.80%	17.70%	72.80%	48.40%

Note: Area in mm^2; thickness in mm.

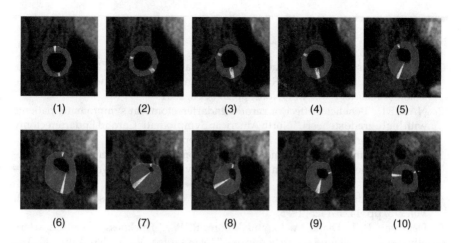

FIGURE 9.14
Thickness maps for images from Figure 9.12.

This table shows that we can easily categorize the different wall shapes into different types based on morphological descriptors. For example, if we use only the *LORatio* as an index to separate the slides, and set the threshold as 20%, slides 1 to 4 are the first group, slides 5 to 9 are the second group, and slide 10 is the third group. These morphological descriptors are a key feature to construct an intelligent database for clinic plaque analysis.

9.7 Conclusion

In this chapter, we presented an overview of the main approaches to characterize carotid plaque morphology. Most of the topics discussed are important and represent broad issues on their own, being covered in several books and in the scientific literature. Nevertheless, we hope that the present chapter can provide the necessary background to understand carotid plaque morphological quantitation analysis.

Acknowledgment

This work was supported in part by grant R01 HL61851 from the NIH.

References

1. Yuan, C., Mitsumori, L. M., Beach, K. W., and Maravilla, K. M., "Carotid atherosclerotic plaque: noninvasive MR characterization and identification of vulnerable lesions," *Radiology*, Vol. 221, No. 2, pp.285–300, 2001.

2. NASCET, "Beneficial effect of carotid endarterectomy in symptomatic patients with high-grade stenosis," North American Symptomatic Carotid Endarterectomy Trial Collaborators, *N. Engl. J. Med.*, Vol. 325, pp. 445–453, 1991.

3. ECST, "Endarterectomy for moderate symptomatic carotid stenosis: interim results from the MRC European Carotid Surgery Trial," *Lancet*, Vol. 347, pp. 1591–1593, 1996.

4. ACAS, "Endarterectomy for asymptomatic carotid artery stenosis," *JAMA*, Vol. 273, pp. 1421–1428, 1995.

5. Dempsey, R. J., Diana, A. L., and Moore, R. W., "Thickness of carotid artery atherosclerotic plaque and ischemic risk," *Neurosurgery*, Vol. 27, No. 3, pp. 343–348, 1990.

6. Iannuzzi, A., Wilcosky, T., Mercuri, M., Rubba, P., Bryan, F. A., and Bond, M. G., "Ultrasonographic correlates of carotid atherosclerosis in transient ischemic attack and stroke," *Stroke*, Vol. 26, No. 4, pp. 614–619, 1995.

7. Joakimsen, O., Bonaa, K. H., and Joakimsen, O., "Reproducibility of ultrasound assessment of carotid plaque occurrence, thickness, and morphology. The Tromso Study," *Stroke*, Vol. 28, No. 11, pp. 2201–2207, 1997.

8. Eliasziw, M., Streifler, J. Y., Fox, A. J., Hachinski, V. C., Ferguson, G. G., and Barnett, H. J., "Significance of plaque ulceration in symptomatic patients with high- grade carotid stenosis. North American Symptomatic Carotid Endarterectomy Trial," *Stroke*, Vol. 25, No. 2, pp. 304–308, 1994.

9. Mitsumori, L. M., Hatsumaki, T. S., Ferguson, M. S., and Yuan, C., "*In vivo* performance of multispectral MR imaging for identifying vulnerable plaques in human carotid arteries," *Circulation*, Vol. 102, No. 18, Suppl. II-252, 2000.

10. Nilsson, N. J., *Problem-Solving Methods in Artificial Intelligence*, McGraw-Hill, New York, 1971.

11. Duncan, J. S. and Ayache, N., "Medical image analysis: progress over two decades and the challenges ahead," *IEEE Trans. Pattern Anal. Mach. Intell.*, Vol. 22, No. 1, pp. 85–106, Jan. 2000.

12. Canny, J., "A computational approach to edge detection," *IEEE Trans. Pattern Anal. Mach. Intell.*, Vol. 8, No. 6, pp. 679–698, Nov. 1986.

13. Mehrotra, R. and Zhan, S. M., "A computational approach to zero-crossing-cased two dimensional edge detection," *Graphical Models and Image Proc.*, Vol. 58, No. 1, pp. 1–17, Jan. 1996.

14. Kass, M., Witkin, A., and Terzopoulos, D., "Snake: active contour models," *Int. J. Computer Vision*, Vol. 1, No. 4, pp. 321–331, 1987.

15. Geiger, D., Gupta, A., Costa, A., and Vlontzos, J., "Dynamic programming for detecting, tracking and matching deformable contours," *IEEE Trans. Pattern Anal. Mach. Intell.*, Vol. 17, No. 3, pp. 294–302, March 1995.

16. Lai, K. F. and Chin, R. T., "Deformable contours: modeling and extraction," *IEEE Trans. Pattern Anal. Mach. Intell.*, Vol. 17, No. 11, pp. 1084–1090, Nov. 1995.

17. Gunn, S. R. and Nixon, M. S., "A robust snake implementation: a dual active contour," *IEEE Trans. Pattern Anal. Mach. Intell.*, Vol. 19, No. 1, pp. 63–68, Jan. 1997.

18. Storvik, G., "A Bayesian approach to dynamic contours through stochastic sampling and simulated annealing," *IEEE Trans. Pattern Anal. Mach. Intell.*, Vol. 16, No. 10, pp. 976–986, Oct. 1994.

19. Xu, G., Segawa, E., and Tsuji, S., "Robust active contour with insensitive parameters," *Proc. Fourth Int. Conf. Computer Vision*, IEEE Computer Society Press, Los Alamitos, CA, pp. 562–566, April 1993.

20. Das, P. P., "An algorithm for computing the number of the minimal paths in digital images," *Patt. Recog. Lett.*, Vol. 9, No. 2, pp.107–116, Feb. 1989.

21. Caselles, V., Kimmel, R., and Sapiro, G., "Geodesic Active Contours," *Int. J. Computer Vision*, Vol. 22, No. 1, pp. 61–79, Feb.–March 1997.

22. Osher, S. J., and Sethian, J. A., "Fronts propagating with curvature dependent speed: algorithms based on Hamilton-Jacobi formulation," *J. Computational Physics*, Vol. 79, pp. 12–49, 1988.

23. Cohen, L. D. and Kimmel, R., "Global minimum for active contour models: a minimal path approach," *Int. J. Computer Vision*, Vol. 24, No. 1, pp. 57–78, 1997.

24. Sethian, J. A., "Fast Marching Methods," *SIAM Review*, Vol. 41, No. 2, pp. 199–235, 1999.

25. Hassanien, E. and Nakajima, M., "Feature-specification algorithm based on snake model for facial image morphing," *IEICE Trans. Information and System*, Vol. E82-D, No. 2, pp. 439–445, Feb. 1999.

26. Mortensen, E. N. and Barrett, W. A., "Interactive segmentation with intelligent scissors," *Graphical Models and Image Proc.*, Vol. 60, No. 5, pp. 349–384, Sept. 1998.

27. Dijkstra, E. W., "A note on two problems in connection with graphs," *Numerische Mathematic*, Vol. 1, pp. 269–271, 1959.

28. Vazquez, L., Sapiro, G., and Randall, G., "Segmenting neurons in electronic microscopy via geometric tracing," *Proc. 1998 Int. Conf. Image Processing*, ICIP98 IEEE Comput. Soc, Los Alamitos, CA, Vol. 3, pp. 814–818, 1998.

29. Sedgewick, R., *Algorithms*, Addison-Wesley, Reading, MA, 1988.

30. Villalobos, L., "The conic curve (computer graphics)," *Computer Graphics World*, Vol. 10, No. 5, pp. 91–94, May 1987.

31. Bookstein, F. L., "Fitting conic sections to scattered data," *Computer Graphics and Image Proc.*, Vol. 9, No. 1, pp. 56–71, Jan. 1979.

32. Fischler, M. A., Tenenbaum, J. M., and Wolf, H. C., "Detection of roads and linear structures in low-resolution aerial imagery using a multisource knowledge integration technique," *Computer Graphics and Image Proc.*, Vol. 15, No. 3, pp. 201–223, March 1981.

33. Martelli, S. "An application of heuristic search methods to edge and contour detection," *Commun. ACM*, Vol. 19, No. 2, pp. 73–83, Feb. 1976.

34. Oh, W. and Lindquist, W. B., "Image thresholding by indicator kriging," *IEEE Trans. Pattern Anal. Mach. Intell.*, Vol. 21, No. 7, pp. 590–597, July 1999.

35. Glagov, S., Zarins, C., Giddens, D. P., and Ku, D. N., "Hemodynamics and atherosclerosis: insights and perspectives gained from studies of human arteries," *Arch. Pathol. Lab. Med.*, Vol. 112, pp. 1018–1031, 1988.

36. Beach, K. W., Hatsukami, T. S., Detmer, P. R., et al., "Carotid artery intraplaque hemorrhage and stenotic velocity," *Stroke*, Vol. 24, pp. 314–319, 1993.

37. Besl, P. J., *Surfaces in Range Image Understanding*, Springer-Verlag, New York, p. 65, 303, 1988.

38. Hatsukami, T. S., Ross, R., and Polissar, N. L., "Visualization of fibrous cap thickness and rupture in human atherosclerotic carotid plaque *in vivo* with

high-resolution magnetic resonance imaging," *Circulation,* Vol. 102, No. 9, pp. 959–964, Aug. 2000.

39. Yuan, C. K., Beach, W., Smith, L. H., and Hatsukami, T. S., "Measurement of atherosclerotic carotid plaque size in vivo using high resolution magnetic resonance imaging," *Circulation,* 98(24), pp. 2666–2671, Dec. 1998.

40. Besl, B. J. and Jain, R. C., "Invariant surface characteristics for 3D object recognition in range images," *Computer Vision, Graphics, and Image Proc.,* Vol. 33, pp. 33–80, 1986.

41. Wang, Y. P., Lee, S. L., and Toraichi, K., "Multiscale curvature-based shape representation using B-spline wavelets," *IEEE Trans. Image Processing,* Vol. 8, No. 11, pp. 1586–1592, Nov. 1999.

42. Kehtaravaz, N. and Defigueiredo, R. J. P., "A 3-D contour segmentation scheme based on curvature and torsion," *IEEE Trans. Pattern Anal. Mach. Intell.,* Vol. 10, No. 5, pp. 707–713, Sep. 1988.

43. Keppel, E., "A approximating complex surface by triangulation of contours lines," *IBM J. Res. Develop.,* Vol. 19, pp. 2–11, 1975.

44. Fuchs, H., Kedem, Z. M., and Uselton, S. P., "Optimal surface reconstruction from planar contours," *Graphics and Image Processing,* Vol. 20, No. 10, pp. 693–702, 1977.

45. Barillot, C., Gibaud, B., Lis, O., Min, L. L., et al., "Computer graphics in medicine: a survey," *CRC Crit. Rev. Biomed. Eng.,* Vol. 15, No. 4, pp. 269–307, 1988.

46. Meyers, D., "Multiresolution tiling," *Computer Graphics Forum,* Vol. 13, No. 5, pp. 325–340, 1994.

47. Unser, M., Aldroubi, A., and Eden, M., "B-spline signal processing. I. Theory," *IEEE Trans. Pattern Analysis and Mach. Intell.,* Vol. 41, No. 2, pp. 821–833, Feb. 1993.

48. Herbert, E., *Geometry and Topology for Mesh Generation,* Cambridge University Press, 2001.

49. David, M., "Multiresolution tiling," *Computer Graphics Form,* Vol. 13, No. 5, pp. 325–340, 1994.

50. Ganapathy, S. and Dennehy, T., "A new general triangulation method for planar contours," *Computer Graphics,* Vol. 16, pp. 69–75, 1982.

51. Kang, X. J., Polissar, N. L., Han, C., Lin, E., and Yuan, C., "Analysis of the measurement precision of arterial lumen and wall areas using high resolution magnetic resonance imaging," *MRM,* Vol. 44, pp. 968–972, 2000.

10

On the Role of Computer Vision
in Intravascular Ultrasound Image Analysis

Petia Radeva

CONTENTS

10.1   Introduction

Heart attack and stroke are the major causes of human death in the Western world; almost twice as many people die from cardiovascular diseases as from all forms of cancer [1]. Every 20 seconds a European citizen experiences a mortal heart attack; every year, 500,000 persons die due to cardiac diseases.

Coronary heart disease (also known as atherosclerosis) is the most common form of heart disease that directly affects the artery and coronary vessels (see Figure 10.1). It involves deposits of fatty substances, cholesterol, cellular waste products, calcium, and fibrin (a clotting material in the blood) in the inner lining of an artery. The build-up that results, called plaque, may partially or totally block the blood's flow through the artery. This can lead to bleeding (hemorrhage) into the plaque or formation of a blood clot (thrombus) on the

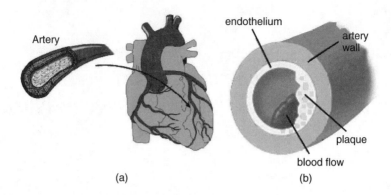

FIGURE 10.1 (See color insert.)
(a) Coronary arteries as an essential part of the heart, and (b) the morphological structure of coronary vessel.

plaque's surface. If either of these occurs and blocks the entire artery, a heart attack or stroke (brain attack) may result.

When patients come for treatment, the disease usually involves focal atherosclerotic lesions in the lumen arteries. Under local anesthesia, an x-ray-guided catheter is inserted into an artery in the patient's leg or arm and a second, balloon-tipped catheter is placed within it. With the help of a guidewire, the balloon catheter is advanced to the area of the blockage and inflated and deflated several times until the blockage is successfully compressed and the narrowed artery is widened.

With the appearance of catheter devices, many heart surgical operations are substituted by interventional procedures that amount to 450,000 per year in Europe. In general, catheter devices are used for the measurement of various physiological flow characteristics (e.g., arterial blood pressure, pressure gradient, and flow velocity or flow rate) as well as for the diagnosis (e.g., x-ray angiogram and intravascular ultrasound) and treatment (e.g., coronary balloon angioplasty) of various arterial diseases.

10.2 Vessel Imaging

Traditional methods for studying human coronary artery disease involve histological evaluation of vessel material and x-ray angiogram. However, these common techniques have significant limitations in the study of vessel dimensions and morphological vessel structure. The histological analysis provides the structural information of the atherosclerotic tissue structure (see Figure 10.2a), but it cannot be used in patients because the tissue specimens are only available at autopsy.

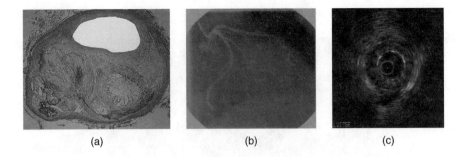

(a)   (b)   (c)

FIGURE 10.2
Main imaging modalities of coronary vessels: (a) histological image, (b) angiogram, and (c) intravascular ultrasound image.

For the past 30 years the angiogram (see Figure 10.2) has been used as a "gold standard" of coronary imaging for vessel diagnosis and coronary pathology treatment [2]. Actually, what we are looking at is a radiographic projection of a column of contrast inside a complex structure, that is, a diseased coronary artery. Given that an angiogram evaluates only a two-dimensional projection of the three-dimensional geometry of the vessel lumen, it cannot provide the rich structural information on the arterial wall that is essential for the detailed evaluation of the mechanistic process during plaque progression and rupture. As a consequence, angiographic assessment of lesion severity, vessel morphology, calcification, and thrombus is subjective and difficult to quantify. The introduction of percutaneous coronary revascularization and the growing appreciation of the pathophysiological and prognostic importance of arterial morphology have led to the realization that angiograms are inherently limited in defining the distribution and extent of coronary wall disease and in accurately measuring stent expansion and irregular lumen [2]. In particular, the angiogram can sometimes be misleading and in many cases underestimates the severity of disease within the artery. On the other hand, because this is a two-dimensional representation in terms of the projective geometry of an obviously three-dimensional structure, numerous x-ray images from different points of view (at least, two) can be used to recreate a three-dimensional picture of the artery centerline [3].

IVUS (intravascular ultrasound) provides a unique two-dimensional *in vivo* vision of the internal vessel walls, determining the extension, distribution, and treatment of different kind of plaques and their possible repercussion on the internal arterial lumen (see Figure 10.2c). The main difference between the intravascular ultrasound and the angiogram images deals with the fact that most of the visible plaque lesions with IVUS are not evident with angiogram. Studies on intravascular echocardiography have shown that a reference vessel segment could have up to 40% of its sectional area occluded because of the plaque, although it appears as normal in the angiogram [4]. Moreover, IVUS uniquely contains rich information about the composition of the internal

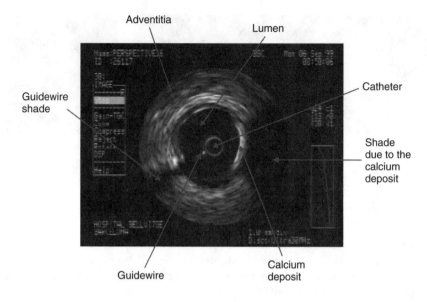

FIGURE 10.3

Intravascular ultrasound image represents a cross-sectional (short axis) plane of the vessel where different morphological structures can be observed: adventitia, lumen, calcium deposit, etc.

lesion (atherosclerotic, fibrotic plaques and thrombus, etc.); in particular, about calcium deposits as the most important isolated predictors to evaluate if a particular lesion will respond to catheter treatment (see Figure 10.3). The possibility of directly visualizing the plaque by IVUS also benefits the receptors of a heart transplant to assure that a heart to be transplanted is not already ill.

10.3   IVUS Acquisition

The progress of ultrasound leads to developing IVUS as a new imaging technique using a catheter over a guidewire, producing ultrasonographic images of the arteries. The IVUS device consists of a catheter, with a sensor on its tip, introduced inside the artery and a console to form, display, and record IVUS movies (see Figure 10.4). The IVUS sensor rotates and emits pulses of ultrasound. When it receives the echoes the tissues return, it generates an image in which the image intensity is a function of the ultrasound impedance of the tissue structures.

IVUS images are acquired during a pull-back of the catheter through the vessel. Using an angiogram-guided process, the catheter is introduced in the vessel to diagnose and determine the position of the vessel lesion. Afterward,

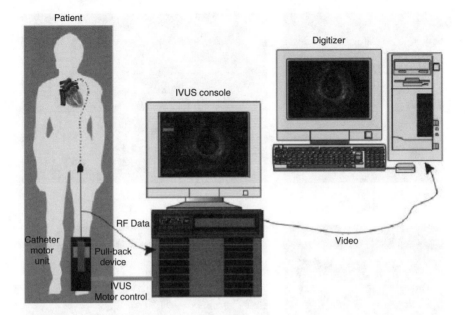

FIGURE 10.4

IVUS device contains a console to form, display, and record IVUS, and a catheter introduced in a patient artery to acquire vessel data. A digitizer (frame grabber) can be connected to the IVUS device to digitize IVUS data and store it in digital format.

a pull-back of the catheter with constant speed (usually, 0.5 mm/sec or 1 mm/sec) is performed, acquiring the IVUS sequence of images. Most IVUS devices are not synchronized to acquire only images during the catheter pull-back. Usually, the device is set to record the IVUS sequence of images and the pull-back is switched on. To know when the pull-back is switched on/off, the physician should indicate it by voice. The IVUS sequence of images is recorded onto an S-VHS tape that can be later digitized by a frame grabber.

The obtained stack/sequence of images define spatio-temporal data that allows one to scan the morphology of the vessel lesion in space. Dark zones correspond to the artery lumen (see Figure 10.3), light zones to the artery wall; and the brightest parts with a dark shadow behind, to calcium plaque (see Figure 10.3). The circle in the center of the image represents the catheter. The guidewire can be seen in some images as a bright spot beside the catheter, followed by a dark shadow.

Using IVUS, physicians can see the lumen interior and visualize a longitudinal picture of the artery constructed by drawing the catheter distally to proximally (see Figure 10.5). Compared to angiograms, where the amount of disease and plaque inside an artery is often underestimated, IVUS shows the composition of the vessel and stent in detail and helps quantify their mutual position.

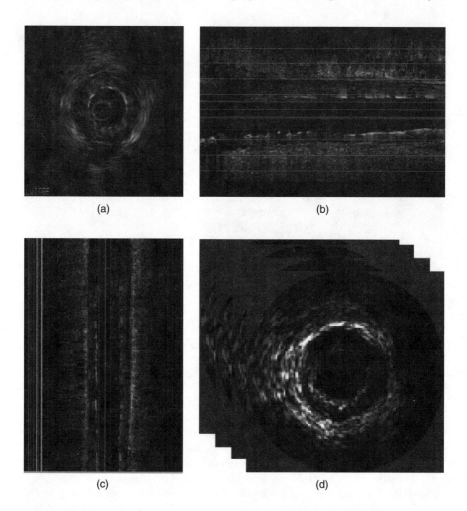

FIGURE 10.5
IVUS data represents a movie of short-axis images (a) and (d). Intersecting IVUS data horizontally (b) or vertically (c) gives a longitudinal picture of the coronary vessel.

10.4   Segmentation of IVUS Images

Due to the amount of information they carry [5, 6], IVUS images are increasing their role in the diagnosis and treatment of several diseases. Quantitative studies using IVUS require the identification of the internal (luminal) and external (medial-adventitial) border in IVUS images (see Figure 10.6) to allow more in-depth knowledge of the true extension of the coronary vessel illness. Today, vessel diagnosis in clinical practice is limited to observation

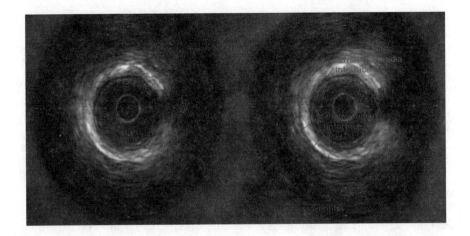

FIGURE 10.6
Original IVUS image (on the left), and the internal and external vessel wall (on the right).

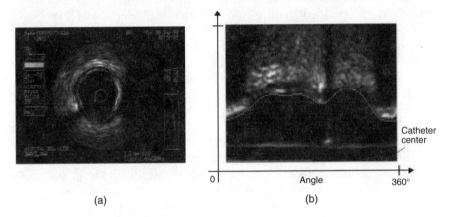

      (a)   (b)

FIGURE 10.7
(a) IVUS image and (b) its polar representation.

and measurements extracted from manually traced vessel walls in the serial IVUS planes. This process is extremely tedious and time-consuming, and data are difficult to reproduce; inter-observer and intra-observer variability is estimated to be 20% [7]. Given the high cost of IVUS analysis and measurement extraction, many automated and semi-automated computer vision techniques have been proposed [7–13].

To achieve more robust and faster results of the segmentation process, a polar representation of IVUS data is usually considered that is a natural representation of ultrasound signals (see Figure 10.7). In this representation, the number of image columns corresponds to the number of sampled angles (usually, 360) of IVUS image, and the number of rows depends on the radius of the circle that contains IVUS data. The final row corresponds to the catheter center. The first column of the polar representation corresponds to the horizontal IVUS data segment, beginning at the center of IVUS data and finishing at the most right IVUS data point.

When the three-dimensional cube of IVUS data should be considered, manual segmentation of vessel borders is a laborious task, taking into account that a pull-back IVUS stack could contain thousands of images. The development of three-dimensional segmentation techniques that take advantage of the similarity between vessel shapes in adjacent IVUS slices has been considered in different works [3, 14–20].

One of the most widely reported semi-automated segmentation approaches used in clinical research was developed by Li et al. [21]. Their method is based on a dynamic programming technique for semi-automated segmentation of longitudinally resampled IVUS image sequences, followed by lumen and media border detection in cross-sectional IVUS images. Another semi-automated method based on dynamic programming for three-dimensional IVUS segmentation was developed by Dawhale et al. [22] for border detection. Given the speckled "nature" of IVUS images, Meier et al. [7] proposed a three-dimensional IVUS segmentation technique that uses a combination of region growing and cost function optimization. The poor quality of the images suggests the use of techniques such as Fuzzy logic [13] guiding an active contour to adjust the inner wall. Escolano et al. [13] have proposed to use circular deformable models guided by a function that had an added term to cope with noise. The rigidity of the shape prevented the template from being misled by dark shadows. Sonka et al. [8] have reported another IVUS segmentation technique based on optimal graph searching combined with a knowledge-based approach to select edge points from the vessel wall.

Most segmentation techniques based on longitudinal views use ECG-triggered video labeling during uniform pull-back of the intracoronary ultrasound transducer [23]. Video frames coinciding with the R-wave of the ECG are automatically labeled and images acquired at the same phase of the cardiac cycle are used for offline spatial reconstruction. This approach minimizes the systolic-diastolic artifacts that are frequently observed in non-triggered, uniform-speed pull-backs. One can see the "curly" appearance of the internal wall of the vessel in the longitudinal view of the IVUS data (Figure 10.5b). Using a ECG-triggered IVUS pull-back device in combination with ECG-gated image acquisition, the problem of cyclic motion artifacts can be overcome [24, 25]. The price to be paid is that IVUS acquisition is much slower, taking into account that each image should be acquired at the same ECG-phase stage (R-wave).

The low signal-to-noise rate of IVUS images makes unsupervised segmentation based on traditional segmentation algorithms (such as edge or ridge/valley detection) fail to achieve the expected results. From most mentioned work on vessel segmentation, it can be concluded that more elaborate segmentation techniques are necessary to achieve robust results. The typical edge point extractor should be substituted by a more elaborate detector of the vessel boundary; as well, a high-level restriction about the shape can be introduced into the segmentation process.

Among the wide variety of image segmentation techniques, deformable models are receiving special attention, primarily in medical imagery, due to their ability to interpret a sparse set of image features (e.g., edge points, region-based descriptors, etc.) and to link them to obtain object contours by applying general assumptions about the contour shape [26–28].

A snake is an elastic curve that evolves from its initial shape and position as a result of the combined action of external and internal forces [29]. The external forces push the snake toward features of the image, whereas internal forces model the elasticity of the curve. In a parametric representation, the snake appears as a curve $u(s) = (x(s), y(s))$, where $s \in [s_0, s_{N-1}]$, and $s_0 = s_N$ for closed curves. Its internal energy is defined as follows [29]:

$$E_{int}(u) = \int \alpha |u_s|^2 \, ds + \int \beta |u_{ss}|^2 \, ds$$

The first term, called the membrane energy, determines the resistance of the deformable model to stretching; and the second term, called the stiffness energy, defines the resistance to model bending. These terms are weighed by the elastic parameters α and β. The external energy is generally defined from a potential field P:

$$E_{ext}(u) = \int P(u(s)) \, ds.$$

A typical potential field for a snake attracted to image edge points is given by [29]:

$$P(u(s)) \propto -|G_\sigma * \nabla I(u(s))| \qquad (10.1)$$

where $I(u)$ represents the intentisity value of image pixels and G_σ is a Gaussian smoothing function of scale σ.

In general, the potential must define a surface which the minima correspond, as accurately as possible, to the image features of interest. The total energy of the snake is the sum of the external and internal energies:

$$E_{snake}(u) = \int E_{int}(u(s)) + E_{ext}(u(s)) \, ds$$

The solution to the problem of detecting the contour is obtained by a minimization of the energy function, which is generally performed using variational principles and finite difference techniques [29]. As a result, a snake with the smallest energy corresponds to the desired object contour.

Practical computations demand discretization over time and space. In finite difference approximations, the curve $u(s)$ is sampled at certain points where computations are done. Methods such as finite elements [30] and B-splines [31] interpret $u(s)$ by means of control points that define the curve shape.

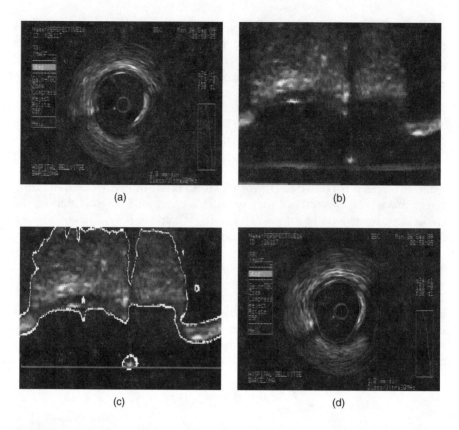

FIGURE 10.8

(a) Original IVUS image, (b) its polar representation, (c) Canny edges and initial snake in red, and (d) final result of segmentation.

These methods allow one to define a high degree of continuity of the curve representation and the external energy of each curve vertex is now evaluated on its corresponding curve patch.

Recently, the snake formulation has proved definite advantages with respect to other segmentation techniques in IVUS data [20]. A snake minimizing its energy inside a dynamic programming framework is applied where internal forces of the snake are in charge of keeping the continuous and smooth shape of the model. Figure 10.8 shows an example of an original IVUS image, its polar representation, Canny's edges and initial snake, and the result of vessel segmentation. Note that a polar representation of the image is used to segment the lumen, taking into account that in this case the snake deforms toward the vessel wall only in the vertical direction. Segmenting the whole sequence of images and interpolating the snake curve allow the recovery of a spatial model of the coronary vessel (see Figure 10.9). When the segmentation is applied to the lumen and the adventitia, a spatial model of both vessel walls is obtained (see Figure 10.10).

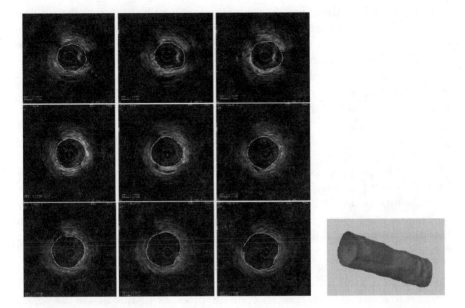

FIGURE 10.9
Segmentation of a sequence of IVUS images (left) and the interpolated spatial model of the coronary vessel (right).

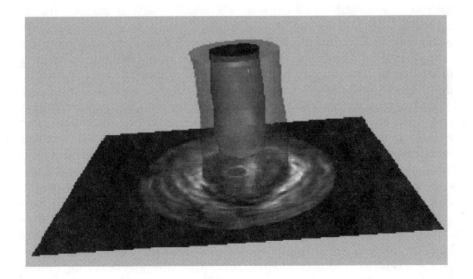

FIGURE 10.10 (See color insert.)
Volumetric model of the coronary vessel obtained by interpolating the segmentation of IVUS images.

The classical formulation of snake approach can be successfully applied in IVUS data when there is no strong plaque inside the vessel. Otherwise, a good initialization of the snake is necessary to avoid snake attraction by image features not belonging to the vessel wall.

Using constraints on the snake shape represents an alternative to the close initialization in order to make the snake more robust in the process of segmentation. Hand-crafted parameterized templates with few degrees of freedom have been used, for example, for modeling features of faces [32]. More general methods, such as Fourier descriptors, have been used for representing shapes in medical images [33]. Alternative approaches based on modal analysis have also been proposed to constrain the model to deform only in ways implied by the training set of shapes [31, 34]. Although shape models convey important information, they do not ensure the desired solution; high-accuracy techniques must make the most of grey-level information too. In line with this idea, authors working on deformable models propose to combine shape models and appearance models [35].

In the case of IVUS images, stronger constraints (such as using an elliptical deformable model) on the segmenting model should be applied to avoid artifacts in the image interpretation due to blood or plaque inside the vessel interior. In [36] the authors present a probabilistic flexible template to separate different regions in the image. In particular, they use elliptic templates to model and detect the shape of the vessel inner wall in IVUS images. On the one hand, the use of probabilities is a good way of reducing the impact of noise. On the other hand, using such a restricted deformable shape makes the model more stable in the presence of artifacts such as shadows due to calcium plaque and the guidewire. An elliptic shape is applied to achieve better adjustment of the model to the inner wall and, at the same time, this shape also gives a direct estimation of the maximum and minimum diameters of the lumen. The only assumption made is that lumen and tissue appear in the image as gray-level pixels generated by two distinct normal distributions.

Let us consider the IVUS image as a function $i(x; y)$ of two variables x and y. The key idea of the method is to compute a first approximation of an elliptical model that has a high probability of being close to the inner wall. This initial ellipse is obtained by means of a binarized image obtained with a fixed threshold. The next step is based on the assumption that lumen and tissue appear in the image as gray-level pixels generated by two distinct normal distributions. Let λ be the value that best separates both distributions. This value can be computed automatically by means of Otsu's method described in [37]. Let us denote by D_r the disk of radius r centered at the initial ellipse and by P the probability of having a dark gray-level inside D_r. In fact, the function $g(r) = P(I(x; y) < \lambda)$ is considered. If one takes disks of increasing radius, the global minimum of $g(r)$ indicates the stopping point having significant echoes. Once the parameter λ has been fixed, the deformation of the ellipse is performed [38]. Let E_{int} denote the interior of the deformable ellipse and E_{ext} its complement in the image. Then, the ellipse approximating the lumen is the global maximum of the function:

$$F = \frac{\int_{E_{int}} I(x, y) \, dxdy}{\int_{E_{int}} dxdy} + \left(1 - \frac{\int_{E_{ext}} I(x, y) \, dxdy}{\int_{E_{ext}} dxdy}\right)$$

where $I(x, y) = \begin{cases} 1, & \text{if } i(x, y) \leq \lambda \\ 0, & \text{otherwise} \end{cases}$

The converged elliptical deformable model can be used as an initialization of a snake that converges to the vessel wall.

In the classical formulation, the snake is an image segmentation technique that uses energy terms defined from gradient features of global interest to find the desired contour [29]. The external energy defines global features of interest that rest specifically in the problem domain. The success of the segmentation of an object is based on the discrimination of locally computed image features and their spatial continuity. Obtaining correct result of the segmentation is intricately tied to the type features sought and the criteria used for discriminating between the extracted features. So, the feature space must be capable of representing any image features of interest. Different authors suggest the combination of the gradient-based potential with valley and crest maps [31, 32]. However, on one hand, the best way of integrating different features remains an open problem and, on the other hand, these features are not yet sufficiently selective. This leads to heuristical combinations that enhance too many feature points that do not belong to the object of interest; meanwhile, others go unnoticed.

Discriminant snakes proposed in [39] are based on the statistics of the image features to increase the *selectivity* of the description of the target object. Instead of an edge detector, discriminant snakes use a bank of Gaussian derivative filters of different scales to construct a generalized description of the object contour. At this point, the description of the target image features is still too general. It is necessary to locally decide (learn) the best way of combining derivative degrees and scales in the description of each contour part by means of a classification vector. Supervised learning in conjunction with discriminant analysis is carried out to characterize each contour patch. Then a classifier is assigned to each snake patch and the external energy is represented by the distance of each snake point to the cluster of its target contour in the corresponding feature space. The discriminant snake approach is of particular interest for segmentation and tracking of objects in temporal or spatial image sequences such as IVUS data. The snake is able to learn the changes in contour features/appearance of new morphological structures inside each image as well as along the image sequence in an adaptive way.

As any image structure can locally be represented as a combination of local image derivatives, the authors apply a convolution of the image by a bank of Gaussian derivative filters to extract the image features [40]. The segmentation approach presented in [39] relies on derivative features computed over multiple spatial orientations that generalize the classical image features (edges, ridges, and valleys). Additionally, the authors consider different scales to a number sufficient for characterizing all possible configurations, and allow the snake to follow the translation of the object of interest in image sequences or, in general, to *see* the object from possible remote locations of the initial contour.

Due to the high dimension of the feature space generated by the bank of filters, a dimensional reduction is necessary to eliminate nondiscriminant filter responses and weight the contribution of the remaining filter responses to the classifier, as described below.

Given the responses of the different filters, the authors define a multi-valued potential as follows:

$$\mathcal{P} : \mathcal{I} \longrightarrow \mathbf{R}^{d_\mathcal{G}}$$
$$(i, j) \longrightarrow (p_1, \ldots, p_{d_\mathcal{G}})$$

where $p_i (i = 1, \ldots, d_\mathcal{G})$ are the results of image convolution with the bank of filters.

Henceforth, the *potential* denotes the responses of filters on the image and the *external energy* refers to what each snake pixel interprets on the multi-valued potential (similarity and distance to target configurations).

On one hand, the relative importance of derivative features depends on the task domain. On the other hand, the human selection needs expert knowledge on image processing and it is prone to error. It seems natural to perform a self-training to reduce the space and weight the features. The authors apply a technique commonly used for dimensionality reduction based on principal component analysis (PCA) and Fisher linear discriminant analysis (FLD) [41, 42].

Linear discriminant functions are used to assign image feature filter responses to one or both populations (target contour configuration vs. no contour). FLD analysis is the optimal solution to this problem if the underlying distributions of the observations are multi-variate normal [43]. The Fisher discriminant function is a scalar function:

$$\mathcal{F}(\mathcal{P}) = \mathcal{V} \cdot \mathcal{P} \tag{10.2}$$

where $\mathcal{V}$ is the learned discriminant classifier and $\mathcal{P}$ is the multi-valued potential.

Applying FLD analysis, the new scalar feature r_j is defined by the following linear transformation:

$$\mathcal{F}_k : \mathcal{P} \longrightarrow \mathbf{R}$$
$$(p_{j1}, \ldots, p_{jd_\mathcal{G}}) \rightarrow r_j = V_k^T \mathcal{P}_j$$

where $V_k \in \mathbf{R}^{d_\mathcal{G}}$ is a vector that projects the features (filter convolutions) of pixel j into the reduced feature space to determine the similarity to the contour class k. To find an optimal projection into a reduced feature space where the distance between samples of class C_k and the remaining samples is maximized, the authors have to obtain the best discriminant function.

After applying PCA to remove correlation between filter responses, the optimal projection V_k is defined as the vector that maximizes the ratio of the determinant of the between-class scatter matrix S_{bc} of the projected samples to the within-class scatter matrix S_{wc} of the projected samples [42, 43]:

$$V_k = \arg\max_{V_k} \frac{|V_k^T S_{bc} V_k|}{|V_k^T S_{wc} V_k|}$$

To drive a snake curve patch toward the contour of interest, each snake pixel must be able to distinguish between its corresponding contour target and other structures (in particular, other parts of the contour or contours of nearby objects). To make the snake more selective, the authors distinguish the configurations of different contour parts. To this end, instead of using the classical definition of potential energy, given in Equation 10.1, to build a distance map, the authors construct feature spaces that yield the relevant feature spaces to characterize all the contour configurations. Different contour configurations imply no edge detection (magnitude and orientation) but projection in the space of filter set and deformation to minimize distance to the target cluster in the feature space.

The global process is described in Figure 10.11. Each patch k of the snake curve has its own classifier $\mathcal{V}_{C_k}$ that defines the image features (target contour representation) it is looking for. The scalar product of the mean feature vector μ_{C_k} of the patch and the classifier vector gives the center of the class $\mathcal{O}_{C_k}$ of points in the feature space that correspond to the target contour representation:

$$\mathcal{V}_{C_k} = V_k$$
$$\mathcal{O}_{C_k} = \mathcal{V}_{C_k}^T \mu_{C_k}$$

The local external energy of the discriminant snake is defined by measuring the similarity of the actual image features $\mathcal{P}_f$ in the current location of the snake to the desired contour configuration in terms of the Mahalanobis distance from the projection of the image feature vectors $\mathcal{P}_f$ to the target class center:

$$D_{C_k} = \left(\mathcal{V}_{C_k}^T(\mathcal{P}_f - \mu_{C_k})\right)^T \left(\mathcal{V}_{C_k}^T(\mathcal{P}_f - \mu_{C_k})\right) = \left(\mathcal{V}_{C_k}^T \mathcal{P} - \mathcal{O}_{C_k}\right)^2$$
$$\mathcal{P}_f = \mathcal{G}_{\mathcal{D}\Sigma} * \mathcal{I}$$

where $\mathcal{I}$ is the original image and $\mathcal{P}_f$ is the multi-valued potential obtained by a convolution of the IVUS image with the bank of filters. As a result, each target contour part generates its own distance map from the constant multi-valued potential. That is, each snake pixel interprets in different way the image filter responses depending of the goal it carries (the contour type

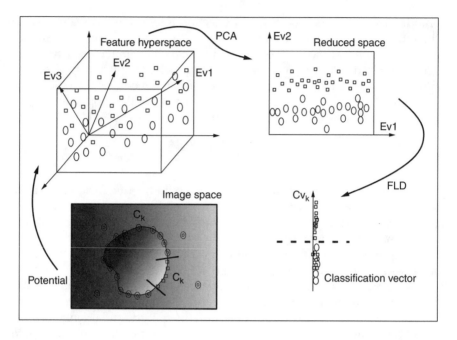

FIGURE 10.11
Procedure for classifying local image structures: a feature space is constructed from the original image that is transformed into a reduced feature space to be classified according to its similarity to the snake target.

it has learned in its previous stage). Figure 10.12 and Figure 10.13 show the result of the segmentation process by discriminant snakes. Note the excellent results of IVUS segmentation although the presence of plaque and variable shape of the vessel.

10.5   Texture Characterization

The ultimate biological behavior of atherosclerotic lesions depends not only on their extent of luminal narrowing but also on their biophysical composition and material properties [44]. Ultrasonic tissue characterization methods may be useful for quantitative delineation of the biophysical composition and organization of normal and pathological vascular tissue.

The low signal-to-noise ratio of IVUS images leads to a need for more elaborate computer vision techniques for tissue characterization. In [45] the authors propose a statistic framework for separating different textured areas over real images by discriminant analysis. For each region prototype (vessel, plaque, etc.), a global statistical model is generated as a set of probability density

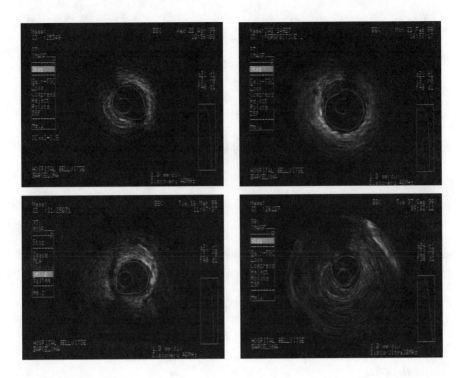

FIGURE 10.12
Results of IVUS segmentation by discriminant snakes.

function attributes from a multi-valued function. This function is generated by means of responses of convolving the image by the bank of Gaussian derivative filters. Linear discriminant analysis is performed to obtain a statistical classifier. Given an input image composed by different texture types, a likelihood map is built where each pixel is projected in a feature space and assigned its Mahalanobis distance to the nearest target region prototypes. A discriminant snake deforms on the likelihood map to delineate regions with similar IVUS texture descriptions according to the learned texture patterns. Figure 10.14 shows the classification of different regions of the coronary vessel: the original IVUS image, its polar representation, a likelihood map where the grey-level corresponds to the Mahalanobis distance between the class representing the plaque and adventitia and the delineated classified regions by a snake. In [3] an automated approach for determining plaque composition is presented that considers different kinds of texture descriptors: gray-level-based texture descriptors, co-occurrence matrix, run-length measures, and fractal-based measures. The determined regions of plaque were classified into three classes: soft plaque, hard plaque, and hard plaque shadow.

In [46] the authors propose to use texture analysis to distinguish between plaque lesions of different composition. Using histological correlation, the

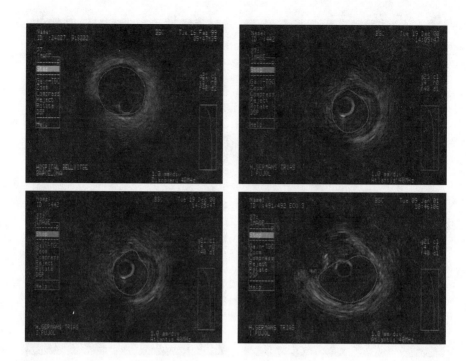

FIGURE 10.13
Results of IVUS segmentation by discriminant snakes.

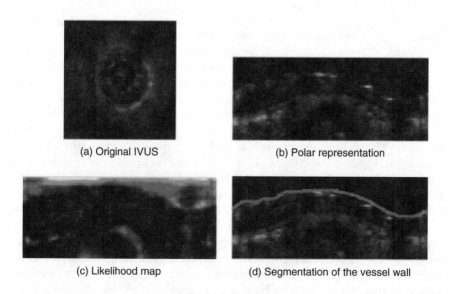

FIGURE 10.14
Classifying and delineation of different regions of IVUS images.

authors consider image regions of calcified, fibrous, and necrotic core plaque from 27 coronary plaques. Different texture descriptors, such as first-order statistics, Haralick's method, Laws' texture energy method, the neighborhood gray-tone difference matrix method, and texture spectrum features, are examined and discriminant analysis is applied to compare them. Self-validation indicated that Haralick's method yielded the most accurate results, with low substitution and cross-validation error rates. The authors apply further optimization to obtain acceptable error rates using only two discriminating features: entropy and inverse difference moment.

10.6   Image-Guided Stent Positioning and Follow-Up

Stents have become the most important advance in mechanical techniques for percutaneous coronary revascularization. They represent a minimum invasive technique to enlarge the vascular lumen, which decreases the risk of complications and restenosis. Intracoronary stenting has emerged as the most powerful tool, due to the better predictability and improved clinical outcome with stent placement as compared to plain balloon angioplasty. However, it soon became apparent that these positive results of coronary placement were threatened by thrombosis of the prosthesis, causing life-threatening acute or subacute complications. Stent thrombosis occurred in up to 16.6% of emergency cases, despite combined anticoagulant therapy [47]. Observations of stents by IVUS revealed that most stents were, in fact, underexpanded.

IVUS information can be critical before any coronary vessel intervention. By measuring the distal reference diameter, the most appropriate size of a balloon or stent is chosen for a given lesion. Therefore, preinterventional IVUS has been shown to be of value before stent placement to assess lesion severity and length, as well as the degree and location of calcification. During the intervention (angioplasty and stenting, and/or rotational atherectomy and stenting), IVUS images contain invaluable information about eventually nonoptimal placement of stents, despite an excellent angiographic appearance. IVUS is used to guide coronary stenting without coagulation [48]. After intervention, in case of necessity, the stent expansion can be improved by IVUS using the cross-sectional area of the artery, reducing in this way the chance of restenosis to 10% or less.

An intracoronary stent is a spiral metallic mesh (see Figure 10.15a) that is implanted inside a vessel to prevent the stenosis effect caused by calcification or growth of the intimal vessel layer. In the IVUS image, the stent can be observed as a set of bright spots that corresponds to the metal struts of the stent (see Figure 10.15b). The stent mesh widens the vessel walls, recovering the necessary lumen for good irrigation. The studies on stents carried out with IVUS show that the appearance in the angiogram of good stent deployment

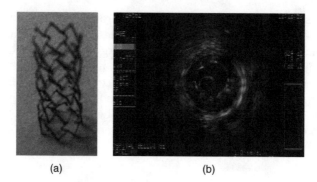

(a)   (b)

FIGURE 10.15
(a) Stent and (b) its visualization in an IVUS image.

can hide two possible problems: incomplete apposition (a portion of the stent is not making pressure on the vessel wall) and incomplete expansion (a portion of the stent remains closed although expansion occurs for the rest of the stent area). Both problems are very significant because they can be worse than the problem they are trying to solve.

Since the first reports of inadequate stent expansion by IVUS, numerous criteria for optimal stent expansion have been suggested [47]. Today, the ultrasound criteria generally accepted are those used in the MUSIC study, which resulted in a low complication and restenosis rate [49]. These criteria compare the stent cross-sectional lumen area with an average reference lumen area before and after the stent site, the stent apposition with respect to the inner vessel wall, and the symmetric stent expansion expressed by the minimal and maximal lumen diameter. To estimate the quality of the stent deployment, the authors in [50] defined criteria by means of three parameters (see Figure 10.16):

1. *Cross-sectional area (CSA).* The ratio of stent minimal CSA to normal reference vessel CSA (average CSA proximal and distal to stent) must be greater than 0.8.

2. *Apposition.* The maximum gap between the stent and the vessel wall must be less than 0.1 mm.

3. *Symmetry.* The ratio of the stent minor axis to the stent major axis must be at least 0.7 mm.

These parameters are usually measured plane by plane in IVUS images and are accessible to the physician in terms of numerical data.

Given that a pull-back acquiring IVUS images can lead to thousands of images, manual evaluation of stent position is tedious and time-consuming, making it impractical. Moreover, the existence of intra-observer and inter-observer variability of morphometric measurements justifies the

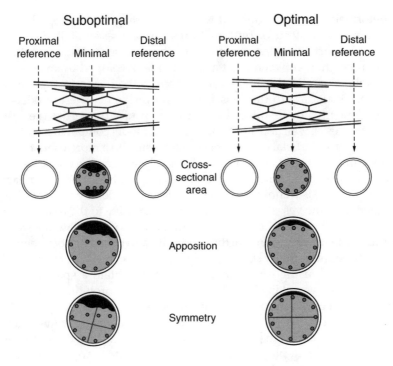

FIGURE 10.16
Three main criteria to estimate the correct expansion of a stent inside a vessel.

development of objective automatic segmentation and measurements of the vessel. Although two-dimensional segmentation can give an idea about the wall morphology and stent position, reliable serial evaluation critically depends on the correct matching of the images of measurement. This problem is avoided using volumetric intracoronary ultrasound, allowing spatial reconstruction for not only area measures but also volumetric estimates of the wall structures. Moreover, three-dimensional reconstruction of a vessel and stent facilitates intervention planning and evaluation of complications before, during, and after intervention.

In [51, 52] the authors propose to use a physics-based technique for three-dimensional reconstruction of stent and vessel inner wall based on deformable models. Their aim was to obtain a spatial reconstruction of both the vessel and the stent from an IVUS volumetric image to provide a tool for correctly estimating stent expansion. As mentioned, deformable models [29, 53] represent physics-based models that allow interpreting sparse image data under general constraint on their shape (smoothness, continuity, approximate model, etc.). Such a global segmentation and reconstruction technique is very important to reconstruct robustly the stent from the appearance of its struts as a sparse set of bright spots in the IVUS images (see Figure 10.15b) as well as to detect the inner wall, given the speckled "nature" of ultrasound images.

A deformable model is defined to interpret image data altogether in the IVUS sequence (instead of by longitudinal or cross-sectional slice-by-slice analysis). In particular, the technique of three-dimensional reconstruction of mutual position between stent and vessel is developed by means of two deformable generalized cylinders that adapt to the image features in IVUS planes corresponding to the vessel wall and the stent. These models have been implemented by B-splines because of their nice properties (i.e., easy to adapt to the vessel wall and stent, local control, model compactness, etc.) [54].

The use of a superficial deformable model results in a more robust segmentation technique that ensures globally smooth surface interpolating image features between image slices. A second advantage of the model compared to other IVUS analysis techniques is that it deforms guided by an *a priori* model of the stent and the vessel that makes it more selective to the image features. The elastic properties of the deformable model help interpolate the stent and vessel image features and ensure the continuity and coherence between image features throughout the IVUS image planes.

As mentioned, using deformable cylinders to obtain a spatial model of the stent and the vessel is of great interest because it provides a more robust technique for segmentation of the stent and vessel. Moreover, once the shapes of the stent and the vessel wall are available, the measurements regarding stent expansion defined in [50] can automatically be extracted to estimate the quality of the stent deployment. To help estimate stent apposition, a color-coded distance map can be offered for a more comprehensive interpretation of the stent deployment in the current IVUS plane (see Figure 10.17). In this map, the color of each pixel indexes the minimum distance to the closest boundary (of the stent or the vessel wall). In particular, reddish spots infer a large distance between stent and vessel. As a result, an easy perception of location of large distances between stent and vessel wall is achieved.

Developing tools for computer-assisted diagnosis of stent expansion is of great interest because the physician is able to determine the images of

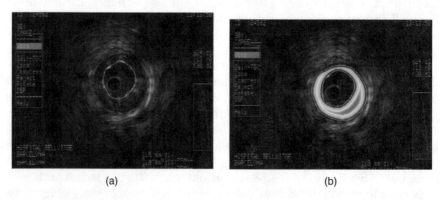

(a)   (b)

FIGURE 10.17 (See color insert.)
(a) Segmenting stent and (b) vessel allows measurement of their mutual position.

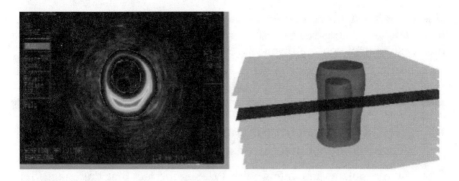

FIGURE 10.18 (See color insert.)
(Left) Visualization of the mutual position between stent and (right) vessel in the IVUS plane and space.

reference lumen area as well as the images of the beginning and end of stent appearance in order to reconstruct the stent and the inner vessel wall. Once both deformable cylinders have been adapted to the stent and to the vessel wall, the physician has a global three-dimensional view of the criteria for correct stent expansion (see Figure 10.18). Note that this view provides a new perspective of IVUS imaging because volumetric information about the place-ment of the stent is not available using just an IVUS sequence (due to its local nature). The physician is able to obtain and visualize the three-dimensional reconstruction of the stent and the inner wall of the vessel in order to make a decision about the optimal intervention and its result. Moreover, interaction with the reconstructed shapes is possible (rotation, zoom, observing a partic-ular IVUS image and its intersection with the reconstructed models, edition of the reconstruction results, etc.). Visualization of the mutual position of image data and the deformable models is crucial in getting confidence in the results of the IVUS analysis.

The IVUS tool allows temporal pursuit of the quality of the stent deploy-ment to study the evolution of the mutual position of stent and vessel wall. This possibility is of high clinical interest because it is still unknown whether or not improper stent expansion occurs gradually. Moreover, a quantitative assessment of the gain in lumen diameter after intervention can be done.

Summarizing, extracting measurements of the stent and vessel from their cylindrical representations in an entire coronary segment provides more detail of the complex vessel architecture and avoids the difficult mental conceptual-ization process. Compared to the approach of segmenting volumetric images slice by slice, the advantage of the deformable models approach is that im-age data from the volume are considered altogether, which leads to higher robustness taking into account the coherence of image features among image planes. This property is crucial, given the difficult interpretation of ultra-sound images. A second advantage of the deformable models approach is that it allows the introduction of general geometric assumptions about the object that is sought (guidance by an approximate model). Additionally, segmentation and reconstruction are unified in a single step, which allows for a direct estimate of volumetric measurements.

10.7   Need for Volumetric Measurements and Real Three-Dimensional Reconstruction of the Vessel

One of the problems in dealing with IVUS is the fact that the images represent a two-dimensional plane perpendicular to the catheter without any depth information. This IVUS property hides the real disease's extension and represents a very unnatural way of conceptualization. The foremost limitation of IVUS in pre- and posttreatment studies is the lesion image correlation in serial studies. This limitation is due to the lack of the third dimension, which gives much more global information about the internal and external vessel structure [55].

The third dimension allows a better knowledge of the vessel, the lumen, and the plaque, visualizing simultaneously multiple sections of the vessel and obtaining a longitudinal perspective [18, 56]. The vessel can be later studied under multiple formats and different cut axes to interpret, in the space, a certain discovery, hardly esteemed from the two-dimensional images (see Figure 10.19). The spatial reconstruction allows a more precise calculation of the size of the stent or the balloon to be implanted and makes easier the selection of better interventional instruments and their sizes. Three-dimensional images are synthesized by the sequential superposition of the two-dimensional ones. This kind of reconstruction presupposes that we are treating the coronary section as a straight line with the catheter transducer in the middle of the IVUS data cube.

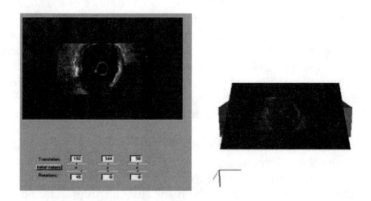

FIGURE 10.19
Dealing with the IVUS data cube allows visualization of data under different angles.

Gathering volumetric vessel information is also a very important point. For this purpose, IVUS data are completed by vessel and stent models to extract volumetric measurements about the vessel structures. According to medical experts, measuring the volume of the lumen before and after an intervention is useful for evaluating the positive and/or negative effects that the intervention has provoked. It helps to decide about further stent or angioplasty balloon interventions.

Extracting volumetric information is very important in evaluating intervention effects. Until now, area and distance calculations in IVUS planes have been the only possible ones carried out with IVUS images. Given a superficial analytical (e.g., B-spline) representation of vessel and stent, it is easy to estimate the distance between them in the images with delineated vessel and stent models. Then we can calculate the area of each model in pixels and infer the intersection area.

The criteria parameters that measure the mutual position between the stent and vessel are defined as planar parameters extracted from IVUS images. However, we should note that the IVUS planes are perpendicular to the catheter trajectory and not necessarily to the vessel. It is easy to see that assuming parallel IVUS planes and perpendicular to the vessel centerline yields to a loss of vessel tortuosity. Figure 10.20 shows an original image from a sequence of IVUS data and the extracted spatial model of the vessel from this sequence. One can note the straight shape of the reconstructed cylindrical model of the vessel wall. This fact can be a source of nonnegligible error of measurements that can be avoided using real three-dimensional reconstructed models of stent and vessel. To this end, IVUS data are not sufficient; we need to segment and reconstruct the vessel curvature from biplane angiograms (see Figure 10.20c and d). Having obtained a real three-dimensional shape of the vessel registering data from IVUS and angiograms, correct volumetric measurements can be estimated that will allow a redefinition of the clinical criteria for stent deployment based on volumetric vessel measurements.

10.8   Angiogram Analysis

An x-ray angiogram is performed to specifically image and diagnose diseases of the blood vessels of the body (e.g., heart, brain, etc.). Traditionally, an angiogram was used to diagnose the pathology of these vessels, such as blockage caused by plaque build-up. However, in recent decades, radiologists, cardiologists, and vascular surgeons have used the x-ray angiogram procedure to guide minimally invasive surgery of the blood vessels and arteries of the heart. In the past several years, diagnostic vascular images are often made using MR, CT, and/or ultrasound while the x-ray angiogram is reserved for therapy.

Angiographic x-ray imaging has grown into its own classification of x-ray imaging over time. The basic principle is the same as a conventional x-ray:

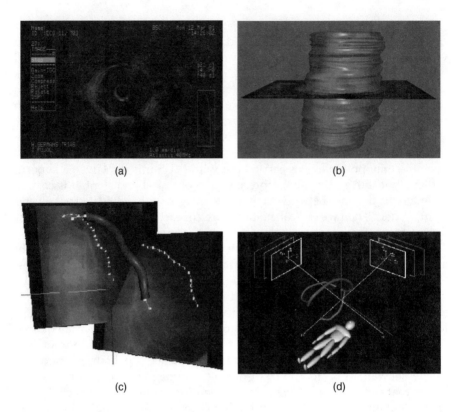

FIGURE 10.20 (See color insert.)
(a) Original IVUS image and (b) spatial model of the vessel extracted from IVUS; (c and d) spatial curvature of vessels recovered from biplane angiograms.

x-rays are generated by an x-ray tube and, as they pass through the body part being imaged, they are attenuated (weakened) at different levels. Figure 10.21 shows a cardiac catheterization laboratory. One can note the position of the fluoroscope device to acquire angiogram images with the image intensifier on the top and the x-ray generator underneath with respect to the patient. These differences in x-ray attenuation are then measured by an image intensifier and the resulting image is picked up by a TV camera. In modern angiogram systems, each frame of the analog TV signal is then converted to a digital frame and stored by a computer in memory and/or on hard magnetic disk. These x-ray "movies" can be viewed in real-time as the angiogram is being performed, or can be stored in a standard medical image format (Dicom) and reviewed later using recall from digital memory.

To acquire an angiogram to examine the blood vessels, the patient is positioned on the examination table by the technologist so that the anatomy of interest is in the proper field of view between the x-ray tube and image intensifier. A specialist in interventional radiology inserts a small tube (catheter)

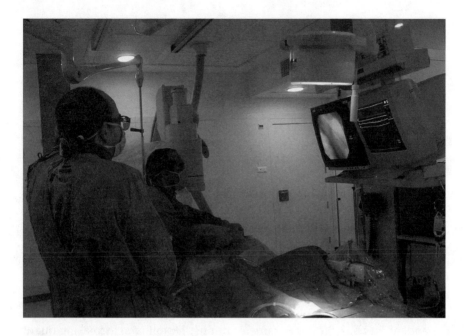

FIGURE 10.21 (See color insert.)
Cardiac catheterization laboratory.

into the blood vessel. During the angiogram, physicians inject streams of contrast agents or dyes into the area of interest using a catheter to create detailed images of the blood vessels in real-time and determine how well the blood moves through the vessels of the body.

Given that conventional x-ray angiography plays a leading role in the detection, diagnosis, and treatment of heart disease, heart attack, acute stroke, and vascular disease that can lead to stroke, a significant amount of work has been done on automatic analysis of angiograms [57–60]. The main areas of research in computer applications for angiograms during the past 15 years have been devoted to geometric and densitometric methods to automate quantitative analysis of coronary arteriograms. The first steps include assessment of coronary lesion severity [57] in individual segments, followed by a growing interest in automated identification and analysis of the entire coronary tree. Over the past few years, attention has been directed to research toward three-dimensional reconstruction from biplane projection [61], to improve measurements of small vessels [62] to mix data coming from different imaging devices [63], and to obtain three-dimensional dynamic models. Figure 10.22 shows the result of automatic borders segmentation of a vessel segment and quantitative estimate of vessel stenosis.

Correct vessel segmentation is a key issue in any automatic analysis task related to angiogram analysis. To extract and use the information present in the coronary image, many conventional methods have been proposed,

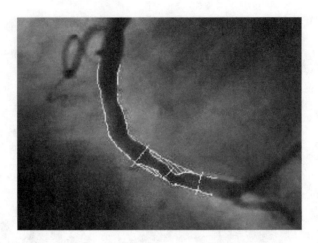

FIGURE 10.22
Automatic segmentation of vessel borders and stenosis evaluation.

although ambiguities and artifacts make the segmentation process highly dependent on heuristics or parameter tuning. Despite the increasing quality of the imaging equipment, the computer analysis task remains nontrivial. Hence, the impact of any improvement in the segmentation step is important. Two main strategies to segment the coronary tree have been reported:

1. Scanning consists of edge or ridge extraction, usually by a mask convolution. The second step implies recognition of the vascular structure by chaining the centerline points while heuristically excluding noise points. Most of the reported image feature detectors are conventional ones: Laplacian of a Gaussian [64], hat transform [65], ridge detector based on level-set theory [66], etc.

2. Tracking begins at an *a priori* known position of the vessel in the image. In a single-pass operation, feature extraction and vessel structure recognition are performed. By its very nature, a tracking strategy is computationally more efficient than scanning. In [67], given a starting point and direction, the authors define a line profile that is extracted some pixels ahead in the fixed direction and then used to compute the centerline of a vessel and the new forward direction for tracking purposes. In [68], the authors extract a curve sampling profile and use it to track the entire tree.

The conventional image feature detectors used in scanning are too general for the purpose of vessel detection in angiogram, bringing too many false responses. On the other hand, tracking strategy relies on simple densitometric features that are not enough to discriminate the vessel appearance.

Moreover, the tracking strategy needs a continuous set of image features, which usually is too strong a constraint for angiograms.

To cope with these shortcomings, the authors in [69] define a physics-based model called eigensnake that integrates the snake technique as a global segmentation and interpolation method combined with statistical image feature learning. Segmentation using snakes is a well-known technique that comprises two steps: feature detection using a scanning method to construct a potential map, followed by an energy minimization of the snake curve toward the minima of the potential (the image features of interest). The object recognition step is built in the curve shape deformation. Taking advantage of this property, the proposal of the authors is to reduce the method to only one step. The idea of this work is to specify the feature detector, depending on the target object and thus avoiding the map construction of conventional snakes. A sound statistical model is introduced to define a likelihood estimate of the grey-level local image profiles, together with their local orientation. This likelihood estimate allows one to define a probabilistic potential field of the snake where the elastic curve deforms to maximize the overall probability of detecting learned image features.

In particular, the eigensnake has defined its external energy as a function of the Mahalanobis distance of the image features located in the snake pixel position to a learned statistical vessel description. The vessel description is obtained from object responses of one-dimensional Gaussian derivative filters over different spatial scales. To obtain a filter response invariant to the vessel orientation, the authors project the filter output along the direction of grey-level variance [70]. Figure 10.23 shows the direction of the first eigenvector

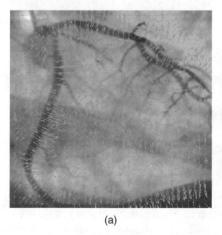

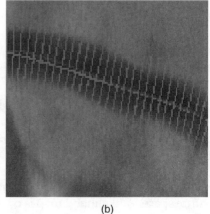

(a)   (b)

FIGURE 10.23 (See color insert.)
(a) Direction of the first eigenvector of the image structure tensor and (b) training vessel profiles oriented in this direction.

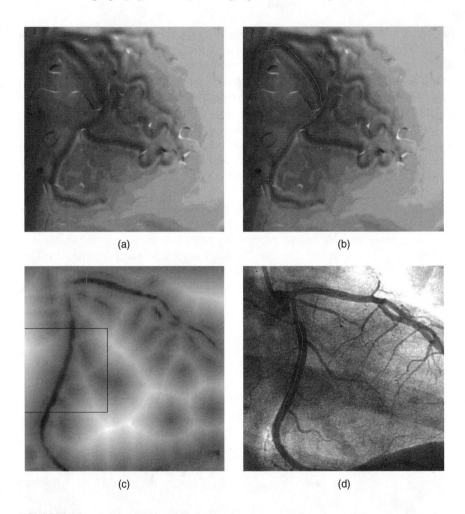

(a)   (b)

(c)   (d)

FIGURE 10.24
(a) The likelihood map of eigensnake and (b) the result of segmentation by eigensnakes on the likelihood map. (c) Improved likelihood map by eigensnakes based on PPCA and (d) the result of the segmentation process by eigensnakes.

of the image structure tensor and training vessel profiles oriented in this direction.

Given that each point of the vessel is represented by a set of filter responses, a dimensional reduction is carried out by means of PCA to define a reduced feature space. A likelihood map is constructed to illustrate the separability of vessel and no-vessel representations (see Figure 10.24a). The snake deforms using as external energy the Mahalanobis distance between the image features in the pixels under analysis and the learned feature projecting them into the reduced space (see Figure 10.24b). This process guides the snake toward the vessel centerlines. As a result, the formulation of eigensnakes allows statistically learning and detecting image features characterizing different appearances of nonrigid, elongated objects. The eigensnake technique has been successfully applied to the segmentation of angiograms presented in [69].

In [71], an improved version of eigensnakes has been presented to address the tracking problem of coronary vessels in angiograms. By means of probabilistic principal component analysis (PPCA), a feature description is obtained from a training set of object profiles. To improve the convergence of snake deformation, the authors enhanced the likelihood map by a physics-based model simulating a dipole-dipole interaction. Figure 10.24c shows the improved version of the potential field of the eigensnake and the results of the segmentation of the eigensnake on the improved potential field. As a result, a new extended local coherent interaction is introduced, defined in terms of an extended structure tensor of the image to give priority to parallel coherence vectors. Additionally, the probabilistic map is combined with the distance map to ensure less dependence on model initialization during its deformation. The approach presented has been applied to analyze and track coronary vessels in angiograms. In Figure 10.25, the snake tracking is illustrated for a set of consecutive angiogram frames.

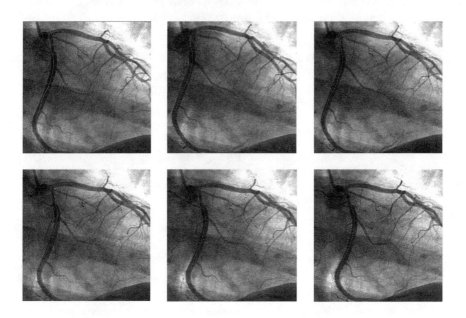

FIGURE 10.25
Tracking by eigensnakes.

10.9   Extraction of Three-Dimensional Measurements from Angiograms

Presently, medical imaging techniques (in particular, angiograms) are not only supposed to give qualitative information, but also quantitative measurements about the objects to be analyzed. Whereas the technique of angiogram was developed to obtain images from the coronary vessels from different views, measurements of the vessels became necessary very soon thereafter. This is the case with the determination of stent size. When the selected stent is too large, the vessel becomes too rigid, and the lesion is not treated. Obtaining the length of stenosis is of vital importance for the success in this kind of intervention. To obtain these measurements, a view of the affected vessel is taken and the length of the lesion is inferred. The imprecision in the system calibration, as well as the foreshortening due to the view, make these measurements inexact and unreliable. To cope with this, it is necessary to address the problem of a three-dimensional reconstruction of the vessel from two x-ray views (see Figure 10.26).

There are two main approaches to reconstruct the vessel centerline in space:

1. *Bottom-up strategy*: the user marks the corresponding points in angiograms, and their three-dimensional point is recovered and marked by the user (see Figure 10.27),

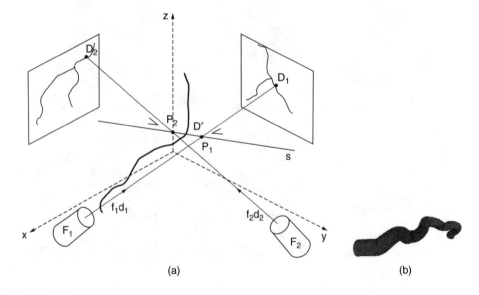

(a)   (b)

FIGURE 10.26
Defining corresponding projection points in x-ray images allows recovery of the vessel curvature.

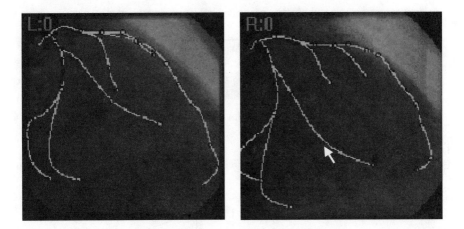

FIGURE 10.27 (See color insert.)
A bottom-up strategy to reconstruct vessel centerline is based on user-defined corresponding points in x-ray images.

2. *Top-down strategy*: a three-dimensional curvilinear model is considered that deforms in space so that its projections approximate the vessel in the x-ray images as well as possible.

Different works have been presented in the literature that follow the bottom-up strategy. Dumay et al. [72] describe a method for the reconstruction of a point using two views. Wahle et al. [73] address three-dimensional reconstruction of skeletons of the coronary tree from biplane views. Wunderlich et al. [74] present a procedure to obtain the length of a lesion after its reconstruction from biplane angiograms.

Now consider the problem of three-dimensional reconstruction of vessel centerlines following the bottom-up strategy.

Given an angiogram device (see Figure 10.21), the angles by which the left-right movement of a system can be defined with respect to the patient determine the rotational angles. The angles by which the movement of a system can be defined toward the head of the patient (cranial (CR) direction) or the feet (caudal (CA) direction) determine the angulation angles. With the imaging equipment, the heart can be displayed under x-ray exposure from a left anterior oblique (LAO) view to a right anterior oblique (RAO) view, with either a cranial or caudal angulation. Rotational angles are denoted by α and angulation angles by β. For the frontal and lateral rotation angles, $\alpha > 0$ represent LAO views and $\alpha < 0$ represent RAO views; angulation angles $\beta > 0$ represent caudal views and $\beta < 0$ represent cranial views. Both rotational degrees of freedom are shown in Figure 10.28a and b.

The projection axes of both systems intersect in the *isocenter* [72]. Once fixed at position i of the fluoroscope, the acquisition parameters are predetermined

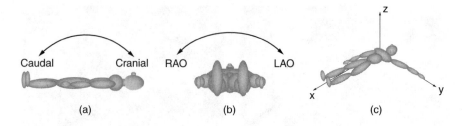

FIGURE 10.28
(a) Orientation of global coordinate system, and rotational degrees of freedom: rotation (b) and angulation (c).

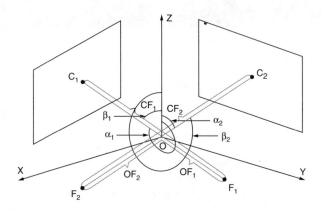

FIGURE 10.29
Acquisition parameters $(F_iC_i, \alpha_i, \beta_i)$ for two x-ray projections.

before the image acquisition process. They include the distance from the x-ray source to the image intensifier F_iC_i, angles of rotation α_i, and angulation β_i (see Figure 10.29). For a three-dimensional reconstruction, a global reference system is defined with origin at the isocenter O, X-axis in the direction of the patient bed toward the patient legs, Y-axis in the plane of the bed perpendicular to the X-axis oriented toward the left hand of the patient, and the Z-axis perpendicular to the bed plane and oriented to form a right-handed system (in the direction of the patient nose) (see Figure 10.28c). Moreover, local reference systems on both image planes are defined to allow for conversion from an image point to the global reference system (see Figure 10.30).

The equations to calculate the local reference system of a given image i are [72]:

$$\vec{k}_i = (0, -\cos\alpha_i, \sin\alpha_i)^T$$
$$\vec{c}_i = (\sin\beta_i, \sin\alpha_i \cos\beta_i, \cos\alpha_i \cos\beta_i)^T$$
$$\vec{l}_i = \vec{k}_i \times \vec{c}_i, \text{ where } i = 1, 2$$

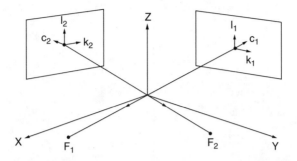

FIGURE 10.30
Global reference system (x,y,z) with the projection planes and their local systems.

A data point in the image matrix with coordinate pair (x, y) is transformed into a pair of real coordinates (x_k, y_k) in the projection plane by:

$$x_k = c_{cal}x \quad \text{and} \quad y_l = c'_{cal}y$$

Here, c_{cal} is the calibration factor and c'_{cal} is the calibration factor corrected by the pixel aspect ratio.

To assist in the process of determining corresponding points from both x-ray projections, a general constraint from projective geometry is applied. It is based on the fact that given a point D_1 in one x-ray image, its corresponding point in the other x-ray image should belong to the epipolar line (the projection of the ray $F_1 D_1$ onto the second x-ray image). Figure 10.31 shows the projection of a ray to a point from the first x-ray image into the second x-ray image. Hence, we are now able to identify a given point in one image plane in the other image by projecting the epipolar line corresponding to that point in the other projection plane (see Figure 10.32). The epipolar line in the second projection plane of a point D_1 from the first projection plane is computed from:

$$v\overrightarrow{F_1 F_2} + \mu\overrightarrow{F_1 D_1} + \overrightarrow{OF_1} = x_k \vec{k}_2 + y_l \vec{l}_2 + \overrightarrow{OC_2}$$

The line $y_l(x_k)$ is represented in the image matrix as $y(x)$ by applying the inverse transform of Equation 10.3.

Having determined the corresponding points D_1 and D_2 in both x-ray images, the spatial location of their three-dimensional point can be computed using the back-projection process. The spatial position of this point is computed by a simple intersection of the lines with vector representation:

$$\overrightarrow{OF_1} + \tau\overrightarrow{F_1 D_1} \quad \text{and} \quad \overrightarrow{OF_2} + \sigma\overrightarrow{F_2 D_2}$$

Both parameters τ and σ are solved from any two of the three equations of the vector components by elimination of the other parameter [72].

The bottom-up approach has several shortcomings. First, in many cases it is difficult to determine corresponding points. Second, even when the user is

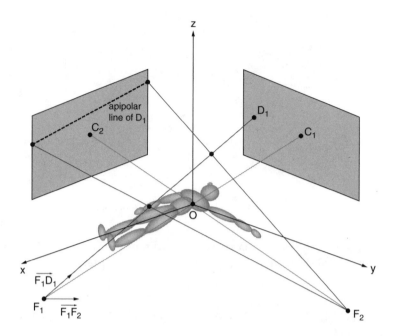

FIGURE 10.31
Illustration of the epipolar line.

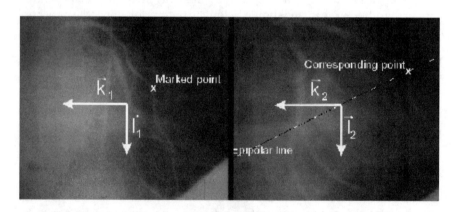

FIGURE 10.32
Epipolar line assists in determining the corresponding points in both x-ray images.

helped by the epipolar line in matching points in different views, measurement error in the calibration parameters makes the epipolarity constraint fail. Third, the curve is directly interpolated among marked points. As shown in Figure 10.33, the error in three-dimensional reconstruction can be deduced from the fact that the projection rays F_1D_1 and F_2D_2 constructed from both

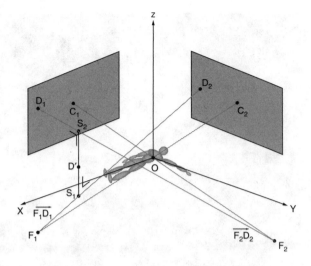

FIGURE 10.33
Due to the lack of precision in the fluoroscope acquisition parameters, the projection rays corresponding to the same point projected in both angiograms frequently do not intersect.

projections of the same three-dimensional point do not intersect. In these cases, the authors in [72] propose to use the closest three-dimensional point D' to the projection rays leading to an approximate solution of the three-dimensional reconstruction problem.

To improve three-dimensional reconstruction of the vessel centerline, in [75] the authors adopt a different approach to achieve three-dimensional vessel reconstruction from biplane images by means of deformable models. These authors propose to apply a top-down strategy: an elastic curve in the space deforms to adapt its projections to the vessels in the images. The user initializes the curve by a few points in the zone of the vessel to be reconstructed. Then, the curve deforms until its complete adaptation to the vessels in the images. This new kind of deformable curve is called a biplane snake. The authors studied the known shortcoming of point-based three-dimensional vessel reconstruction consisting of no intersection of projective beams and illustrated that by using biplane snakes, the reconstruction error is minimal.

Biplane snakes have been successfully applied to three-dimensional reconstruction of the vessel/lesion (see Figure 10.34). Note that length measurements of the lesion from just one x-ray image are prone to error due to the projective distortion of the vessel/lesion segment. Only a real three-dimensional reconstruction of the vessel/lesion segment can give exact three-dimensional measurements about the lesion to assist the cardiologist in his/her choice of the correct therapeutical intervention.

Furthermore, biplane snakes allow three-dimensional reconstruction of other therapeutical devices, such as the balloon during angioplasty (see

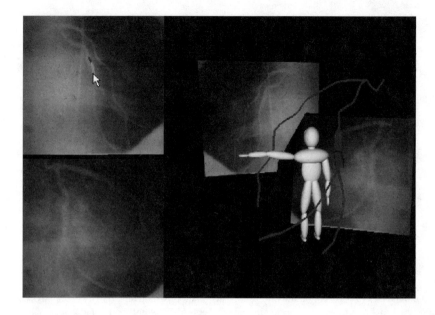

FIGURE 10.34 (See color insert.)
Three-dimensional reconstruction of the vessel by biplane snakes allows real three-dimensional measurements.

Figure 10.35). Such a three-dimensional reconstruction can be very useful before the stenting therapy to provide a global picture of the coronary scene [3].

Three-dimensional reconstruction of vessel centerlines can be applied to the entire coronary tree (see Figure 10.36). Furthermore, if the three-dimensional reconstruction process is applied to sequential angiogram sequences, dynamic parameters can be extracted about the motion of vessels in order to locally describe the motion of different zones of the heart. This dynamic information can be compared/coupled with information from other image modalities (e.g., nuclear magnetic resonance) to complete the computer-assisted diagnostic tools. Figure 10.37 shows the reconstructed coronary tree where a color map is applied to differentiate the dynamics of different vessel segments. The red color means high velocity of vessel segment while the blue color means more static vessel parts.

10.10   IVUS and Angiogram Registration

IVUS images represent cross-sectional pictures of the vessel in planes perpendicular to the catheter trajectory during its pull-back. Therefore, when observing an intravascular ultrasound stack of images, it is difficult to figure

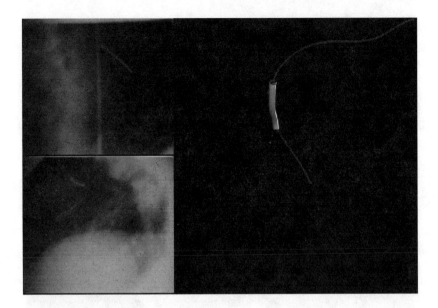

FIGURE 10.35
Three-dimensional reconstruction of the balloon by biplane snakes.

out the image position with regard to the vessel parts and ramifications, and misclassification or misdiagnosis of lesions is possible. This fact leads to the need for computer vision techniques to fuse the information from angiograms and intravascular ultrasound images to define the correspondence of every ultrasound image with a corresponding point of the vessel in the angiograms. Both methods (IVUS and angiogram) provide a lot of information about the internal and external shapes of the coronary vessels, respectively, as well as about vessel therapy (e.g., stent, etc.). The fusion of all this information will allow physicians to interact with the real extension and distribution of the disease in the space, making easier the arduous task of having to imagine it. Fusing angiographic and IVUS information has been considered in different works [76–78].

The focus of this section is to discuss a method to find the spatial placement of the IVUS image planes to guide vessel exploration.

To locate IVUS images in space a three-dimensional reconstruction of the catheter trajectory is necessary. For this purpose, registration of the catheter in two views of angiograms before and after the pull-back of the IVUS catheter should be performed. Moreover, to ensure precise three-dimensional reconstruction of the catheter from both x-ray views, minimal spatial displacement of the catheter should occur during the process of acquisition of multiple views of x-ray images. A biplane x-ray system provides two views of the catheter at the same time and provides conditions for a precise three-dimensional reconstruction of the catheter. However, today many hospital

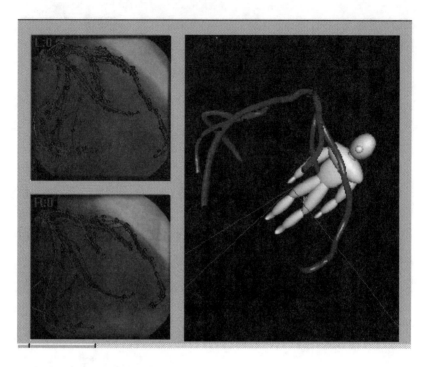

FIGURE 10.36 (See color insert.)
Vessel segmentation of angiogram sequences (on the left) and three-dimensional reconstruction of the coronary tree (on the right).

environments are still equipped with mono-plane x-ray devices (Figure 10.21). Considering the general case, given a mono-plane x-ray image system, ECG-gated x-ray images should be used and the patient should be asked to hold his breath during an instantaneous x-ray image acquisition in order to keep minimal spatial displacement of the catheter corresponding to both x-ray projections.

At this stage, the cardiologist locates the catheter head position before and after the pull-back in both angiogram views, and two, three-dimensional points are reconstructed. Note that these points represent the location in space of the center of the first and last IVUS images. Figure 10.38 shows two views of the catheter after finishing the pull-back. Once located, the position of the catheter head in one x-ray projection, the epipolar line, suggests the position of the catheter head in the other view. A local histogram-based image enhancement can be applied to the angiograms (see Figure 10.38) to emphasize the appearance of catheter position.

The reconstruction of the whole trajectory of the catheter consists of two steps: (1) detection/segmentation of the catheter projection from both x-ray views, and (2) reconstruction of its trajectory in space.

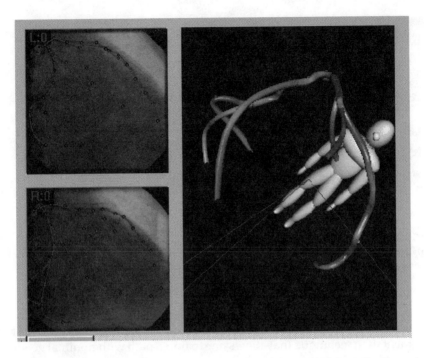

FIGURE 10.37 (See color insert.)
Spatial and dynamic model of the coronary tree: red color means high dynamic properties while blue color means static vessel segments.

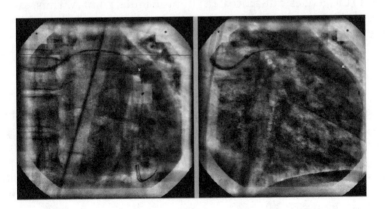

FIGURE 10.38
Locating the catheter head after the IVUS pull-back.

The catheter appears in the angiograms as a fine wire that makes it different in appearance compared to the vessel. Therefore, standard segmentation techniques based on vessel border extraction or eigensnakes are not robust or are time-consuming. In [78] the authors propose to apply the fast marching

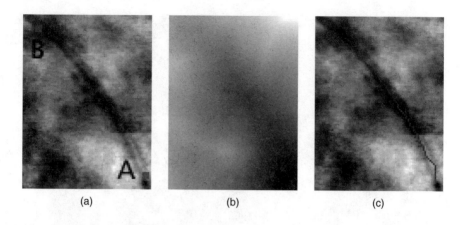

(a)   (b)   (c)

FIGURE 10.39
(a) Preprocessed x-ray image, (b) surface of minimal action, and (c) geodesic path between points A and B defining the catheter trajectory during the IVUS pull-back.

algorithm on the gray-level angiogram acquired without contrast dye to detect the catheter in a fast and robust way. The fast marching algorithm is a fast segmentation technique that allows one to find a path with minimal geodesic distance between two points of an image [79]. The fast marching algorithm as a segmentation algorithm is based on level set theory. A surface of minimal action (SMA) is constructed as a level set of curves L where the level corresponds to the geodesic distance $C\{L\}$ from an initial point A. Thus, each point (p from the SMA) U has a value $U(p)$ equal to the integral minimal energy of the geodesic path P starting from the initial point A and ending at point p:

$$U(p) = inf_{C\{L\}=p} \int \tilde{P} ds$$

The level sets construction can be considered a front propagation weighted by image cost (in our case, bright pixels provoke "resistance" of the front propagation). Beginning from a point A, front propagation (level set construction) is performed until the front reaches point B. It can be shown that the path of minimal geodesic distance from point B to A can be constructed by following the normal direction of the level sets, beginning from this passing through point B (see Figure 10.39).

When both projections of the catheter have been obtained, M equidistant points from one of the projections are chosen. Their corresponding points are the intersections of the corresponding epipolar lines and the detected catheter projection in the other x-ray view. Once defined, the corresponding points from both angiograms, their three-dimensional points are reconstructed and interpolated by a spatial B-spline curve [54] that represents the three-dimensional reconstruction of the catheter path done between the

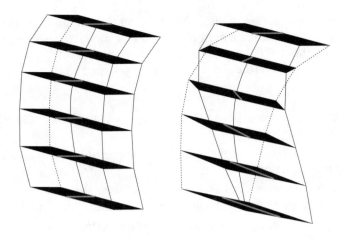

FIGURE 10.40
Orientation of IVUS planes: IVUS data cube should take into account the curvature of catheter trajectory (on the left) and twisting/rotation around the catheter path (on the right).

beginning and the end of the pull-back. Note that this spatial curve represents the trace of the centers of the IVUS images.

As a result, considering two projections with the catheter stopped before the pull-back begins and another two images at the end of the catheter pull-back, we can create a curve model of the pull-back situating one model's extreme at the position of the IVUS catheter before the pull-back beginning and, using the projections taken at the end of the pull-back, situate the ending extreme of the model coinciding with the last position of the catheter during its pull-back.

The next step is to place each IVUS plane in space to allow later reconstruction of vessel tortuosity. The position of each IVUS image is determined by IVUS catheter trajectory. The last IVUS image is positioned at the curve's extreme, corresponding to the ending of the pull-back, perpendicular to the curve, and the other images are situated along the curve at a distance given by the pull-back speed and the image discretization.

Special attention should be given to the image orientation/rotation around the catheter path (see Figure 10.40). First works presented in [77] apply geometrical constraints for the IVUS image location in space. For this purpose, the normals and binormals of the three-dimensional curve should be calculated. Using B-splines to represent the catheter trajectory, the Frenet triangle $(\vec{t}, \vec{n}, \vec{b})$ is analytically calculated, where $\vec{t}$ is the curve tangent, $\vec{n}$ is the curve normal, and $\vec{b}$ is the curve binormal of the B-spline catheter model. Taking into account that the IVUS image plane is perpendicular to the catheter, it means that it coincides with the normal plane defined by the normal and binormal of the catheter model. Thus, considering the distance the catheter head has moved from the endpoint of the catheter model (computed from IVUS data) and the three-dimensional length of the catheter model (computed from the angiograms data), the IVUS plane is located in space.

When dealing with the Frenet frame approximation, some problems arise:

1. The normal vector is not defined for linear segments or at inflection points.

2. The normal vector flips abruptly to the opposite direction around an inflection point.

3. For three-dimensional trajectories, the normal vectors can rotate excessively around the tangent vectors, causing unwanted twists.

4. The geometric approximation does not model the physical phenomena caused by the movement of the probe.

To solve all these problems and those concerned with physical laws ruling the movement of the catheter, in [80] the authors propose a dual method based on geometrical and computer vision techniques. The two main problems they address are the right position of the image planes in three-dimensional space and their accurate orientation. To solve the first problem, a sweeping-based method is proposed based solely on geometrical constraints. This method allows one to cope with the first three problems due to conventional approaches being based on the Frenet frame. To minimize the rotational transformation between two consecutive planes, the normal and binormal vectors of the previous IVUS plane are projected on the actual one, applying the following formulae:

$$\vec{n}_i = \vec{n}_{i-1} - \vec{t}_i * (\vec{n}_{i-1} \cdot \vec{t}_{i-1})$$

$$\vec{b}_i = \vec{t}_i \times \vec{n}_i$$

As a consequence, the result is a set of image planes with the right position but still there is no warranty that we have a correct image orientation. Image orientation can be changed due to physical causes (e.g., catheter/vessel friction effect) or physiological reasons (e.g., diastole/systole motion). Due to the difficult modeling of all these processes, to solve the image rotation problem, angular cross-correlation between consequent IVUS images can be used. Figure 10.41 shows consecutive IVUS frames and a graphic of the estimated rotation between them by cross-correlation procedure. The green line shows the estimated rotation and the blue one shows the estimated error. From the graphic it can be seen that the estimated rotation graphic shows resemblance with the blood pressure and ECG data. However, it is still a research issue to prove this relation. The rotation estimate based on image cross-correlation can be very time-consuming, which can make the calculation impractical.

Another observed motion effect is the axial movement of the intravascular ultrasound probe during the cardiac cycle [81]. The authors gave approximate

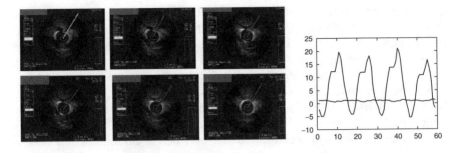

FIGURE 10.41
Rotational estimate between IVUS images.

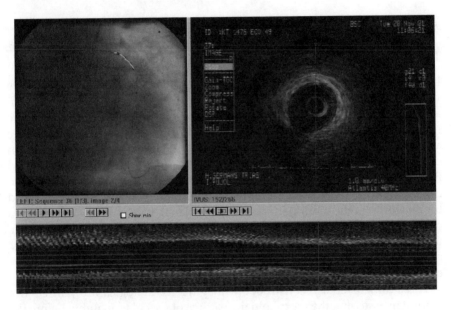

FIGURE 10.42
Registration of angiogram and IVUS data: the red point in the angiogram (top left) corresponds to the IVUS transverse plane (top right) and to the blue line in the longitudinal view of IVUS data (bottom).

estimates of the longitudinal transducer motion that can reach 1.5 mm with a variance of 0.8 mm. There is no analytical solution to control such movement and sort IVUS images. ECG-gated acquisition devices could avoid this shortcoming but make the IVUS procedure last several times longer.

Once oriented IVUS images are placed along the three-dimensional curve of the catheter model that is described during the catheter pull-back, the correspondence between IVUS and angiogram data is determined (see Figure 10.42). This allows the user to define corresponding data between angiograms and IVUS data. As a result, complete information about the vessel is obtained, including (1) information about the external view of the vessels, distance to ramifications, lesions, stents, and other anatomic parts of the heart using angiograms; and (2) information about the internal shape of the vessel (e.g., its morphological structure, vessel wall thickness and composition, plaque, calcium deposits, etc.) from IVUS data.

In summary, fusing IVUS and angiogram data is of high clinical interest to help physicians locate in IVUS data and decide which lesion is observed, how long it is, how far from a bifurcation or another lesion, etc. Automatic tools to estimate and show the correspondence between IVUS images and vessels in angiograms are of high clinical interest and it is a topic of further research by different teams working on IVUS and angiogram registration.

10.11   IVUS for Abdominal Aorta Aneurysm Analysis

Intravascular ultrasound images are proving their importance for coronary vessels. However, one should not think that cardiology is the only useful application of these images. Given their excellent properties (intraoperative images as well as providing morphological information about tissue structure and composition), IVUS images are generating increasing clinical interest in diagnosis and therapy of abdominal aortic aneurysms. It has been reported that determination of fixation sites and assessing dimensional information by cinefluoroscopy and angiography were limited by inaccuracies produced by image magnification, parallax, and uniplanar views. IVUS was used to determine the morphological features of vascular structures (i.e., calcium, thrombus), to perform real-time observation of the expansion of devices (e.g., graft), and to ensure firm fixation of balloon-expanded stents before the procedures of vascular anatomy were completed.

Three-dimensional reconstruction imaging technologies are particularly helpful in assessing the morphologic features of vascular anatomy before the intervention and at follow-up intervals. Moreover, three-dimensional IVUS provides a similar real-time perspective *during* the procedure [82]. Therefore, the problem of segmentation, three-dimensional reconstruction, and registration of fluoroscopy and IVUS images is relevant to the abdominal aorta aneurysm diagnosis and therapy. Figure 10.43 shows the result of applying deformable models (discriminant snakes) for segmenting IVUS images to obtain a spatial model of the abdominal aorta. Figure 10.44 and Figure 10.45 show the results of three-dimensional reconstruction of the abdominal aorta by segmenting IVUS and x-ray images and registration of their data. Both figures show the two x-ray projections with the segmented catheter trajectory on the left, and the three-dimensional model and the IVUS image on the right. The red point in the angiograms corresponds to the shown IVUS image on the right.

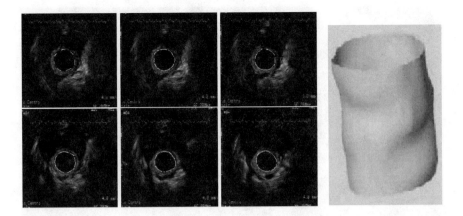

FIGURE 10.43
Segmentation and reconstruction of spatial model of abdominal aorta by discriminant snakes.

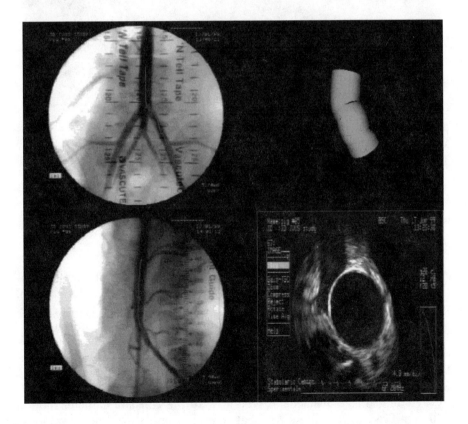

FIGURE 10.44
Three-dimensional reconstruction of abdominal aorta from IVUS and x-ray images.

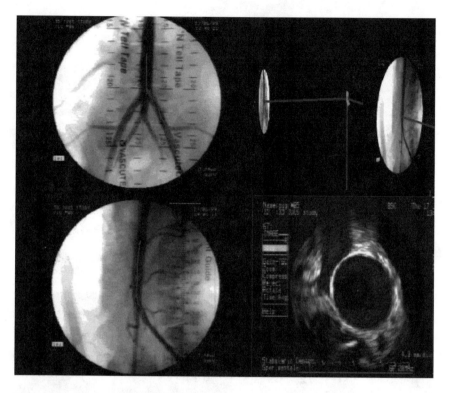

FIGURE 10.45
Mutual position of x-ray images and three-dimensional reconstructed model of the abdominal aorta obtained from IVUS and x-ray images.

10.12   Conclusions

As a conclusion, several factors including problems related specifically to intravascular ultrasound as well as general limitations of the three-dimensional reconstruction can affect the quality of the IVUS analysis, in particular vessel three-dimensional reconstruction. Both lumen and plaque volumetric measurements showed short-term biological variablity during repeated pull-back of the same coronary segment [83]. The quality of the basic intravascular ultrasound images is crucial; the image resolution is under continuous improvement by commercial IVUS device producers. Improving image quality, avoiding image artifacts, as well as assuring constant catheter motion will significantly contribute to a better understanding of and developing more robust image processing and computer vision techniques. At the same time, more clinical studies on IVUS are necessary to elucidate the important problems and real advantages of diagnosis and therapy IVUS images. On the other hand, although experts from image processing and computer vision have presented a lot of interesting and valuable work, there is still not enough transference of research studies into clinical practice. There are a lot of still open problems and questions in IVUS analysis and, in to our opinion, image devices technologists, physicians, and computer vision researchers should continue to work together to achieve really valuable computer-assisted tools for precise diagnosis and therapy by IVUS in an effort to further determine its clinical importance and its routine clinical use. Definitely, IVUS analysis is an interdisciplinary field of research as proved by several works published by such interdisciplinary teams.

References

1. P. Kearney, I. Starkey, and G. Sutherland. Intracoronary ultrasound: current state of the art, *Br. Heart J.*, 73(2), 1995.
2. A. Colombo, P. Hall, et al. Intravascular stenting without anticoagulation accomplished with intravascular ultrasound guidance, *Circulation*, 91(2), 1676–1688, 1995.
3. X. Zhang, C. R. McKay, and M. Sonka. Tissue characterization in intravascular ultrasound, *IEEE Trans. Med. Imag.*, 17(6), 889–899, 1998.
4. J. K. Morton. *The Cardiac Catheterization Handbook*, Mosby-Year Book, Inc., 1998.
5. F. De Man, I. De Scheerder, M. C. Herregods, J. Piessens, and H. De Geest. Role of intravascular ultrasound in coronary artery disease: a new gold standard? Beyond angiography, in *Intravascular Ultrasound: State-of-the-art XX Congress of the ESC*, Vol. 1, August 1998.
6. D. Hausmann, A. J. S. Lundkvist, G. Friedrich, K. Sudhir, P. J. Fitzgerald, and P. G. Yock. Lumen and plaque shape in atherosclerotic coronary arteries assessed by *in vivo* intracoronary ultrasound, in *Beyond Angiography. Intravascular Ultrasound: State-of-the-art XX Congress of the ESC*, Vol. 1, August 1998.
7. D. Meier, R. Cothren, D. Vince, and J. Cornhill. Automated morphometry of coronary arteries with digital image analysis of intravascular ultrasound, *Am. Heart J.*, 133, 681–690, 1997.
8. M. Sonka, X. Zhang, M. Siebes, et al. Segmentation of intravascular ultrasound images: a knowledge-based approach, *IEEE Trans. Med. Imag.*, 14, 719–732, 1995.
9. C. J. Bouma, W. J. Niessen, K. J. Zuiderveld, E. J. Gussenhoven, and M. A. Viergever. Evaluation of segmentation angorithms for intravascular ultrasound images, *Visualisation Biomed. Computing*, pp. 203–212, 1996.
10. J. Vandenberg, G. Liersch, H. Hanna, and J. Cameron. Fully automated media and lumen boundary detection in intravascular ultrasound images, in *Proc. IEEE Southwest Symp. Image Analysis and Interpretation*, pp. 71–75, 1996.
11. B. Solaiman, R. Debon, F. Pipelier, J.-M. Cauvin, and C. Roux. Information fusion: application to data and model fusion for ultrasound image segmentation, *IEEE Trans. Biomed. Eng.*, 46(10), 1171–1175, October 1999.

12. A. Mojsilovic, M. Popovic, N. Amodaj, R. Babic, and M. Ostojic. Automatic segmentation of intravascular ultrasound images: a texture-based approach, *Ann. Biomed. Eng.*, 25, 1059–1071, 1997.

13. F. Escolano, M. Cazorla, D. Gallardo, and R. Rizo. Deformable templates for plaque thickness estimation of intravascular ultrasound sequences, in *Proc. VII Nat. Symp. Pattern Recognition and Image Analysis*, Vol. 1, April 1997.

14. W. Li, J. G. Bosch, Y. Zhong, W. J. Gussenhoven, H. Rijsterborgh, J. C. H. Reiber, and N. Bom. Semiautomatic frame-to-frame tracking of the luminal border from intravascular ultrasound, in *Computers in Cardiology*, pp. 353–356, 1992.

15. J. Hu and X. Hu. Approach to automatic segmentation of 3-D intravascular ultrasound images, in *Proc. IEEE Nucl. Sci. Symp. on Medical Imaging Conf.*, Vol. 3, pp. 1461–1464, 1995.

16. R. J. Frank, D. D. McPherson, K. B. Chandran, and E. L. Dove. Optimal surface detection in intravascular ultrasound using multi-dimensional graph search, in *Computers in Cardiology*, pp. 45–48, 1996.

17. C. Von Birgelen, A. van der Lugt, A. Nicosia, G. S. Mintz, E. J. Gussenhoven, E. de Grey, and P. J. de Feyter. Computerised assessment of coronary lumen and atherosclerotic plaque dimensions in three-dimensional intracoronary ultrasound correlated with histomorphometry, *Am. J. Cardiol.*, 78, 1202–1209, 1996.

18. C. von Birgelen, C. Di Mario, W. Li, J. C. Schuurbiers, S. J. Slager, P. J. de Feyter, J. R. Roelandt, and P. W. Surreys. Morphometric analysis in three-dimensional intracoronary ultrasound: an *in vitro* and *in vivo* study performed with a novel system for the contour detection of lumen and plaque, *Am. Heart J.*, 132, 516–527, 1996.

19. R. Shekhar, R. M. Cothren, D. G. Vince, S. Chandra, J. D. Thomas, and J. E. Corhnill. Three-dimensional segmentation of luminal and adventitial borders in serial intravascular ultrasound images, *Computerised Medical Imaging and Graphics*, 23, 299–309, 1999.

20. J. D. Klingensmith, R. Shekhar, and D. G. Vince. Evaluation of three-dimensional segmentation algorithms for the identification of luminal and medial-adventitial borders in intravascular ultrasound images, *IEEE Trans. Med. Imag.*, 19(10), 996–1011, 2000.

21. W. Li, E. Gussenhoven, Y. Zhong, et al. Validation of quantitative analysis of intravascular ultrasound images, *Int. J. Cardiac Imaging*, 6, 247–254, 1991.

22. P. Dawhale, D. Wilson, and J. Hodgson. Volumetric intracoronary ultrasound: methods and validation, *Cathet., Cardiovasc. Diagn.*, 33, 296–307, 1994.

23. C. Von Birgelen, G. S. Mintz, P. J. de Feyter, N. Bruining, A. Nicosia, C. Di Mario, P. W. Serruys, and J. R. T. Roelandt. Reconstruction and quantification with three-dimensional intracoronary ultrasound, *Am. Heart J.*, 18, 1056–1067, 1997.

24. N. Bruining, C. von Birgelen, C. Di Mario, et al. Dynamic three-dimensional reconstruction of IVUS images based on ECG gated pull-back device, in *Computers in Cardiology*, pp. 633–636, 1995.

25. C. Von Birgelen, G. S. Mintz, A. Nicosia, et al. ECG-gated intravascular ultrasound image acquisition after coronary stent deployment facilitates on-line three-dimensional reconstruction and automated lumen quantification, *J. Am. Colleague on Cardiol.*, 1997.

26. P. Radeva, J. Serrat, and E. Martí. A snake for model-based segmentation, in *Proc. Int. Conf. Computer Vision-ICCV'95*, June 1995.

27. T. McInerney and D. Terzopoulos. Deformable models in medical image analysis: a survey, *Med. Image Anal.*, 1(2), 91–108, 1996.
28. J. Pardo, D. Cabello, and J. Heras. A snake for model-based segmentation of biomedical images, *Patt. Recog. Lett.*, 18(14), 1529–1538, 1997.
29. M. Kass, A. Witkin, and D. Terzopoulos. Snakes: active contours using finite elements to control local shape, in *Int. Conf. Computer Vision*, pp. 259–268, 1987.
30. L. D. Cohen and I. Cohen. Finite-element methods for active contour models and balloons for 2-d and 3-d images, *IEEE Trans. Patt. Anal. Mach. Intell.*, 15(11), November 1993.
31. A. Blake and M. Isard. *Active Contours*, Springer-Verlag, 1998.
32. A. Yuille, P. Hallinan, and D. Cohen. Feature extraction from faces using deformable templates, *Int. J. Computer Vision*, 8(2), 1992.
33. L. H. Staib and J. S. Duncan. Boundary finding with para-metrically deformable models, *IEEE Trans. Patt. Anal. Mach. Intell.*, 14(11), 1061–1075, 1992.
34. T. F. Cootes, C. J. Taylor, D. H. Cooper, and J. Graham. Active shape models—their training and application, *Computer Vision and Image Understanding*, 61(1), 38–59, January 1995.
35. A. Lanitis, C. J. Taylor, and T. F. Cootes. Automatic face identification system using flexible appearance models, *Image and Vision Computing*, 13(5), 393–401, 1995.
36. D. Gil, P. Radeva, and J. Saludes. Segmentation of artery wall in coronary IVUS images: a probabilistic approach, in *Proc. 15th Int. Conf. Pattern Recognition*, 4, 2352–2355, May 2000.
37. N. Otsu. A threshold selection method from gray-level histogramsedical engineering, *IEEE Trans. Systems, Man and Cybernetics*, 9(1), 62–65, January 1979.
38. R. Fletcher. *Practical Methods of Optimization*, John Wiley & Sons, 1987.
39. X. Pardo and P. Radeva. Discriminant snakes for 3d reconstruction in medical images, in *Proc. 15th Int. Conf. Pattern Recognition*, May 2000.
40. R. Rao and D. Ballard. Natural basis functions and topographic memory for face recognition, in *Proc. Int. Joint Conf. Artificial Intelligence*, pp. 10–17, 1995.
41. M. Turk and A. Pentland. Eigenfaces for recognition, *J. Cognitive Neurosci.*, 3(1), 71–86, 1991.
42. P. N. Belhumeur, J. P. Hespanha, and D. J. Kriegman. Eigenfaces vs. fisherfaces: recognition using class specific linear projection, *IEEE Trans. Patt. Anal. Mach. Intell.*, 19(7), 711–720, July 1997.
43. R. O. Duda and P. E. Hart. *Pattern Classification and Scene Analysis*, John Wiley & Sons, 1973.
44. S. A. Wickline, J. G. Miller, D. Recchia, A. M. Sharkey, S. L. Bridal, and D. H. Christy. Beyond intravascular imaging: quantitative ultrasonic tissue characterization of vascular pathology, in *Proc. Ultrasonics Symp.*, 1994.
45. P. Radeva and J. Vitria. Region-based approach for discriminant snakes, in *Proc. Int. Conf. ICIP*, Thesaloniki, Greece, 2001.
46. D. G. Vince, K. J. Dixon, R. M. Cothren, and J. F. Cornhill. Comparison of texture analysis methods for the characterisation of coronary plaques in intravascular ultrasound images, *Computerised Medical Imaging and Graphics*, 24(4), 221–229, 2000.
47. N. C. Hermann, M. Buchbinder, M. W. Cleman, et al. Emergent use of balloon expandable coronary artery stenting for failed percutaneous transluminal coronary angioplasty. *Circulation*, 82, 812–819, 1992.
48. P. N. Ruygrok and P. W. Serruys. Intracoronary stenting: from concept to custom, *Circulation*, 94, 1996.

49. H. Mudra, M. Sunamura, H. Figulla, et al. Six month clinical and nagiographic out-come after IVUS guided stent implantation, *J. Am. Colleague Cardiology*, 29(171A), 812–819, 1997.

50. D. Robert and M. D. Safian. Coronary stents, in *The New Manual of Interventional Cardiology*, pp. 459–518, Malaga, Spain, 1998.

51. C. Cañero, O. Pujol, P. Radeva1, et al., in *Optimal Stent Implantation: Three-Dimensional Evaluation of the Mutual Position of Stent and Vessel via Intracoronary Echocardiography*, in *Proc. Int. Conf. Comp. Cardio.*, Hannover, Germany, 1999.

52. P. Radeva, C. Cañero, J. J. Villanueva, et al. 3d reconstruction of a stent by deformable models, in *Proc. Int. Conf. IASTED*, Malaga, Spain, 2001.

53. S. Menet, P. Saint-Marc, and G. Medioni. B-snakes: implementation and applica-tion to stereo, in *DARPA Image Understanding Workshop*, 1990.

54. B. A. Barsky, R. H. Bartels, and J. C. Beatty. *An Introduction to Splines for Use in Computer Graphics and Geometry Modeling*, Morgan Kaufmann, 1987.

55. O. Pujol. Model-Based Three Dimensional Interpolation of IVUS Images, Masters thesis, Computer Vision Center, 1999.

56. C. von Birgelen, C. Slager, C. Di Mario, P. J. de Feyter, and W. Serruys. Volumetric intracoronary ultrasound: a new maximum progression-regression of atheroscle-rosis, *Atherosclerosis*, 118 Suppl., 1995.

57. J. Reiber and P. Serruys. *Progress in Quantitative Coronary Arteriography*, Kluwer Academic, 1994.

58. A. Klein, F. Lee, and A. Amini. Quantitative coronary angiography with deformable spline models, *IEEE Trans. Med. Imag.*, 16(5), 468–482, October 1997.

59. K. Kitamura, J. M. Tobis, and J. Sklansky. Estimating the 3-d skeletons and trans-verse areas of coronary arteries from biplane angiograms, *IEEE Trans. Med. Imag.*, 7(3), 173–187, September 1988.

60. L. van Tran, R. C. Bahn, and J. Sklansky. Reconstructing the cross sections of coronary arteries from biplane angiograms, *IEEE Trans. Med. Imag.*, 11(4), 517–529, December 1992.

61. A. C. M. Dumay. Image Reconstruction from Biplane Angiographic Projections, Ph.D. thesis, *Technische Universiteit Delft, The Netherlands*, 1992.

62. M. Sonka, G. Reddy, and S. Collins. Adaptive approach to accurate analysis of small diameter vessels in cineangiograms, *IEEE Trans. Med. Imag.*, 16, 87–95, 1997.

63. G. Prause, X. Zhang, S. DeJong, C. R. McKay, and M. Sonka. Semiautomated segmentation and 3D reconstruction of coronary trees: biplane angiography and intravascular ultrasound data fusion, in *Proc. SPIE*, Vol. 2709, 1996.

64. R. Poli, G. Coppini, M. Demi, and G. Valli. An artificial vision system for coronary angiography, in *Proc. Int. Conf. Computers in Cardiology*, pp. 17–20, 1991.

65. X. Zhan, S. M. Collins, and M. Sonka. Tree pruning strategy in automated detection of coronary trees in cineangiograms, in *Proc. Int. Conf. Image Process-ing ICIP–95*, pp. 656–659, 1995.

66. A. Lopez, R. Toledo, J. Serrat, and J. Villanueva. Extraction of vessel centerlines from 2d coronary angiographies, in *8th Spanish Conf. on Pattern Recognition and Image Analysis*, 1, 489–496, 1999.

67. Y. Sun. Automated identification of vessel contours in coronary arteriograms by an adaptive tracking algorithm, *IEEE Trans. Med. Imag.*, 8, 78–88, 1989.

68. K. Barth, B. Eicker, and J. Seissl. Automated biplane vessel recognition in digital coronary angiograms, in *Proc. SPIE. Medical Imaging IV, Image Processing*, 1233, 266–274, 1990.

69. R. Toledo, X. Orriols, P. Radeva, X. Binefa, J. Vitria, C. Cañero, and J. J. Villanueva. Eigensnakes for vessel segmentation in angiography, in *Proc. 15th Int. Conf. Pattern Recognition*, May 2000.
70. J. Weickert. Coherence-enhancing diffusion of colour images, *Image and Vision Computing*, 17, 1999.
71. R. Toledo, X. Orriols, P. Radeva, X. Binefa, J. Vitria, C. Cañero, and J. J. Villanueva. Tracking elongated structures using statistical snakes, in *Proc. Int. Conf. Computer Vision and Pattern Recognition*, 2000.
72. A. C. M. Dumay, J. H. C. Reiber, and J. J. Gerbrands. Determination of optimal angiographic viewing angles: basic principles and evaluation study, *IEEE Trans. Med. Imag.*, 13(1), March 1994.
73. W. Wahle, H. Oswald, G. Schulze, J. Beier, and E. Fleck. 3-D reconstruction, modelling and viewing of coronary vessels, in *Proc. Int. Conf. CAR'91*, pp. 669–676, 1991.
74. W. Wunderlich, F. Fischer, H.-R. Arntz, H.-P. Schultheiss, and A. Morguet. Development and clinical evaluation of an online procedure for lesion length measurement in coronary intervention, in *Proc. Int. Conf. Computers in Cardiology*, September 1999.
75. C. Cañero, P. Radeva, R. Toledo, J. J. Villanueva, and J. Mauri. 3d curve reconstruction by biplane snakes, in *Proc. 15th Int. Conf. Pattern Recognition*, May 2000.
76. C. J. Slager, J. J. Wentzel, J. C. H. Schuurbiers, et al. True 3-dimensional reconstruction of coronary arteries in patients by fusion of angiography and IVUS (ANGUS) and its quantitative validation, *Circulation*, pages 511–516, August 2000.
77. A. Wahle, G. P. M. Prause, S. C. DeJong, and M. Sonka. Geometrically correct 3-D reconstruction of intravascular ultrasound images by fusion with biplane angiography—methods and validation, *IEEE Trans. Med. Imag.*, 18(8), 686–699, 1999.
78. D. Rotger, P. Radeva, C. Cañero, J. J. Villanueva, et al. Corresponding IVUS and Angiogram Image Data, *Proc. Int. Conf. Computers in Cardiology*, Rotterdam, The Netherlands, 2001.
79. L. D. Cohen and R. Kimmel. Global minimum for active contour models: a minimal path approach, *Int. J. Computer Vision*, 24(1), 57–78, August 1997.
80. O. Pujol, C. Cañero, P. Radeva1, et al. Three Dimensional Reconstruction of Coronary Tree Using Intravascular Ultrasound Images, *Proc. Int. Conf. Computers in Cardiology*, Hannover, Germany, 1999.
81. A. Arbab-Zadeh, A. N. DeMaria, W. F. Penny, R. J. Russo, B. J. Kimura, and V. Bhargava. Axial movement of the intravascular ultrasound probe during the cardiac cycle: implications for three-dimensional reconstruction and measurements of coronary dimensions, *Am. Heart J.*, 138(5), 865–872, November 1999.
82. R. A. White, C. E. Donayare, I. Walot, et al. Preliminary clinical outcome and imaging criterion for endovascular prosthesis development in high-risk patients who have aortoiliac and traumatic arterial lesions, *J. Vasc. Surg.*, 24(4), October 1996.
83. P. Dawhale, Q. Rasheed, J. Berry, and J. Hodgson. Quantification of lumen and plaque volume with ultrasound: accuracy and short term variability in patients, *Circulation*, 90, I-164, 1990.

11

Clinical Applications Involving Vascular Image Segmentation and Registration

Stephen Aylward and Elizabeth Bullitt

CONTENTS

11.1 Introduction

Blood vessels both aid and impede medical procedures. For example, angiogenesis increases bleeding and the risk of complications during tumor resection. Yet, vascular networks provide pathways for a growing number of minimally invasive procedures such as tumor embolization. The publication of this book and the rapid expansion of the use of vascular interventional radiology are indicative of the increasing importance of *vascular images*, that is, images that detail the location and geometry of a patient's vasculature. Vascular images play an important role in every phase of clinical care: disease detection and diagnosis, as well as treatment planning, guidance, and assessment. This chapter discusses computer-based methods for vascular images that help clinicians appreciate vascular images in a timely manner.

Computer-based image analysis methods generally focus on image segmentation and registration. Vessel *segmentation*, that is, the delineation of vessels in an image, enables vessel visualization and quantification. For example, vascular segmentation enables intracranial vessel visualization for surgical path planning and automated stenosis quantification. Vessels can also serve as an excellent set of dense landmarks for image *registration*, that is, identifying corresponding points between two images and defining how one image should be rotated, translated, and possibly warped to best match another image. Registering images taken over time helps localize anatomic changes for cancer detection, treatment monitoring, and augmenting intra-operative images with detailed preoperative images for surgical guidance.

Vessel segmentation and registration, however, are long-standing challenges for medical image analysis researchers [1–20]. Even with advanced contrast agents and scanners, image analysis methods must cope with the fact that many vessels (1) exist at or below the spatial resolution of most clinical scanners, (2) may be poorly differentiated from their background due to contrast timing, and (3) may appear to be discontinuous due to flow characteristics and scanner noise. This chapter reviews a variety of segmentation and registration methods with respect to these three difficulties.

This chapter also presents examples of the clinical utility of select vascular image segmentation and registration methods [19, 21–24]. While these examples focus on three areas of vascular anatomy — intra-cranial vasculature, the abdominal aorta, and liver vasculature — the methods presented can nevertheless be more broadly applied. Furthermore, many vessel segmentation methods [8, 21] not only improve the visualization and quantification of vessels, but also enable the characterization of their *interconnectedness*, that is, their arrangment as a vascular network. By selectively coloring or hiding one or more segmented vessels based on their interconnections, clinicians can simulate intravascular procedures such as the passage of a catheter or the change in flow resulting from the embolization of a particular arterial branch; clinical hypotheses can be interatively tested, refined, and communicated. In the near future, we expect such *procedural vascular visualizations* to drive the specifications of new clinical hypotheses and techniques. Consider the vascular image analysis application shown in Figure 11.1. Two CT scans of the same patient were taken at different times after the release of a contrast agent. Those scans selectively captured the portal and hepatic vascular networks of the patient's liver. The liver vessels in those scans were segmented; the branching patterns of those networks were then extracted to characterize the function of the segmented vessels; the vessel models were then registered; and in Figure 11.1 they are being viewed simultaneously for living donor liver tranplant planning.

To date, most medical image segmentation and registration research has focused on processing images that are tuned to discriminate between tissues, that is, *tissue images*. For an excellent overview of statistical segmentation methods, the reader is encouraged to consult the synopsis provided by Duda et al. [25]. An excellent review of methods for registering tissue images is provided by Hill [26]. It is beyond the scope of this chapter to detail the state-of-the-art of tissue image segmentation and registration.

In this chapter, Section 11.3 discusses the primary methods for vascular image display: volume rendering and surface rendering. Section 11.4 and Section 11.5 present select methods for vascular image segmentation and

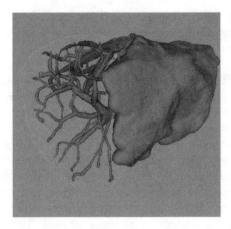

FIGURE 11.1 (See color insert.)
Portal and hepatic vein segmentations taken from two contrast CT scans are shown simultaneously for living donor liver transplant planning.*

registration, illustrate their roles in vascular image display, and emphasize their utility for procedural visualizations. Special attention is given to multiscale segmentation and registration methods based on vessel centerlines because this class of methods offers insensitivity to image noise and can extract vessels near the resolution of an image. This chapter concludes with a discussion of future applications of vascular image analysis with special emphasis on using vascular images for intra-operative guidance. Each section has information relevant to clinicians and researchers. However, the next section, on vascular image acquisition, is probably most relevant to both groups. It is critical for clinicians and researchers to realize that acquisition protocols for images intended for computer-based medical image analysis are likely to be different from the protocols being used to generate images for human review.

11.2   Vascular Image Acquisition Requirements

The complex interplay of image resolution in time and space is inherent to photography as well as medical imaging. Subject movement, shutter speed, contrast agent uptake, lighting, radiation dose, film speed and grain, and the film development process are intertwined in many ways. Traditional imaging

---

* The medical data used to generate this and all of the other images in this chapter were acquired in and provided by the Department of Radiology at The University of North Carolina at Chapel Hill.

protocols balanced these parameters to favor human review of the resulting images. In particular, human visual processing speeds and spatial and gray-scale acuity drove the balance. A new balance must be sought to support computer analysis. For example, for three-dimensional medical image analysis, the balance shifts to produce data sets with *isotropic voxels*, that is, having the same physical size in x, y, and z dimensions. Images with isotropic voxels typically have a massive number of slices so as to match the slice thickness with the in-plane resolution. This multitude of slices cannot be reviewed in a timely manner without computer assistance. In general, for two- and three-dimensional medical image acquisition, computer analysis introduces more stringent requirements on existing acquisition parameters, such as contrast timing and intensity homogeneity; very few computer-based analysis methods are as robust as the human visual system. The parameters, quality, and consistency of the images to be processed will determine whether an analysis method can be devised and applied in a few minutes using existing techniques or instead requires extensive research, method development, and hours to compute. The successful integration of computer-based analysis into a clinical environment depends on the acceptance of new acquisition protocols as well as the acceptance of the computer methods.

This section provides details regarding the major issues involved in the acquisition and processing of two- and three-dimensional vascular images for computer analysis. This section is intended as an overview of the common requirements for these data as well as the computational power required to process them. Specific applications will often add to these requirements. The good news is that existing commercial CT, MR, fluoroscopy, ultrasound, and other image acquisition devices can provide images that meet most of these requirements. For those cases in which suitable images cannot be acquired or in which the retrospective analysis of less-suitable images is necessary, preprocessing methods can often be employed to generated sufficient images from less-suitable images. We provide illustrations of select preprocessing methods.

11.2.1 Two-Dimensional Vascular Imaging via Projection

The major difficulty with two-dimensional vascular images is projection overlap. Consider Figure 11.2. The digital subtraction angiogram captures the intracranial arteries distal to a patient's right carotid artery. It is problematic to distinguish branchings from crossings, to determine which vessels are in front of others, to decide if a vessel is directed toward or away from the x-ray source, or to identify if smaller vessels may exist in front or behind the larger vessels. One technique to aid in the resolution of projection-depth ambiguities is to capture a sequence of projection images during contrast release; however, ambiguities due to overlap and a lack of out-of-plane information will remain. Additionally, because stenoses and aneurysms may only be visible when projected from specific points of views, unfortunate

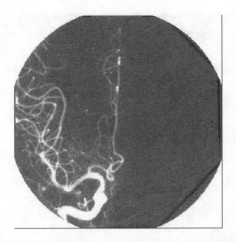

FIGURE 11.2
This x-ray digital subtraction angiogram of intracranial vasculature poorly conveys the three-dimensional structure of the vascular network. It is difficult to distinguish vessel crossings from branches. Depth information is absent. Small vessels may be completely obscured by larger ones. Such images do, however, enable the detection of aneursyms and stenoses, the tracking of catheters, and the visualization of "downstream" vascularity for embolization guidance.

point-of-view selection, or overlapping vessels may make any two-dimensional vascular image formed via projection clinically suspect.

In addition to these general issues with two-dimensional images, many device- and application- dependent two-dimensional vascular image analysis issues exist. For example, the image intensifiers used to acquire digital subtraction x-ray angiograms are often distorted by gravity. Consider Figure 11.3. A precisely machined grid of fine wires was imaged in a clinical x-ray fluoroscopic machine to illustrate the spatial distortions present in its images. By rotating the machine with respect to the direction of gravity, the shape and strength of this distortion will change. For certain registration algorithms it may be necessary to correct for these distortions. Imaging grid phantoms such as the one shown help quantify and therefore calculate the corrections for these distortions.

To provide out-of-plane information and thereby resolve many of the difficulties associated with two-dimensional vascular image analysis, multiple two-dimensional angiograms can be acquired from different points of view. The vessels in those images can then be segmented; and by establishing correspondence between, that is, registering, those segmentations, their three-dimensional positions can be triangulated and three-dimensional vascular models can be formed. In biplane angiography, this model formation process is traditionally performed mentally by clinicians; see Figure 11.4. Much medical image analysis research has focused on explicitly segmenting and registering multiple angiograms to form and display three-dimensional vascular

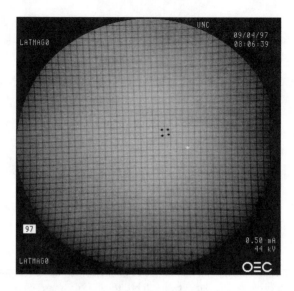

FIGURE 11.3

This fluoroscopic image of a carefully machined regular grid of wires illustrates the spatial distortion induced by the acquisition process, that is, the wires appear to bend inward near the left and right edges of the image. Much of the apparent bending results from the effect of gravity on the image intensifier.

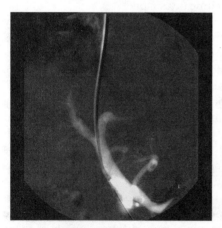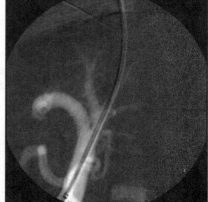

FIGURE 11.4

During a transjugular intrahepatic portosystemic shunt placement, a long needle is guided down the jugular and into a hepatic vein. The needle is forced through the liver and into a portal vein so that a shunt can be inserted to enable blood to flow through cirrhotic livers. This procedure is guided using biplane fluoro to capture the position of the needle with respect to the portal vein. Shown are anterio-to-posterio and lateral digital subtraction angiograms that depict a patient's portal veins. Establishing correspondence between these images is difficult but enables the three-dimensional triangulation of the vessels, needles, and other instruments in the images.

models on a computer [27–29]. The most difficult step in this process is identifying corresponding points in both scans. Researchers have investigated two computer-based approaches for resolving correspondence ambiguities. (1) Vascular models can be formed from pre-operative three-dimensional data, registered with the intra-operative biplane angiograms, and thereby used to resolve correspondence in biplane images [5]. (2) Building upon the fact that establishing correspondence is easier if the points-of-view of two images are close, other researchers have developed three-dimensional vessel models by rapidly moving c-arms through partial or full circles (i.e., *rotational angiography*) and then reconstructing the vasculature in three dimension from the multiple scans [27, 28]. Both approaches utilize vessel segmentation and registration methods. The rotational angiography approach is essentially a three-dimensional acquisition technique. Issues surrounding three-dimensional acquisition are discussed next.

11.2.2   Three-Dimensional Vascular Imaging

To enable the computer analysis of three-dimensional vascular images, two existing clinical requirements are emphasized: (1) resolution in time and space, and (2) avoiding intensity inhomogeneities and noise. These issues are common in medical image acquisition for human review; but as mentioned previously, higher levels of compliance are required for accurate and consistent computer-based medical image analysis.

11.2.2.1   *Three-Dimensional Resolution in Space and Time*
For computer-based three-dimensional medical image analysis, localizing an image's features in time and space is of utmost importance. The spatial resolution requirements refer to the need for high-resolution (i.e., small), isotropic voxels. Time resolution is essential when contrast agents are used so that the desired vascular structures are well distinguished. The role of these requirements is given below.

The need for most computer-based image analysis methods to rely strictly on the information in an image to perform its analyses motivates the need for high-resolution, isotropic voxels. Human readers are able to process coarse images because humans incorporate previous experience and anatomic knowledge into their analyses. Few computer-based methods have reached that level of sophistication. Computer-based image analysis systems generally seek points, curves, or surfaces in an image. Such structures are located using first- and second-derivative image intensity measures. As a rule of thumb, we have found that such measures are rotationally invariant if a maximum of a three-to-one ratio exists between the in-slice point spacing and the slice thickness. Furthermore, given a three-to-one ratio, such measures are accurate to a scale of about 1.5 times the in-slice point spacing. For details on such scaled measures and their role in medical image analysis, see [30]. For example, if it is necessary to model the centerline of vessels with 2-mm diameters, then if a three-to-one ratio must be used, the spatial resolution should be, at most, 1 mm × 1 mm within a slice and the slice thickness should be less than 3 mm. Changing the in-plane resolution to 0.75 mm × 0.75 mm will not significantly add to the quality of the three-dimensional model formed. Decreasing the slice thickness will add to the quality. Consider Figure 11.5. The high-resolution in-plane appearance of a slice masks the fact that the slice

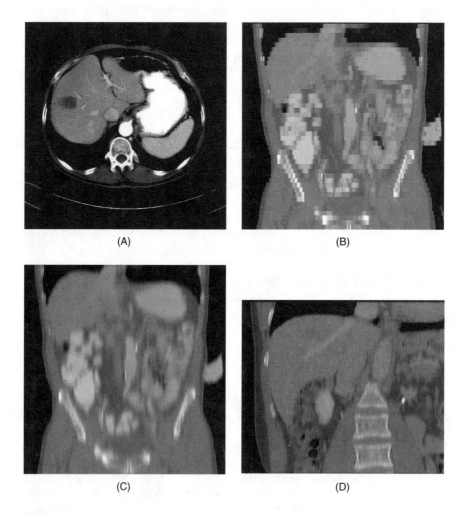

(A)   (B)

(C)   (D)

FIGURE 11.5
Three-dimensional medical images must have nearly isotropic voxels to provide sufficient data for three-dimensional model formation. (A) In-plane resolution is misleading. (B) The reslicing of the volume containing the slice in (A) illustrates the true coarseness of the data. (C) B-spline interpolation can be used to create isotropic voxels after image acquisition, but missing details cannot be reconstructed in this manner. (D) High-resolution, nearly isotropic voxels are available from modern scanners for computer-based three-dimensional medical image analysis.

thickness causes small features to be lost or their across-plane positions to be undefined.

Another motivation for isotropic voxels is computation time. If the computer analyses require the calculation of image intensity derivatives, then if the data are not isotropic, those calculations become as much as three times slower to mathematically account for the anisotropy.

Many preprocessing methods have been developed to resample an image to create isotropic voxels, including B-spline interpolation and shape-based interpolation [31].

An example of the effect of B-spline interpolation is shown in Figure 11.5. The data across slices is used to smoothly approximate data in intervening slices. The figure illustrates the difficulty with this popular approach — boundaries are blurred in the intervening slices. To combat this blurring, shape-based interpolation was developed; the objects and boundaries in an image are segmented in the coarse data and used to constrain the interslice interpolation so that the boundaries remain sharp between slices. However, when the anisotropy is large, the utility of any interpolation scheme is limited. Information not present, such as the position of a small feature within the depth of a slice, can never be resolved via interpolation. Most modern scanners, however, do provide isotropic voxels at high resolution. The two slices in Figure 11.6 clearly indicate the increase in resolution provided by modern scanners. The first image is from a 1.5T magnetic resonance machine and is at a 1 mm × 1 mm × 3 mm resolution. The second is from a 3T magnetic resonance machine and is at 0.6 mm × 0.6 mm × 0.6 mm resolution. The slices are shown using the same point size to emphasize the resolution difference. A larger number of small vessels is clearly visible in the high-resolution image.

The ability to detect smaller vessels in high-resolution isotropic images is, however, of limited utility if the relevant vessels cannot be distinguished from the irrelevant vessels. Once again, human reviewers can use past experience and anatomic knowledge to quickly focus on desired vessels and mentally prune irrelevant vessels, but those skills are difficult to impart to a computer method. The conspicuity of desired features (e.g., the ability to distinguish arteries from veins) in a three-dimensional vascular image is generally dependent on the delay between the release of a contrast bolus and the time and duration of the image's acquisition. In Figure 11.7, for example, the appreciation of the arteries is confounded by the visibility of veins. Research is underway to aid in the differentiation of segmented arteries and veins and is reported in Section 11.4 of this chapter.

Contrast timing is not the whole story regarding vessel conspicuity in medical images being analyzed by computers. It is also important for the intensity characteristics of the desired vessels to be consistent throughout the image. Achieving this consistency is a matter of achieving a uniform intensity bias field, consistent contrast uptake, and minimal intensity noise. These imaging features are discussed next.

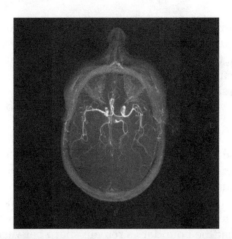

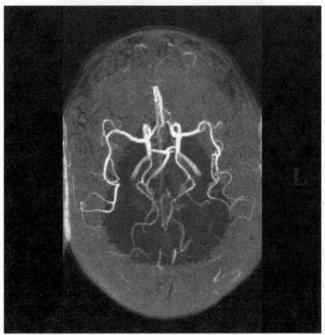

FIGURE 11.6
The maximum intensity projections of two magnetic resonance angiograms are shown. The top projection is from a 1.5T scanner and was acquired using 1 mm × 1 mm × 3 mm voxels. The bottom projection is from a 3T scanner and was acquired using 0.6 mm × 0.6 mm × 0.6 mm voxels. The projections are shown using the same number of voxels per inch to emphasize the increased number of voxels recorded by the 3T scanner. A larger number of small vessels are clearly visible in the 3T data.

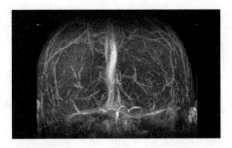

FIGURE 11.7
This volume rendering (maximum intensity projection) of the intracranial vasculature of a patient illustrates the importance of contrast agent timing. This acquisition protocol captured arteries and veins. It is difficult to visually distinguish between the two networks. If the task is to detect small aneurysms, this protocol is inappropriate.

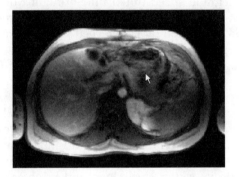

FIGURE 11.8
This abdominal MR scan illustrates a strong intensity inhomogeneity. An intensity threshold appropriate for segmenting the contrast-enhanced liver vessels in the middle of the image is inappropriate for segmenting the liver vessels near the top and bottom of the image.

11.2.2.2 Intensity Inhomogeneities, Contrast Uptake, and Noise

An *intensity inhomogeneity* is a spatially varying intensity bias across a two- or three-dimensional image; that is, the image will appear bright in one region and dim in another [32, 33]. Intensity inhomogeneities are most commonly associated with MR images in which they arise due to RF field inhomogeneities and poor coil alignment. However, intensity inhomogeneities are also evident in x-ray images such as mammograms due to x-ray heel effects and in CT images due to beam hardening. Acquistion protocols and scanner technologies are improving, and these spatially varying biases generally do not interfere with human review; however, even subtle inhomogeneities must be considered by computer-based analysis systems. These inhomogeneities may cause the accuracy of intensity-based segmentation methods to vary throughout an image. These inhomogeneities may also cause systematic errors in intensity-based registration methods. Figure 11.8 is an abdominal

MR image. Its intensity inhomogenity is evident as bright regions in the anterior and posterior of the patient's data.

Image processing methods have been developed to retrospectively reduce the effect of intensity inhomogeneities in MR images [32, 33]. Some of the most successful versions of these correction methods segment the images into tissue classes in order to estimate a bias correction field that induces consistent statistical tissue characteristics throughout a volume [33]. A method that retrospectively corrects the bias fields in MR angiograms has recently been developed and is illustrated in Figure 11.9.

Even with the removal of intensity inhomogeneities, spatial variations may still be present in an image. For example, if a large vascular network must be captured, even an ideally timed contrast bolus may be non-uniformly distributed throughout that network. Additionally, within and across vessels, blood flow velocity variations due to laminar flow can disrupt contrast agent distribution and degrade speed-tuned time-of-flight MR angiography. An excellent review of contrast agent distribution and flow rate factors is given in the papers and dissertation by Hoogeveen [10]. An example of flow rate variations inducing an irregular intensity profile within a vessel in a time-of-flight MR angiogram is shown in Figure 11.10. Time-of-flight MR angiography is tuned to respond maximally to fluid flowing at a particular speed. Any fluid flowing faster or slower than that speed will produce a weaker response. Blood flows rapidly down the center of a vessel and more slowly near the vessel's wall. This MR was tuned to find fluid flowing slower than the blood was flowing at the center of the carotid and yet faster than the blood was flowing along the edges of the carotid. Therefore, the vessel's intensity profile is dim along its center and edges, and brighter at a certain radial distance from the center where the blood was moving at the tuned speed. These irregular intensity profiles can complicate vessel segmentation and registration.

Of course, random noise also exists in vascular images, and a variety of pre-processing methods are available to reduce its effect. Many of these methods essentially attempt to remove the high-frequency spikes within the data. Such smoothing, however, may unsharpen (blur) the edges within an image. A more sophisticated and valid method for noise removal is variable conductance diffusion (VCD) [34]. This is an edge-preserving smoothing method. Variations on VCD that preserve tubes (vessels) in an image have also been developed [35]. A demonstration of edge-preserving VCD is given in Figure 11.11 — the intensities internal to the liver have been smoothed but the liver's edges remain sharp. The difficulty with edge-preserving smoothing is specifying a sensitive and specific metric to define "edges" in an image. Resolution, intensity homogeneity, and the ability of an imaging device to associate different intensities with different tissues factor into the edge detection metric and thereby the utility of VCD. Additionally, VCD can be computationally expensive, requiring multiple iterations over the data to produce effective results. Many of the other methods mentioned in this section can also require

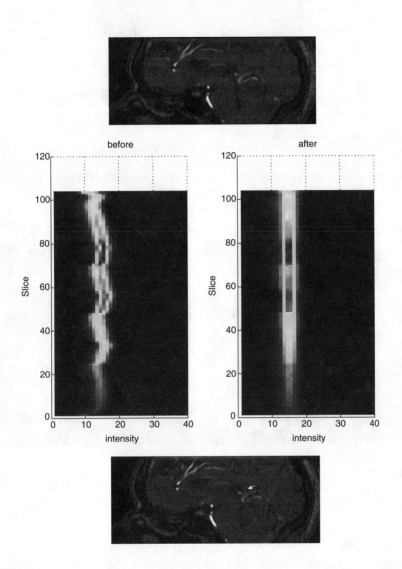

FIGURE 11.9

Top: A cut-through, axially acquired MR angiogram reveals *venetian-blind* artifacts (i.e., the wide horizontal bands of varying intensity) that are associated with the slabs that comprise the volume. Within the slabs, smoothly varying intensity inhomogeneities exist. The first two-dimensional histogram depicts the slice-by-slice changes in intensity frequency in the volume. The venetian-blind and smoothly varying bias fields are obvious as discrete jumps and smooth changes in the cluster of intensities associated with vessels. The second histogram was calculated in the same manner but using the corrected MRA (bottom image). The inhomogeneities have been eliminated. Vessel intensity statistics are consistent throughout the volume.

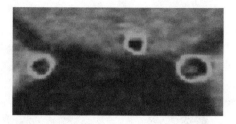

FIGURE 11.10 (See color insert.)
An enlargment of a region of an axial time-of-flight MRA slice. Artificial coloring is used to emphasize the different intensities within the carotids, which indicate different flow rates within them. These cross-sectional intensity variations complicate vessel segmentation and may confound vessel registration methods.

(A)   (B)

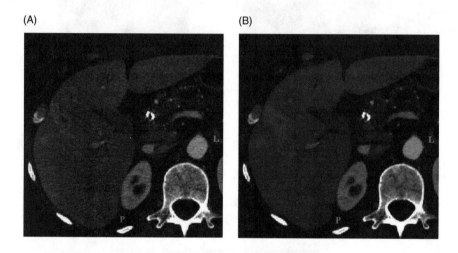

FIGURE 11.11
(A) Before and (B) after variable conductance smoothing has been applied to make the intensities within the liver more homogeneous while preserving the sharpness of the edges of the liver.

extensive computer memory and processing time, especially when processing the large, high-resolution data sets inherent in three-dimensional vascular image analysis. These computational demands are detailed next.

11.2.3 Computational Demands

Advances in vascular imaging have increased the standard of care for planning, delivering, and assessing vascular interventional, tumor resection, partial-organ transplant, and many other clinical procedures. One of the initial advances was an increase in image quality (resolution and anatomic specificity) such that clinically effective, computer-based image analysis methods could be developed. More recent advances have increased image quality to the point that fully utilizing the detail available in the images (1) places extreme processing speed and memory demands on the hardware executing the methods and (2) enables of development of highly complex computer methods. For example, high-gradient MR and multi-detector CT machines can produce $512 \times 512 \times 440$ voxel data sets that require 230 megabytes of memory; multiple CT and MR scans are being acquired from a single contrast bolus; and perfusion, diffusion, and other MR protocols are being used more frequently in clinics.

Regarding ever-increasing processing speed and memory requirements, there are two classic computer science solutions: "more powerful" processors and parallel computing. Using "more powerful" processors is valid when computational power and computing requirements are expected to increase simultaneously. While this expectation has been met for word processors and other office productivity software, there are indications that this expectation is unwarranted for medical image analysis software. The amount of information that must be simultaneously considered by physicians appears to be quickly outpacing the processing capabilities of readily available computer equipment. Parallel computing, however, offers hope. For this discussion we have broadened the definition of parallel computing to include many of its variants: fine-grain parallelism (multi-processor machines), data streaming through a single processor, and distributed (multiple, networked computer) solutions. Many medical image analysis methods are, in fact, extremely well suited for most forms of parallel processing (e.g., [21]).

The maturation of the fields of medical image acquisition and analysis, as well as the apparent need for parallel computation, have lead to the development of increasingly complex image analysis methods. Researchers are learning how to devise methods that consider more detail within and across images and how to incorporate anatomic and expert knowledge [36, 37]. These methods generally utilize a similar set of basic image processing modules (building blocks), and it is those modules that must be explicitly programmed to parallelize a method. These modules form a *software library*, but the required number of modules and the need to optimize the implementation of these modules make them difficult to program and debug. Additionally, if different individuals develop methods using different sets of software modules, then the resulting methods may not be able to interoperate or be easily exchanged or compared. These difficulties are alleviated by the establishment of a standard set of modules for medical image analysis method development. The National Library of Medicine has established a public domain software library for medical image analysis, the Insight Toolkit. It is available from http://www.itk.org. Unfortunately, as stated by Professor Andrew Tanenbaum in his *Computer Networks* book, "The nice thing about standards is that there are so many to choose from" [38]. The ultimate acceptance of the Insight Toolkit remains to be proven, but it is a viable tool for medical image analysis researcher and users today.

In conclusion, the necessary two- and three-dimensional data, the software libraries, and the computational power for effectively specifying medical image analysis methods are available; all that remains are the design and implementation of segmentation and registration methods to bring computer-based vascular image analysis to clinicians. This, however, is not a trivial task. Not only must a common language be developed between clinicians and developers to enable ideas to flow, but the time and complexity of each other's tasks must also be understood so that the real problems of medical image analysis can be identified and realistic solutions and timeframes established. Fred Brooks, who led the development of the IBM 360 operating system, describes computer method development as fun for several reasons: "First there is the sheer joy of making things.... Second is the pleasure of making things that are useful to other people.... Third is the fascination of fashioning complex puzzle-like objects of interlocking moving parts and watching them work in subtle cycles, playing out the consequences of principles built-in from the beginning. ... Fourth is the joy of always learning, which springs from the non-repeating nature of the task.... Finally, there is the delight of working in such a tractable medium. The programmer, like the poet, works only slightly removed from pure thought-stuff" [39]. However, that tractable medium can also be an algorithm developer's downfall. Its pliable nature means that well over half of a method's development time will probably be spent on debugging and testing, and developing a friendly user interface may increase overall product delivery time by a factor of nine. Truly, the time to develop a method may frequently seem inordinate, but the potential benefits are enormous. Some of the successes in medical image segmentation and registration methods and their applications are presented later in this chapter. First, we present how the original and processed (e.g., segmented) medical image data can be viewed.

11.3   Displaying Vascular Volume Images

To display a volume of data on a computer screen so as to simulate a three-dimensional object, there are two techniques: volume rendering and surface rendering. It is critical to understand their strengths and weaknesses prior to using them to make clinical decisions [40].

11.3.1   Volume Rendering

The most common form of three-dimensional medical image display is volume rendering. Volume rendering simulates rays passing through a volume of data and striking the computer screen. Volume rendering methods are differentiated based on how they accumulate the intensities encountered by

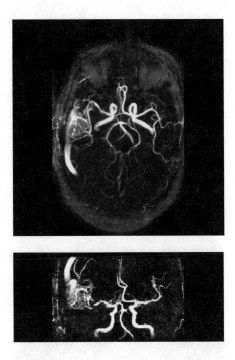

FIGURE 11.12
Such maximum intensity projection (MIP) renderings of intracranial vasculature are common outputs of MR scanners. Intensity window and level settings are preset to segment the vessels from the background.

each ray. Clinicians are quite familiar with maximum intensity projection volume rendering (see Figure 11.12). When certain MRA protocols are run on MR scanners, the scanners automatically generate a sequence of such MIP images from different points of view to convey the three-dimensional arrangement of the vessels in the recorded volume. Without renderings from multiple points of view, MIP renderings can be as difficult to interpret as two-dimensional vascular images formed via projection (see Section 11.2.1 and Figure 11.13).

Most volume rendering research has focused on developing ray integration functions that provide more three-dimensional information, increase realism, and decrease computation time. The state-of-the-art for vascular image volume rendering is provided by a commercial system: Vitrea by Vital Images, Inc., Minneapolis, MN. This system uses a ray integration function that heavily weights the intensity of the last "important" point it encountered in the volume. Its default rendering of the abdominal aortic aneurysm originally shown in Figure 11.13 is displayed in Figure 11.14. Human preference for such images is unquestionable. The Vital Images rendering clearly provides significant three-dimensional detail from a single point of view. Furthermore, the hardware on which this system runs allows the user to interactively adjust

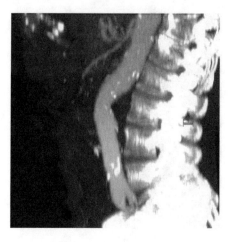

FIGURE 11.13
An MIP of an abdominal aortic aneurysm as captured by contrast CT data. The three-dimensional configuration of the aneurysm is difficult to determine from this single point of view. Hounsfield values simplify the selection of intensity window width and level settings.

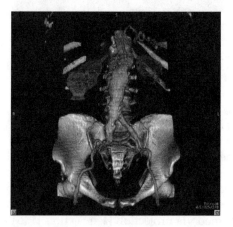

FIGURE 11.14 (See color insert.)
This vivid depiction of an abdominal aortic aneurysm was generated on a commercial medical image volume rendering system (Vitrea by Vital Images, Inc.). The user can interactively change the point of view. The points shown and the colors in the image were assigned to the CT data using preset thresholds based on Hounsfield units. These thresholds can be interactively modified. The volume can be trimmed or a region of interest hand-segmented.

the point of view — providing a very convincing kinetic depth perception effect. Additionally, the user can update the intensity window widths and levels used to designate what is "important"and assign colors to the recorded CT values. These thresholds, just like the threshold used to distinguish vessels from background in MIP renderings, are, in fact, segmentation methods; they are global thresholding methods.

Global thresholding is one of the most basic forms of segmentation. Every point in an image is determined to be part of an object of interest, or not, based on its recorded intensity value. The user of the segmentation system or the physics of the acquisition device (e.g., via Hounsfield units) determines the threshold values. Global thresholding is effective for select CT and MRA visualization applications, but global thresholding has severe limitations. For example, intensity alone is often insufficient to distinguish an object of interest from surrounding objects; for example, thresholds are unable to distinguish vessels from skull near the base of the brain in contrast CT data. Additionally, slightly changing a threshold value may drastically change the apparent shape and size of an object as surrounding points are included or excluded — determining the "correct" threshold can be problematic. Furthermore, as mentioned in the previous section, intensity inhomogeneities, laminar flow, and contrast timing can cause a threshold to be valid only for one small region of an image at a time.

To reduce global thresholding's susceptibility to spatially varying distortions, most visualization packages allow a user to trim a volume to a small rectangular region of interest or to coarsely outline the object to specify an arbitrarily shaped region of interest. Such region-of-interest specification is another form of segmentation and in its extreme produces hand segmentations of the object of interest. There are many difficulties with hand segmentation: significant time may be required, anatomic expertise is required, and hand segmentation suffers from high intra- and inter-user variability. The time requirements and the probability for error make hand segmentation infeasible for intracranial and liver vascular network analysis. Nonetheless, it is arguably the *de facto* state-of-the-art in the clinic for segmentation. Hand segmentation has found clinical use in three-dimensional analysis of abdominal aortic aneurysm (AAA), in liver segmentation for partial liver transplant planning, in tumor tracking to monitor drug therapies, and in many other applications. Also, even hand segmentation enables the next form of visualization for medical image display: surface rendering.

11.3.2 Surface Rendering

Surface rendering techniques simulate light rays bouncing off a surface and striking the computer screen [41]. This technique is used to generate the photorealistic computer images used in movies, the three-dimensional stereo graphics visualizations used in virtual reality systems, and the fanciful fast-action scenes favored by computer game developers. As a result of its popularity and prevalence in the entertainment industry, the hardware required to rapidly generate and interact with surface renderings already exists on most personal computers. Using standard PC hardware it is possible to rapidly change a surface's color, texture, illumination, and transparency.

Obscuring surfaces can quickly be removed from a scene. For medical applications, these capabilities translate to being able to illustrate vascular connectivity by color and being able to remove irrelevant vessels from view. However, the difficulty with surface rendering is that it requires the specification of a surface.

Surface delineation is the focus of segmentation, and it is particularly difficult for many anatomic data sets. Most critically, a surface implies a sharp boundary, and the location or even the existence of such a boundary may simply not be supported by the recorded data. Additionally, in many medical situations, a lack of boundary sharpness may be the deciding factor for making a diagnosis; for example, to distinguish benign and malignant tumors. As a result, a user's *preference* to view a surface rendering must be tempered by its potential effect on his or her *performance*. Depending on the clinical task, segmentation should perhaps be limited to specifying regions of interest for volume rendering. Luckily, boundary sharpness is rarely critical to the analysis of vessels in an image, and so for the remainder of our discussion we focus on segmentation methods and assume that surface rendering the results is appropriate. The following taxonomy of segmentation has global intensity thresholding at its foundation.

11.4   Vascular Image Segmentation

One of the most common adaptations of global thresholding is *connected components* [24]. Connected components refers to a class of methods that augment intensity thresholding with the requirement that the points belonging to an object of interest must be continuous; that is, they must be linked together by other object points having appropriate intensities in the volume. The behavior of this method is intuitive. It is illustrated in Figure 11.15 and in Figure 11.16. Variations on this method follow up with pruning and smoothing techniques (via morphological operators) to clip small structures and fill in holes due to intensity noise. These extensions, however, may cause small vessels to be clipped from a vascular network segmentation or noise to be included. Additionally, this method remains sensitive to intensity inhomogeneities and obscuration by undesired structures that abut the desired object and have similar intensity values. This obscuration is evident in the images: in Figure 11.15, segmenting the AAA via connected components also causes the spine and two ribs to be segmented; in Figure 11.16, the intracranial aneursym is only partially segmented due to flow effects and neighboring vessels that obscure the view of its neck.

To compensate for intensity inhomogeneities, spatially adaptive threshold methods have been developed [19]. These methods use localized statistical measures to monitor the subtle changes in intensity within an object as it is represented throughout a volume. It notes when the mean intensity of an

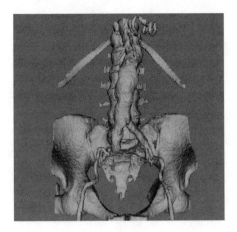

FIGURE 11.15
From contrast CT abdominal images, connected components can be applied to segment the bright objects in the image. A typical result is shown here. Regretfully, because this AAA and the spine abut, they are grouped as a single object. However, such segmentations can still speed the measurement of the length and cross-sectional area of the AAA for stent planning.

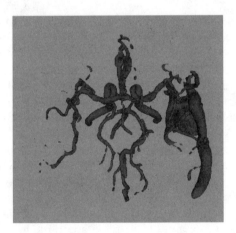

FIGURE 11.16 (See color insert.)
In this image, connected components has been applied to segment the vasculature in a ToF MRA volume image. This segmentation can be interactively viewed on standard PC hardware. Embolization planning is facilitated; however, connected components was not able to segment the small vessels in the image.

object's points becomes darker or brighter, and adapts its thresholds accordingly. These methods have had good clinical success for localizing the neck of an aneurysm and automatically planning optimal digital subtraction angiogram points-of-view to visualize the neck [19]. For vascular images in our lab, we have instead chosen to focus on preprocessing methods to correct

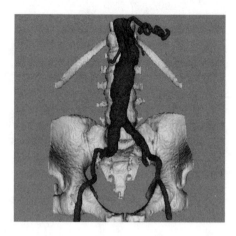

FIGURE 11.17 (See color insert.)
By integrating smoothness and connectedness constraints into segmentation via adaptive surface or boundary evolution (shown here) methods, an AAA that abuts the spine can still be segmented from the spine. The spine was still included in this visualization to provide anatomic reference. By isolating the AAA, stent planning is fast and accurate.

for slab and other intensity inhomogeneities inherent in MR angiograms (see Section 11.2.2.2). Neither approach, however, prevents adjoining structures from being included with the vascular segmentations. Both methods are still susceptible to noise, and neither can extract smaller vessels.

To compensate for adjoining structures, boundary evolution and level set methods have been developed and are now beginning to be used in clinical vascular image analysis tasks [13]. This is a very active area of medical image analysis research. Most variants of this class of methods begin with a rough estimate of the boundary of the object of interest and then iteratively refine that boundary toward the nearest edges in the volume while maintaining a user-defined degree of smoothness. An example of our method for boundary evolution is illustrated in Figure 11.17 for our AAA data. The AAA is distinguished from the spine, but in this illustration the spine is still rendered (using connected components) to provide anatomic reference. By focusing on boundary features using first- and second-derivative measures instead of intensity features at the scale of the image, these methods are inherently insensitive to intensity inhomogeneities [30].

Boundary evolution segmentations also enabled a new set of clinical tasks to be addressed: vessel cross-sectional area estimation. Stenoses and aneurysms are defined with respect to their effect on the expected width of the vessel. Via segmentation it is no longer necessary to measure diameters by hand and assume that such measures accurately represent the cross-sectional area of the blood vessel; a plane can be automatically oriented normal to the centerline of a segmented blood vessel, and the vessel points in that plane can be automatically counted and used to accurately measure cross-sectional area.

Similarly, by reslicing an image normal to a vessel's centerline, the ideal length of a stent or shunt can be quickly determined. Furthermore, these solid-object representations have been used by researchers to model the flow of blood through a vessel [8]. These fluid dynamic models have reached a level of detail that enables the modeling of the elastic properties of the vessel walls and the particle/fluid behavior of blood. Such models support the detection of turbulent flow and thereby the potential locations for calcium buildup [42].

Boundary evolution approaches, however, will not work for smaller vessels, that is, when the radius of the vessel of interest approaches the resolution of the image. These small vessels exist at nearly the same scale as the noise in the images. Looking for one edge of one of these vessels would require measurements at or below the actual resolution of the data; and if interpolation was used to create isotropic voxels, the situation is worse due to edge blurring. These difficulties led to the investigation of features that could be measured at larger scales in order to segment vessels. Vessel centerlines are one such feature.

11.4.1 Dynamic-Scale Centerline and Radius Representations

The contents of this section partially overlap with the journal article by Aylward, S. and Bullitt, E., "Initialization, Noise, Singularities, and Scale in Height Ridge Traversal for Tubular Object Centerline Extraction," IEEE Transactions on Medical Imaging, 21(2), pp. 61–75 Feb. 2002, Refer to that article for additional details.

Blood vessels, bronchi, bowels, ducts, or nerves in two- and three-dimensional medical data and other anatomic objects are tubular; that is, they have nearly circular cross sections, smoothly varying radii, and possibly follow tortuous paths and branch.

We will show that vessel centerlines can be used to segment small as well as large vessels in the presence of noise, irregular intensity profiles, intensity inhomogeneities, and contrast uptake variations. These methods have been in extensive use in multiple research labs and clinical sites and are beginning to be incorporated into commercial products. Centerline extraction methods perform well compared to many other techniques because the centerline of a vessel can (must) be localized by looking along a broader local extent than can be used to localize a vessel's edge. By incorporating a larger extent of an image into its localization process, small noise and intensity profile irregularities interfere relatively less, the measures remain above the resolution of the image, and second-order image information can be used to provide additional insensitivities to intensity inhomogeneities. Once a centerline has been extracted, it serves to stabilize width estimation and other quantifications.

We have devised a novel centerline and radius modeling method that operates via dynamic-scale ridge traversal. Ridge methods operate by considering an N-dimensional image to be a surface in an (N+1)-dimensional space by mapping intensity to height. In these (N+1)-dimensional spaces, tubular object centerlines will exist as one-dimensional height ridges on the

N-dimensional surfaces. To quantify the general capabilities of dynamic-scale ridge traversal for centerline extraction, we identified three criteria that are common to most medical imaging applications. Those criteria are described next.

Speed. As noted previously in this chapter, high-resolution, isotropic data sets can contain millions of points of data and occupy hundreds of megabytes of memory. Our goal is to automatically process such vascular images within 30 minutes, thereby making our approach applicable to all but the most urgent-care clinical situations. The presented method is able to extract a centerline passing through 20 voxels in approximately 0.3 sec on a 733-MHz Pentium III PC running Windows 2000. A patient's intracranial vasculature captured by MRA can be modeled in less than 15 min.

Accuracy. Critical to any tubular object segmentation method is the robust handling of image noise, branch points, and widths approaching the inner scale of the data. As mentioned previously, interventional radiologists require the definition of 1-mm feeding vessels for the embolization of tumors and arteriovenous malformations, and yet many MR angiograms are acquired using $1 \times 1 \times 1$-mm voxels. Even in noisy images, our dynamic-scale method can accurately extract the centerlines of 1-voxel-wide tubes: average error is less than 0.5 voxel, branch points are consistently passed, and the full length of a centerline is consistently extracted.

Automation. The performance of many of the extraction methods presented thus far in this chapter are highly dependent on the initial specification of multiple parameter values, in particular, thresholds. Automation is greatly facilitated if a method has few parameters and if it is insensitive to the initial value of those parameters. The minimal information required to designate a centerline of interest is a localization of the tube in image space $x' \in \Re^N$ and scale space σ'. Using the dynamic-scale ridge traversal method, centerline extraction accuracy is not statistically significantly dependent on the values of x' and σ'.

First, we introduce the criteria we have established for a point to be considered on a height ridge. Second, we emphasize the importance of scale to ridge formation and traversal. Third, we introduce the ridge traversal for centerline extraction: from a seed point x' and seed scale σ', a local ridge point is found, and its ridge is traversed via a step-maximize procedure. Fourth, we detail how our dynamic-scale ridge traversal method uses multi-scale heuristics and tube radius estimation to improve the speed, accuracy, and ease of automation of ridge traversal.

11.4.1.1 Ridge Criteria

Without loss of generality, we assume that tubes of interest appear brighter than the background and exist in three-dimensional data. That is, we assume that centerlines are intensity ridges. Via a sign change, these methods can track intensity valleys. Via blurring and filtering, these methods can be applied to extract tubular objects that do not have central extrema, are defined by texture, or are differentiated from their surroundings by other image features. These methods have also been applied to two- and four-dimensional data. We define:

I	an N-dimensional volume of data
x	a point in $\Re^N$ on a one-dimensional ridge in I
σ	the scale at which measures in I at x are made; that is, a scale at which the ridge exists
∇I	the gradient vector of I at x
$\vec{t}$	the ridge's tangent direction at x

We seek maximum convexity height ridges; therefore, the directions normal to the ridge are well approximated by the N − 1 most negative eigenvalued eigenvectors of the Hessian matrix at x, and the ridge tangent direction is well approximated by the remaining eigenvector. We define:

$\vec{v_1}, \vec{v_2}, \vec{v_3}$	the eigenvectors of the Hessian of I at x
$\alpha_1, \alpha_2, \alpha_3$	the eigenvalues of $\vec{v_1}, \vec{v_2}, \vec{v_3}$ with vectors and values ordered such that $\alpha_1 \leq \alpha_2 \leq \alpha_3$

Therefore, we test that we are on a ridge (not a valley or a saddle) by verifying that the local Hessian has N − 1 negative eigenvalued eigenvectors:

$$\alpha_1 \leq \alpha_2 < 0 \tag{11.1}$$

(This condition is relaxed in our dynamic-scale implementation.)

We test that we are on a local N − 1 dimensional extreme (at a ridge) by confirming that the projection of the gradient at x onto the N − 1 directions normal to the ridge is equal to zero [43]:

$$\vec{v_1} \bullet \nabla I = 0 \quad \text{and} \quad \vec{v_2} \bullet \nabla I = 0 \tag{11.2}$$

In Equation 11.2, we test for equal-to-zero using:

$$\sum_{i=1}^{N-1} (\nabla I \bullet \vec{v_i})^2 < 0.0001 \tag{11.3}$$

This test for zero enforces orthogonality of the normals and the gradient at places of large gradient and thereby precisely localizes the ridge; but as the gradient magnitude goes toward zero, indicating a broad ridge, less orthogonal directions are allowed. This tolerance is often acceptable; but when a tube becomes dim and its borders diffuse relative to its background (as occurs where blood vessels feed capillary beds), the ridge traversal should terminate. In these situations, the faint tubular structure often appears more elliptical than circularly symmetric; to terminate traversal in such situations without introducing an application dependent threshold, we introduce another criterion: we verify that the a tubular object has a nearly circular cross section using the ratio of the eigenvalues in the directions normal to the ridge:

$$\frac{\alpha_2}{\alpha_1} \geq 1 - \epsilon \tag{11.4}$$

This ratio is equal to one when the tube's cross section is symmetric. We allow for $\epsilon = 0.5$ to allow for cross-section intensity patterns that deviate from circular and resemble an ellipse with a 2:1 ratio between the lengths of the major and minor axis.

11.4.1.2 *The Importance of Scale*

In these calculations, our experience and the teachings of others [30] have indicated that the critical parameter for making measures in images is the scale at which those measures (e.g., the intensity, gradient, and Hessian of I at x) are calculated. For intensity ridge traversal, using scaled measures is particularly important.

1. Scaled measures may be needed to create a central intensity ridge in a tubular object. As mentioned previously in this chapter (Section 11.2), intensity ridges inherently exist along the central tracks of many tubular objects in many types of medical images. For example, vessels in time-of-flight (TOF) MRA data often have central intensity ridges. However, blurring may be necessary to create intensity ridges along the centers of other tubes in other data. For example, blood vessels in CT data will often have uniform intensity profiles.

2. Scale is necessary to designate the tube of interest. Without the specification of a scale, it may be unclear, for example, if the user seeks to define a blood vessel within an arm, the arm, or the entire torso of the person imaged.

3. Scale provides insensitivity to image noise. Measures made at larger scales (i.e., with larger apertures) are less affected by high-frequency variations in the data.

These three benefits of scale make central intensity ridges of tubular objects stable. Intensity ridges will persist along the centerlines of tubular objects for a wide range of scales, image resolutions, amounts of image noise, changes in imaging parameters and modalities, contrast density, uptake rates, and intensity inhomogeneities. However, too much blurring may cause neighboring objects to bias local calculations and may smooth the curves along an intensity ridge.

Consider Figure 11.18. When this simulated tube in a noisy image is viewed as a surface, the tube cannot be discerned. Via blurring, the tube becomes

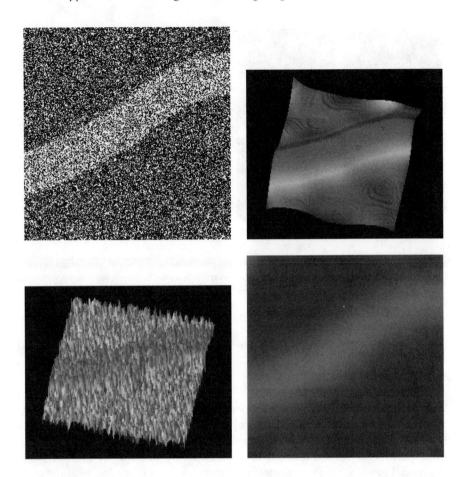

FIGURE 11.18

Two-dimensional images can be viewed as two-dimensional surfaces in three dimensions. For three-dimensional vascular image segmentation, the three-dimensional image is operated upon as if it were a three-dimensional surface in four dimensions. The left column shows that noise corrupts the appearance of a ridge along the simulated vessel's centerline. The right column shows that, via blurring (i.e., multi-scale analyses), the effect of noise is reduced and a centerline is clearly visible.

obvious. For the disk shown in Figure 11.19, the center estimate remains stable for a wide range of scales above the noise in the image, extending beyond the radius of the tube and yet not incorporating neighboring objects.

11.4.1.3 Modeling a Tube

Forming a centerline-based model of a tube consists of three steps: designating a centerline for extraction, traversing that centerline, and then estimating the radius along that centerline. We have also developed and will illustrate results from a probabilistic boundary evolution method that refines a tubular

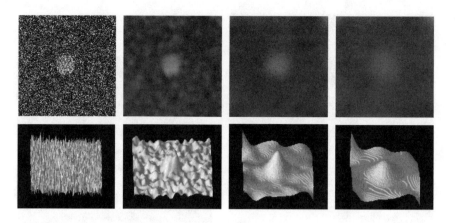

FIGURE 11.19
Dynamic-scale centerline extraction for vessel segmentation is fast, accurate, and robust because the centerline of a tube in three dimensions remains stable for a wide range of scales. Shown from left to right: (top row) image at the resolution of the image and then blurred with a Gaussian with $\sigma = 5, 15$, and 25 pixels; (bottom row) visualizations of the two-dimensional images as two-dimensional surfaces by mapping intensity to height.

boundary estimate to match the cross-sectional shape of a vessel as captured in an image.

11.4.1.3.1 Step 1: Automatic Vessel Designation

Appropriate heuristics for automatically designating tubes of interest for extraction are usually application dependent; but, in general, such heuristics are complicated if extraction initiation has many parameters or if the initial parameter values strongly affect the quality or quantity of the center-line model generated. The minimum parameters necessary for designating a tube-of-interest include:

x' the "seed point" that designates the image-space location of the tube of interest

σ' the "seed scale" that designates the approximate size (location in scale space) of the tube of interest

Only approximate initial values for these minimal parameters are needed; that is, the gradient ascent from x' should lead to the centerline of interest. The simplicity of these requirements facilitates automation.

To find the local centerline from our initial seed point x', making measures at scale σ', we:

1. Perform a line search to reach the point that is locally maximal in the gradient direction; that is, the point is a one-dimensional maximum.

2. From that one-dimensional maximum, we expand our search to find a local $(N-1)$-dimensional maximum. We use the $N-1$ most

negative eigenvalued eigenvectors of the Hessian at the one-dimensional maximum as the basis of our search space.

3. The ridge criteria are tested at that local (N−1)-dimensional maximum. If they are satisfied, that local maximum becomes our initial ridge point x_0.

4. If they fail, the N−1 most negative eigenvalued eigenvectors of the Hessian at that point are used to find a new local (N−1)-dimensional maximum.

5. If the ridge criteria at that new (N−1)-dimensional maximum also fail, our method reports that a local ridge cannot be found.

6. Otherwise, that new local maximum is used as our initial ridge point x_0.

In the default ridge-following implementation, σ_0 is set equal to σ'. The dynamic-scale ridge-following method estimates the radius of the object at x_0 and uses that estimate for σ_0.

11.4.1.3.2 Step 2: Dynamic-Scale Centerline Modeling

Once a centerline has been found, our ridge traversal method uses an iterative, optimal-scale, step-maximize procedure. Dynamic-scale heuristics are used to continue a traversal past local singularities and branch points.

Given an initial ridge point x_0, the ridge will extend in the positive $\overrightarrow{t_0}$ and negative $-\overrightarrow{t_0}$ tangent directions. Each direction is traversed independently. At the ith point x_i traversed on a ridge, the approximate tangent direction $\overrightarrow{t_i}$ is defined as $\overrightarrow{v_3}$, the maximum eigenvalued eigenvector of the Hessian at x_i. The direction of ridge traversal is maintained by multiplying $\overrightarrow{v_3}$ by the sign of the dot-product of $\overrightarrow{v_3}$ and the previous tangent direction $\overrightarrow{t_{i-1}}$:

$$\overrightarrow{t_i} = \text{sign}(\overrightarrow{v_3} \bullet \overrightarrow{t_{i-1}}) \overrightarrow{v_3} \qquad (11.5)$$

The approximate normal directions at x_i defined by default as $\overrightarrow{v_1}$ and $\overrightarrow{v_2}$ specify an (N−1)-dimensional plane that the local ridge passes through. Under the assumption of smoothness, if that normal plane is shifted by a small amount β in the tangent direction (see Figure 11.20), the ridge should continue to pass through that shifted normal plane — the ridge will exist as a local maximum in that shifted normal plane. The ridge criteria are tested at that (N−1)-dimensional maximum; and if the criteria are met, that maximum becomes the next ridge point x_{i+1}. Otherwise, heuristics are applied to determine if the termination is premature. First, however, we discuss the incorporation of scale optimization into this process.

As an optimal-scale method, the scale used during traversal is a function of the radius of the tube at the point being traversed. Specifically, during traversal, the traversal scale is set to the object's local radius. Application-specific knowledge of image noise and centerline tortuosity can be used to

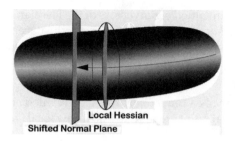

FIGURE 11.20
The step-maximize centerline traversal process: eigenvectors of the local Hessian matrix approximate the tangent and normal directions of the ridge being traversed. Shifting the normal plane in the tangent direction is used to focus the search for the next ridge point.

specify alternative mappings from object radius to scale, but we have found such tuning unnecessary. Additionally, based on the assumed smoothness of vessels, the tube's local radius is determined only every 10 voxels using a tolerance of 0.1 voxel. As a result, the speed of traversal is minimally affected.

Another important parameter of this iterative traversal process is β, the distance the normal plane is shifted per step. Appropriate values for β (and "same direction" and "close") are dictated by the assumed smoothness of the tube. For our implementations, β is 0.2 voxel. For some applications in which the tubes are generally much larger than the inner scale of the data, it may be beneficial to use an adaptive step size β_i that is proportional to the local scale of the tube σ_i ("same direction" and "close" thresholds should also be adapted).

Both the traversal scale and β are adapted by our dynamic-scale heuristics to provide insensitivities to local discontinuities such as image noise, singularities, and the difficulties previously mentioned as being common to vascular images. We have developed four recovery heuristics to attempt to continue ridge traversal past these discontinuities. Two of the heuristics are intuitive: (1) we smooth the tangent directions during traversal to reduce the effects of small scale noise; and (2) at places of high curvature as measured by the rate of change in the ridge tangent, we reduce the step size β. We also address singularities (such as may occur at branch points) in the images. At these points, the image data contain intensities that more closely resemble a sphere than a tube. All three eigenvalues of the local Hessian become negative, and the ordering of the eigenvectors with respect to the previous ridge point's tangent and normal directions may change. So, (3) we detect eigenvector swapping and reorient them by determining which eigenvector best matches the previous tangent direction. Addtionally, because singularities are nongeneric in image data, local perturbations to the image data cause those points to be displaced or destroyed. Therefore, (4) if a valid ridge point is not found after the application of the above recovery techniques, image perturbation is employed: σ is slightly decreased, β is slightly increased, and then the step-maximize process is retried. If a second discontinuity is encountered within the next 2 voxels, a second recovery is not attempted, and the radius of the tube along the centerline is then precisely estimated.

11.4.1.3.3 Step 3: Radius Estimation

We estimate the local radius of the tube by finding a local maximum of a medialness function at x_i:

$$\sigma_i = \operatorname{argmax}_\rho(M(x_i, \overrightarrow{t_i}, \rho)) \tag{11.6}$$

Our medialness function $M(\cdot)$ uses an adaptive convolution kernel. The kernel is a ring centered about x, aligned with the normal plane at x, and at a distance ρ from x. The ring is implimented using paired spherical operators of size 0.25ρ aligned radially about x at a distance of 0.75ρ and 1.25ρ. The inner spheres of the kernel ring have a positive sign and the outer spheres have a negative sign (Figure 11.21). To increase the stability of the medialness response in the presence of image noise and neighboring objects (including branches), the radial direction that produces the weakest convolution response is eliminated from the kernel's convolution sum. In that manner, the kernel is adaptive.

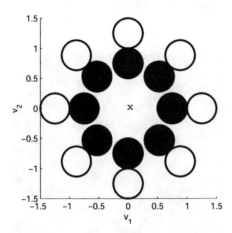

FIGURE 11.21
A rendition of the kernel used to estimate a tubular object's radius. Kernel is aligned normal to the centerline; inner circles represent positive spheres; outer circles represent negative spheres; spheres bound the radius being tested; and sphere radius (i.e., the kernel's aperture) is proportional to the radius being tested.

11.4.1.3.4   Speed, Accuracy, and Automation

We have performed extensive simulated data, phantom data, and clinical data evaluations of our vessel modeling method. This section provides only the briefest summary of some of those studies. In this section we quantify and compare the speed (time to extract a centerline), accuracy (difference from ideal centerline), and automation (ability to extract long centerlines and pass branch points).

We created a $100 \times 100 \times 100$-voxel, isotropic data set containing a tortuous, branching, tubular object. The object's centerline passes through 350 voxels. At its ends, the tube's radius is 4.0 voxels. In the middle, at the branch point, the radius is 0.5 voxel. A rendering of the explicit surface of the object is shown in Figure 11.22. The background intensity is 100, and the object's cross-sectional intensities have a parabolic profile ranging from 150 at the object's edge to 200 at the object's middle. This profile is typical of contrast MRA and TOF MRA for small vessels [10].

Gaussian noise having standard deviations η of 20, 40, and 80 (Figure 11.23) was added to the image. The $\eta = 20$ data are representative of the noise levels in MR and CT data. The $\eta = 40$ data more closely resemble the noise magnitude of ultrasound data. The $\eta = 80$ data were chosen to explore the methods' performance on worst-case data.

Regarding speed, the dynamic-scale ridge traversal method requires approximately 0.3 sec to follow a 20-voxel extent of the centerline of the 0.5 to 4.0 voxel radius tube. Given the prevalence of 0.5 to 2 voxel radius vessels (1 to 4 mm in diameter) in intracranial MRA images ($1 \times 1 \times 1$-mm voxel size), it is quite easy to process an intracranial MRA data set in 15 min.

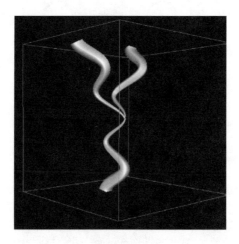

FIGURE 11.22
A rendering of the mathematically defined surface of the tortuous, branching object used in the simulated-data Monte Carlo experiments.

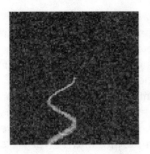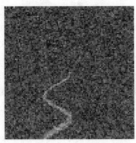

FIGURE 11.23
A slice (x-vs.-z at y = 50) along the center of the tube in the simulated data with three different levels of Gaussian noise added. Noise standard deviations are (left) $\eta = 20$, (middle) $\eta = 40$, and (right) $\eta = 80$. The noise-free background value is 100, and the noise-free tubes have parabolic intensity profiles: value of 150 at edges and 200 along the middle.

To quantify the accuracy and automation, Monte Carlo experiments were conducted using 200 random starting points x', three initial scale values ($\sigma' = 1.0$, 2.0, and 4.0), and three different levels of image noise ($\eta = 20$, 40, and 80). Six measures were made:

1. *Average error*: mean distance between a point on the extracted ridge and its closest ideal centerline point.

2. *Maximum error*: maximum distance between each point on the extracted ridge and the closest ideal centerline point.

3. *Percent of points within 0.5 voxel*: percent of points on the extracted ridge within 0.5 voxel of their closest ideal centerline point.

4. *Percent of points within 1 voxel*: percent of points on the extracted ridge within 1 voxel of their closest ideal centerline point.

5. *Average percent length*: percent of points in the extracted ridge. Extraction using a noise-free image produced 800 points, so this number is reported as a percentage of 800. This number is strongly correlated with the percent of branch points crossed (measure 6).

6. *Percent of branch points crossed*: percent of the 200 extractions that spanned the z-dimension from slice 47 to slice 53 — these slices bound the branch point.

Regarding accuracy, there are several conclusions that were drawn from these studies. The most significant of these is that for the $\eta = 20$ and $\eta = 40$ data, the average error was less than 1 voxel, the maximum error was about 2 voxels, about 90% of the extracted points were within 1 voxel of the ideal; and for the $\eta = 20$ data, on average over 90% of the ideal centerline was traversed by the dynamic-scale method (it consistently crossed the difficult, inner-scale branch point nearly 90% of the time). The most surprising result is the success of ridge traversal on the extraction of tubes from the extremely noisy $\eta = 80$ data. The average centerline point error was about 1 voxel, with approximately 70% of the extracted centerline points within 1 voxel of the ideal centerline. The branch point was passed less than half of the time, but most extractions covered the full extent of the branch upon which they fell.

Automation was measured as the percent of times the branch point was crossed and the dependence of the method's performance on σ'. We tested the Null Hypothesis that there was no difference between the mean performance of the system for different σ' values. Levels of significance and power were calculated. The results were conclusive. The dynamic-scale method supports automated centerline extraction; that is, the dynamic-scale method demonstrated no statistically significant performance dependence on the seed scale. Additionally, the method requires few seed points; that is, nearly 90% of the time for the $\eta = 20$ data and over 50% of the time for the $\eta = 40$ data, the optimally difficult branch point was crossed.

Clearly, all of these simulated data experiments support the use of the dynamic-scale implementation. The next section demonstrates that the dynamic-scale method is also applicable to clinical data. Subsequently we show that it is an effective basis for vascular image registration.

11.4.2   Clinical Applications of Vascular Segmentation

Vascular segmentation and visualization research seeks to reduce the time spent planning a procedure, increase the accuracy and consistency of the plans made, enable the simultaneous consideration of more detailed and a wider variety of information, and eventually lead to the design of new procedures. One of the first clinical applications of vascular segmentation methods (outside of cardiology) was in neurosurgery. Intracranial vasculature poses unique challenges for segmentation; in particular, the range of vessel widths, the importance of detailed (near or at the resolution of the scanner) representations, and the massive inter-patient variability of the distribution and interconnections of the network. Returning to the MRA data that has been shown via volume rendering (Figure 11.12) and via connected components (Figure 11.16), the utilization of segmentations augmented with branching/interconnectedness information enables the depiction shown in Figure 11.24. The information important to planning the treatment of this AVM (arteriovenous malformation) is clearly visible. The AVM has been segmented using connected components due to its irregular shape. The vessels have been segmented using our dynamic-scale centerline and radius technique. Those segmentations have been surface rendered and colored according to their connectedness and relevance to the AVM.

As Figure 11.24 illustrates, perhaps the most important outcome of vessel segmentation is not the improved visualization of the individual vessels but the ability to manipulate the vessels as objects in the visualization, that is, procedural visualizations. Via procedural visualizations, clinical hypotheses

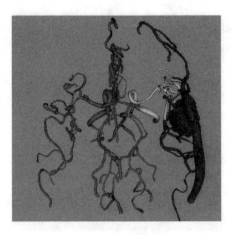

FIGURE 11.24 (See color insert.)
The MRA AVM previously depicted in Figure 11.12 and Figure 11.16 is shown here using centerline and radii vessel models, connected component AVM models, and colorings that portray the connectedness of vessels with respect to the AVM. The information content of this image (compared to the information in the other figures) is arguably much more directed to the clinical task at hand: embolization planning.

can be interactively tested, refined, and communicated. Such manipulations require the accurate reconstruction of the branching pattern of the vessels [8]. This has been the focus of Bullitt's work [6, 23]. Her method takes any set of segmented vessels and their source image data and reconnects the vessels based on supporting image findings. Nearly all of the remaining images in this chapter benefit from including interconnectedness information. An excellent illustration of the benefit of such information is presented in Figure 11.25. These models were formed from a TOF MRA volume image of a patient with an arteriovenous malformation (AVM). One form of treatment for these vascular tumors is embolization, and the difficulty with that procedure is determining the feeding arteries and draining veins of the nidus. It is important to identify all of the feeding arteries and to block their flow, and yet it is critical to not interrupt blood flow to viable tissue (which would induce a stroke). Such illustrations of vessel connectedness have sped and increased the accuracy of such embolization plans. Furthermore, with Bullitt's software it is possible to simulate the passage of a catheter and only render distal vasculature, thereby providing an interactive visualization that exactly reflects the important functional information needed to test embolization hypotheses.

These segmentation and interconnectedness extraction techniques are also applicable to other organs and multiple other vascular imaging modalities. We have found them to be particularly helpful for living related donor partial liver transplant planning, including adult-to-adult living donor partial liver transplantation. We have devised an interactive tool that semi-automatically

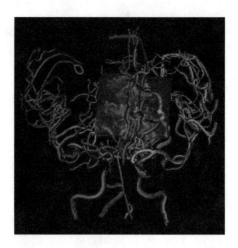

FIGURE 11.25 (See color insert.)
This figure is a clear illustration of the power of segmentation when the form of the segmentation (here centerlines and radii) enables functional information also to be captured and displayed. Specifically, coloring is used to illustrate what distal trees are being fed by the right and left carotids and the basilar. Additionally, the AVM is segmented but then volume rendered to allow the fuzzy borders of the nidus to be fully appreciated.

segments the liver parenchyma via connected components, automatically segments the vessels within the liver, and then forms vascular trees that correspond to the portal and hepatic venous systems within the liver. Those trees can be viewed independently or color coded. Ultimately, the transplant surgeons can interact with those segmentations in three dimensions to determine cutting plans to resect a lobe of the liver while maintaining blood vessel patency for transplantation into a recipient. An example visualization from a partial liver transplant plan is shown in Figure 11.26.

During liver transplant procedures and the planning and delivery of other liver procedures, three-dimensional ultrasound is often used to acquire up-to-date information. Our vascular segmentation techniques can be applied to three-dimensional ultrasound data as is shown in Figure 11.27. We show in the next section how such segmentations can also be used to drive vascular image registrations. In that manner, intra-operative three-dimensional ultrasound images can be registered with pre-operative liver CT data for surgical guidance.

Partial lung transplant planning can also benefit from tubular segmentations. All of the anatomic structures shown in Figure 11.28 are centerlines and radius models of lung vessels and bronchi generated from noncontrast scans from a multi-detector CT system.

It is important to note that the same dynamic-scale centerline and radius segmentation software was used to generate all of the visualizations in the clinical cases presented in this section. The method is truly independent of

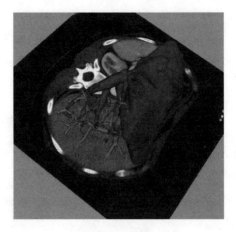

FIGURE 11.26 (See color insert.)
From CT images taken with contrast, the liver parenchyma is segmented via connected components and the vessels are segmented using dynamic-scale centerline and radius modeling. Segmented vessels are then reconstructed into vascular trees corresponding to the portal and hepative venous systems. Transplant surgeons interact with these visualizations to specify a cutting path for lobe resection. Here, a portion of the liver to be donated is shown. Vascular patency can be verified. Vessel cross-sectional areas can be compared with those of the recipient to estimate risk of thrombosis.

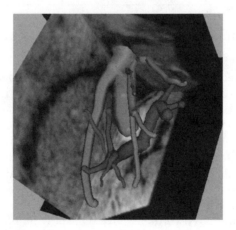

FIGURE 11.27 (See color insert.)
The dynamic-scale centerline and radius vessel segmentation system is robust such that without modification it can be used to extract vessel from three-dimensional ultrasound data.

imaging modality. Many other groups are working on developing related methods and extensions to this approach for segmentation [7]. Additionally, centerline and radius segmentations form an effective basis for vascular image registration [21].

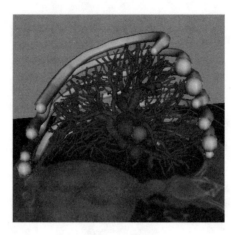

FIGURE 11.28 (See color insert.)
The vessels, bronchi, and ribs depicted in this figure were segmented using the dynamic-scale centerline and radius method. Such visualizations can be rapidly interacted with on a standard PC using inexpensive graphics cards (designed for running computer games). Such visualizations are effective for partial lung transplant planning.

11.5   Vascular Image Registration

Vessels are an ideal basis for medical image registration. Vessels are well distributed throughout most organs and therefore capture deformations within organs, whereas organ surfaces and anatomic landmarks (traditional registration features) are often poorly correlated with internal deformations. Additionally, compared to surfaces and landmarks, tubes are defined by integrating over larger image regions and therefore are less sensitive to image noise, are often better differentiated from the surrounding tissue, and thereby can be easily registered across data from multiple imaging devices.

The specific task of aligning vascular images, however, has several complications, such as having to compensate for vascular network changes and nonrigid deformations. Nevertheless, we will show that for multiple modalities, centerline and radius vascular image registration methods are able to produce registrations with sub-voxel consistency in less than 1 minute despite these difficulties.

There are three basic approaches to image registration. They are as follows. *Image-image registration* methods such as mutual-information optimization methods are favored for registering tissue images. These methods, however, are not well suited for registering vascular images. The sparseness of tubes in most vascular images prohibits the use of sampling to speed the calculation of mutual information and other voxel-matching metrics [44]. These methods are also poorly suited to handling the alignment ambiguities of tubes and the vascular network changes and nonrigid deformations of vascular images. For example, we have applied normalized mutual image information registration strategies to intracranial MR angiograms; we found that initialization is very critical to the successful registration of those vascular images. In fact, without an initial hand-registration of the data, the system often failed. However, other groups are developing modified mutual information metrics that may handle vascular images and, in particular, MR/three-dimensional ultrasound registration [45, 46].

Feature-feature registration methods have been heavily investigated for tissue images and several such methods have been developed for vascular images. This class of methods includes iterative closest point [47, 48] and landmark-based techniques [49]. This class also includes two-dimensional/three-dimensional registration methods that attempt to determine how to project vessel centers from a three-dimensional image so as to best match the vessel centers in a two-dimensional image formed via x-ray projection through the same anatomy [22] (see Figure 11.29). Recently, a three-dimensional/three-dimensional feature-based registration technique was published [16]

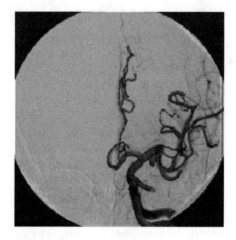

FIGURE 11.29 (See color insert.)
Trigeminal neuralgia is characterized by extreme pain on one side of the patient's face. It can be treated by ablating the corresponding nerve but this requires the insertion of a needle through the same opening in the skull that the carotid artery passes through. By performing a feature-based three-dimensional-to-two-dimensional registration of the preoperative MRA with intraoperative biplane digital subtraction angiograms, the three-dimensional position of the needle can be reconstructed and shown in correspondence with the patient's orientation on the table and with respect to the patient's vasculature and anatomy captured in the preoperative CT. The procedure is made safer for the patient.

that uses closest-point pairings of the brightest (by threshold) voxels in MRA and Doppler three-dimensional ultrasound data to quantify their alignment. That method rigidly registers these data in 5 to 10 minutes; work is still needed to meet intra-operative speed requirements.

The remaining set of registration methods are *feature-image registration* methods, and they are arguably ideal for vascular image registration. We will show that by incorporating multi-scale ridge and radius measures into the feature-image match metric, accurate and consistent patient-specific vascular image registrations can be attained across modalities and despite local, nonrigid deformations. Some of the hierarchical registration work of van den Elsen also falls into this category [50]. There has also been research into fitting generic models to multiple images from the same patient; most often, this is for the purpose of segmentation but how to align those images could also be deduced. However, the inter-patient variability of the vasculature of nearly every organ (except perhaps the coronary arteries) prohibits the use of generic models for vascular image registration. The details of our patient-specific model to image matching process are given next.

11.5.1   Vascular Model-to-Image Matching

In vascular image registration, a registration metric is used to quantify how well a rotation matrix and offset vector align two vascular images. The metric presented here is based on the fact that vessel centerlines are scaled intensity ridges in the image; therefore, when two vascular images are aligned, the centerline points in one will map to bright points in the other. The method's speed comes from the use of coarse-to-fine registration strategies that are directly enabled by dynamic-scale tube models and the model–image match metric. Additionally, because this method is insensitive to local, nonrigid deformations, it enables the visualization and quantification of the effects of such deformations, that is, changes in the number, size, and location of tubes. For medical applications, such quantifications and visualizations can be critical in tracking tumor and lesion changes/movement during and after surgical procedures.

Because when two vascular images are aligned, the centerline points in one will map to bright points in the other, our vascular image registration metric is a weighted sum of the scaled intensities of the target image at the transformed points of the centerlines of the vessel models formed from a source image. As a rigid registration technique, a point x in the model is transformed to a point y in the target image via multiplication with a rotation matrix and the addition of a translation vector, that is, $y = xR + \overrightarrow{o}$, where R is a Euler matrix with parameters α, β, γ as rotations about the $z, y,$ and x-axes, respectively, and with offsets $\overrightarrow{o} = [o_x, o_y, o_z]$.

$$F(R, \overrightarrow{o}) = \frac{1}{\sum_{i=1}^{n} w_i} \sum_{i=1}^{n} w_i \, I_{\kappa\sigma_i}(x_i R + \overrightarrow{o}) \qquad (11.7)$$

Our metric is controlled by the sampling of the centerlines (x_i and n), the scaling (κ_{σ_i} = standard deviation of the Gaussian kernel used to blur the data) of the image data I, and the weighting w_i of the centerline points x_i. Via these parameters, coarse-to-fine registration optimization algorithms are possible. Extensive analyses and visualizations of the parameter space of our registration metric are provided in the published article in the appendix [3]. In summary, sampling, scaling, and weighting operate as follows.

Sampling. We have performed experiments that show that our method is not sensitive to the number of samples n if the x_i are carefully chosen. For example, to calculate the value of the metric and its derivatives, our optimization strategy only uses one tenth to one twentieth of the centerline points extracted during height–ridge traversal. Additionally, the number of samples used is further reduced, and yet the quality of the metric is actually improved by rejecting any points whose circularity or medialness (see Section 11.4.1 on vessel extraction) is less than 0.2; that is, points are rejected if the local vessel's cross section has an orientation bias or is poorly differentiated from the background. As expected, if additional points are used, the accuracy of the metric will increase along with the computation time. Based on this trade-off, our optimization strategy increases n to implement a coarse-to-fine registration heuristic.

Scaling. If a tube is differentiated from its background by contrast, an intensity ridge will exist along that tube's center for a range of scales proportional to the radius of the tube. By default (and for all experiments presented in this chapter), the local scaling of the image is equal to the radius of the tube ($\kappa = 1$). However, by increasing the scale beyond the radius of the tube (i.e., by using $\kappa > 1$), the intensity ridge will persist and the spatial range for which that point is the local maximum will increase (barring neighboring objects).

Weighting. As a final technique for smoothing the metric surface, the sample points are weighted based on their radius. The vessel extraction system is capable of capturing vessels whose radius is near the inner scale of the data. While effective for understanding the vascular anatomy, the points on these vessels exist at such a relatively small scale that they have small capture radius and are affected by image noise. We therefore demote the contribution of these points via a weighting function. Again, a coarse-to-fine registration strategy could be implemented by equalizing the weighting during optimization to increase the contribution of smaller vessels when in the vicinity of the local maximum.

The utility of this metric is further supported by a modified optimization process. Because of intensity irregularities along a centerline, derivatives of the metric may induce shifts along a vessel, whereas ideally, shifts will only be produced across a vessel; for example, horizontal tubes will be limited to inducing vertical shifts. Therefore, at each centerline point, we limit the local intensity's gradient to the direction normal to the tube in the original data. Additionally, we compensate the rotation and translation updates for the favored orientation of the tubes in a network so that the transformation parameters' gradients do not have an orientation bias (if most tubes are horizontal, the system should not be unduly biased toward vertical transformations). Furthermore, we implement a multi-scale coarse-to-fine gradient ascent registration optimization strategy by increasing the sampling of the tube's centerlines during optimization.

As a result of these metric optimization modifications, the vessel model-to-image registration strategy is fast and requires only minimal correspondence between the vascular networks in the images. Additionally, it is insensitive to local deformations and operating across imaging modalities.

Regarding speed, the metric and its optimization strategy are fast. The speed of the system is determined by the complexity of the vascular models, not the size of the images, and vessel centerlines are relatively sparse in any image. Also, the coarse-to-fine subsampling speeds the registration process without degrading (and even potentially improving) the final registration accuracy. We are able to perform three-dimensional/three-dimensional liver model-to-liver image registrations in approximately 6 sec.

Registering vascular images despite apparent changes in the vascular network across images, local deformations in spatial locations of the vessels, and differing modalities are the clinical strengths of our method. These qualities are discussed specifically in the next section, which focuses on the clinical utility of vascular image registration.

11.5.2 Clinical Applications of Registration

One potential use of vascular image registration is to fuse images taken at different contrast timings so that more complete vascular descriptions can be generated. Such registration requires that the method be insensitive to the fact that only a few of the vessels in the model may actually be present in the data. To illustrate our method's ability to register images in which few vessels coexist, and to illustrate the generation of large vascular networks from different timed images, we register arterial-phase contrast CT images of a liver with venous-phase contrast CT images of the same liver. A bolus of contrast is released and 30 sec later, the arterial phase image that captures the portal venous network is taken. Another 30 sec are then allowed to pass and a venous phase image that captures the hepatic venous system is acquired. Because the patients hold their breath to different depths between scans and because patients move between scans, vascular registration is required. The vessels from two scans and their registrations are shown in Figure 11.30.

In general, vascular image registration is needed to register different phase contrast images of the abdomen such as these. Because, for example, the liver has moved with respect to the spine between the scans, if a volumetric registration method (such as mutual information registration) is applied, the result is often that the spine is aligned, but the liver remains misaligned. Vascular registration is driven by the vessel models from the source image; thus, it can easily be focused on the liver.

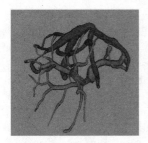 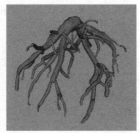 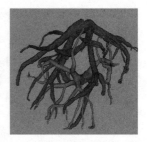

FIGURE 11.30 (See color insert.)
Left and middle: The vessels extracted from the arterial and venous phase contrast CT images from a potential liver donor. The first scan captures the portal network and some of the hepatic network. The second captures the hepatic network. Despite few corresponding vessels, the portal models can be registered with the hepatic image (the hepatic models are only shown for illustration; they are not used during registration). Right: After registration, the models from both scans can be fused to get a single complete view of the liver vasculature. These models drive the definition of liver lobes resected during transplantation.

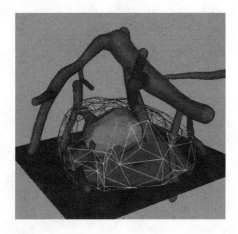

FIGURE 11.31 (See color insert.)
A small section from a lung CT image volume containing a tumor. The tumor was modeled using connected components. The vessels were modeled using dynamic-scale centerlines and radii. The tumor was then artificially enlarged (shown in wireframe) and the data was rotated and translated and then given to be registered with the prior vascular models. Despite the enlarged tumor obscuring multiple vessels, the final registration was excellent. Tumor growth can be detected and quantified.

Lung cancer detection is another application that can benefit from vessel registration. A chest CT scan was cropped to a lesion of interest and the vessels were extracted. The lesion was then enlarged to simulate growth, which obscured neighboring vessels, and then the data were translated and rotated. The results after registration are shown in Figure 11.31.

Finally, we show that vascular image registration can be performed despite localized spatial distortions such as those that result from embolizations. In fact, via registration, the location and extent of those deformations can be quantified. Such measures are useful for tracking treatment effectiveness, treatment side effects, and tumor growth. Knowing the prevalence of nonlinear deformations in medical data, we have quantified the vascular registration's ability to perform well when nonlinear deformations are present [3]. These quantifications involved Monte Carlo simulations, registration parameter space analyses, and visualizing local vascular misalignments. Consider the difficult task of registering MRA scans acquired from pretreatment, postradiation, and postembolization therapy of a patient with an arteriovenous malformation. The vascular models from pretreatment were extracted and aligned with postradiation data. A visualization of the vascular models from both volumes after alignment is shown in Figure 11.32. There is good correspondence between vessels on the image on the left; but on the right, near the AVM, multiple vessels are misaligned and others are missing due to nonrigid deformations that occurred as a result of treatment. The potential of such visualizations are only beginning to be realized. Other conclusions and such future applications are discussed next.

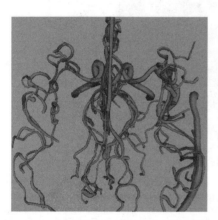 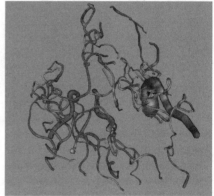

FIGURE 11.32 (See color insert.)
Two visualizations of the effect of radiation and surgery on intracranial vessels containing a tumor (an AVM). Left: Pre- and posttreatment vessels are shown registered. On the image right, near the treatment site, there are local vascular displacements. The large wireframe vessel is missing in the posttreatment image. Right: Shading encodes the distance from pre-treatment vessels to nearest postsurgery vessels. The ends of some vessels are colored because of differences in extraction. Long, bright vessels indicate areas of large anatomic change; the tumor bears the majority of the effects of treatment. Visualizations of such vascular changes help physicians determine treatment effectiveness.

11.6 Conclusion and Future Work

Vascular imaging is undergoing explosive growth in disease detection and diagnosis, and in treatment planning, delivery, and assessment. Vascular interventionalists use blood vessels as minimally invasive conduits to precisely deliver treatments throughout the body. Partial-organ transplant procedures are often driven by the vasculatures of the donor and the recipient so as to maintain patency and minimize the risk of thrombosis. The development of computer methods to assist with the analysis of vascular images, however, poses new challenges for medical image analysis researchers.

In this chapter we have discussed several vascular image segmentation and registration methods and presented clinical applications that use them. Segmentation and registration are critical to the development of effective computer-assistance systems for existing clinical tasks. Eventually, these methods will drive the development of new clinical procedures for disease detection, diagnosis, intervention, and outcome assessment.

Consider Figure 11.33. Using a CT- and ultrasound-compatible vascular phantom, the vessels can be extracted from the CT and registered in 6 sec with three-dimensional ultrasound scans [3, 21]. The green and blue balls are corresponding features visible in the CT and ultrasound scan that were not used during registration. They are aligned within 2.3 mm of each other. This simulation depicts a possible future application of vascular image segmentation and

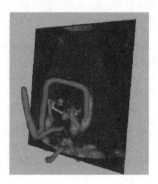

FIGURE 11.33 (See color insert.)
A vascular model was extracted from a CT scan of a liver phantom and then registered with intra-operative 3D ultrasound scans of the phantom. In that manner, lesions seen on pre-operative CT can be transcribed into the intra-operative 3D ultrasound data. Lesions not seen directly on the 3D ultrasound data can still be treated using ultrasound guided radio-frequency ablation. In these data, targets seen on the CT data (white blobs) are aligned with their locations in the ultrasound data (dark blobs) to an average error of 2.0 mm and maximum error of 2.8 mm.

registration: mimimally invasive procedure guidance. By registering preoperative vascular models with intra-operative, three-dimensional ultrasound data, lesions seen only on the preoperative data can be accurately transcribed to the intra-operative ultrasound and thereby treated percutaneously. Potentially, any markings made on preoperative data can be localized by the surrounding vasculature and registered with intra-operative ultrasound images. Surgical plans can be made to appear within the intra-operative ultrasound images. Surgical paths can be carried out exactly as planned. It will be possible to carry out new procedures percutaneously or intravascularly. The potential of this one application of vascular image segmentation and registration is huge, and vascular image analysis researchers are on the cusp of numerous other, equally effective breakthroughs. This truly is an exciting time for this rapidly growing field.

References

1. N. Alperin, D. N. Levin, and C. A. Pelizzari, "Retrospective registration of x-ray angiograms with MR images by using vessels as intrinsic landmarks," *Journal of Magnetic Resonance Imaging,* Vol. 4, pp. 139–144, 1994.
2. S. Aylward, E. Bullitt, S. M. Pizer, and D. Eberly, "Intensity ridge and widths for tubular object segmentation and registration," in *IEEE Workshop on Mathematical Methods in Biomedical Image Analysis,* 1996, pp. 131–138.
3. S. Aylward, S. Weeks, and E. Bullitt, "Analysis of the parameter space of a metric for registering 3d vascular images," in *MICCAI,* Utrecht, The Netherlands, October 2001, p. 8.
4. S. Aylward and E. Bullitt, "Initialization, noise, singularities, and scale in height ridge traversal for tubular object centerline extraction," *IEEE Transactions on Medical Imaging,* Vol. 21, No. 2, pp. 61–75, February 2002.
5. E. Bullitt, A. Liu, S. Aylward, M. Soltys, J. Rosenman, and S. Pizer, "Methods for displaying intracerebral vascular anatomy," *American Journal of Neuroradiology,* Vol. 18, pp. 417–420, March 1997.
6. E. Bullitt, S. Aylward, K. Smith, S. Mukherji, M. Jiroutek, and K. Muller, "Symbolic description of intracerebral vessels segmented from MRA and evaluation by comparison with x-ray angiograms," *Medical Image Analysis,* Vol. 5, pp. 157–169, 2001.
7. A. F. Frangi, W. J. Niessen, R. M. Hoogeveen, T. Van Walsum, and M. A. Viergever, "Model-based quantitation of 3-d magnetic resonance angiographic images," *IEEE Transactions on Medical Imaging,* Vol. 18, No. 10, pp. 946–956, October 1999.
8. G. Gerig, T. Koller, G. Szekely, C. Brechbuhler, and O. Kubler, "Symbolic description of 3-d structures applied to cerebral vessel tree obtained from MR angiography volume data," in *Information Processing in Medical Imaging '93: Lecture Notes in Computer Science 687,* 1993, pp. 94–111.
9. K. Haris, S. N. Efstraatiadis, N. Maglaveras, C. Pappas, J. Gourassas, and G. Louridas, "Model-based morphological segmentation and labeling of coronary

angiograms," *IEEE Transactions on Medical Imaging,* Vol. 18, No. 10, pp. 1003–1015, October 1999.

10. R. M. Hoogeveen, C. J. G. Bakker, and M. A. Viergever, "Limits to the accuracy of vessel diameter measurement in MR angiography," *Journal of Magnetic Resonance Imaging,* Vol. 8, 1998.

11. T. Koller, G. Gerig, G Szekely, and D. Dettwiler, "Multiscale detection of curvilinear structures in 2-d and 3-d image data," in *Proceedings of the 5th International Conference on Computer Vision,* Boston, MA, 1995, pp. 864–869, IEEE Computer Society Press.

12. C. Lorenz, I. C. Carlsen, T. M. Buzug, C. Fassnacht, and J. Weese, "Multi-scale line segmentation with automatic estimation of width, contrast, and tangential direction in 2d and 3d medical images," in *CVRMed-MRCAS '97,* J. Troccaz, E. Grimson, and R. Mosges, Eds., 1997, pp. 233–242, Springer-Verlag.

13. L. M. Lorigo, O. Faugeras, W. E. L. Grimson, R. Keriven, R. Kikinis, and C. F. Westin, "Co-dimension 2 geodesic active contours for MRA segmentation," in *Information Processing in Medical Imaging '99: Lecture Notes in Computer Science 1613,* 1999, pp. 126–139.

14. Y. Masutani, T. Schiemann, and K. H. Hohne, "Vascular shape segmentation and structure extraction using a shape-based region-growing model," in *Proceedings of Medical Image Computing and Computer-Assisted Intervention, Lecture Notes in Computer Science 1496,* 1998, pp. 1242–1249.

15. T. McInerney and D. Terzopoulos, "Topology adaptive deformable surfaces for medical image volume segmentation," *IEEE Transactions on Medical Imaging,* Vol. 18, No. 10, pp. 840–850, October 1999.

16. B. C. Porter, D. J. Rubens, J. G. Strang, J. Smith, S. Totterman, and K. J. Parker, "3d registration and fusion of ultrasound and mri using major vessels as fiducial markers," *IEEE Transactions on Medical Imaging,* Vol. 20, No. 4, 2001.

17. P. Reuze, J. L. Coatrieux, L. M. Luo, and J. L. Dillenserger, "A 3-d moment based approach for blood vessel detection and quantification in MRA," *Technology and Health Care,* Vol. 1, pp. 181–188, 1993.

18. Y. Sato, S. Nakajima, H. Atsumi, T. Koller, G. Gerig, S. Yoshida, and R. Kikinis, "3d multi-scale line filter for segmentation and visualization of curvilinear structures in medical images," in *CVRMed-MRCAS '97,* J. Troccaz, E. Grimson, and R. Mosges, Eds., 1997, pp. 213–222, Springer-Verlag.

19. D. L. Wilson and J. A. Noble, "An adaptive segmentation algorithm for time-of-flight MRA data," *IEEE Transactions on Medical Imaging,* Vol. 18, No. 10, pp. 938–945, October 1999.

20. P. J. Yim, P. L. Choyke, and R. M. Summers, "Gray-scale skeletonization of small vessels in magnetic resonance angiography," *IEEE Transactions on Medical Imaging,* Vol. 19, No. 6, pp. 568–576, June 2000.

21. S. Aylward, J. Jomier, J. P. Guyon, and S. Weeks, "Intra-operative 3d ultrasound augmentation," in *IEEE International Symposium on Biomedical Imaging,* July 2002, p. 4.

22. E. Bullitt, A. Liu, S. Aylward, C. Coffey, J. Stone, S. Mukherji, and S. Pizer, "Registration of 3d cerebral vessels with 2d digital angiograms: clinical evaluation," *Academic Radiology,* Vol. 6, pp. 539–546, 1999.

23. E. Bullitt, S. Aylward, E. Bernard, and G. Gerig, "Technical report: computer-assisted visualization of arteriovenous malformations on the home PC," *Neurosurgery,* Vol. 48, pp. 576–583, 2001.

24. L. Soler, H Delingette, G. Malandain, N. Ayache, C. Koehl, J. M. Clement, O. Dourthe, and J. Marescaux, "An automatic virtual patient reconstruction from CT-scans for hepatic surgical planning," in *Medicine Meets Virtual Reality*, J. D. Weswood, Ed., IOS Press, 2000, pp. 316–322.

25. R. O. Duda, P. E. Hart, and D. G. Stork, *Pattern Classification*, 2nd edition, John Wiley & Sons, 2001.

26. D. Hill, P. Batchelor, M. Holden, and D. Hawkes, "Medical image registration," *Physics in Medicine and Biology*, Vol. 46, 2001.

27. K. M. Andress, "Evidential reconstruction of vessel trees from rotational angiograms," in *International Conference on Image Processing*, Vol. 3, October 1998, pp. 385–389.

28. N. Niki, Y. Kawata, H. Satoh, and T. Kumazaki, "3d imaging of blood vessels using x-ray rotational angiographic system," in *Nuclear Science Symposium and Medical Imaging Conference*, Vol. 3, November 1993, pp. 1873–1877.

29. A. Wahle, H. Oswald, and E. Fleck, "3d hard-vessel reconstruction from biplane angiograms," *IEEE Computer Graphics and Applications*, Vol. 16, No. 1, pp. 65–73, 1996.

30. T. Lindeberg, *Scale-Space Theory in Computer Vision*, Kluwer Academic, Dordrecht, Netherlands, 1994.

31. G. J. Grevera and J. K. Udupa, "An objective comparison of 3-d image interpolation methods," *IEEE Transactions on Medical Imaging*, Vol. 17, No. 4, pp. 642–652, 1998.

32. M. Styner, C. Brechbuhler, G. Szckely, and G. Gerig, "Parametric estimate of intensity inhomogeneities applied to mri," *IEEE Transactions on Medical Imaging*, Vol. 19, No. 3, pp. 153–165, March 2000.

33. W. M. Wells III, W. E. L. Grimson, R. Kikinis, and F. A. Jolesz, "Adaptive segmentation of MRI data," *IEEE Transactions on Medical Imaging*, Vol. 15, No. 4, pp. 429–442, 1996.

34. B. M. ter Haar Romeny, *Geometry-Driven Diffusion in Computer Vision*, Computational Imaging and Vision, Kluwer, 1994.

35. Y. Du, D. Parker, and W. Davis, "Improved vessel visualization in MR angiography by nonlinear anisotropic filtering," *Journal of Magnetic Resonance Imaging*, Vol. 5, pp. 353–359, 1995.

36. A. Kelemen, G. Szekely, and G. Gerig, "Elastic model-based segmentation of 3d neuroradiological data sets," *IEEE Transactions on Medical Imaging*, Vol. 18, No. 10, pp. 828–839, October 1999.

37. S. M. Pizer, D. S. Fritsch, P. A. Yushkevich, V. E. Johnson, and E. L. Chaney, "Segmentation, registration, and measurement of shape variation via image object shape," *IEEE Transactions on Medical Imaging*, Vol. 18, No. 10, pp. 851–865, October 1999.

38. A. S. Tannenbaum, *Computer Networks*, Prentice Hall, 1989.

39. F. P. Brooks Jr., *Mythical Man-Month*, 2nd edition, Addison Wesley, 1995.

40. R. Shahidi, B. Lorensen, R. Kikinis, J. Flynn, A. Kaufman, and S. Napel, "Surface rendering versus volume rendering in medical imaging: techniques and applications," in *Visualization 1996*, November 1996, pp. 439–440.

41. J. D. Foley, A. van Dam, S. K. Feiner, and J. F. Hughes, *Computer Graphics: Principles and Practice*, 2nd edition, Addison-Wesley, 1990.

42. D. Mori and T. Yamaguchi, "Construction of the cfs model of the aortic arch based on mr images and simulation of the blood flow," in *Medical Imaging and Augmented Reality*, June 2001, pp. 111–116.

43. D. Eberly, *Ridges in Image and Data Analysis,* Vol. 7 of *Computational Imaging and Vision,* Kluwer Academic, Dordrecht, 1996.
44. A. Collignon, F. Maes, D. Delaere, D. Vandermeulen, P. Suetens, and G. Marchal, "Automated multi-modality image registration based on information theory," in *Information Processing in Medical Imaging,* Y. Bizais, C. Barillot, and R. Di Paola, Eds. 1995, pp. 263–274, Kluwer Academic.
45. A. Roche, X. Pennec, G. Malandain, and N. Ayache, "Rigid registration of 3d ultrasound with mr images: a new approach combining intensity and gradient information," *IEEE Transactions on Medical Imaging,* vol. 20, no. 10, pp. 1038–1049, 2001.
46. A. P. King, J. Blackall, G. Penney, and D. Hawkes, "Tracking liver motion using 2d ultrasound and a surface based statistical shape model," in *MMBIA,* December 2001.
47. P. J. Besl and N. D. McKay, "A method for registration of 3d shapes," *IEEE Transactions on Pattern Analysis and Machine Intelligence,* Vol. 14, pp. 239–256, 1992.
48. Y. Ge, C. R. Maurer Jr, and J. M. Fitzpatrick, "Surface-based 3-d image registration using the iterative closest point algorithm with a closest point transform," in *SPIE Medical Imaging: Image Processing,* 1996.
49. I. Dryden and K. Mardia, *Statistical Shape Analysis,* Wiley, New York, 1998.
50. Petra A. van den Elsen, Evert-Jan D. Pol, Thilaka S. Sumanaweera, Paul F. Hemler, Sandy Napel, and John R. Adler, "Grey value correlation techniques used for automatic matching of ct and mr brain and spine images," in *Visualization in Biomedical Computing,* Richard A. Robb, Ed., Rochester, MN, 1994, Vol. 2359, pp. 227–237, SPIE.

12

A Note on Future Research in Vascular and Plaque Segmentation

Jasjit S. Suri, Sameer Singh, Swamy Laxminarayan, Roberto M. Cesar Jr.,
Herbert F. Jelinek, Petia Reveda, Badrinath Roysam, Charles V. Stewart,
Kenneth H. Fritzsche, James Williams and Huseyin Tek

CONTENTS

12.1 Future of Skeleton- and Non-Skeleton-Based Segmentation Techniques

Three-dimensional segmentation of vasculature is indeed challenging. We hope to see the geometric techniques fused with regularizers to improve vessel segmentation. Alone, geometric techniques such as level sets are not sufficient. We hope to see more articles in the future on the following topics:

1. Generic angiography imaging for white- and black-blood angiography
2. Fast three-dimensional arterial and venous tree reconstruction
3. Artery–vein separation
4. Volumetric vessel tree reconstruction using artery–vein separation

0-8493-1740-1/03/$0.00+$1.50
© 2003 by CRC Press LLC

12.2   The Future of Retinal Fundus Vasculature

Previous work in our laboratories concentrated on vessel segmentation of fluorescein angiograms obtained from the Albury Eye Clinic, as described in Chapter 5. Our current research aims at providing an assessment tool for community health workers for identification of neovascularization within the optic fundus associated with diabetes using red-free images from non-mydriatic cameras. Community health workers do not use fluorescein for enhancement of vessels for visualizations and, most often, do not have digital cameras available to capture images. Therefore, assessment of the optic fundus is complicated due to the lower resolution of the images obtained from SLR or Polaroid cameras and a smaller field of view obtained from the nonmydriatic camera. We concentrated on two aspects: (1) segmentation of the images obtained from nonmydriatic cameras and captured with a 30-mm SLR camera followed by scanning these photos at 300 dpi for segmentation, and (2) analysis of the vessel patterns to obtain values associated with diverse morphological attributes of the vessel pattern.

Because automated analysis is aimed at being used by nonspecialist health workers, it is advantageous to obtain an optimal set of values of variables used for the segmentation in order to minimize operator-required adjustments. Once the vessels have been segmented, they are analyzed using a set of morphological parameters that allow classification of the pattern and comparison between normal and pathology.

We found that several factors had to be considered for optimal segmentation. Our main consideration was that the technique had to be robust between different images, without being too sensitive to the initial parameters. This was achieved using wavelet filters; more specifically, a Morlet filter, which provides maximum sensitivity for edge detection and direction of vessels. Wavelets are also ideal because they can deal with a large variation in the input images, as is the case with optic fundus photographs that may include microaneurysms, lipid deposits, or over- and underexposure. We have applied the segmentation technique to 58 images using the same parameter settings with good results. The adaptive thresholding steps provided a means of fine-tuning the output by sequentially moving to an optimal segmentation and removing noise in the process. Postprocessing the images was important because it led to the removal of small spurious branches and smoothed the vessel branching pattern. In the last part of the segmentation procedure we included mathematical morphology because it is ideal for dealing with two-dimensional images to perform a postprocessing role. Postprocessing included the conversion of the segmented images to binary skeletons. Some instabilities in the skeletonization algorithm using Matlab were noted and need to be addressed. Skeletonization of images produced 1-pixel-wide blood vessel segments but introduced additional pixels at crossover points and branch points. Provided that this processing error is equal across all images, it does not influence the results apart from possibly increasing some of the morphological feature values. However, this processing error creates difficulty when comparing images that have not been skeletonized using Matlab. It is thus desirable to improve the skeletonization procedure, for example, by considering the multi-scale skeletons approach [2]. The advantage of this approach is that it has an intrinsic parameter, namely the scale, that can be used to cope with small branches that appear due to noise.

Several feature parameters were investigated, including the fractal dimension, area, perimeter, circularity, and correlation dimension. We extended the wavelet shape features approach by applying the wavelet entropy to the characterization of the segmented vessels. This feature provides information on shape complexity and is therefore useful in characterizing optic fundus vessel patterns.

Future development should consider detecting and removing the optic disk artifacts (i.e., false branches), as well as detecting and characterizing microaneurysms. Because of the great flexibility in controlling and changing the analyzing wavelet shape, as discussed in Chapter 9, it is felt that both tasks can be performed using Morlet wavelets, which would lead to a fully integrated approach for analyzing fundus images.

To obtain an indication of how successful the segmentation was, we had an independent assessor evaluate the segmented networks. We found that the main shortfalls were inclusion of the optic disk perimeter, joining of aligning vessels, and exclusion of some smaller vessels in proximity to the macula. Special care must be taken in improving the segmentation technique with respect to these problems and operator intervention may be needed.

To overcome the problems associated with segmentation, we are fine-tuning the algorithms and developing a two-step quality measure that automatically detects problems with aquisition of the image by the operator and problems with the segmentation. For the former we aim to include a registration algorithm that runs in real-time and provides feedback to the operator as to whether the posterior pole is correctly positioned within the frame and has appropriate brightness for analysis and comparison. This step is vital as images that do not show the posterior pole but are from the periphery will have a different vessel pattern and therefore cannot be used for analysis. For the detection of segmentation errors, an option for operator intervention is included. This is intended for advanced users only. Segmentation errors occur when there is extensive hemorrhage or differences in brightness across the fundus.

The use of fractal analysis in detecting neovascularization has been reported in many articles [3, 4, 6]. Because we are interested in automating the identification of diabetic retinopathy by the use of feature parameters, we included fractal analysis and compared our results using nonmydriatic images and the box-counting method with that previously reported for fluorescein angiograms. Our fractal analysis results were comparable to results previously published [3]. We also applied the correlation dimension analysis but incorporated a novel procedure to obtain the region of interest to determine the fractal dimension and therefore could not compare these results with those published previously. A preliminary report has been presented using the local connected fractal analysis [5] as there is some disagreement among researchers as to which method (box-counting, mass-radius, or correlation dimension) is more appropriate [4]. Future studies should shed more light on these questions.

We extended the correlation dimension analysis by investigating alternative approaches to obtain the final dimension estimate [7]. The use of the zero-crossing of the wavelet was implemented to create an automatic technique for fitting a line to the correlation dimension log-log plot without the need for user intervention. There is an interesting variation of the algorithm that should be investigated in future studies. In such an approach, a series of line segments should be fitted to each segment between a pair of consecutive zero-crossings and the slope of each line properly calculated. This idea can be better understood from the example in Figure 12.1, based on the correlation dimension analysis of a triadic Koch curve, whose original log-log plot is shown in Figure 12.1a. The obtained one-dimensional wavelet transform and the corresponding zero-crossings are indicated in Figure 12.1b and the respective fitted lines in Figure 12.1c. The latter shows the log-log segments marked at the extremities with an "o". A histogram of these slopes is then obtained and the correlation dimension can be estimated from this histogram, for example, as the mean, median, or the mode of the histogram. In our experiments, we have used the median, which is less sensitive to outlier values (e.g., values that are too large) that sometimes appear. In the present example, the histogram is shown in Figure 12.1d.

In this study we observed that the log-log zero-crossings often produced too small subsegments with very different slopes, which negatively affected the estimation of the correlation dimension slope. Future work will address this problem based on results published in [8].

Another equally interesting research direction is to explore the whole histogram of slopes to characterize the vessel branching pattern instead of estimating a single slope by using the mean or the median. This could be done by comparing images based on the Battacharaya distance between the respective histograms of slopes [9]. The main advantage of such an approach is that it would take all the histogram information into account, thus circumventing the necessity of defining a statistical measure (e.g., mean, median, etc.) to characterize it.

Our results were promising, with the majority of vessel patterns segmented successfully. Several shortcomings such as inclusion of parts of the optic disk perimeter are now being addressed. Finally, important projects to be carried out from the reported work are to apply the technique to digital images, which generally have much better resolution, to compare the results obtained from the two different images acquisition methods (i.e., nonmydiatric cameras and fluorescein angiographic images), and to explore the segmentation method

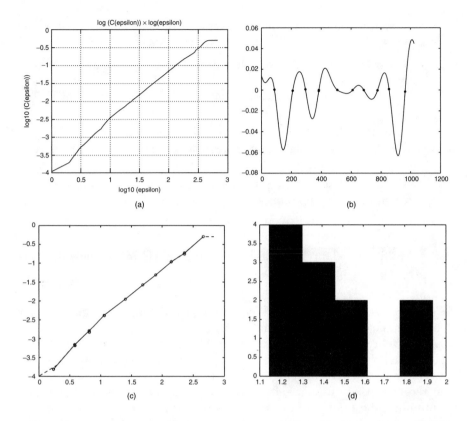

FIGURE 12.1
(a) Log-log plot obtained from the correlation dimension procedure of a triadic Koch curve; (b) resulting one-dimensional wavelet transform using the third derivative of the Gaussian as mother wavelet (the zero-crossings are indicated by "0"); (c) line fitted to the line segments defined by each pair of consecutive zero-crossings; (d) histogram of slopes of the fitted line segments.

and morphological features in classification tasks using more than one class (e.g., neovascularization present vs. control). It would also be highly interesting to consider experiments involving temporal images (e.g., neovascularization in different temporal stages).

12.3 The Future of Model-Based Retinal Angiography

Based on our prior experience, trends in computing technology, and requirements of current and emerging applications, future research in retinal image segmentation is quite likely to evolve in several different directions:

- Real-time computing-oriented algorithm design
- Algorithms driven by parallel computing considerations
- Algorithm designs driven by speed-insensitive applications such as offline registration, change detection, clinical trials image analysis support, remote reading centers, and fundamental research including angiogenesis
- Algorithm designs driven by detailed noise modeling, especially when imaging at high frame rates while attempting to minimize the illumination level, and hence patient discomfort
- Algorithm designs based on more realistic, physics-based models for the retinal imaging process
- Algorithm designs driven by emerging imaging modalities such as scanning laser ophthalmoscopy
- Multiple-modality data-based algorithms, including multi- and hyper-spectral imaging technologies

The work of Shen et al. [19] has set the stage for vessel tracing algorithms whose primary end-goal is *not* the vessel traces, but rather the extraction of just-sufficient vessel-related information from an image for accomplishing a specific task such as registration, keeping in mind the constraints imposed by real-time system design. Figure 12.2 illustrates an extreme example from our recent work. In this case, the tracing algorithm was designed explicitly to minimize the amount of tracing that is performed. In this case, successful registration was accomplished with the extraction of 162 seed points, 336 trace points, 7 grid boxes being traced, and 4 detected landmarks.

Real-time systems require algorithms to be not only efficient, but also highly predictable in terms of overall performance. This includes the need for predictable use of resources such as CPU cycles, input/output devices, and memory. As CCD technology improves, the number of pixels and number of bits/pixel continue to grow, placing a severe burden on computing systems. The amount of computing needed depends on the density of vasculature in an image and the quality of the imaging, both of which vary significantly. For handling such variable computational loads in a real-time environment, there has been growing interest in the use of imprecise computation frameworks [20]. An imprecise computation is a task with two parts: a mandatory part that must be fully executed and an optional part that can be computed to the extent possible given the computational resources. A "correctness function" is defined to measure the quality (e.g., precision) of the system output as a function of time (processor cycles). Computation beyond the mandatory part results in a monotonic increase of the correctness. Therefore, the precision of the final output is related to the amount of computation.

Much work has been done on detailed physics-based modeling of the retinal imaging process, and much remains to be done [21–24]. These increasingly

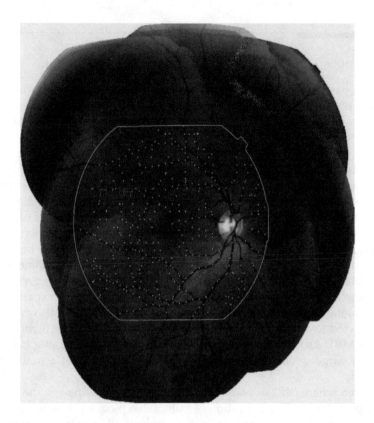

FIGURE 12.2
Results of transforming several individual images into a single "mosaic" image, which in turn is traced with an exploratory vessel identification algorithm to identify the blood vessel.

realistic models offer the potential, at least in principle, to lead to improved vessel segmentation performance. As computing speeds continue to improve, it should be possible to incorporate these models into evermore sophisticated and robust vessel segmentation algorithms.

One aspect of detailed physics-based modeling is the issue of imaging noise. As frame rates are increased to improve tracking and spatial referencing to support clinical procedures (such as laser retinal surgery) and high-precision perimetry, the amount of light available per pixel effectively goes down for a fixed quantum efficiency of the sensor–electronics combination. This calls for algorithms that are designed with sophisticated models based perhaps on Poisson point process models.

Finally, detailed physics-based modeling will be required to handle emerging and future retinal imaging modalities. These modalities may incorporate faster and more adaptive scanning systems, and multiple imaging wavelengths [25]. These models will likely result in new vessel segmentation and tracing algorithms as well.

12.4   Future Directions in MRI of Atherosclerotic Plaque

Over the past decade, significant advances have been made in our understanding of the pathology of atherosclerosis. The belief in the cardiovascular
field is that our aim should be the accurate diagnosis and treatment of those
plaques that are likely to cause thromboembolic events leading to heart attacks
or stroke. A comprehensive histopathological definition of such "vulnerable
plaque" has emerged and is nicely summarized by Virmani et al. [1].

As described in this book (Chapters 7, 8, and 9), MRI is capable of identifying
and quantifying vulnerable plaque. The tools that were presented represent
the current state-of-the-art. To date, these MRI tools are largely developmental, with the emphasis on validating the techniques rather than applying them.
Significant technical and clinical progress can still be made in this field to further our understanding of the diagnosis and treatment of atherosclerosis. First
of all, MR plaque imaging is currently limited to a number of research centers
and research subjects. This technique should be (and can be) expanded into
more imaging centers and clinical use. Multi-center clinical trials will need to
be conducted to evaluate the reproducibility and variability of features identified by MRI. As these validation steps proceed, plaque imaging is likely to
witness a surge in clinical and scientific investigations that actually utilize
these tools.

One area where MRI of plaque is likely to have an impact is the study of
plaque progression. The definition of vulnerable plaque is based on examining autopsy specimens taken from patients who died of heart attacks or other
cardiovascular-related causes. This type of examination provides a one-time
shot of the disease process. Conclusions regarding progression are therefore
based on comparing plaques that appear to be more or less advanced. There is
a clear need to use noninvasive imaging techniques to prospectively examine
progression of individual atherosclerotic plaques. Such studies will provide
valuable information on the relationship of plaque burden, morphology, and
composition to plaque vulnerability, and the development of clinical symptoms. The carotid artery, serially viewed by MRI, is likely to serve as a testbed
for the current theories regarding plaque progression.

A second application of plaque MRI that is likely to emerge is screening
candidates for surgery. Currently, carotid endarterectomy is indicated by percent stenosis alone. Patients with moderate stenosis in the carotid artery are
left with no option for aggressive treatment. A study is needed to determine
if other indicators of vulnerable plaque beyond percent stenosis can be used
to refine the selection of surgical candidates.

A third and perhaps the most significant area where the techniques for
plaque MRI are likely to be applied is in clinical drug trials. An increasing
number of compounds aimed at stabilizing and/or shrinking atherosclerotic
plaques are expected to be proposed. Pharmaceutical companies require a
technique to objectively and quantitatively measure the impact of drugs on

plaque. Imaging the effect of drugs on carotid plaque is likely to be the key first step in evaluating such drugs in the near future.

MRI of carotid plaque is thus likely to figure prominently in many studies of atherosclerosis to come. These studies, however, merely scratch the surface of MRI's potential. In the future, MRI of atherosclerosis is expected to be applied to vessels beyond the carotid arteries and to appear in regular clinical use. To reach this potential, a number of technological and image processing advances are necessary.

12.4.1 Advances in MRI Technology

The spatial resolution used in current techniques is adequate for characterizing carotid atherosclerosis. Improved resolution, however, is still desired for finer structures of a plaque such as the fibrous cap thickness and for smaller arteries such as coronaries. Such improvement is expected with the use of higher-field, whole-body scanners such as commercially available 3T or 4T machines. Improvement may also be obtained through the adoption of three-dimensional data acquisition, especially the combination of three-dimensional FSE technique with DIR or QIR.

In addition, for imaging lesions within coronary arteries, fast imaging strategies are needed to stop the motion of the heart and provide sufficiently high resolution to show coronary plaque structure. At present, imaging techniques are nearly up to the challenge, as shown in Figure 12.3. If the remaining obstacles to coronary imaging can be overcome, MRI of atherosclerotic plaque will have achieved the foremost goal in the evaluation of coronary artery disease.

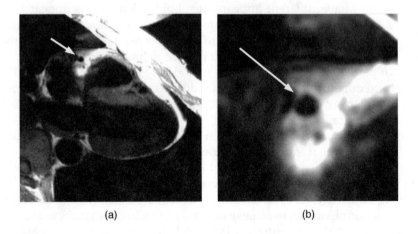

(a)   (b)

FIGURE 12.3
Images of a coronary artery in a normal volunteer: (a) oblique DIR FSE MRI of the heart shows (b) a cross-sectional view of the right coronary artery (arrow).

12.4.2   Advances in Image Processing

The image processing tools described in Chapters 8 and 9 provide the basic needs for quantitatively analyzing MRI of atherosclerosis. As such, they are entirely suitable for scientific study of the disease. For clinical applications, however, increased automation, reliability, and repeatability are needed. Thus, MRI of atherosclerotic plaque also poses a challenge to the image processing community. Ultimately, tools are needed that will allow the clinician to rapidly extract the most significant features from plaque images. This will permit the techniques described here to make the jump to regular practice.

12.5   The Future of Ultrasound Angiography

During the past two decades we have witnessed great advances in cardiac imaging. Advances in microprocessor technology as well as improved scanner hardware led to developing sophisticated imaging devices for rapid processing of extremely large quantities of data applied for the acquisition, processing, and formation of images of the coronary lumen and plaque. IVUS as a new and unique imaging tool for tomographic assessment of lumen area, plaque size, distribution, and composition provides new insights into the diagnosis of and therapy for coronary disease.

Providing a detailed picture of vessel structure and morphology allows for the development of new diagnostic and therapeutic methodology. IVUS images allow one to study the process of plaque formation and temporal and spatial distribution and to extract planar measurements about area and diameters of lumen and vessel that are basic to the exploration of the process of positive and negative remodeling of the vessel. With IVUS, different lesions and plaques have different appearances: lipid-laden lesions appear hypoechoic, fibromuscular lesions generate low-intensity echoes, and fibrous or calcified tissues are echogenic (calcium causes acoustic shadowing). Furthermore, IVUS commonly detects occult disease in angiographically "normal" sites. In particular, an *in vivo* arterial remodeling is possible due to IVUS to detect and quantify changes in vascular dimensions during the development of atherosclerosis, a fact often invisible in angiography. In ambiguous lesions, ultrasound permits lesion quantification.

The problem of vessel and lumen delineation is a tedious and time-consuming task that introduces a significant amount of imprecision during manual segmentation of hundreds of images. As a consequence, this problem has received attention from researchers in computer vision community. Although different works have been presented, there is not available a robust segmentation algorithm to achieve optimal results (more than 98%) of correct vessel segmentation for different IVUS catheters, or different patients with different morphological structures [20]. Still, from the different algorithms presented, one can conclude that only a well-designed vessel model with appropriate elastic properties and robust interpretation of image features can help to solve the problem of automatic segmentation and extraction of planar vessel measurements from IVUS images.

As mentioned, IVUS images contain rich information about the morphological structure of the vessel that can prove difficult for visual interpretation from IVUS images. Automatic IVUS analysis can be of significant help in assisting image interpretation and removing expert subjectivity. Given that the problem of automatic tissue characterization is even more complex than vessel delineation, robust statistical techniques for classification are necessary when there is a significant amount of data from different patients and different plaque structures, in order to develop the automatic tools to help physicians in clinical practice.

In addition to being a good diagnostic tool, the IVUS imaging technique is an excellent intraoperative tool to assist in vessel therapy. The mechanisms of action of interventional devices have been elucidated using IVUS, and ultrasound can be used to select the most suitable interventional device. Additionally, IVUS has proven to be a valuable tool for evaluating the effect of brachytherapy. As a conclusion, new and emerging applications for IVUS are continuing to evolve for the purposes of intraoperative diagnosis and therapy that are impossible with other imaging devices. It is a challenge for the team of cardiologists and vascular interventionists to define exactly the physiological phenomena related to the coronary diseases that are observable in IVUS images as well as to estimate the benefit, feasibility, and robustness of applying the IVUS technique compared to other imaging devices when studying these phenomena.

The recent appearance of IVUS images led to ambiguous terminology and various alternative synonyms for similar structures and measurements. Accordingly, the current expert consensus committee was commissioned by the American College of Cardiology, in collaboration with the European Society of Cardiology, to provide a framework for the standardization of nomenclature, methods of measurements, and reporting of IVUS results. The committee has sought to provide a logical and consistent approach to IVUS analysis to assist both clinicians and investigators [25].

Correct use and analysis of IVUS data is a direct consequence of image quality. Image quality is partially described by two important factors: spatial resolution and contrast resolution. To obtain the correct ultrasound image of objects, two principal spatial factors are very important: resolution in the axial direction (parallel to the beam and primarily a function of wavelength) and the lateral direction (perpendicular to the beam and the catheter, and a function of wavelength and transducer size, known as aperture). These characteristics depend on the ultrasound frequency of IVUS transducer. Contrast resolution is the distribution of the gray scale of the reflected signal and is often referred to as the dynamic range. Commercial companies providing

IVUS catheters are working hard on obtaining high-resolution images. Still, due to the nature of the ultrasound image, any improvement in this direction represents a significant benefit in interpreting IVUS images. On the other hand, a real challenge and still a field not explored to its full extent by image processing people is to include knowledge on IVUS image formation in the process of image processing, which will definitely make image analysis techniques more robust and will ease the process of extracting important vessel data.

Another important characteristic of IVUS images is the principle of distributing ultrasound waves. As an ultrasound pulse encounters a boundary between two tissues, the beam will be partially reflected and partially transmitted. The degree of reflection depends on the difference between the mechanical impedance of the two materials. As the wave passes through many tissue interfaces, the energy is attenuated as a function of the tissue characteristics, the energy scattering by small structures, and absorption by tissue. Only a small percentage of emitted signal returns to the transducer to be converted to electrical energy and sent to the external signal processing for amplification, filtering, scan-conversion, user-controlled modification, and graphic presentation. As one can note, the process of formation of the IVUS image sequence is a complex process where still a lot of improvement in signal emitting and receiving as well as processing toward image formation is expected. In particular, computer vision people will face different shortcomings regarding IVUS image formation [26].

Image non-uniform rotational distortion (NURD) and motion artifacts. This shortcoming is common in mechanical catheter systems and results from mechanical binding of the drive cable that rotates the transducer. A distinct motion artifact can result from an unstable catheter position. If the vessel moves before a complete circumferential image is created, a cyclic deformation is obtained. Image processing algorithms should take into account this shortcoming to avoid wrong image processing results. Moreover, such algorithms could help IVUS devices detect and correct vessel data extraction.

Image artifacts such as ring-down, blood speckle, and near-field artifacts. These artifacts are usually observed as bright halos of variable thickness surrounding the catheter, are produced by acoustic oscillations in the transducer, and result in high-amplitude ultrasound signals obscuring the area immediately adjacent to the catheter. The phenomenon of blood speckle is due to the fact that the intensity of the blood speckle increases as transducer frequency increases and as blood flow velocity decreases. This can limit the ability to differentiate lumen from tissue and, in particular, soft plaque neointima and thrombosis. A trend in IVUS image analysis is to develop robust and fast computer-based imaging algorithms that can suppress or differentiate blood speckle from tissue.

Obliquity, eccentricity, and problems of vessel curvature. Most current imaging techniques assume that the vessel is circular, that the catheter is located in the center of the artery, and that the transducer is parallel to the long axis of the vessel. Both transducer obliquity and vessel curvature can produce an image giving the false impression that the vessel is elliptical. This fact is especially important in large vessels and can result in overestimation of dimensions and a reduction in image quality. This phenomenon occurs because the amplitude of an echo wave reflected from an interface depends on the angle at which the beam strikes the interface. As a consequence, lower image quality and errors in interpretation are more likely when the IVUS catheter is not parallel to the vessel wall. Because transducer producers cannot assure that the strongest signals obtained when the catheter is coaxial within the vessel and when the beam strikes the target at a 90° angle, algorithms for IVUS analysis should take this phenomenon into account. To address this shortcoming, three-dimensional vessel reconstruction is necessary combining IVUS images with other imaging modality (usually, angiography [27, 28]). Presented algorithms for three-dimensional reconstruction should achieve not only the necessary robustness, but also the real-time execution in order to be applicable in clinical practice. Three-dimensional reconstruction of vessel is of high clinical interest in assessing the spatial configurations of plaques, dissections, and stents and in performing basic measurements.

Problem of spatial orientation of IVUS data. Until recently there was no absolute posterior, anterior, left, and right orientation possible in IVUS images. However, some systems can be electronically rotated to produce a constant orientation using landmarks, such as the circumflex, to appear in a certain direction. Electronic rotation of the image is an electromagnetic aid in the interpretation, *not* a definite standard. Angiographic images can be very useful to provide essential landmarks in facilitating image interpretation and comparisons. The development of different image-processing and mechanical guidances for image orientation will be very important for the correct orientation by physicians inside IVUS data.

In addition to the information extracted directly from IVUS images (planar measurements, morphological analysis), IVUS data allow one to extract volumetric estimates of the vessel and its structures. It is obvious that only real volumetric data will avoid artifacts and errors in planar measurements, due to the position between vessel and images, and will allow one to define objective rules for diagnosis and therapy based on spatial relations of vessel parts and therapeutic devices. Given that volumetric analysis includes different problems — segmentation of vessel in IVUS and angiography, fusion of IVUS and angiography data, and spatial orientation of IVUS data — a significant effort is expected by the computer vision community to achieve and prove the robustness of real-time algorithms. Nevertheless, we feel that volumetric analysis will gain further importance and become a routine technique if the interest, effort, and technical developments in the field are sustained.

Complementary to geometric information about the vessel, the three-dimensional vessel model extracted by IVUS represents a good basis for assessment of hemodynamic consequences of coronary disease using shear stress calculations in the framework of computational fluid dynamics [29]. It was concluded that initiation and growth of atherosclerotic plaque can be correlated with the flow reversal and separation as well as relatively wall shear and oscillating shear stresses. It will be a challenge for computer vision and mechanics researchers to explore the relation between the three-dimensional geometry and morphology of the vessel, as well as its cross-sectional changes and vessel motion, and their relation to the contraction of cardiac muscles and relaxation during cardiac cycles that have substantial impact on vessel hemodynamics.

12.6   Future Directions in Plaque and Aneurysm Assessment

In this section we present our view of future directions in vascular imaging technology. Let us first present what we consider the important issues in vascular imaging. Specifically, the following are some of the areas where we see the postprocessing role expanding in the near future:

1. Quick detection of vascular pathologies, preferably from noninvasive imaging modalities
2. Robust determination of the severity of these pathologies to guide a treatment decision
3. Accurate treatment planning
4. Treatment simulations to reduce human errors during interventions
5. Follow-up monitoring of pathologies after surgery or during drug therapy

To illustrate the future directions, we consider two types of pathologies: namely, plaques and aneurysms. Specifically, plaques are often considered to be the most important area of vascular imaging, especially for cardiovascular imaging. Similarly, aneurysms are a significant health problem. Aortic abdominal aneurysm rupture is the 13th leading cause of death in the United States. We believe that developments in these areas are a good representation of developments in other blood vessel diseases.

In vascular imaging, detection and classification of plaques are probably the most important task because they can cause severe health problems, such as heart attack and stroke. Plaques are often classified as stable and unstable (*or vulnerable*). Plaques are associated with the accumalation of lipids in the arterial walls. Plaque formation can cause narrowing and decreased blood flow through the arteries. The degree of blood flow blockage, *stenosis degree* due to a plaque, determines whether an intervention procedure such as angioplasty or stent deployment is necessary. In this area, we believe that fast, multi-row CT scanners will be competitive with x-ray angiography in the accurate evaluation of plaques in coronary arteries. In addition, rapid developments in CT technology make us believe that it will be possible to use CT in interventions such as graft deployments.

Traditionally, it has been believed that the larger-sized plaques are more dangerous and need more attention. However, recent findings show that the scenario is not simple; that is, small plaques may be quiescent for years and then suddenly rupture, often leading to death [12]. Unfortunately, it is still not known why these plaques, often called *vulnerable* or *unstable*, suddenly rupture. For example, when plaques in carotid arteries create more than 60% stenosis, it is usually deemed necessary to operate on them to prevent possible a stroke [11]. However, only one in twenty patients with such a high degree of stenosis experience stroke; thus, large number of patients are operated on while there is, in fact, no stroke risk. Thus, factors other than the degree of stenosis play important roles in detecting high-risk plaques. A similar scenario exists in coronary arteries. A rupture-prone plaque in coronary arteries often appears small enough to be considered insignificant. Thus, one of the major goals of current vascular imaging research is and will be to detect these insignificant plaques with their micro-anatomic characteristics to assess their risk of rupture.

Although distinguishing between stable plaques and vulnerable plaques is difficult, recent findings show that information obtained from plaque surface characteristics, plaque volume, plaque internal structures, and functional characteristics such as inflammatory features can be successfully used to detect these dangerous plaques. In noninvasive imaging modalities, MR has the advantage over other modalities in that it differentiates between components in the plaque, such as calcium, lipid, the fibrous cap, thrombus [18]. However, some limitations include long acquisition times, the high cost factor, and its ineligibility for patients with metal prostheses. While it is not clear if CT data provides information on detecting vulnerable plaques, it is a fast imaging modality and has sufficient spatial resolution to image soft plaques in the coronary arteries.

In addition to noninvasive imaging modalities, several new invasive imaging techniques have been developed to measure certain plaque characteristics. Specifically, angioscopy and intravascular ultrasound techniques provide information about the surface of plaque and some limited information on its structural properties. Intravascular thermography exploits the fact that vulnerable plaques have a higher temperature due to inflammation; thus, this technique measures the blood-free temperature of plaques. Several new invasive imaging modalities, such as optical coherence tomography (OCT), near-infrared (NIR) spectroscopy, photonic spectroscopy, etc., go beyond creating an image of plaque and provide information on its chemical and molecular structure.

Thus, detecting vulnerable plaques may be possible by combining information obtained from these invasive imaging modalities along with the popular noninvasive ones (e.g., MR and CT). Other possibilities include the development of contrast agents for CT and MR that may provide information about the structural composition of plaques and functional characteristics (e.g., inflammation).

12.6.1 Aneurysms

Aneurysms form at arteries when artery walls become weaker due to disease, injury, or high blood pressure. The worst happens when they rupture, which often causes death. In this section, we focus on aortic abdominal aneurysms (AAA) because they are the most common ones. In fact, AAA rupture is the 13th leading cause of death in the United States. Approximately, 200,000 people, mostly over 65 years old, are diagnosed with AAAs each year. It is believed that there are approximately 1.5 million Americans with aneurysms. The current AAA treatment market is believed to be $1.2 billion. This is expected to grow, due to an aging U.S. population and an increasing proportion of elderly patients.

12.6.1.1 Diagnosis of AAAs

Several types of imaging modalities can be used to detect AAAs [16]. Ultrasound may be the right choice for the initial diagnosis of AAAs due to its low cost and minimally invasive nature. However, it is quite difficult to make accurate measurements on ultrasound images of aneurysms. While angiography is currently the gold standard for demonstrating vascular structures, we expect that its popularity will steadily decline due to its invasive nature and measurement errors. Aneurysms can be easily detected from contrast-enhanced MR and CT data. In addition, accurate measurements of the aneurysm and neighboring vascular structures are possible from CE-CTA/MRA data. The advantages of MRA over CTA include: (1) no iodinated contrast medium is necessary; (2) no radiation dosage is necessary; and (3) no bone removal is necessary for visualization of vascular structures. Similarly, the advantages of CTA over MRA include: (1) it provides good details of calcification on arteries (e.g., common iliac arteries, thrombus, and other plaques on the inner walls of artery); and (2) there is no restriction of ferromagnetic endoprotheses for follow-up studies. Thus, we believe that CTA and possibly MRA will be the major imaging modalities for AAAs.

12.6.1.2 Assessment of the AAA Rupture Risk

Quantification of aneurysms is necessary for determining the risk of rupture. For example, if the size of aneurysm is greater than 5 cm, the risk of rupture increases significantly, thus suggesting treatment. The maximum diameter of an aneurysm can be easily ascertained from cross-sectional views on MRA and CTA. However, the volume of an aneurysm may be a better measurement for determining the severity of the aneurysm. Unlike maximum diameter measurements, volume measurements in MRA and CTA is much more difficult due to the requirement of accurate three-dimensional segmentation [10, 17]. Ideally, a use-friendly segmentation algorithm should be used to determine the volume. The segmentation of an aneurysm in CTA data is more difficult due to the presence of thrombus.

Recently, it was argued that the "5 cm criterion" for determining rupture risk is not sufficient. Other factors such as asymmetry and wall stress should also be considered. Specifically, Vorp et al. [15] investigated the effect of maximum diameter and asymmetry on the aneurysm wall and noted that asymmetry also plays an important role in the assessment of rupture risk. In addition, Raghavan et al. [13] proposed that rupture occurs when the mechanical stress acting on the wall exceeds the wall tissue strength. Specifically, first, aneurysm boundaries from six patients were segmented via simple thresholding combined with an edge detection. Second, the finite element method was used to determine the wall stress distribution. Another important measure is the vessel wall shear stress created by pulsatile flow of blood [14]. In addition, the determination of vessel wall size via higher-resolution imaging techniques such multi-detector CT will contribute to the accuracy of the risk assessment.

12.6.1.3 *Treatment Options*

Abdominal aortic aneurysms can be surgically treated either with traditional open surgery or with a minimally invasive repair such as endovascular grafting. The endovascular graft treatment has, in general, better morbidity and mortality rates than typical open surgery. In addition, it is less painful and patients have shorter hospital stays. However, only 30 or 40% of patients with abdominal aortic aneurysms are eligible for endovascular graft treatment. Specifically, the structure of the aorta and its neighboring arteries and risk factors for open surgery determine which method is best for each patient. We expect that there will be more advanced grafts, which will then increase the ratio of patients who are eligible for endovascular treatment.

12.6.1.4 *Endovascular Graft Treatment Planning*

Accurate geometric measurement of the aneurysm and its neighboring arteries is the first important step in endovascular graft planning. Specifically, the following measurements should be made accurately and efficiently [16]: (1) max/min diameter of the aneurysm neck, (2) tortuosity or angulations of aneurysm neck, (3) max/min diameter of aneurysm sack, (4) max/min diameter of common iliac and external iliac arteries, (5) length of aneurysm neck, (6) distance from renal artery to bifurcation of aorta, (7) length of the right and left common iliac arteries, and (8) angulations, tortuosity, and calcification of the iliac arteries. That is, accurate segmentation and subsequent geometric modeling of the aorta with aneurysm are necessary for endovascular graft treatment planning.

12.6.1.5 Simulations of Endovascular Graft Treatment

Once the model of the aorta with aneurysm is constructed from medical data, better visualization can be done via surface shaded display. In addition, it may be important to simulate the navigation and deployment of a stent graft on a computer before the real operation takes place in order to minimize any unexpected complications during the operation. Also, this simulation software can be used to train doctors for the endovascular graft treatment. We expect that fast, multi-row CT scanners equipped with such advanced postprocessing algorithms will play an important role in the simulations of such interventions.

12.6.1.6 Patient Follow-Up Studies

Unfortunately, the mid- and long-term effects of endovascular graft treatments are still not well known. Thus, life-long follow-up studies are necessary to monitor for leaks, endograft failure, changes in aneurysm neck, movement of graft, changes in the shape of the graft, etc. The need for accurate evaluation of the aneurysm and the endograft after the operation will continue to drive research into advanced segmentation algorithms and improvements in the quality of images produced by the scanners.

12.6.2 Conclusions

We believe that accurate atherosclerotic plaque detection and classification will be the one of the most important areas in vascular imaging research, especially in cardiac imaging, in the coming years. Specifically, fast, multi-row CT scanners will play an important role in the detection and treatment of calcified, stable plaques. For example, accurate stenosis evaluation in the coronaries from CT data will be competitive with x-ray angiography. In addition, it will be possible to use CT data during the interventions, such as endovascular graft deployment. MR imaging has the potential to be a leader among the noninvasive imaging modalities for distinguishing vulnerable (dangerous) plaques from the stable ones. However, the reliable detection of vulnerable plaques in the near future may still depend on combining information acquired from several imaging modalities. Also, we expect to see new MR contrast agents that will allow longer imaging times so that it will be possible to acquire high-resolution images for plaque characterization based on a global vascular scout image.

The other area that will experience significant improvement is the postprocessing of vascular data. Segmentation of vascular pathologies for quantification and generation of computer models will be available due to more advanced algorithms and also easier due to the improvements in the image quality from scanners. Accurate computer models of pathologies will be needed for diagnosis and treatment planning. In addition, computer simulation of treatments will be crucial in assessing the risk associated with an intervention and for physician training. Furthermore, accurate and fast segmentation of vascular pathologies, and also endovascular grafts after interventions or drug treatments, will be important in monitoring the success/failure of such treatments. New three-dimensional postprocessing algorithms are and will continue to be vital for the interpretation of CT data where the number of images slices has already become too large for a radiologist to analyze in a reasonable amount of time using conventional two-dimensional methods.

Acknowledgments

Roberto M. Cesar Jr. is grateful to FAPESP (99/12765-2) and to CNPq (300722/98-2, 468413/00-6). Herbert F. Jelinek was in receipt of a CSU small grant (A5141739605). The authors also wish to acknowledge the contribution of Graeme Frauenfelder, who provided the nonmydriatic images and to the West Australian Lions Clinic for providing the Polaroid and Zeiss images. J. LaNauze from the Albury Eye Clinic provided expert advise. Finally, Jorge J. G. Leandro and Emerson L. N. Tozette helped with the programs and bibliographic review.

References

1. Virmani, R., Kolodgie, F. D., Burke, A. P., Farb, A., and Schwartz, S. M., Lessons from sudden coronary death: a comprehensive morphological classification scheme for atherosclerotic lesions, *Arterioscler. Thromb. Vasc. Biol.*, Vol. 20, No. 5, pp. 1262–1275, 2000.
2. Costa, L. F. and Estrozi, L. F., "Multiresolution shape representation without border shifting," *Electronics Lett.*, Vol. 35, No. 21, pp. 1829–1830, 1999.
3. Daxer, A., "Characterisation of the neovascularisation process in diabetic retinopathy by means of fractal geometry: diagnostic implications," *Graefe's Arch. Clin. Exp. Ophthalmol.*, Vol. 231, pp. 681–686, 1993.
4. Landini, G., Murray, P., and Misson, G., "Local connected fractal dimensions and lacunarity analysis of 60 degree fluorescein angiograms," *Invest. Ophthalmol. Vis. Sci.*, Vol. 36, pp. 2749–2755, 1995.
5. McQuellin, C. and Jelinek, H., "Characterisation of fluorescein angiograms of retinal fundus using mathematical morphology: a pilot study," in *Proc. 5th Int. Conf. Ophthalmic Photography*, 2002 (accepted).
6. Family, F., Masters, B., and Platt, D., "Fractal pattern formation in human retinal vessels," *Physica D*, Vol. 38, pp. 98–103, 1989.
7. Grassberger, P. and Procaccia, I., "Characterization of strange attractors," *Physical Rev. Lett.*, Vol. 50, No. 5, pp. 346–349, 1983.
8. Struzik Z. R., Dooijes, E. H., and Groen F. C. A., "Fitting the generic multi-parameter crossover model: towards realistic scaling estimates," in M. M. Novak and T. G. Dewey, Eds., *Fractal Frontiers*, World Scientific, Vol. 3, pp. 163–180, 1997.

9. Theodoridis, S. and Koutroumbas, K., *Pattern Recognition*, 1st ed., Academic Press, 1999.

10. Fiebich, M. T., Engelmann, R., McGilland, J., and Hoffman, K., "Computer assisted diagnosis in CT angiography of abdominal aortic aneurysms," *Medical Imaging: Image Processing, Proc. of SPIE*, 3034, 86–94, 1997.

11. Geroulakos, G. and Sabetai, M. M., "Review: ultrasonic carotid plaque morphology," *Arch. Hellenic Med.*, Vol. 17, No. 2, 141–145, 2000.

12. Naghavi, M., Khan, M. R., Mohammadi, R. M., Willerson, J. T., and Casscells, S. W., "New developments in the detection of vulnerable plaque," *Curr. Atheroscler. Rep.*, Vol. 3, No. 2, 125–135, 2001.

13. Raghavan, M. L., Vorp, D., Federle, M. P., Makaroun, M. S., and Webster, M. W., "Wall stress distribution on three-dimensionally reconstructed models of human abdominal aortic aneurysm," *J. Vascul. Surg.*, Vol. 31, No. 4, 760–769, 2000.

14. Taylor, C. A., Huges, T. J. R., and Zarines, C. K., "Finite element modelling of three-dimensional pulsatile flow in the abdominal aorta: relevance to atherosclerosis," *Ann. Biomed. Eng.*, Vol. 26, 975–987, 1998.

15. Vorp, D., Raghavan, M. L., and Webster, M. W., "Mechanical wall stress in abdominal aortic aneurysm: influence of diameter and assymetry," *J. Vascul. Surg.*, Vol. 27, No. 4, 326–332, 1998.

16. Whitaker, S. C., "Imaging of abdominal aortic aneurysm before and after endoluminal stent-graft repair," *Eur. J. Radiol.*, Vol. 39, 3–15, 2001.

17. Wink, O., Niessen, W., and Viergever, M. A., "Fast delination and visualization of vessels in 3-D angiographic images," *IEEE Trans. Med. Imag.*, Vol. 19, No. 4, 337–345, 2000.

18. Yuan, C., Mitumori, L. M., Beach, K. W., and Maravilla, K. R., "Carotid atherosclerotic plaque: noninvasive MR and characterization and identification of vulnerable lesions," *Radiology*, Vol. 221, 285–299, 2001.

19. Shen, H., Roysam, B., Stewart, C. V., Turner, J. N., and Tanenbaum, H. L., "Optimal scheduling of tracing compuations for real-time vascular landmark extraction from retinal fundus images," *IEEE Trans. Info. Technol. Biomed.*, Vol. 5, No. 1, 2001.

20. Natarajan, S., *Imprecise and Approximate Computation*, Kluwer Academic Publishers, Boston, MA, 1995.

21. Denninghoff, K. and Smith, M., "Optical model of the blood in large retinal vessels," *J. Biomed. Optics*, Vol. 5, No. 4, pp. 371–374, 2000.

22. Smith, M., Denninghoff, K., Lompado, A., and Hillman, L., "Effect of multiple light paths on retinal vessel oximetry," *Appl. Optics*, Vol. 39, No. 7, pp. 1183–1193, 2000.

23. Roberts, D., "Analysis of vessel absorption profiles in retinal oximetry," *Med. Phys.*, Vol. 14, pp. 124–130, 1987.

24. Brinchmann-Hansen, O. and Heier, H., "Theoretical relations between light streak characteristics and optical properties of retinal vessels," *Acta Opthalmologica*, 33–37, 1986.

25. Klingensmith, J. D., Shekhar, R., and Vince, D. G., "Evaluation of three-dimensional segmentation algorithms for the identification of luminal and medial-adventitial borders in intravascular ultrasound images," *IEEE Trans. Med. Imag.*, Vol. 19, No. 10, 996–1011, 2000.

26. Mintz, G. S., Nissen, S., et al., "American College of Cardiology clinical expert consensus document on standards for acquisition, measurement and reporting

of intravascular ultrasound studies (IUUS)," *J. Am. Coll. Cardio.*, Vol. 37, No. 5, 1478–1492, 2001.

27. Slager, C. J., Wentzel, J. J., Schuurbiers, J. C. H., et al., "True 3-dimensional reconstruction of coronary arteries in patients by fusion of angiography and IVUS (ANGUS) and its quantitative validation," *Circulation*, August, 511–516, 2000.

28. Cañero, C., Radeva, P., Toledo, R., Villanueva, J. J., and Mauri, J., "3D curve reconstruction by biplane snakes," *Proc. 15th Intl. Conf. on Pattern Recognition*, Barcelona, Spain, May 2000.

29. Wahle, A., Mitchell, S., Ramaswamy, Sh., Chandran, K., and Sonka, M., "Visualizations of human coronary arteries with quantification results from 3-D and 4-D computational hemodynamics based upon virtual endoscopy," *Proc. Computer-Assisted Radiology and Surgery* 2001, Elsevier, 2001.

Index

N

O